TEXTBOOK OF
THE CERVICAL SPINE

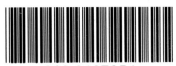

TEXTBOOK OF THE CERVICAL SPINE

Francis H. Shen, MD

Warren G. Stamp Endowed Professor
Division Head, Spine Division
Director, Spine Fellowship
Co-Director, Spine Center
Department of Orthopaedic Surgery
University of Virginia Health Science Center
Charlottesville, Virginia

Dino Samartzis, DSc

Warden, Hornell Hall
Assistant Professor
Director of Clinical Spine Research
Department of Orthopaedics and Traumatology
Deputy Director
Laboratory and Clinical Research Institute for Pain
Li Ka Shing Faculty of Medicine
The University of Hong Kong
Hong Kong

Richard G. Fessler, MD, PhD

Professor
Department of Neurosurgery
Rush University Medical Center
Chicago, Illinois

ELSEVIER
SAUNDERS

3251 Riverport Lane
Maryland Heights, Missouri 63043

TEXTBOOK OF THE CERVICAL SPINE   ISBN: 978-1-4557-1143-7

Library of Congress Cataloging-in-Publication Data

Textbook of the cervical spine / [edited by] Francis H. Shen, Dino Samartzis, Richard G. Fessler.
   p. ; cm.
Includes bibliographical references and index.
ISBN 978-1-4557-1143-7 (hardcover : alk. paper)
I. Shen, Francis H., editor. II. Samartzis, Dino, editor. III. Fessler, Richard G., editor.
[DNLM: 1. Cervical Vertebrae. 2. Spinal Diseases. WE 725]
RD768
616.7'3--dc23
                                        2014012927

Senior Content Strategist: Don Scholz
Content Development Specialist: Margaret Nelson
Publishing Services Manager: Patricia Tannian
Senior Project Manager: Sharon Corell
Book Designer: Brian Salisbury

Printed in China
Last digit is the print number: 9 8 7 6 5 4 3 2 1

To my daughter, Mia, whose smile and laughter make me realize that there is no greater joy than having children, and to my parents who continue to astound and impress me each and every day.

F.H.S.

First and foremost, I would like to dedicate this textbook to my parents, Steve and Joanna. I want to thank them for giving me a "blessed" life, immense love, and the precious, special gift of always believing in me and supporting my passions. I also dedicate this to my beautiful wife, Imelda, for giving me an unparalleled love and for enduring all my late nights being hard at work. Lastly, I dedicate this project to my colleagues and friends in the spine community who with their wonderful smiles and kind words have fueled my desires and interests to pursue a career among this multi-colored canvas of spine. In particular, I dedicate this to Dr. Spiros Stamelos and Dr. Howard S. An who gave me my "first steps" in orthopaedics and spine, and who "always" served as a rock of support and inspiration. To all – family, friends, and colleagues – I remain eternally grateful for having you in my life and making it more meaningful on a daily basis.

D.S.

This text is dedicated to my wife, Carol, whose lifelong companionship has made my journey worthwhile.

R.G.F.

CONTRIBUTORS

Kuniyoshi Abumi, MD, DrMedSci
Director, Vice President
Sapporo Orthopaedic Hospital
Center for Spinal Disorders
Sapporo, Japan

Tim E. Adamson, MD
Surgeon
Carolina Neurosurgery and Spine Associates
Medical Director
Carolina Center for Specialty Surgery
Charlotte, North Carolina

Todd J. Albert, MD
Surgeon-in-Chief, Medical Director, and Korein-Wilson
    Professor of Orthopedic Surgery
Hospital for Special Surgery
New York, New York

Christopher P. Ames, MD
Professor
Neurological Surgery
University of California, San Francisco
San Francisco, California

Howard S. An, MD
The Morton International Endowed Chair
Professor of Orthopaedic Surgery
Director of Spine Surgery and Spine Fellowship Program
Department of Orthopaedic Surgery
Rush University Medical Center
Chicago, Illinois

D. Greg Anderson, MD
Professor
Departments of Orthopaedic and Neurological Surgery
Rothman Institute
Thomas Jefferson University
Philadelphia, Pennsylvania

Vincent Arlet, MD
Professor of Orthopedic Surgery
Department of Orthopedic Surgery
University of Pennsylvania
Philadelphia, Pennsylvania

Paul M. Arnold, MD
Professor of Neurosurgery
Department of Neurosurgery
University of Kansas Medical Center
Director
Spinal Cord Injury Center
University of Kansas Hospital
Kansas City, Kansas

Casey C. Bachison, MD
Fellow
Orthopaedic Surgery of the Spine
Department of Orthopaedic Surgery
William Beaumont Hospital
Royal Oak, Michigan

Raghav Badrinath, BS
Medical Student
Yale School of Medicine
New Haven, Connecticut

Jun Seok Bae, MD
Department of Neurological Surgery
Wooridul Spine Hospital
Seoul, South Korea

Kelley Banagan, MD
Assistant Professor
Orthopaedics
University of Maryland
Baltimore, Maryland

Rahul Basho, MD
Midwest Orthopedic Specialists
Director of Spine Surgery
Hannibal Regional Hospital
Hannibal, Missouri

Ulrich Batzdorf, MD
Professor Emeritus
Department of Neurosurgery
David Geffen School of Medicine at UCLA
Los Angeles, California

Carlo Bellabarba, MD
Professor
Orthopaedics and Neurological Surgery
University of Washington School of Medicine
Director
Orthopaedic Spine Service
Orthopaedics and Sports Medicine
Harborview Medical Center
Seattle, Washington

Edward C. Benzel, MD
Chairman
Department of Neurosurgery
Center for Spine Health
Cleveland Clinic
Cleveland, Ohio

Justin E. Bird, MD
Assistant Professor
Orthopaedic Oncology and Spine Surgery
The University of Texas MD Anderson Cancer Center
Houston, Texas

Bronek M. Boszczyk, PD Dr.med
Consultant Spinal Surgeon and Head of Service
Centre for Spinal Studies and Surgery
Queen's Medical Centre
Nottingham University Hospitals
Nottingham, Great Britain

Richard J. Bransford, MD
Associate Professor
Department of Orthopaedics and Sports Medicine
University of Washington School of Medicine
    and Harborview Medical Center
Seattle, Washington

Jacob M. Buchowski, MD, MS
Professor of Orthopaedic and Neurological Surgery
Department of Orthopaedic Surgery
Director
Center for Spinal Tumors
Washington University Orthopaedics
Washington University School of Medicine
St. Louis, Missouri

Clinton J. Burkett, MD
Spine Fellow
Department of Neurosurgery
University of Virginia School of Medicine
Charlottesville, Virginia

Jens R. Chapman, MD
HansJoerg Wyss Professor and Chairman
Department of Orthopaedic Surgery and
    Sports Medicine
Joint Professor of Neurological Surgery
University of Washington School of Medicine
    and Harborview Medical Center
Seattle, Washington

Jason Pui Yin Cheung, MBBS, MRCS(Edin), MMedSc
Clinical Assistant Professor
Department of Orthopaedics and Traumatology
The University of Hong Kong
Pokfulam, Hong Kong

Norman Chutkan, MD
Professor of Orthopaedic Surgery
Department of Orthopaedic Surgery
Georgia Health Sciences University
Augusta, Georgia

Giac Consigilieri, MD
Medical Director of Neurosurgery
Santa Rosa Memorial Hospital
Santa Rosa, California

Chris A. Cornett, MD
Assistant Professor of Orthopaedic Surgery
University of Nebraska Medical Center
Medical Director of Physical and Occupational Therapy
The Nebraska Medical Center and Bellevue
    Medical Center
Omaha, Nebraska

Bradford L. Currier, MD
Director
Spinal Fellowship Program
Professor of Orthopedics
Mayo Clinic College of Medicine
Rochester, Minnesota

Nader S. Dahdaleh, MD
Assistant Professor
Department of Neurosurgery
Northwestern University Feinberg School of Medicine
Chicago, Illinois

Mihir J. Desai, MD
Resident Physician
Department of Orthopaedic Surgery
Emory University
Atlanta, Georgia

Vedat Deviren, MD
Associate Professor
Orthopaedic Surgery
University of California, San Francisco
San Francisco, California

Ashvin Kumar Dewan, MD
Housestaff
Orthopaedic Surgery
The Johns Hopkins School of Medicine
Baltimore, Maryland

Shah-Nawaz M. Dodwad, MD
Resident Physician
Department of Orthopaedics
The Ohio State University
Columbus, Ohio

Denis S. Drummond, MD
Emeritus Chair
Orthopaedic Surgery
The Children's Hospital of Philadelphia
Emeritus Professor
Orthopaedic Surgery
University of Pennsylvania School of Medicine
Philadelphia, Pennsylvania

Jason C. Eck, DO
Assistant Professor
Department of Orthopedic Surgery
University of Massachusetts
Worcester, Massachusetts

Richard G. Fessler, MD, PhD
Professor
Department of Neurosurgery
Rush University Medical Center
Chicago, Illinois

Eric Feuchtbaum, MD, MBA
Resident Physician
Department of Orthopaedic Surgery
Washington University School of Medicine
St. Louis, Missouri

Jeffrey S. Fischgrund, MD
Chairman
Department of Orthopaedic Surgery
Beaumont Health System
Royal Oak, Michigan

Mark P. Garrett, MD
Neurosurgeon
Division of Neurological Surgery
Barrow Neurological Institute
St. Joseph's Hospital and Medical Center
Phoenix, Arizona

Sanjitpal S. Gill, MD
Adjunct Assistant Professor
Bioengineering
Clemson University
Clemson, South Carolina
Orthopaedic Spine Surgery
Pelham Medical Center
Greer, South Carolina

Joseph P. Gjolaj, MD
Assistant Professor
Department of Orthopaedics and Rehabilitation
University of Miami Miller School of Medicine
Miami, Florida

Panagiotis Glavas, MD
Assistant Professor
Division of Orthopaedic Surgery
CHU Sainte-Justine
University of Montréal
Montréal, Canada

Ziya L. Gokaslan, MD
Department of Neurosurgery
The Johns Hopkins School of Medicine
Baltimore, Maryland

Gregory Grabowski, MD
Assistant Professor
Orthopaedic Surgery
Department of Orthopaedic Surgery and Sports Medicine
University of South Carolina School of Medicine
Columbia, South Carolina

Jonathan N. Grauer, MD
Associate Professor
Department of Orthopaedics and Rehabilitation
Yale University School of Medicine
New Haven, Connecticut

Yoon Ha, MD
Fellow
Department of Neurological Surgery
University of California, San Francisco
San Francisco, California

Melvin D. Helgeson, MD
Chief
Pediatric and Spine Surgery Service
Department of Orthopaedics
Walter Reed National Military Medical Center
Bethesda, Maryland

Joshua E. Heller, MD
Assistant Professor
Neurological Surgery
Thomas Jefferson University
Philadelphia, Pennsylvania

Faisal R. Jahangiri, MD, CNIM, D.ABNM, FASNM
Consultant
Clinical Neurophysiology
Division of Neurology
Department of Medicine
King Abdulaziz Medical City
King Fahad National Guard Hospital
Riyadh, Saudi Arabia

Iain H. Kalfas, MD, FACS
Head
Section of Spinal Surgery
Department of Neurosurgery
Cleveland Clinic
Cleveland, Ohio

James D. Kang, MD
Professor of Orthopaedic and Neurological Surgery
UPMC Endowed Chair in Spine Surgery
Vice Chairman
Department of Orthopaedic Surgery
Director of Ferguson Laboratory for Spine Research
University of Pittsburgh School of Medicine
Pittsburgh, Pennsylvania

Jaro Karppinen, MD, PhD
Professor
Institute of Clinical Sciences
University of Oulu
Oulu, Finland

Christopher K. Kepler, MD, MBA
Assistant Professor
Department of Orthopaedic Surgery
Thomas Jefferson University
Philadelphia, Pennsylvania

Safdar N. Khan, MD
Assistant Professor
Department of Orthopaedics
The Ohio State University
Columbus, Ohio

A. Jay Khanna, MD, MBA
Professor
Departments of Orthopaedic Surgery and Biomedical
    Engineering
The Johns Hopkins School of Medicine
Baltimore, Maryland
Division Chief
Johns Hopkins Orthopaedic and Spine Surgery-National
    Capital Region
Bethesda, Maryland

Frank La Marca, MD
Clinical Assistant Professor
Department of Neurosurgery
University of Michigan
Ann Arbor, Michigan

Sang-Ho Lee, MD, PhD
Department of Neurosurgery
Wooridul Spine Hospital
Seoul, South Korea

Sang-Hun Lee, MD, PhD
Associate Professor
Orthopaedic Surgery
Spine center
Kyung Hee University Hospital at Gangdong
Seoul, South Korea

Xudong Joshua Li, MD, PhD
Department of Orthopaedic Surgery
University of Virginia
Charlottesville, Virginia

Isador H. Lieberman, MD
Director
Scoliosis and Spine Tumor Center
Texas Back Institute
Plano, Texas

Moe R. Lim, MD
Associate Professor
Department of Orthopaedics
University of North Carolina–Chapel Hill
Chapel Hill, North Carolina

**Gabriel Liu, MB Bch BAO, MSc, FRCSI,
FRCSEd(Orth), FAMS (Orth)**
Associate Professor
University Spine Center
National University Health System
National University of Singapore
Singapore

Steven C. Ludwig, MD
Associate Professor of Orthopaedics
Chief of Spine Surgery
Department of Orthopaedics
University of Maryland
Baltimore, Maryland

**Keith DK Luk, MCh(Orth), FRCSE, FRCSG, FRACS,
FHKAM(Orth)**
Tam Sai-Kit Professor in Spine Surgery
Chair Professor and Chief Division of Spine Surgery
Department of Orthopedics and Traumatology
The University of Hong Kong
Pokfulam, Hong Kong

Jeffrey T.P. Luna, MD
Staff Orthopaedic Surgeon
Trinity Regional Medical Center
Fort Dodge, Iowa

John P. Malloy, DO
Director
Division of Spine Surgery
East Coast Orthopaedics
Pompano Beach, Florida

Rex A.W. Marco, MD
Professor
Department of Orthopaedic Surgery and Oncology
University of Texas
Houston, Texas

Arnold H. Menezes, MD
Professor and Vice Chairman
Department of Neurosurgery
University of Iowa
Iowa City, Iowa

M. David Mitchell, BS, MS, MD
Clinical Professor
Department of Orthopedics
Medical University of South Carolina
Charleston, South Carolina
Orthopedic Surgeon
Spine Center
Orthopaedic Associates
Spartanburg, South Carolina

Camilo A. Molina, MD
Department of Neurosurgery
The Johns Hopkins School of Medicine
Baltimore, Maryland

Ahmad Nassr, MD
Consultant
Assistant Professor
Department of Orthopedics
Mayo Clinic College of Medicine
Rochester, Minnesota

Abimbola A. Obafemi, MD
Department of Orthopaedics
University of Maryland
Baltimore, Maryland

Daniel K. Park, MD
Assistant Professor
Department of Orthopaedic Surgery
William Beaumont Hospital
Royal Oak, Michigan

Paul Park, MD
Associate Professor
Departments of Neurological and Orthopaedic Surgery
University of Michigan
Ann Arbor, Michigan

Frank M. Phillips, MD
Professor
Department of Orthopaedic Surgery
Spine Fellowship Co-Director
Rush University Medical Center
Chicago, Illinois

Shayan Rahman, MD
Neurosurgeon
Kaiser Permanente Foundation–Los Angeles Medical
    Center
Los Angeles, California

S. Rajasekaran, MS, FRCS, MCH, FACS, PhD
Chairman
Department of Orthopaedics and Spine Surgery
Ganga Hospital
Coimbatore, India
Adjunct Professor of Orthopaedic Surgery
Tamilnadu Medical University
Chennai, India

Conor Regan, MD
Wake Orthopaedics
Raleigh, North Carolina

Dike Ruan, MD
Professor of Orthopedic Surgery
Department of Orthopaedics
Navy General Hospital
Beijing, China

Dino Samartzis, DSc
Warden, Hornell Hall
Assistant Professor
Director of Clinical Spine Research
Department of Orthopaedics and Traumatology
Deputy Director
Laboratory and Clinical Research Institute for Pain
Li Ka Shing Faculty of Medicine
The University of Hong Kong
Hong Kong

Benjamin F. Sandberg, MD
Resident
Department of Orthopaedic Surgery
University of Minnesota
Minneapolis, Minnesota

Rick C. Sasso, MD
Professor
Chief of Spine Surgery
Clinical Orthopaedic Surgery
Indiana University School of Medicine
Indiana Spine Group
Indianapolis, Indiana

Justin K. Scheer, BS
Medical Student
University of California, San Diego
San Diego, California

Daniel M. Sciubba, MD
Department of Neurosurgery
The Johns Hopkins School of Medicine
Baltimore, Maryland

William R. Sears, MBBS, FRACS
Professor
Neurosurgery and Spinal Injuries
Royal North Shore Hospital
Sydney, Australia

Dave J. Seecharan, MD
Resident Physician
Department of Neurosurgery
University of Kansas Medical Center
Kansas City, Kansas

Christopher I. Shaffrey, MD
Harrison Distinguished Professor
Department of Neurological and Orthopaedic Surgery
University of Virginia School of Medicine
Charlottesville, Virginia

Francis H. Shen, MD
Warren G. Stamp Endowed Professor
Division Head
Spine Division
Director
Spine Fellowship
Co-Director
Spine Center
Department of Orthopaedic Surgery
University of Virginia Health Science Center
Charlottesville, Virginia

Wun-Jer Shen, MD
Director
Po-Cheng Orthopaedic Institute
Kaohsiung, Taiwan
Professor
Department of Orthopaedics
Shandong Provincial Hospital affiliated with
    Shandong University
Jinan, Shandong, China

Adam L. Shimer, MD
Associate Professor
Department of Orthopaedic Surgery
University of Virginia
Charlottesville, Virginia

Zachary A. Smith, MD
Assistant Professor
Department of Neurosurgery
Northwestern University-Feinberg School of Medicine
Chicago, Illinois

Volker K.H. Sonntag, MD
Emeritus
Division of Neurological Surgery
Barrow Neurological Institute
St. Joseph's Hospital and Medical Center
Phoenix, Arizona

James A. Stadler III, MD
Resident Physician
Department of Neurological Surgery
Northwestern University–Feinberg School of Medicine
Chicago, Illinois

Geoffrey E. Stoker, MD
Department of Orthopaedic Surgery
Washington University School of Medicine
St. Louis, Missouri

Oliver M. Stokes, MB BS, MSc, FRCS (Tr&Orth)
Consultant Spinal Surgeon
Royal Devon and Exeter NHS Foundation Trust
Exeter, United Kingdom

Jani Takatalo, MD
Institute of Clinical Sciences
University of Oulu
Oulu, Finland

Katsushi Takeshita, MD
Professor
Department of Orthopaedics
Jichi Medical University
Shimotsuke, Tochigi, Japan

Tony Y. Tannoury, MD
Assistant Professor of Orthopaedic Surgery
Boston University School of Medicine;
Director of Spine Services
Boston Medical Center
Boston, Massachusetts

Fernando Techy, MD
Assistant Professor of Clinical Orthopaedics and
    Spine Surgery
University of Illinois at Chicago
Chicago, Illinois

Khoi Than, MD
Chief Resident
Department of Neurosurgery
University of Michigan
Ann Arbor, Michigan

Lauren A. Tomlinson, BS
Clinical Research Coordinator
Division of Orthopaedic Surgery
The Children's Hospital of Philadelphia
Philadelphia, Pennsylvania

Jonathan Tuttle, MD
Assistant Professor
Departments of Neurosurgery and Orthopaedics
Georgia Regents University
Augusta, Georgia

Alexander R. Vaccaro, MD, PhD
Professor and Vice Chairman
Department of Orthopaedic Surgery
Thomas Jefferson University and Hospitals
Philadelphia, Pennsylvania

Dachuan Wang, MD, PhD
Associate Professor of Spine Surgery
Department of Orthopaedics
Shandong Provincial Hospital Affiliated to
    Shandong University
Jinan, China

Hai-Qiang Wang
Assistant Professor
Department of Orthopaedics
Xijing Hospital
Fourth Military Medical University
Xi'an, China

Jeffrey C. Wang, MD
Chief
Orthopaedic Spine Service
Co-Director USC Spine Center
Professor of Orthopaedic Surgery and Neurosurgery
USC Spine Center
Los Angeles, California

Brian C. Werner, MD
Resident Physician
Department of Orthopaedic Surgery
University of Virginia
Charlottesville, Virginia

Adam S. Wilson, MD
Resident
Department of Orthopaedic Surgery
University of Virginia
Charlottesville, Virginia

Albert P. Wong, MD
Resident Physician
Neurological Surgery
Northwestern University–Feinberg School of Medicine
Chicago, Illinois

Hee Kit Wong, MBBS,
M. Med(Surg), FRCS(Glas), MCh(Orth)Liv, FAMS
Professor and Head
Department of Orthopaedic Surgery
Yong Loo Lin School of Medicine
National University of Singapore
Chairman
University Orthopaedic and Hand Reconstructive
    Microsurgery Cluster
National University Health System
Head
University Spine Centre
National University Health System
Singapore

Albert S. Woo, MD
Assistant Professor
Plastic Surgery
Chief
Pediatric Plastic Surgery
Director,
Cleft Palate-Craniofacial Institute
Washington University School of Medicine
St. Louis, Missouri

Moshe M. Yanko, MD
Department of Orthopaedics
University of Maryland
Baltimore, Maryland

Byung M. (Jason) Yoon, MD, PhD
Resident Physician
Department of Neurosurgery
Stanford University
Palo Alto, California

S. Tim Yoon, MD, PhD
Associate Professor
Orthopedic Surgery
Emory University
Atlanta, Georgia

Clinical practice has greatly changed. Previously, it was a system led by doctors, but now it is a system shared by doctors, patients, and third parties (public and payers). The development of the computer has promoted the concept of evidence-based medicine, which has enabled evaluation of the quality of medical care. Medical care has been standardized, and now it should convince patients and other people. "Medical care experienced by the individual doctor" has been changed to "medical care with everyone convinced."

Spine surgery has been part of this rapid change, and the cervical spine field is no exception. The changes are found in every aspect: development of basic science, rapid progress of diagnostic techniques including imaging studies, and introduction of multi-dimensional evaluation in analyzing outcomes such as the shift from "evaluation by doctors" to "evaluation by patients" and pursuit of minimally invasive surgery.

This textbook is composed of chapters written by leading professionals in each field of cervical spine surgery, who are clinically working in this changing time.

Furthermore, it includes all the aspects from basics to clinical practice and is organized pathologically. It provides us practical information for treating patients. It also provides useful information for surgery: state-of-the-art techniques, emerging technologies, and complications. The chapter on complications explains how to avoid and manage complications, which is very helpful for clinical doctors.

Each chapter includes a preview that provides a synopsis and the important points of the chapter. It is very well organized, and we can clearly understand all the aspects of cervical spine surgery in a short time.

I assure you this textbook is beneficial for both specialists and residents. For specialists, it is a good tool for evaluating the current situation of the cervical spine field and for learning cutting-edge surgery techniques. For residents, it provides a solid foundation in cervical spine surgery and useful learning direction.

Shin-ichi Kikuchi, MD, PhD
President of Fukushima Medical University
Fukushima, Japan

Drs. Shen, Samartzis, and Fessler have produced an outstanding textbook that is relevant for cervical spine surgeons all over the world. This is a comprehensive textbook covering anatomy, pathology, and surgical technique, as well as the latest advances in the field. As such, it is an outstanding reference source for all spine surgeons, including those in training. The authors of this book are some of the most well-recognized cervical spine surgeons in the world and thought leaders in the field. That they are also from many different countries expands the scope and comprehensive nature of the book. The topics covered include everything from rare pathologies such as tuberculosis of the cervical spine, a rarity in North America, to more common topics such as cervical myelopathy. I believe that this work is destined to become an important reference work in the field.

I sincerely congratulate Drs. Shen, Samartzis, and Fessler for their excellent textbook.

K. Daniel Riew, MD
Mildred B. Simon Distinguished Professor
    of Orthopedic Surgery
Professor of Neurological Surgery
Chief, Cervical Spine Surgery
Director, Orthopedic and Rehab Institute
    for Cervical Spine Surgery
Washington University Orthopedics
Barnes-Jewish Hospital
    and Washington University School of Medicine
President, Cervical Spine Research Society 2012-2013
Chair, AOSpine International Research Commission
    2012-2015

During the past two decades, our knowledge of spine functional anatomy and biomechanics advanced significantly. Complex neuroradiologic techniques were introduced that allow us to appreciate the pathological changes and disease characteristics. Moreover, the effects of surgery on spine functions and stability can be visualized in detail. The surgical technique was elaborated; neuromonitoring and intraoperative imaging became more reliable. All these advancements influenced the management principles of spine diseases, rendering it safer and more efficient.

On the other side the industry provides more sophisticated and fancy solutions that may influence the decision-making process. In order to help the patient, the surgeon should have a clear idea what he or she wants to achieve and how to do it.

The current textbook, edited by Drs. Shen, Samartzis, and Fessler, will certainly help the reader in finding answers to many issues. Special chapters cover the more general aspects, such as applied spine anatomy, neuro-imaging, and neuromonitoring. Still, the main focus and strength of the textbook is the in-depth presentation of the spinal diseases—degenerative, traumatic, neoplastic, and infectious/inflammatory—and the related management options and surgical techniques. This textbook is a valuable addition to spine literature, and I would definitely recommend it.

Madjid Samii, MD, PhD
Founder and President
International Neuroscience Institute
Hannover, Germany

PREFACE

The practice of medicine is ever expanding, and the art and science of surgery are no different. Advances in spine surgery in particular continue to evolve at an ever-increasing rate. The complex anatomy of the craniocervical and cervicothoracic junction, combined with the intimate relationship to the vertebral artery, spinal cord, and nerve roots to the spine, along with the mobile nature of the cervical segments, makes management of pathologies of the cervical spine uniquely different than in any other parts of the neuroaxis.

The editors have been extremely fortunate to have assembled an internationally renowned, multidisciplinary group of specialists. *Textbook of the Cervical Spine* includes the experience and expertise of both neurosurgical and orthopaedic spine specialists, not only from North America, but also from South America, Europe, and Asia. As a result, this textbook is well suited to serve as a reference for both orthopaedic and neurosurgical residents and fellows in training, and also for the practicing spine surgeons who are continually working to expand their knowledge. It also serves as a ready reference for the non-operative health care provider who is interested in better understanding conditions of the cervical spine.

Textbook of the Cervical Spine has been organized into eight main sections. The first section focuses on the core basics, including anatomy, surgical approaches, and evaluation of the cervical spine. In sections two through four, we organized the chapters to focus on specific pathologic conditions. In the fifth through seventh sections, we strive to cover both classic and newer surgical techniques that can be applied across a wide range of pathologies. In the eighth and final section, we attempt to cover complications and their management options. The reader will find that, throughout the textbook, the authors have included tips and tricks, while attempting to point out more subtle pearls and pitfalls for each of the specific topic being addressed.

Enjoy.

Francis H. Shen, Charlottesville, Virginia, USA

Dino Samartzis, Hong Kong, China

Richard G. Fessler, Chicago, Illinois, USA

CONTENTS

VIDEO CONTENTS

TEXTBOOK OF
THE CERVICAL SPINE

SECTION 1

Basics

Cervical Spine Anatomy

1

Shah-Nawaz M. Dodwad, Safdar N. Khan, and Howard S. An

Chapter Synopsis
An expert understanding of cervical anatomy is critical to a spine surgeon operating in this region. An understanding of this anatomy is essential for surgical technique and diagnosis of pathologic processes. This chapter is a review of cervical spine osteology, ligaments, muscles, and neurovascular structures.

Important Points
The ringlike structures of the atlas (C1) and axis (C2) are unique as compared with C3 to C7 vertebral bodies.

The junction between the spinous process and the lamina is important during spino-laminar wiring to avoid injury to the spinal cord.

The posterior neural arch fuses at 3 years of age, and the anterior arch fuses at 7 years of age; these features should not be confused with fracture lines.

The major stabilizing ligament of C1 and C2 is the transverse ligament.

Understanding the various anatomic relationships of the spinal ligaments and muscles is essential.

The suboccipital triangle contains the vertebral artery, the suboccipital nerve (dorsal rami of C1), and the suboccipital venous plexus.

The posterior triangle is bounded anteriorly by the sternocleidomastoid (SCM) muscle and posteriorly by the trapezius muscle.

The anterior triangle is formed by the SCM posteriorly, the midline of the neck anteriorly, the mandible inferiorly, and the sternal notch at the apex.

The vertebral artery usually enters the transverse foramen at C6.

Between the vertebral canal bone and the dura mater is the epidural space, which contains fat, internal venous plexus, and loose connective tissue. The epidural space can harbor infection or hematoma that can cause neurologic compromise.

Injury to the sympathetic chain results in Horner syndrome, which consists of the triad of miosis (pupillary constriction), ptosis (drooping eyelid), and anhidrosis (lack of sweat) on the ipsilateral side of the face.

To optimize outcomes after cervical spine surgery, the surgeon must select an appropriate patient and surgical procedure and must be technically able to perform the operation precisely. The surgical technique requires the surgeon to use the correct approach and carefully carry out the dissection to minimize complications. Thus, an expert understanding of cervical spine anatomy is essential to a surgeon operating in this region, as well as an understanding of the underlying spinal disorder. This chapter explores cervical spine osteology, ligamentous structures, intervertebral disks, muscles, neurovascular configuration, and other adjacent soft tissue elements.

Osteology

In the sagittal plane, the curvature of the spine at birth is concave anteriorly and is termed the primary curve. In response to head elevation and ambulation, the compensatory cervical and lumbar secondary curvatures develop and are concave posteriorly in the sagittal plane (Fig. 1-1). Normally, the cervical spine contains seven vertebrae with C1 to C8 spinal nerves.

The atlas or C1 is unique and has no body, thus resulting in its ringlike appearance (Fig. 1-2). Rather than having a body, the atlas has an anterior tubercle, which serves

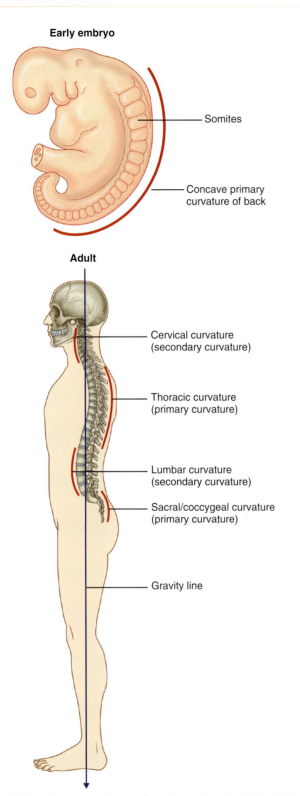

Early embryo

Somites

Concave primary curvature of back

Adult

Cervical curvature (secondary curvature)

Thoracic curvature (primary curvature)

Lumbar curvature (secondary curvature)

Sacral/coccygeal curvature (primary curvature)

Gravity line

FIGURE 1-1 Curvatures of the vertebral column. (From Drake RL, Vogl W, Mitchell AWM: *Gray's anatomy for students,* ed 2, Philadelphia, 2010, Elsevier.)

as an attachment for the longus colli muscle. The rectus capitis posterior minor muscle and the suboccipital membrane attach at the posterior tubercle. The obliquus capitis superior muscle originates from the transverse process of C1 and inserts into the base of the occipital bone. The oblique capitis inferior muscle originates from the

transverse process of C1 and inserts into the spinous process of C2. The transverse processes contain the foramen transversarium or transverse foramen, through which the vertebral arteries pass. C1 has three ossification centers: the body and each neural arch (lateral mass). The posterior neural arch fuses at the age of 3 years, and the anterior arch fuses at 7 years of age.[1,2] The lateral masses are located at the junction of the anterior and posterior arch. The concave superior facet of the lateral mass articulates above with the occipital condyle, and the flatter inferior facet of the lateral mass articulates below with C2 or the axis.[3,4] Just posterior to the lateral mass is the groove for the vertebral artery. The atlanto-occipital articulation is reinforced by the cephalic extensions of the anterior longitudinal ligament (ALL) and ligamentum flavum, respectively termed the anterior and posterior atlanto-occipital membranes at this level. The atlanto-occipital articulation primarily permits extension and flexion, as well as lateral flexion.[5]

The axis or C2 is also unique, in part because of the odontoid process or dens (Fig. 1-3). The dens protrudes superiorly to articulate with the posterior aspect of the atlas as a synovial joint. At the point of constriction where the dens meets the axis lies the transverse ligament. The transverse ligament holds the dens in place by spanning the anterior arch of the atlas and is the primary stabilizing structure of the atlantoaxial articulation.[6] The cruciform ligament is created from the cephalad and caudal projections of the transverse ligament. Arising from the sides of the dens and projecting to the medial aspect of the occipital condyles, the alar ligaments are additional stabilizers to the atlantoaxial articulation. The apical ligament is the residual portion of the notochord and connects the apex of the dens to the anterior aspect of the foramen magnum.[7] The bifid spinous process of the axis is where the rectus capitis posterior major and obliquus capitis inferior muscles attach. From posterior to anterior, the comparatively large pedicle projects medially and superiorly. At the age of 4 years, the dens begins to fuse to the ossific nucleus of C2 and can mistakenly be identified as a fracture, rather than a physiologic feature. Fifty percent of cervical spine rotation occurs at the atlantoaxial articulation. In the upper cervical region, the spinal canal diameter is larger compared with the lower cervical region. The sagittal diameters of the spinal canal at C1 and C2 are approximately 23 and 20 mm, respectively. In accordance with Steel's rule of thirds, the total spinal canal at the level of the axis is approximately 3 cm in sagittal diameter. The dens occupies approximately 1 cm, and the spinal cord occupies approximately 1 cm, thereby leaving approximately 1 cm of free space for the spinal cord before compression.[8] The atlantoaxial articulation primarily permits rotation.[9]

The C3 to C6 vertebrae are similar to each other, and they consist of a body, transverse processes, and pedicles (Fig. 1-4). Their caudally projecting spinous processes are bifid. The oval body is small compared with the more caudal vertebrae. The superior end plate of the body is concave and the inferior end plate is convex in the coronal plane. The coronal diameter of the body is larger than the sagittal diameter. The vertebral body is lipped inferiorly on the anteroinferior border. The uncinate process

Atlas (CI vertebra) and axis (C2 vertebra)

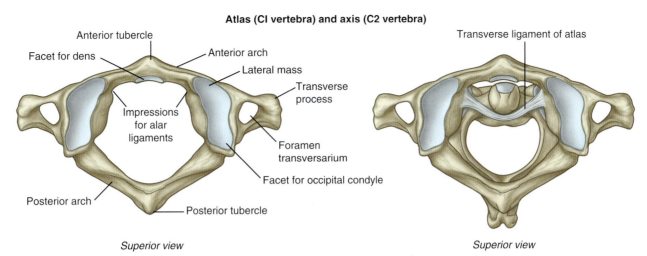

FIGURE I-2   **The atlas.** (From Drake RL, Vogl W, Mitchell AWM: *Gray's anatomy for students,* ed 2, Philadelphia, 2010, Elsevier.)

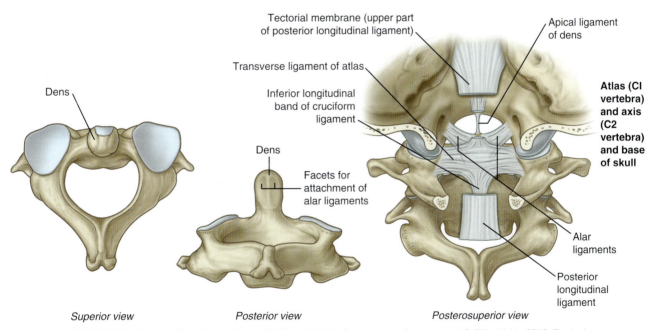

FIGURE I-3   **The axis.** (From Drake RL, Vogl W, Mitchell AWM: *Gray's anatomy for students,* ed 2, Philadelphia, 2010, Elsevier.)

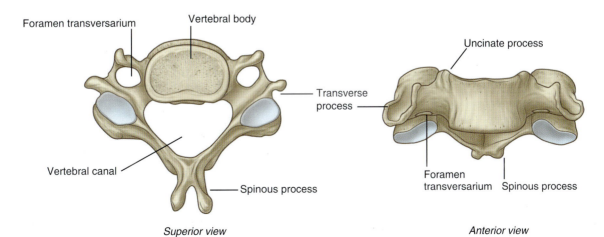

FIGURE I-4   **Typical cervical vertebra.** (From Drake RL, Vogl W, Mitchell AWM: *Gray's anatomy for students,* ed 2, Philadelphia, 2010, Elsevier.)

projects upward from the lateral surface of the superior aspect of the vertebral body. The uncinate process contours to the lateral surface of the inferior aspect of the cephalad vertebral body, to form the uncovertebral joints or joints of Luschka, which prevent vertebral body posterior translation and excessive lateral flexion. From C2 to C6, the average width and depth of the vertebral body are 17 and 15 mm, respectively. At C7, these measurements increase to approximately 20 and 17 mm, respectively.[10] The range for midsagittal vertebral heights is 11 to 13 mm.

The transverse process projects laterally from the superior aspect of the vertebral body to form the anterior and posterior tubercles at its distal aspect. The anterior tubercle is a costal element. The carotid tubercle is the C6 anterior tubercle and is a prominent surgical landmark. The spinal nerve courses between the anterior and posterior tubercles in the inferiorly projecting spinal nerve groove or costotransverse lamella.

The transverse processes contain the foramen transversarium that allows passage of the vertebral artery and venous system. These vessels pass lateral to the vertebral bodies, medial to the tubercles, and anterior to the spinal nerves. The vertebral arch is formed by the confluence of the lamina and the pedicle. The pedicles project posterolaterally from the vertebral body at an angle of 30 to 45 degrees.

The junction between the spinous process and the lamina is important during spinous process wiring. In this situation, if the wire penetrates beyond the spinolaminar line, it may injure the spinal cord. The lamina merges into the lateral mass laterally. The lateral mass lies between the superior and inferior articular processes. The superior articular process of the caudal vertebral body articulates with the inferior articular process of the adjacent cephalad vertebral body to form the facet joint. Encapsulated by a capsular ligament and lined by synovium, the facet joint is a true synovial joint that contains articular cartilage and menisci. As age-related degeneration occurs, the cartilage thins, and irregularly thickened subarticular cortical bone forms osteophytes that can cause nerve impingement.[11] The cervical facet joints have four distinct types of menisci.[12] Proprioceptive and pain receptors richly innervate the facet joints, a feature that in part explains cervical pain in facet disorders. The sagittal orientation of the facet joint at the level of the cervical spine is approximately 45 degrees compared with the more vertical coronal orientation of the lumbar facet joints.[13]

This facet orientation facilitates flexion and extension in the cervical spine. The facet joint line appears relatively horizontal with rounded edges when it is observed from the posterior aspect. The interfacet distance varies from 9 to 16 mm, with an average of 13 mm.[14] For this reason, screw hole distances of 13 mm are used in the many lateral mass plate-screw systems.

The spinal canal is triangular, with the apex posterior and rounded edges. The lateral width of the spinal canal is larger than the sagittal width at all levels. The normal sagittal widths of the cervical canal at C3 to C6 are 17 to 18 mm, and the width at C7 is 15 mm.[10] The C7 spinal canal has the smallest cross-sectional area, compared with the largest cross-sectional area located at C2. Slightly increasing from C3 to C7, the average width and height of the pedicle are approximately 5 to 6 and 7 mm, respectively.[10]

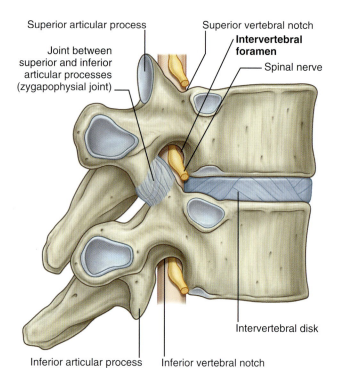

FIGURE 1-5 Intervertebral foramina. (From Drake RL, Vogl W, Mitchell AWM: *Gray's anatomy for students*, ed 2, Philadelphia, 2010, Elsevier.)

The C2 pedicle is larger, with an average height and width of 10 and 8 mm, respectively. From C3 to C7, the sagittal plane pedicle angle decreases from 45 to 30 degrees. The spinal nerve exits from the intervertebral foramen, which is bounded by the vertebral body and intervertebral disk anteriorly, by the facets posteriorly, and by adjacent level pedicles superiorly and inferiorly (Fig. 1-5). The spinal nerves pass through the cervical foramina, which are approximately 9 to 12 mm in height and 4 to 6 mm in width.[15,16] Because of the 45-degree oblique orientation of the foramina, oblique imaging is needed to assess the intervertebral foramina. Caution is advised during anterior exposure of the cervical spine because dissection on the inferior half of the vertebral body and uncovertebral joints that is too far lateral risks injury to the spinal nerve and vertebral artery around the intervertebral foramen. Iatrogenic vertebral artery injury has an incidence of 0.3%.[17]

The C7 vertebra is unique in that it represents a transition point between the more mobile cervical spine and the rigid thoracic spine. The large bony posterior prominence of the C7 spinous process identifies it as the vertebra prominens. The C7 spinous process is not bifid. Occasionally, cervical ribs are found at C7 that can compress the subclavian vasculature or brachial plexus and cause neurovascular symptoms, such as ischemic pain, numbness, tingling, and weakness. This cervicothoracic junction is a transitional area where C7 is similar to T1 and T2. The facet joint between C7 and T1 is similar to the thoracic facet articulation, and the lateral mass of C7 is thinner compared with the upper cervical levels. When performing transpedicular procedures at the C7, T1, and T2, it is important to remember some average measurements. The diameters of the pedicles of C7, T1, and T2 are approximately 5.2, 6.3, and 5.5 mm, respectively. Medial angulations are 34, 30, and 26 degrees, respectively.

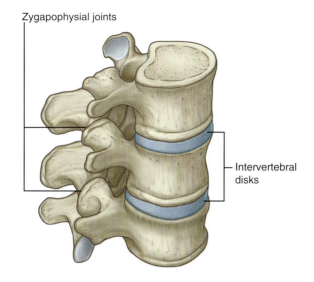

Zygapophysial joints

Intervertebral disks

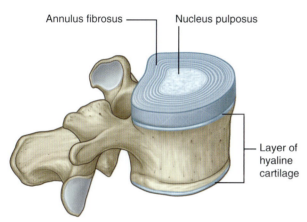

Annulus fibrosus — Nucleus pulposus

Layer of hyaline cartilage

FIGURE I-6   Intervertebral joints. (From Drake RL, Vogl W, Mitchell AWM: *Gray's anatomy for students*, Philadelphia, 2005, Elsevier.)

Intervertebral Disks and Ligaments

Intervertebral disks are avascular structures present between adjacent vertebral bodies, except at the occipitoatlantal and the atlantoaxial junctions. Each disk has an outer layer called the annulus fibrosus and an inner portion called the nucleus pulposus (Fig. 1-6). The junction of the disk with the vertebral body is lined by the cartilaginous end plates. In addition to the ligamentous structure and facet joints, the annulus fibrosus adds to motion segment stability. A motion segment is defined as two adjacent vertebral bodies and the intervertebral disk between them. The nucleus pulposus originates from the notochord and functions as a shock absorber. With age, the margin between the annulus fibrosus and the nucleus pulposus becomes blurred.[18] After the age of 50 years, the nucleus pulposus becomes difficult to identify because it becomes fibrocartilaginous in structure, similar to the annulus fibrosus. The annulus fibrosus is composed of concentric rings with obliquely oriented fibers to form a lamella. Fibers of each lamella are oriented perpendicular to the adjacent lamella. The fibers of the posterior portion of the disk are more vertical than oblique, thus partially explaining the relative frequency of radial tears seen in practice.

The cervical disks increase in height from 0.3 to 0.7 inches from birth to adolescence.[19] Disk height grows more slowly than does vertebral body height. One third of the length of the spine is related to the disks at birth. The disks account for one fifth of total spinal length after the age of 7 years. In the coronal plane, the superior surface of the disk is concave and the inferior surface is convex to conform to the adjacent vertebral bodies. Anteriorly, the disks are thicker than posteriorly to facilitate the lordotic curvature of the cervical spine. Movement in the coronal plane is limited by the uncinate process; however, the disks allow for some anteroposterior translation. Posterolateral disk herniations are fewer in frequency, likely secondary to the posterolateral location of the uncinate process. Although radial tears in the posterior aspect of the disk may be more clinically relevant, concentric, transverse, and radial tears also do occur in the cervical disks.[20]

The cartilaginous end plate is composed of hyaline cartilage and is located adjacent to the subchondral bone. One function of the end plate is to serve as a barrier to nucleus pulposus pressure on the vertebral body to limit protrusion. In addition, the end plate serves as the growth plate and is responsible for endochondral ossification. Furthermore, the end plates permit diffusion of nutrients from the subchondral bone to the disk and serve as insertion points for the inner fibers of the annulus.

The ALL and the posterior longitudinal ligament (PLL) are confluent with the outer fibers of the annulus (Fig. 1-7). The ALL runs from the base of the skull as the anterior atlanto-occipital membrane and continues inferiorly to the sacrum on the anterior aspect of all the vertebral bodies and disks. The ALL is wider and thinner over the disks and narrower and thicker over the concave vertebral bodies. The PLL is contiguous with the tectorial membrane and extends inferiorly to the sacrum within the spinal canal along the posterior aspect of the disks and vertebral bodies. Similar to the ALL, the PLL is wider over the disks and narrower over the bodies.[4] The PLL has two layers, of which the deeper layer sends fibers to the annulus fibrosus and the intervertebral foramina.[21] The ALL also has a deep layer that sends fibers to the annulus fibrosus that continue until they merge with the PLL at the intervertebral foramina.[21] The superficial layer of the PLL envelops the dura mater, nerve roots, and vertebral artery as a connective tissue layer.

The ligamentum flavum connects adjacent lamina from the axis to the sacrum (Fig. 1-8). It runs obliquely from the anterior aspect of the cephalad lamina to the superior margin of the caudal lamina. For this reason, it is easier to begin dissection of the ligamentum flavum from the inferior portion of the lamina. The ligamentum flavum continues laterally to the intervertebral foramina. It is composed primarily of elastic fibers that lose their elastic properties with age. During extension, the lack of elasticity may cause anterior buckling of the ligament into the spinal canal, with resulting spinal cord compression. Veins exit through a midline gap in the ligamentum flavum.

The interspinous ligament connects adjacent spinous processes (Fig. 1-9). This ligament runs between the ligamentum flavum anteriorly and the supraspinous ligament posteriorly. In the cervical region, the interspinous ligament is thin and not well developed. It attaches in an

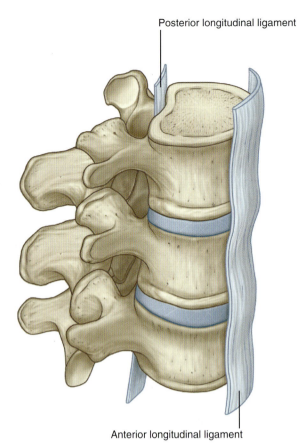

Posterior longitudinal ligament

Anterior longitudinal ligament

FIGURE 1-7   Anterior and posterior longitudinal ligaments of the vertebral column. (From Drake RL, Vogl W, Mitchell AWM: *Gray's anatomy for students,* ed 2, Philadelphia, 2010, Elsevier.)

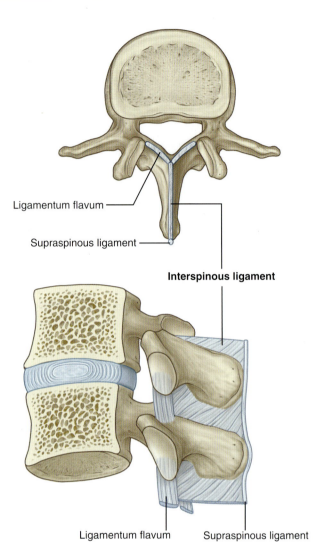

Ligamentum flavum

Supraspinous ligament

Interspinous ligament

Ligamentum flavum   Supraspinous ligament

FIGURE 1-9   Interspinous ligaments. (From Drake RL, Vogl W, Mitchell AWM: *Gray's anatomy for students,* ed 2, Philadelphia, 2010, Elsevier.)

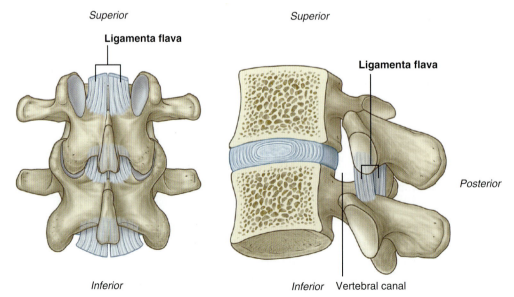

Superior

Ligamenta flava

Inferior

Superior

Ligamenta flava

Posterior

Inferior   Vertebral canal

FIGURE 1-8   Ligamenta flava. (From Drake RL, Vogl W, Mitchell AWM: *Gray's anatomy for students,* ed 2, Philadelphia, 2010, Elsevier.)

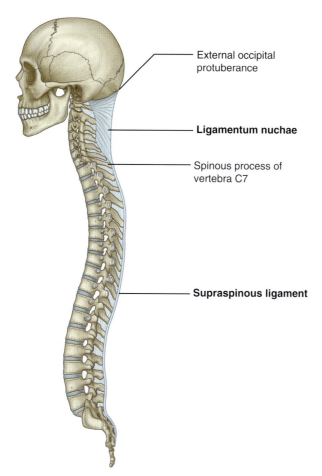

FIGURE 1-10   Supraspinous ligament and ligamentum nuchae. (From Drake RL, Vogl W, Mitchell AWM: *Gray's anatomy for students*, ed 2, Philadelphia, 2010, Elsevier.)

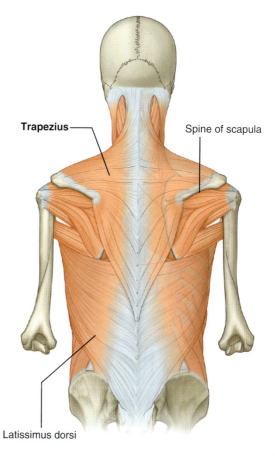

FIGURE 1-11   Trapezius muscle. (From Drake RL, Vogl W, Mitchell AWM: *Gray's anatomy for students*, Philadelphia, 2005, Elsevier.)

oblique direction from the posterosuperior aspect of the caudal spinous process to the anteroinferior aspect of the adjacent cephalad spinous process.

The supraspinous ligament connects the posterior tips of the spinous processes (Fig. 1-10). Because no supraspinous ligament is present at this level, the ligamentum nuchae becomes the extension of the supraspinous ligament.[7] The ligamentum nuchae extends from the external occipital protuberance to C7 and serves as an attachment point for adjacent muscles.

Muscles and Fascia

The posterior cervical musculature is divided into three groups: superficial, intermediate, and deep. The superficial group contains the trapezius muscle, which is innervated by the eleventh cranial nerve or spinal accessory nerve (Fig. 1-11). The trapezius originates from the ligamentum nuchae and external occipital protuberance, continues to the spinous process of T12, and inserts onto the scapular spine, acromion, and lateral third of the clavicle. The trapezius muscle is responsible for elevating, adducting, and depressing the scapula.

The muscles in the intermediate layer are the splenius capitis and splenius cervicis (Fig. 1-12). These muscles originate from the spinous processes of the cervicothoracic vertebrae and insert onto the transverse processes of upper cervical vertebrae and base of the occipital bone. When contracting bilaterally, they cause neck extension, and when contracting unilaterally, each muscle causes ipsilateral lateral flexion.

The posterior deep muscles are innervated by the posterior primary rami, and their blood supply is from the deep cervical vessels. The deep layer contains the superficial and deep erector spinae muscles. From lateral to midline, the deep erector spinae muscles include the iliocostalis cervicis, longissimus capitis, longissimus cervicis, and spinalis cervicis (Fig. 1-13). The semispinalis cervicis, multifidus, and rotatores are the transversospinales muscles of the posterior spine that represent the deep erector spinae muscles (Fig. 1-14). These muscles originate from transverse processes and insert on spinous processes in an oblique fashion, crossing a specific number of spinal segments.

In the upper cervical region, suboccipital muscles attach from the occiput to the atlas and axis (Fig. 1-15). The posterior primary rami innervate these muscles. The rectus capitis posterior major muscle originates from the spinous process of the axis and inserts into the inferior nuchal line of the occiput. The rectus capitis posterior minor muscle originates from the posterior tubercle of

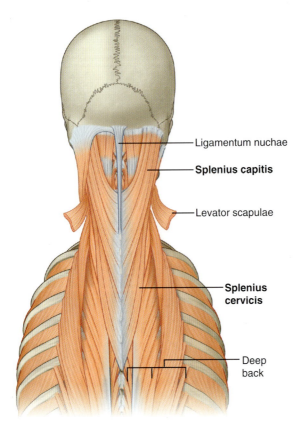

Ligamentum nuchae

Splenius capitis

Levator scapulae

Splenius cervicis

Deep back

FIGURE 1-12 Deep group of back muscles: spinotransversales muscles (splenius capitis and splenius cervicis). (From Drake RL, Vogl W, Mitchell AWM: *Gray's anatomy for students*, ed 2, Philadelphia, 2010, Elsevier.)

the atlas and inserts into the occiput. The obliquus capitis inferior muscle originates from the spinous process of the axis and inserts onto the transverse process of the atlas. The obliquus capitis superior muscle originates from the transverse process of the atlas and inserts between the superior and inferior nuchal lines onto the occiput. The suboccipital triangle is formed by the borders of the rectus capitis posterior major and the obliquus capitis superior and inferior muscles. The suboccipital triangle contains the vertebral artery, the suboccipital nerve (dorsal rami of C1), and the suboccipital venous plexus. These muscles are involved in producing the finer movements of extension of the neck and head.[4]

The anterolateral cervical muscles consist of the platysma, sternocleidomastoid (SCM), hyoid muscles, strap muscles of the larynx (omohyoid, thyrohyoid, sternohyoid, and sternothyroid), scalenes, longus colli, and longus capitis (Figs. 1-16 and 1-17). The platysma, the most superficial muscle, extends from the pectoralis major and deltoid fascia and continues medially and superiorly over the clavicle to attach to the mandible, the muscles of the lip, and the skin of the lower part of the face (Fig. 1-18). When contracting, the platysma muscle causes depression of the lip and lower jaw, as well as a wrinkling of the overlying skin. At the angle of the mandible and deep to the platysma, the external jugular vein can be seen descending.

The SCM muscle lies deep to the platysma and has two heads of origination: the sternum and medial clavicle. The SCM inserts onto the mastoid and superior nuchal line (Fig. 1-19). If only one SCM contracts, it causes the head

to tilt toward the ipsilateral side and the chin to rotate to the contralateral side. If both SCM muscles contract, they cause neck flexion. The SCM is innervated by the spinal accessory nerve and C2 spinal nerve. SCM contracture is involved in the pathogenesis of torticollis.

The group of muscles that attach to the hyoid include the digastric, stylohyoid, mylohyoid, geniohyoid, and omohyoid (Fig. 1-20; see Fig. 1-16). The sternohyoid and sternothyroid comprise the strap muscles of the larynx. These muscles are important as landmarks during the anterior approach to the cervical spine because they do not directly control cervical motion.

The longus colli and longus capitis muscles lie anterior to the cervical spine and are part of the prevertebral musculature. The longus colli originates from the anterior tubercles of the transverse processes of C3 to C6 and spans from C1 to T3 in an oblique fashion to insert onto the anterior aspect of the atlas. Originating from the anterior tubercles of the transverse processes of C3 to C6, the longus capitis muscle attaches on the inferior surface of the basilar part of the occipital bone. Deep to the longus capitis, the rectus capitis anterior muscle originates from the lateral mass of the atlas to insert into the base of the occipital bone. The rectus capitis lateralis originates from the transverse process of the atlas and inserts onto the inferior surface of the jugular process of the occiput. Originating from the anterior tubercles of the transverse processes of C3 to C6, the scalenus anterior muscle inserts onto the first rib. The scalenus medius muscle originates from the posterior tubercles of the transverse processes of C2 to C7 and its insertion is on the first rib. Thoracic outlet syndrome can occur from compression of the subclavian artery or brachial plexus between the scalenus anterior and scalenus medius muscles. Although anatomic variability exits, typically the scalenus posterior is described to originate from the posterior tubercles of the transverse process of C4 to C6 and inserts onto the lateral superior surface of the second rib.

The musculature of the neck is also organized into anatomic triangles that are important landmarks during the anterior approach to the cervical spine. The posterior triangle is bounded anteriorly by the SCM and posteriorly by the trapezius muscle. The posterior triangle is further divided by the omohyoid muscle into the upper occipital triangle and lower supraclavicular triangle.[4] The anterior triangle is formed by the SCM posteriorly and the midline of the neck anteriorly. The base is bounded by the mandible, and the sternal notch is the apex. The anterior triangle is further subdivided into four triangles: (1) the submental triangle, (2) the muscular or submandibular triangle, (3) the digastric triangle, and (4) the carotid triangle (Fig. 1-21).

The anterior neck contains fascia that invests the muscles and viscera in separate compartments that can be used to aid in guiding the surgical dissection. The superficial fascia lies between the skin and deep fascia and contains fat and areolar tissue. It envelops the platysma muscle, external jugular vein, and cutaneous sensory nerves. Deep to the superficial fascia lie the three layers of the deep fascia: the outer investing layer fascia, the middle cervical fascia, and the prevertebral fascia. The outer layer of the deep fascia extends the trapezius muscle, continues anteriorly over the posterior triangle, and divides to encircle the SCM muscle. The middle layer of the deep

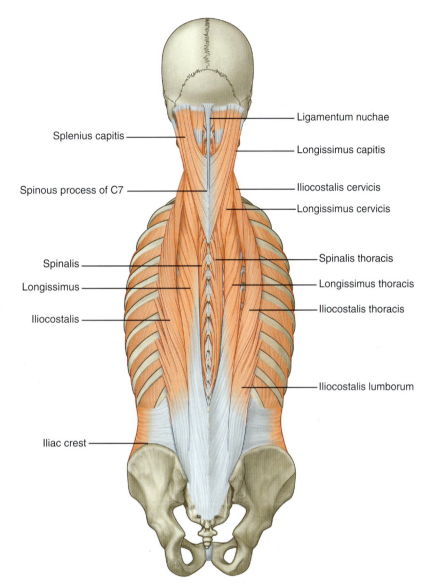

Splenius capitis

Ligamentum nuchae

Longissimus capitis

Spinous process of C7

Iliocostalis cervicis

Longissimus cervicis

Spinalis

Spinalis thoracis

Longissimus

Longissimus thoracis

Iliocostalis

Iliocostalis thoracis

Iliocostalis lumborum

Iliac crest

FIGURE 1-13   Deep group of back muscles: erector spinae muscles. (From Drake RL, Vogl W, Mitchell AWM: *Gray's anatomy for students*, ed 2, Philadelphia, 2010, Elsevier.)

cervical fascia encloses the omohyoid and strap muscles and continues laterally to the scapula. The thyroid gland, larynx, trachea, pharynx, and esophagus are enclosed by the visceral fascia of the deeper aspect of the middle layer. The alar fascia is often described as part of the prevertebral fascia and extends posterior to the esophagus and encloses the carotid sheath laterally. The contents of the carotid sheath are the carotid artery, internal jugular vein, and vagus nerve. The scalenus muscles, longus colli muscles, and ALL are associated with the deepest layer of the deep fascia known as the prevertebral fascia.

Neurovascular Structures

The major neurologic structures of the cervical spine are the spinal cord and nerve roots. The spinal cord emerges from the foramen magnum at the base of the skull from the medulla oblongata to approximately L2 (Fig. 1-22). The maximal cervical cord circumference is at C6 and is

approximately 38 mm, to accommodate the increased neurologic structures to the upper extremity from the brachial plexus.[4] The spinal cord contains butterfly-shaped inner gray matter and an outer circumferential layer of white matter, seen with magnetic resonance imaging (Fig. 1-23).[22] The white matter is divided into the posterior, lateral, and anterior columns and primarily contains myelinated axons and glia. In the posterior column, immediately adjacent to the posterior median sulcus, is the fasciculus gracilis, and lateral to that is the fasciculus cuneatus; these structures are responsible for proprioception, vibration, and fine touch. The lateral column contains the descending motor lateral corticospinal tract, which controls ipsilateral limb movement. The lateral spinothalamic tract is also located in the lateral column, where these tracts cross through the ventral commissure to the contralateral side of the cord to deliver sensory pain and temperature. The anterior column contains other descending tracts and the anterior spinothalamic tract, which is responsible for deep touch. The efferent

Text Continued on p. 15

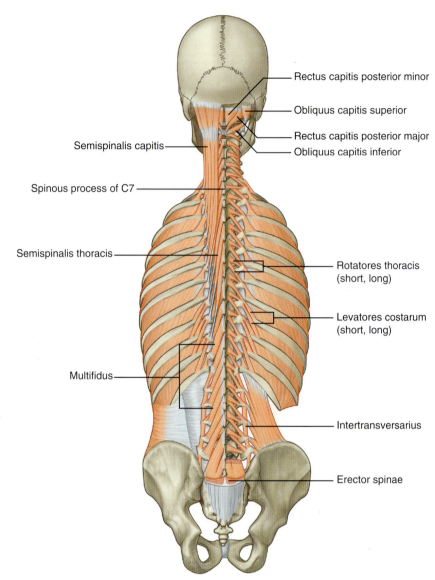

Rectus capitis posterior minor

Obliquus capitis superior

Rectus capitis posterior major

Obliquus capitis inferior

Semispinalis capitis

Spinous process of C7

Semispinalis thoracis

Rotatores thoracis
(short, long)

Levatores costarum
(short, long)

Multifidus

Intertransversarius

Erector spinae

FIGURE 1-14   Deep group of back muscles: transversospinales and segmental muscles. (From Drake RL, Vogl W, Mitchell AWM: *Gray's anatomy for students,* ed 2, Philadelphia, 2010, Elsevier.)

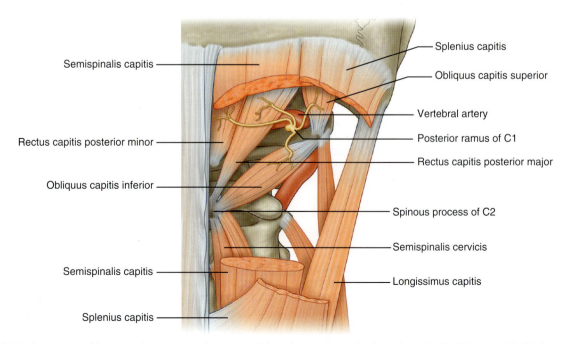

Semispinalis capitis

Splenius capitis

Obliquus capitis superior

Vertebral artery

Posterior ramus of C1

Rectus capitis posterior minor

Rectus capitis posterior major

Obliquus capitis inferior

Spinous process of C2

Semispinalis cervicis

Semispinalis capitis

Longissimus capitis

Splenius capitis

FIGURE 1-15   Deep group of back muscles: suboccipital muscles and the suboccipital triangle. (From Drake RL, Vogl W, Mitchell AWM: *Gray's anatomy for students,* ed 2, Philadelphia, 2010, Elsevier.)

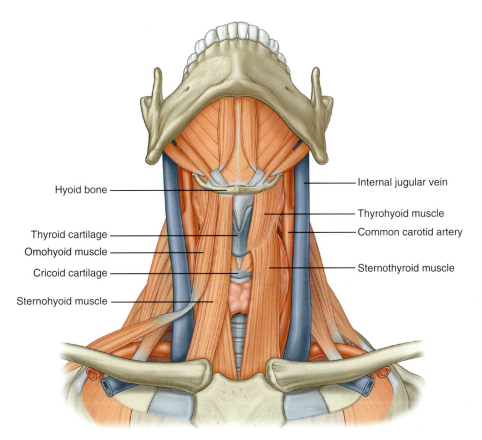

FIGURE 1-16   Infrahyoid muscles. (From Drake RL, Vogl W, Mitchell AWM: *Gray's anatomy for students,* ed 2, Philadelphia, 2010, Elsevier.)

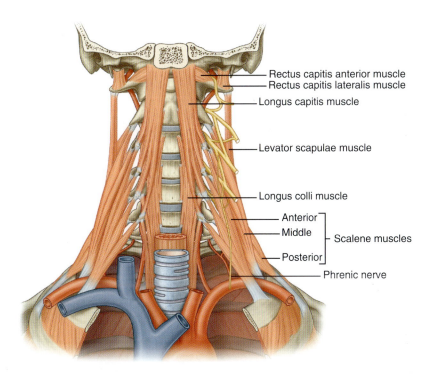

FIGURE 1-17   Prevertebral and lateral muscles supplied by the cervical plexus. (From Drake RL, Vogl W, Mitchell AWM: *Gray's anatomy for students,* ed 2, Philadelphia, 2010, Elsevier.)

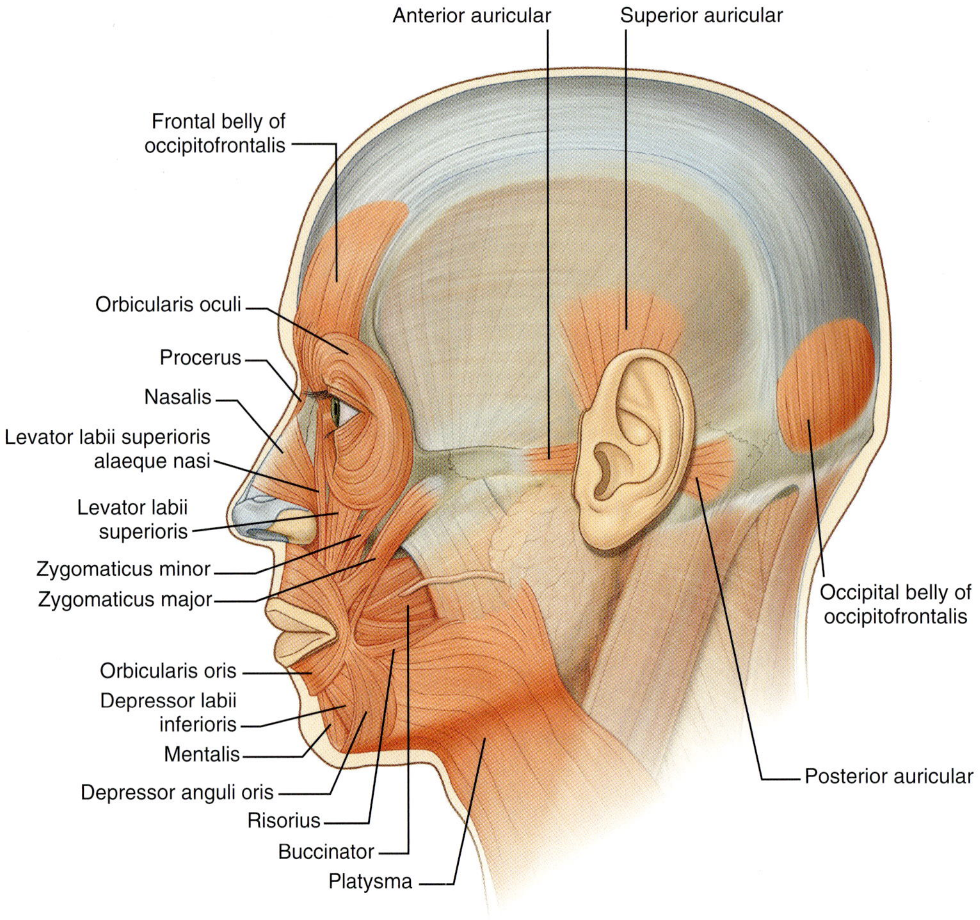

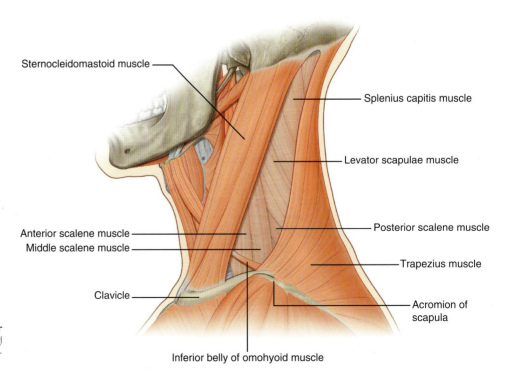

Anterior auricular

Superior auricular

Frontal belly of
occipitofrontalis

Orbicularis oculi

Procerus

Nasalis

Levator labii superioris
alaeque nasi

Levator labii
superioris

Zygomaticus minor

Zygomaticus major

Orbicularis oris

Depressor labii
inferioris

Mentalis

Depressor anguli oris

Risorius

Buccinator

Platysma

Occipital belly of
occipitofrontalis

Posterior auricular

FIGURE 1-18 Facial muscles. (From Drake RL, Vogl W, Mitchell AWM: *Gray's anatomy for students,* ed 2, Philadelphia, 2010, Elsevier.)

Sternocleidomastoid muscle

Splenius capitis muscle

Levator scapulae muscle

Anterior scalene muscle

Middle scalene muscle

Posterior scalene muscle

Trapezius muscle

Acromion of
scapula

Clavicle

Inferior belly of omohyoid muscle

FIGURE 1-19 Muscles of the superior triangle of the neck. (From Drake RL, Vogl W, Mitchell AWM: *Gray's anatomy for students,* ed 2, Philadelphia, 2010, Elsevier.)

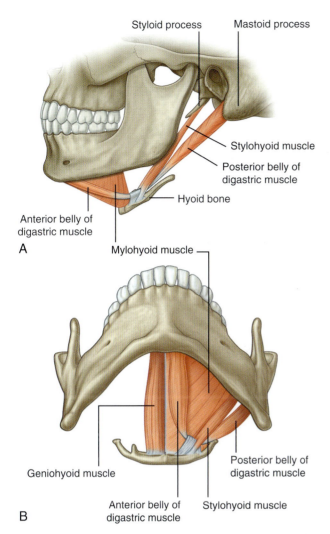

Styloid process

Mastoid process

Stylohyoid muscle

Posterior belly of
digastric muscle

Hyoid bone

Anterior belly of
digastric muscle

A

Mylohyoid muscle

Geniohyoid muscle

Posterior belly of
digastric muscle

Anterior belly of
digastric muscle

Stylohyoid muscle

B

FIGURE 1-20 Suprahyoid muscles. **A,** Lateral view. **B,** Inferior view. (From Drake RL, Vogl W, Mitchell AWM: *Gray's anatomy for students,* ed 2, Philadelphia, 2010, Elsevier.)

neural cell bodies and internuncial neurons are located in the gray matter. The anterior horn of the gray matter contains the somatomotor neurons. The posterior horn of the gray matter contains somatosensory neurons. The intermediolateral horn contains the visceral center of the gray matter. The central ependymal canal is located in the middle of the spinal cord and is an extension of the ventricular system to allow a channel of cerebrospinal fluid (CSF).

The spinal cord is enveloped by the meninges, which are made up of three layers: pia mater, arachnoid mater, and dura mater (Fig. 1-24). The pia is the closest layer to the spinal cord, followed by the arachnoid, followed by the dura. The dura is continuous at the foramen magnum with the inner layer of the cranial dura. The denticulate ligaments project from the pia laterally at positions in between exiting spinal nerves and attach to the arachnoid and dura to serve as motion stability for the spinal cord. The denticulate ligaments, in addition to the CSF, provide cushioning and motion stability of the spinal cord.

Between the vertebral canal bone and the dura mater is the epidural space, which contains fat, internal venous plexus, and loose connective tissue. The epidural space can harbor infection or hematoma that can cause neurologic compromise. The internal venous plexus facilitates propagation of infection or neoplasm. The CSF, spinal vasculature, and nerve rootlets are contained within the subarachnoid space located between the pia and the arachnoid.

The ventral lateral sulcus of the spinal cord is where the ventral motor rootlets exit. The lateral longitudinal sulcus of the spinal cord is where the dorsal sensory rootlets enter. At each level, six to eight rootlets leave the spinal cord laterally to be bathed in the CSF of the lateral subarachnoid space. The rootlets merge and form the dorsal and ventral roots. These become a nerve root at each level by entering a narrow envelope of arachnoid and passing through the dura. These nerve roots continue approximately 10 degrees inferiorly in the axial plane and 45 degrees anterolaterally in the coronal plane. Anteroinferiorly to the uncovertebral joint lies the anterior root. The posterior root lies next to the superior articular process. As the nerve root enters the intervertebral foramina, it passes above the corresponding level of the pedicle, except for the C8 nerve root, which passes below the C7 pedicle (Fig. 1-25). In the medial aspect of the foramen, the nerve root is located at the inferior portion of the superior articular process. As the nerve root courses laterally, it assumes a more inferior position just above the pedicle.[23]

Normally, the neural foramen is approximately 9 to 12 mm in height, 4 to 6 mm in width, and 4 to 6 mm in length and is bounded superiorly and inferiorly by pedicles (see Fig. 1-5).[16] The anterior border of the foramen is the uncinate process, the posterolateral aspect of the intervertebral disk, and the inferior portion of the vertebral body above the disk level. The posterior margin of the foramen includes the facet joint and superior articular process of the caudal vertebral body. The nerve root occupies approximately one third of the foramen, although this space significantly decreases in the degenerative spine. At rest, the nerve roots are located in the caudal half of the foramen; however, when the neck is fully extended, the foramen size is decreased, and the nerve roots assume a more superior position within the foramen.[7] Fat and small veins are present in the superior half of the foramen.[24]

The dorsal root ganglion (DRG) contains the efferent cell bodies and is located in the dorsal root, between the vertebral artery and a small concavity in the superior articular process. The DRG is seen as an enlargement on the dorsal root in the distal aspect of the intervertebral foramen.[25] The spinal nerve is formed just distal to the DRG, as the confluence of the ventral and dorsal roots (Fig. 1-26). At this point, the spinal nerve divides into the dorsal primary ramus and the ventral primary ramus. Gray rami from the sympathetic cervical ganglion join the ventral primary rami. The ALL, outer annulus fibrosis, and anterior vertebral body are innervated by the ventral nerve plexus, which has contributions from the interconnections among the gray rami, the perivascular plexus around the vertebral artery, and the sympathetic trunk.[26,27] The gray rami and perivascular plexus of the vertebral artery give rise to the sinuvertebral nerves, which

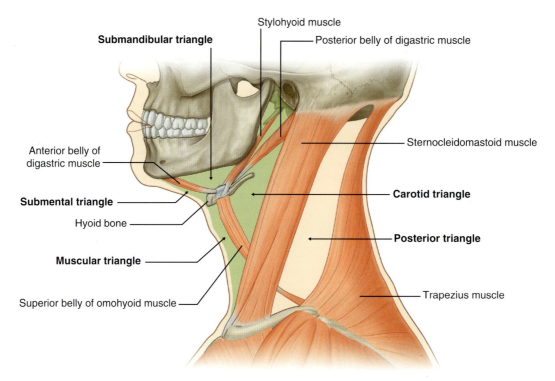

FIGURE 1-21   Borders and subdivisions of the anterior triangle of the neck. (From Drake RL, Vogl W, Mitchell AWM: *Gray's anatomy for students*, ed 2, Philadelphia, 2010, Elsevier.)

contribute to the dorsal nerve plexus, as well as innervate two or more disks or motion segments. The posterior part of the annulus, the ventral part of the dura, and the PLL are innervated by the dorsal nerve plexus.

Above the posterior arch of the atlas and posteromedial to the lateral mass, between the vertebral artery and the posterior arch, exits the suboccipital nerve or first cervical nerve. Motor fibers to the deep muscles of the suboccipital triangle originate from the posterior primary ramus of the first cervical nerve. The first and second cervical nerve anterior primary rami form a loop that sends fibers to the hypoglossal nerve.

The cervical plexus is located anterolateral to the levator scapulae and scalenus medius muscles, adjacent to C1 to C3, and contains the ventral primary rami of C1 to C4 (Fig. 1-27). The skin and muscles such as the rectus capitis anterior and lateralis, longus capitis and cervicis, levator scapulae, and scalenus medius receive contributions from the cervical plexus. The SCM and trapezius muscles are also supplied by loops and branches of the cervical plexus. The ansa cervicalis is a loop of nerves of the cervical plexus that is composed of the superior and inferior roots. The superior root of the ansa cervicalis consists of fibers from C1 and C2. The inferior root of the ansa cervicalis consists of fibers from C2 and C3. Posterior to the lateral mass, the C2 nerve can be seen lying on the lamina of the axis. Approximately 2 cm below the external occipital protuberance and 2 to 4 cm from midline, the posterior primary ramus of the greater occipital nerve penetrates the trapezius muscle. The skin of the nuchal region has cutaneous branches of the posterior primary rami of C2 to C5. The greater occipital nerve is the largest cutaneous nerve in this area. As a branch of the anterior cervical plexus, the lesser occipital nerve runs superolaterally to

the greater occipital nerve. Approximately 1 cm medial from the midline and more inferiorly, the posterior primary ramus of C3 or third occipital nerve penetrates the trapezius muscle. The first cervical nerve has no cutaneous branches; however, the other posterior primary rami of cervical nerves send motor fibers to the deep muscles and sensory fibers to the skin. The brachial plexus is composed of the anterior primary rami of C5 to T1. The cervical plexus is composed of the anterior primary rami of C1 to C4.

One vertebral artery branches from each subclavian artery to become the major blood supply of the cervical spine (Fig. 1-28). Although variations of the vertebral artery course exist, this vessel usually enters the transverse foramen at C6 and courses superiorly until C1.[28] At the atlas, the vertebral artery bends around the lateral mass and posterior arch of C1 through the vertebral artery groove to pass through the posterior atlanto-occipital membrane into the foramen magnum to join the contralateral vertebral artery to become the basilar artery. At the level of the foramen magnum, the vertebral arteries give rise to the single anterior spinal artery, which supplies the majority of the spinal cord except the posterior columns, which are supplied by the two posterior spinal arteries (Fig. 1-29).[29] The vertebral arteries and ascending cervical arteries give rise to radicular arteries or medullary feeder arteries that also supply blood to the spinal cord.[29] Segmental arteries branch off the vertebral artery and are present at each level to supply the vertebrae and surrounding tissues. Although the presence of the medullary feeder arteries is variable, these vessels are more common on the left at C3 and C6 and on the right at C5 and T1.[4] The posterior spinal arteries arise from the branches of the vertebral arteries called the posterior

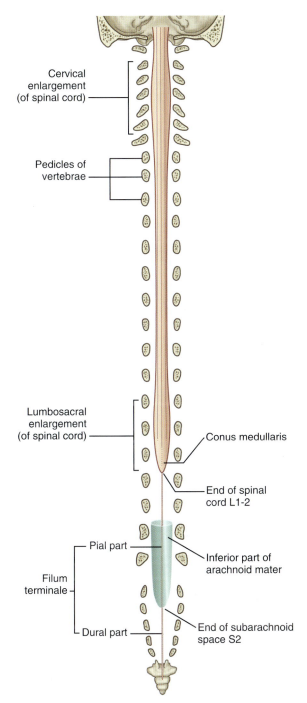

FIGURE 1-22 Spinal cord. (From Drake RL, Vogl W, Mitchell AWM: *Gray's anatomy for students,* ed 2, Philadelphia, 2010, Elsevier.)

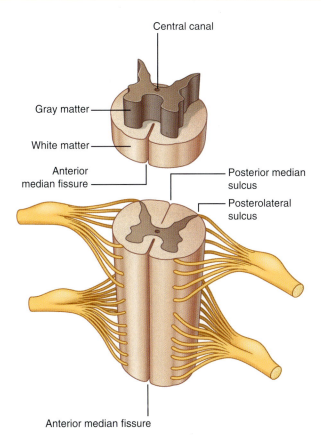

FIGURE 1-23 Features of the spinal cord. (From Drake RL, Vogl W, Mitchell AWM: *Gray's anatomy for students,* ed 2, Philadelphia, 2010, Elsevier.)

sinuses in the epidural space comprise the venous system of the spinal canal. The venous plexus lies just medial to the pedicles over the midsection of the vertebral bodies. The space between the PLL and the posterior aspect of the vertebral body contains the basivertebral sinus.

Related Structures

During the anterior approach to the cervical spine, knowledge of the carotid artery is essential. The carotid sheath invests the internal carotid artery, common carotid artery, internal jugular vein, and vagus nerve and adheres to the thyroid sheath and fascia under the SCM. The carotid sheath is attached to the bone around the jugular foramen and the carotid canal proximally and continues into the thorax distally. Superficial to the internal jugular vein in the carotid sheath lies the ansa cervicalis. The cervical sympathetic trunk lies in the posteromedial aspect of the sheath. During dissection, the carotid artery can be gently retracted or palpated for pulsation. The thoracic duct lies outside the carotid sheath and behind the left common carotid artery, internal jugular vein, and vagus nerve, and it terminates at the junction of the left internal jugular and subclavian veins. The thoracic duct, encountered during the left-sided approach to the lower cervical spine, lies anterior to the subclavian artery, vertebral artery, thyrocervical trunk, and prevertebral fascia, which separates the duct from the phrenic nerve and scalenus anterior muscle.

inferior cerebellar arteries. The posterior spinal arteries course down the posterolateral aspect of the spinal cord to form the transversely arranged plexiform channels on the dorsum of the cord.

The vertebral artery is located just lateral to the uncinate process in line with the middle one third of the vertebral body. Failure to remember this during the anterior cervical approach can cause vertebral artery injury. In addition, severe cervical spondylosis can cause impingement of the vertebral artery by an osteophyte.[28]

Three veins posteriorly and three veins anteriorly return venous blood from the spinal cord. The valveless

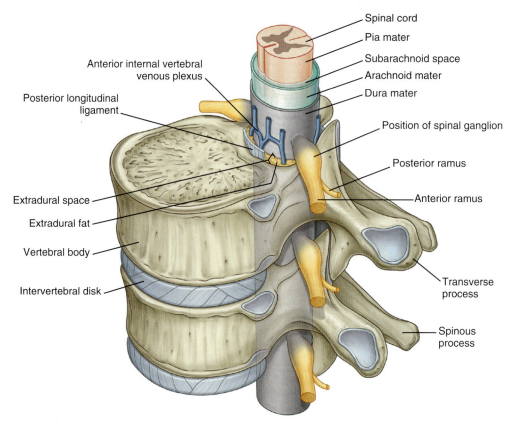

Spinal cord
Pia mater
Subarachnoid space
Arachnoid mater
Dura mater

Anterior internal vertebral
venous plexus

Posterior longitudinal
ligament

Position of spinal ganglion

Posterior ramus

Anterior ramus

Extradural space

Extradural fat

Vertebral body

Intervertebral disk

Transverse
process

Spinous
process

FIGURE 1-24   Vertebral canal. (From Drake RL, Vogl W, Mitchell AWM: *Gray's anatomy for students,* ed 2, Philadelphia, 2010, Elsevier.)

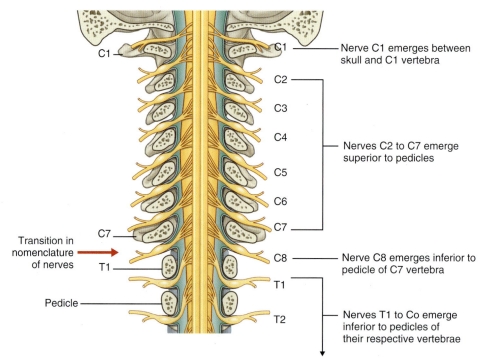

C1

C1

C2

C3

C4

C5

C6

C7

C7

Transition in
nomenclature
of nerves

T1

Pedicle

C8

T1

T2

Nerve C1 emerges between
skull and C1 vertebra

Nerves C2 to C7 emerge
superior to pedicles

Nerve C8 emerges inferior to
pedicle of C7 vertebra

Nerves T1 to Co emerge
inferior to pedicles of
their respective vertebrae

FIGURE 1-25   Nomenclature of the spinal nerves. (From Drake RL, Vogl W, Mitchell AWM: *Gray's anatomy for students,* ed 2, Philadelphia, 2010, Elsevier.)

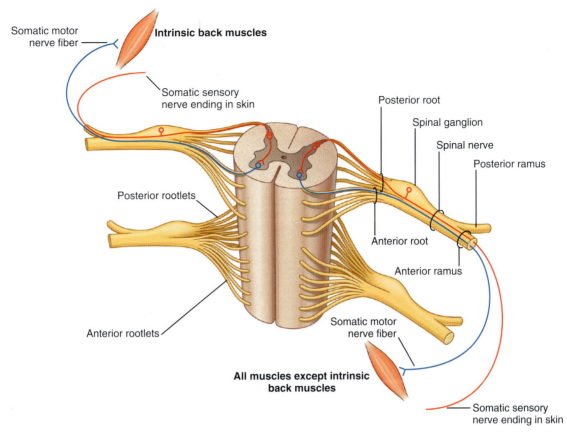

FIGURE 1-26   Basic organization of a spinal nerve. (From Drake RL, Vogl W, Mitchell AWM: *Gray's anatomy for students*, ed 2, Philadelphia, 2010, Elsevier.)

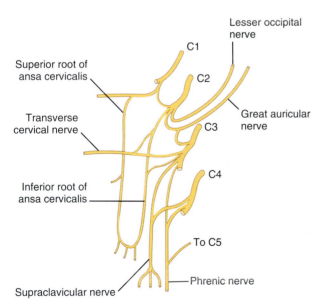

FIGURE 1-27   Cervical plexus. (From Drake RL, Vogl W, Mitchell AWM: *Gray's anatomy for students*, ed 2, Philadelphia, 2010, Elsevier.)

The phrenic nerve lies on the anterior surface of the scalenus anterior muscle and is primarily supplied by C4, but it also receives contributions from C3 and C5 and innervates the diaphragm. The spinal accessory nerve lies behind the posterior margin of the SCM between the greater and lesser auricular nerves. The trapezius and SCM muscles are innervated by the spinal accessory nerve and cervical plexus. Caution must be used during the anterolateral approach to the cervical spine to avoid damage to the phrenic and spinal accessory nerves.

The larynx is responsible for vocalization, breathing, and protection for aspiration. Intrinsic muscles of the larynx are innervated by the recurrent laryngeal nerve, except for the cricothyroid muscle, which is innervated by the external laryngeal branch of the superior laryngeal nerve of the vagus nerve. The anterior thyroid cartilage is located at C4 to C5, and the cricoid cartilaginous ring is located at C6, which can be used for surgical landmarks. Traveling along with the superior thyroid artery, the superior laryngeal nerve is a branch of the inferior ganglion of the vagus nerve that, when damaged, may result in hoarseness, but often produces only minor symptoms such as easy fatiguing of the voice. All laryngeal muscles except the cricothyroid are innervated by the inferior laryngeal nerve, which is a recurrent branch of the vagus nerve. On the left side, the recurrent laryngeal nerve is protected in the left tracheoesophageal groove as it loops under the arch of the aorta. On the right side, the recurrent nerve continues around the subclavian artery and passes posteromedially to the side of the trachea and esophagus, thus putting this nerve at risk of injury in this location. When working at C6 or caudally, the recurrent laryngeal nerve should be located and protected. The inferior thyroid artery is the best guide to the location of this nerve. The area where

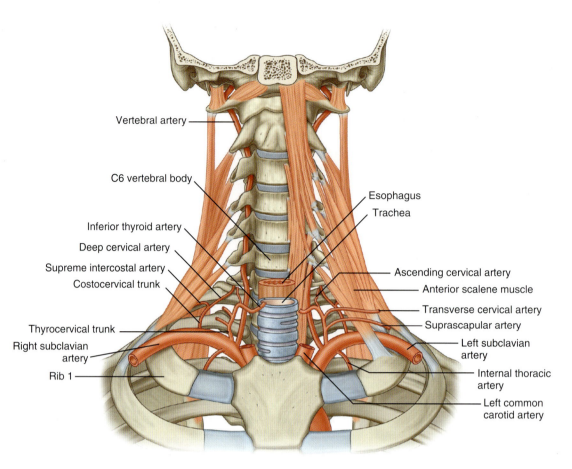

FIGURE 1-28 Vasculature of the root of the neck. (From Drake RL, Vogl W, Mitchell AWM: *Gray's anatomy for students,* ed 2, Philadelphia, 2010, Elsevier.)

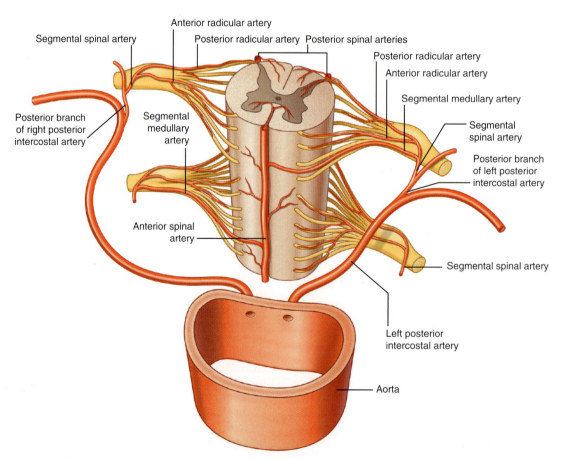

FIGURE 1-29 Segmental blood supply of the spinal cord. (From Drake RL, Vogl W, Mitchell AWM: *Gray's anatomy for students,* ed 2, Philadelphia, 2010, Elsevier.)

the inferior thyroid artery enters the lower pole of the thyroid is usually where the nerve is seen entering the tracheoesophageal groove. Approximately 1% of time, the right inferior laryngeal nerve may be nonrecurrent where it travels directly from the vagus nerve and carotid sheath to the larynx.[30]

One sympathetic chain is present on each side of the vertebrae on the anterior aspect of the transverse processes and is associated with the posterior aspect of the carotid sheath. The cervical ganglia are paravertebral, containing preganglionic and postganglionic autonomic fibers responsible for the cervical sympathetic system. Preganglionic fibers arise from the intermediolateral gray column of the spinal cord segments T1 to T5. White rami communicantes leave the ventral roots of corresponding thoracic nerves to ascend in the trunk. The three ganglia are named the superior, middle, and inferior cervical ganglia. The largest is the superior cervical ganglion, located on the transverse process of C2 to C3. The smallest is the middle cervical ganglion, located on the transverse process of C6 to C7. Between the transverse process of C7 and the neck of the first rib lies the inferior ganglion. The cervicothoracic or stellate ganglion results when the inferior cervical ganglion and the first thoracic ganglion fuse. Injury to the sympathetic chain results in Horner syndrome, which consists of the triad of miosis (pupillary constriction), ptosis (drooping eyelid), and anhidrosis (lack of sweat) on the ipsilateral side of the face. Subperiosteal dissection is performed to avoid damage to the sympathetic chain.

The esophagus runs posterior to the trachea and anterior to the cervical vertebrae and longus colli muscles, with the recurrent laryngeal nerve ascending in the groove between the trachea and the esophagus. Gentle retraction must be used to decrease the risk of nerve injury.

Conclusions

In summary, this chapter reviews cervical anatomy that is essential while operating on the cervical spine. Attention to detail and meticulous dissection is essential to avoid potential pitfalls. Only through a clear knowledge of normal anatomy can the spine surgeon understand pathoanatomy as it relates to symptoms and surgical intervention.

REFERENCES

1. Herman MJ, Pizzutillo PD: Cervical spine disorders in children, *Orthop Clin North Am* 30:457–466, 1999. ix.
2. Ogden JA: Radiology of postnatal skeletal development. XI. The first cervical vertebra, *Skeletal Radiol* 12:12–20, 1984.
3. Daniels DL, Williams AL, Haughton VM: Computed tomography of the articulations and ligaments at the occipito-atlantoaxial region, *Radiology* 146:709–716, 1983.
4. Parke WW, Sherk HH: Normal adult anatomy. In Sherk HH, Dunn EJ, Eismont FJ, et al.: *The cervical spine*, Philadelphia, 1989, Lippincott, pp 11–32.
5. Panjabi M, Dvorak J, Crisco J 3rd, et al.: Flexion, extension, and lateral bending of the upper cervical spine in response to alar ligament transections, *J Spinal Disord* 4:157–167, 1991.
6. Fielding JW, Cochran GB, Lawsing JF 3rd, Hohl M: Tears of the transverse ligament of the atlas: a clinical and biomechanical study, *J Bone Joint Surg Am* 56:1683–1691, 1974.
7. Rauschning W: Anatomy and pathology of the cervical spine. In Frymoyer JW, editor: *The adult spine*, Philadelphia, 1991, Lippincott Williams & Wilkins, pp 907–929.
8. Ebraheim NA, Lu J, Yang H: The effect of translation of the C1-C2 on the spinal canal, *Clin Orthop Relat Res*(351)222–229, 1998.
9. Steinmetz MP, Mroz TE, Benzel EC: Craniovertebral junction: biomechanical considerations, *Neurosurgery* 66:7–12, 2010.
10. Panjabi MM, Duranceau J, Goel V, et al.: Cervical human vertebrae: quantitative three-dimensional anatomy of the middle and lower regions, *Spine (Phila Pa 1976)* 16:861–869, 1991.
11. Fletcher G, Haughton VM, Ho KC, Yu SW: Age-related changes in the cervical facet joints: studies with cryomicrotomy, MR, and CT, *AJNR Am J Neuroradiol* 11:27–30, 1990.
12. Yu SW, Sether L, Haughton VM: Facet joint menisci of the cervical spine: correlative MR imaging and cryomicrotomy study, *Radiology* 164:79–82, 1987.
13. Bland JH: *Disorders of the cervical spine*, Philadelphia, 1987, Saunders.
14. An HS, Gordin R, Renner K: Anatomic considerations for plate-screw fixation of the cervical spine, *Spine (Phila Pa 1976)* 16(Suppl):S548–S551, 1991.
15. Czervionke LF, Daniels DL: Cervical spine anatomy and pathologic processes: applications of new MR imaging techniques, *Radiol Clin North Am* 26:921–947, 1988.
16. Czervionke LF, Daniels DL, Ho PS, et al.: Cervical neural foramina: correlative anatomic and MR imaging study, *Radiology* 169:753–759, 1988.
17. Burke JP, Gerszten PC, Welch WC: Iatrogenic vertebral artery injury during anterior cervical spine surgery, *Spine J* 5:508–514, 2005; discussion 514.
18. Bland JH, Boushey DR: Anatomy and physiology of the cervical spine, *Semin Arthritis Rheum* 20:1–20, 1990.
19. Yeager VL, Cooper MH: Surgical anatomy of the cervical spine surrounding structures. In Young PH, editor: *Microsurgery of the cervical spine*, New York, 1991, Raven Press, pp 1–17.
20. Sether LA, Yu SW, Haughton VM, Wagner M: Ruptures of the anulus fibrosus of cervical intervertebral discs studied by cryomirotomy and magnetic resonance, *Clin Anat* 2:1–8, 1989.
21. Hayashi K, Yabuki T, Kurokawa T, et al.: The anterior and the posterior longitudinal ligaments of the lower cervical spine, *J Anat* 124:633–636, 1977.
22. Czervionke LF, Daniels DL, Ho PS, et al.: The MR appearance of gray and white matter in the cervical spinal cord, *AJNR Am J Neuroradiol* 9:557–562, 1988.
23. Daniels DL, Hyde JS, Kneeland JB, et al.: The cervical nerves and foramina: local-coil MR imaging, *AJNR Am J Neuroradiol* 7:129–133, 1986.
24. Flannigan BD, Lufkin RB, McGlade C, et al.: MR imaging of the cervical spine: neurovascular anatomy, *AJR Am J Roentgenol* 148:785–790, 1987.
25. Pech P, Daniels DL, Williams AL, Haughton VM: The cervical neural foramina: correlation of microtomy and CT anatomy, *Radiology* 155:143–146, 1985.
26. Bogduk N: The clinical anatomy of the cervical dorsal rami, *Spine (Phila Pa 1976)* 7:319–330, 1982.
27. Groen GJ, Baljet B, Drukker J: Nerves and nerve plexuses of the human vertebral column, *Am J Anat* 188:282–296, 1990.
28. Rickenbacher J, Landolt AM, Theiler K: *Applied anatomy of the back*, Berlin, 1982, Springer.
29. Dommisse GF: The blood supply of the spinal cord: a critical vascular zone in spinal surgery, *J Bone Joint Surg Br* 56:225–235, 1974.
30. Sanders G, Uyeda RY, Karlan MS: Nonrecurrent inferior laryngeal nerves and their association with a recurrent branch, *Am J Surg* 146:501–503, 1983.

2 Approaches to the Upper Cervical Spine

Nader S. Dahdaleh and Arnold H. Menezes

CHAPTER PREVIEW

Chapter Synopsis	The upper cervical spine encompasses the area spanning the occiput, the atlas (C1), the axis (C2), and the C2-C3 motion segment. The authors discuss four main approaches to the upper cervical spine: the dorsal or posterior, the posterolateral transcondylar, the transoral transpalatopharyngeal, and the transcervical extrapharyngeal. The indications for, applications of, and descriptions of each approach are reviewed.
Important Points	Selection of the appropriate approach, technique, and construct depends on the patient's age, pathologic process, bony anatomy, and alignment.
Clinical and Surgical Pearls	Knowledge of the anatomy and course of the vertebral artery through adequate preoperative imaging is key to avoiding injury during dissection and determining the appropriate construct during dorsal and far lateral exposures.
	The far lateral exposure offers minimal neural traction and cerebrospinal fluid–tight dural closure while allowing for placement of instrumentation.
	The transoral approach offers excellent exposure to midline anterior structures and pathologic processes in the upper cervical spine with less dissection compared with the extrapharyngeal approach.
	The incidence of dreaded postoperative infections associated with the transoral approach can be reduced by meticulous preoperative, intraoperative, and postoperative preparation and care.
Clinical and Surgical Pitfalls	The vertebral artery is at risk during posterior and posterolateral exposures.
	Bleeding from the voluminous suboccipital venous plexus is also a risk during these exposures.
	The hypoglossal nerve is at risk of injury during extrapharyngeal exposures.

The upper cervical spine is defined by the area encompassing the occiput, the atlas (C1), the axis (C2), and the C2 to C3 motion segment. The anatomic complexity of this region is related to the uniqueness of the bony anatomy of each of these segments and the relation to neural and vascular structures. A comprehensive and detailed knowledge of this intriguing region is key not only to surgical management of the protean disorders affecting this area but also to avoidance of complications.

Selection of the appropriate approach, technique, and construct depends on the patient's age, pathologic process, bony anatomy, and alignment (Fig. 2-1).

Surgical Approaches and Techniques

Dorsal (Posterior) Approach

The dorsal or posterior approach is the most common approach to the upper cervical spine. Through this exposure, atlantoaxial and occipitocervical decompression and fusions can be accomplished. The indication for atlantoaxial fusions is C1 and C2 instability, whereas the indications for occipitocervical fusion include occipitocervical instability and C1-C2 fusion failure. In adults, trauma, tumors, and rheumatoid arthritis are the primary causes of occipitocervical and atlantoaxial instability. In children, congenital abnormalities, Down syndrome,

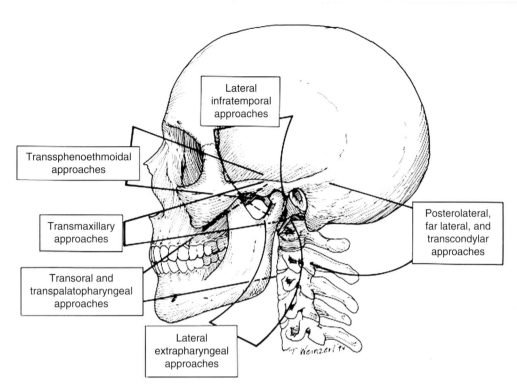

Lateral
infratemporal
approaches

Transsphenoethmoidal
approaches

Transmaxillary
approaches

Posterolateral,
far lateral, and
transcondylar
approaches

Transoral and
transpalatopharyngeal
approaches

Lateral
extrapharyngeal
approaches

FIGURE 2-1 Illustration demonstrating different approaches to the upper cervical spine with the extent of exposure for each approach. (Courtesy of Arnold H. Menezes, MD.)

Klippel-Feil syndrome, and various causes of basilar invagination and impression lead to instabilities in this area.[1,2] Bony components alone or in combination with ligamentous attachments (primarily the transverse and alar ligaments) can be affected by all these processes, with resulting instability.

General Consideration in Dissection

Exposure is achieved through a midline incision from the inion to the C4 spinous process down to the deep cervical fascia. The occiput and the C2 spinous process are identified early during the dissection. Incising through the avascular ligamentum nuchae aids in keeping the dissection midline and avoids unnecessary muscle bleeding.

The points of insertion of suboccipital musculature are the posterior arch of C1, the spinous process, and the lamina of C2. These muscles are detached through subperiosteal dissection with monopolar electrocautery in a mediolateral direction. Dissection beyond 12 mm is transitioned to bipolar cutting current or dissection with a Freer elevator in a subperiosteal fashion, by staying ventral to the suboccipital fascia. This procedure should be done carefully because the vertebral artery courses around the lateral mass of C1 medially in the superior aspect of the posterior arch of C1. Another vascular structure of concern is the suboccipital venous plexus behind the occiput-C1 and C1-2 interspace.

Occipitocervical Fusion

Occipitocervical fusion can be semirigid or rigid. Semirigid fixation includes contoured loop and wire instrumentation. This procedure is supplemented with a postoperative halo vest or a molded rigid orthosis. Rigid fixation encompasses rod and screw fixation. Selection of

the type of instrumentation is dictated by the patient's age, disease process, and associated bony anatomy.

In young patients (3 to 6 years of age), semirigid fixations are employed to allow for additional growth and remodeling. Moreover, the small size of the spine and the incomplete ossification in these patients render rod and screw constructs infeasible. Intraoperative traction to improve and maintain alignment is critical. Thus, the authors most often use crown halo traction resting on a Mayfield headrest, rather than the Mayfield three-point pin headrest for positioning.

Occipitoatlantoaxial Fixation Using Autograft and Wire or Cable

After awake intubation, the patient is positioned prone on the operating table. The head is placed in the cerebellar headrest. Attention should be paid to ensure that no pressure is placed on the eyes. Between 5 and 7 pounds of traction is maintained throughout the operation for satisfactory alignment of the craniocervical junction.

A lateral radiograph using a C-arm fluoroscope is obtained to confirm that appropriate occipitocervical alignment has been maintained.

Subperiosteal electrocautery is used to expose the occipital bone and the dorsal upper cervical spine in a subperiosteal fashion. A notch is placed inferiorly and superiorly on each lamina at its junction with the facet, and a hole is drilled through each side of the occipital bone lateral to the foramen magnum. Titanium cables are passed in a sublaminar fashion and from the occipital trephines to the foramen magnum, to gain occipital purchase. These cables have the advantage of being more pliable yet have equivalent strength compared with wire.

Autologous bone is harvested from the rib or iliac crest, with the former having the advantages of a lower

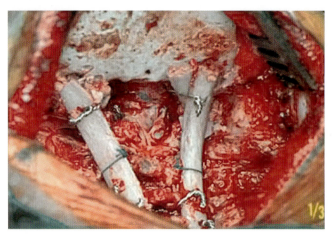

FIGURE 2-2 Intraoperative image demonstrating occipitocervical fusion in a 6-year-old child with Down syndrome who presented with craniocervical dislocation. The construct consisted of the bilateral interlaminar rib graft fusion that extends to the occiput.

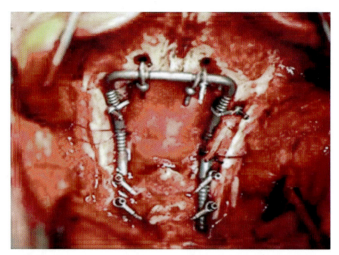

FIGURE 2-3 Intraoperative image demonstrating occipitocervical fusion using a titanium loop and cables with a rib graft in a 12-year-old patient who had undergone transoral odontoid resection for basilar invagination. Posterior fossa decompression was also accomplished.

complication rate, improved strength, and less donor site pain.[3] The graft is notched adjacent to the lamina, and notch or a hole is placed in the rostral end for the occipital cable. The graft is then secured to the recipient laminar surface, or the occipital bone, or both, and the cables are tightened. Postoperatively, patients are immobilized in a custom-made occipitocervical brace for 5 to 6 months (Fig. 2-2).

Occipitoatlantoaxial Fixation Using Rod or Loop and Wire

This semirigid fusion technique offers immediate stabilization. Its advantages are ease of use, a low incidence of neurologic complications, and the ability to place the instrumentation even after wide decompression.

With the same previously described exposure, the titanium loop is placed against the dorsal occipitocervical articulation, and it is custom contoured to the occipitocervical articulation. Cables secure the loop at the points of fixation to the occiput, as well as at the dorsal aspects of the lamina from C1 to C2. The construct should extend to two or three levels below the area of instability. In cases of axial instability, the loop can be designed to incorporate C3 as well. The titanium cables are tightened to 30 pounds of torque pressure at the occiput and C2, whereas at C1 and C3, 15 to 20 pounds of torque pressure is applied. Rib grafts are placed medial to the instrumentation to contact bony surfaces and are secured in place with suture (Fig. 2-3).

Occipitoatlantoaxial Fixation Using Screw Plate and Rod

Occipitocervical fusion using plate and rod instrumentation provides the most rigid construct with higher fusion rates and fewer reported implant failures.[4] Modern occipital plates allow multiple bicortical points of fixation to the midline keel. Moreover, polyaxial screw heads located more laterally on the plate allow easy accommodation of both bent and hinged rod systems.

Patient positioning and exposure are similar to the standard dorsal approach to the upper cervical spine described earlier. Preoperative identification of the location of the torcula and the transverse sinus and of bone

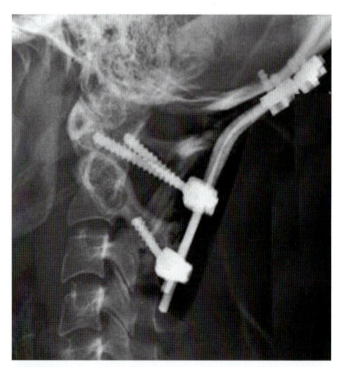

FIGURE 2-4 Lateral radiograph demonstrating occiput-C2 fusion, with an occipital plate, C1 lateral mass screws, and C2 pars interarticularis screws. The rib graft can be seen anterior to the rods. This was accomplished for a patient with craniocervical instability secondary to os odontoideum.

thickness at the proposed area of plate placement is crucial. While the plate is held opposing the proposed position, screw placement is conducted through penetration of the outer cortex with either an awl or a high-speed electric or pneumatic drill. This is followed by hand drilling. The trajectory is then tapped, and the screw is placed. After the occipital plate is secured, various options for atlantoaxial arthrodesis are available. These include C1 and C2 transarticular screws and C1 lateral mass screws combined with C2 pars interarticularis, pedicle, or laminar screws (Fig. 2-4).

C1 to C2 transarticular screw fixation is technically demanding, with potential serious complications. Determination of the course of the vertebral artery is crucial through preoperative computed tomography and magnetic resonance imaging (MRI). The point of entry is usually 3 mm cranial to the C2-C3 facet joint and 3 mm medial to the lateral border of the C2 inferior facet. The steep superior angulation aiming at the anterior tubercle of C1 requires that the incision be extended to the T1 or T2 level. An alternative way to avoid a long incision is to perform a stab incision at that level approximately 2 cm lateral to the midline and, through a trocar with an obturator, introduce a high-speed drill or an awl to decorticate the entry point.

A straight-up or mild medial angulation trajectory though the pars interarticularis is then created with a hand drill until the C1-C2 joint is encountered. Penetration of this joint is completed with a high-speed drill, and advancement into the lateral mass of C1 on the lateral radiographic view is continued. Identifying the medial border of the pars interarticularis with a Freer elevator or a dissector and keeping the drill just lateral to the Freer elevator or dissector avoids medial violation of the pedicle. Care should be maintained not to stray too laterally and thus place the vertebral artery at risk.

If transarticular screw placement is not possible because of unusual bony anatomy or malalignment or because the vertebral artery is in the way of the trajectory, or if the surgeon prefers, then C1-C2 arthrodesis through C1 lateral mass screws combined with C2 pars interarticularis or laminar screws can be employed. Placement of C1 lateral mass screws requires dissection conducted in a subperiosteal fashion along the inferior edge of the posterior arch of C1 with a Freer or Penfield elevator. After retracting the C2 nerve root inferiorly, the medial and lateral borders of the C1 lateral mass are defined. The point of entry for the screw is in the middle, frequently coinciding with an emissary vein. With a hand drill, the trajectory for placement is superior and slightly medial, aiming at the tubercle of C1. Lateral violation places the carotid arteries in jeopardy.

The point of entry for a C2 pars interarticularis screw is approximately 5 mm superior to the C2-C3 facet joint and 3 mm medial to the lateral border of the inferior facet of C2. The medial border of the C2 pedicle is identified with the use of subperiosteal dissection, thus freeing the atlantoaxial membrane from the bony attachment. The trajectory is drilled using a hand drill 25 degrees cranially and 15 to 25 degrees medially. If the pars interarticularis and pedicles are small, C2 laminar screw placement remains another option.

The translaminar screw can provide solid fixation without placing the vertebral artery at risk, although ventral penetration of the lamina can place the spinal cord at risk. A hole is created with a high-speed drill at the junction of the spinous process and the lamina. A trajectory is drilled using a hand drill in the contralateral lamina. This maneuver is followed by tapping the trajectory and placing the screw. A more complete description of the technique is described in Chapter 41.

After securing all instrumentation and achieving satisfactory alignment, the surgeon then places the autograft lateral to the construct. Rib grafts or occipital bone shavings are generally used. Although controversial, in high-risk patients the authors consider the use of recombinant human bone morphogenetic protein. However, caution with regard to potential serious complications should be noted with its use and discussed with the patient. Complications include, but limited to, ectopic bone growth causing compressive lesions, tissue edema, seroma formation, and potential increased cancer risks.[5]

Atlantoaxial (C1-C2) Fixation

Atlantoaxial fixation can be semirigid or rigid. Semirigid fixation encompasses wire or cable constructs combined with autologous grafts and requires external immobilization with a halo vest or, in certain situations, a rigid collar. Rigid fixation encompasses C1-C2 screw rod constructs and transarticular screws and usually requires only rigid collar supplementation.

Atlantoaxial Fixation Using Graft and Cable

Various techniques use graft and cable fixation. These include the original Gallie, interspinous, Brooks, and modified Brooks techniques.[6] Because of their inferior fusion rates compared with screw-rod constructs, these techniques are usually applied to the pediatric population or to patients with anomalous vertebral arteries or small posterior elements.

A standard dorsal approach dissection is employed with exposure of the posterior arch of C1 and the spinous process and lamina of C2. The Gallie technique requires a wire or cable that loops around the spinous process of C2 and the posterior arch of C1 with a graft placed in between them. In a standard Brooks technique, two wires or cables are looped around the posterior arch of C1 and the lamina of C2 on each side while the graft is placed in between them.

Rib or iliac crest autografts are typically the grafts of choice. They are positioned between C1 and C2.

Atlantoaxial Fixation Using Transarticular Screws

This technique provides excellent fixation and fusion rates, although it is demanding and requires expertise. Attention should be paid to the course of the vertebral artery and the bony anatomy. Exposure and placement are described previously in the section on occipitoatlantoaxial fixation using screw plate and rod; however, the initial step of plate placement obviously is skipped (Fig. 2-5).

Atlantoaxial Fixation Using Screws and Rods

C1 lateral mass screw placement combined with either C2 pars interarticularis or laminar screw fixation is described earlier in the section on occipitoatlantoaxial fixation using screw plate and rod (Figs. 2-6 and 2-7).

Posterolateral Transcondylar Approach

Lesions involving the anterolateral upper cervical spine and the lower clivus such as schwannomas, meningiomas, chordomas, and neuroenteric cysts cannot be adequately exposed through a straight dorsal approach. Also known as the extreme lateral transcondylar approach and the extreme lateral and dorsolateral suboccipital condylar approach,[7-9] the posterolateral transcondylar approach

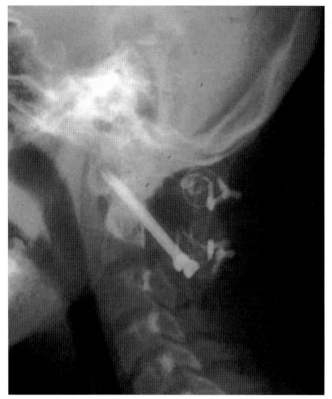

FIGURE 2-5 Lateral cervical radiograph demonstrating bilateral transarticular screws and interlaminal rib graft arthrodesis in a 12-year-old patient with atlantoaxial dislocation and os odontoideum.

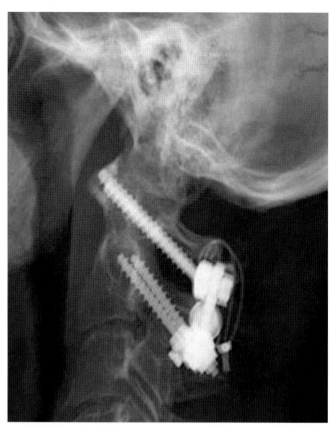

FIGURE 2-6 Lateral cervical radiograph demonstrating atlantoaxial with C1 lateral mass screws and C2 pars interarticularis screws in a male patient. The screw fixation is augmented with interspinous wiring technique and a rib graft.

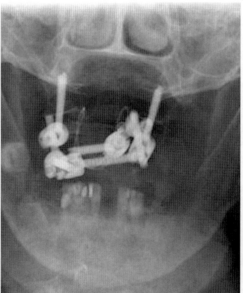

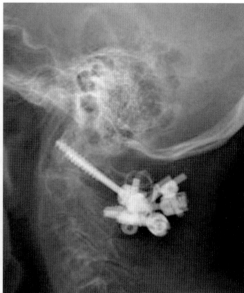

FIGURE 2-7 Open-mouth and lateral radiographs demonstrating C1 lateral mass screws with a C2 translaminar screw construct. Interspinous wiring augments the fusion.

allows for adequate far lateral exposure with minimal neural traction and provides cerebrospinal fluid (CSF)–tight dural closure while allowing for placement of spinal instrumentation in the upper cervical spine, if necessary, in the same setting.[10]

Preoperative planning includes extensive imaging to study the course of the vertebral artery, which can often

be displaced or encased by the tumor. If the patency of the artery is in question, cerebral angiography is advocated to determine whether the artery can be sacrificed should the need arise.

The patient is positioned prone with the head secured to the Mayfield pin headrest and turned slightly to the side of exposure. The incision is started at the ipsilateral

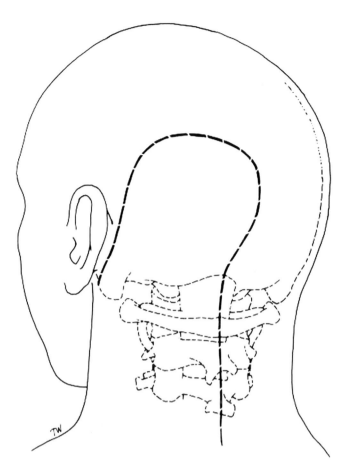

FIGURE 2-8 U-shaped incision for the posterolateral transcondylar approach. (Courtesy of Arnold H. Menezes, MD.)

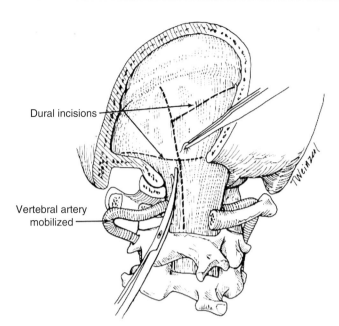

FIGURE 2-9 Dural incisions for the posterolateral transcondylar approach. (Courtesy of Arnold H. Menezes, MD.)

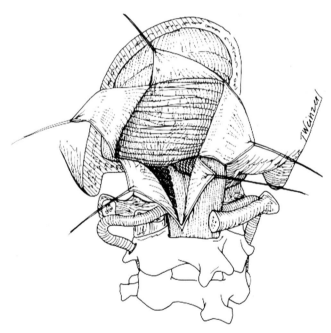

FIGURE 2-10 Exposure after dural opening for the posterolateral transcondylar approach. (Courtesy of Arnold H. Menezes, MD.)

mastoid and extends vertically above the transverse sinus. It then curves toward the midline down to the level of the posterior cervical spine. This completes a U-shaped incision (Fig. 2-8). Splitting of the paraspinous muscle is accomplished with electrocautery, thus exposing the occiput and spinous process of C4. Subperiosteal dissection is then performed to expose the occiput including the foramen magnum lateral to the occipital condyle, the posterior arch of the atlas including the foramen transversarium, and the lamina of C2. The paraspinal muscles are retracted laterally with fishhooks and weights, to avoid placement of self-retaining retractors that would occlude the field of vision.[9]

Occipital craniectomy is performed encompassing the foramen magnum, lateral to the condylar fossa, along the sigmoid and transverse sinuses, then over to the midline to provide a wide exposure. The posterior foramen transversarium of C1 is resected to free the vertebral artery. The vertebral artery is then mobilized to where it enters the atlanto-occipital membrane. The medial third of the occipital condyle is resected to allow exposure to the ventral medulla.

The dural incision extends from the junction of the transverse and sigmoid sinuses, curves inferiorly medial to the vertebral artery, and ends at the level of C2. To enhance the exposure laterally, secondary dural incisions can be made perpendicular to the first (Fig. 2-9). Sectioning of the dentate ligaments at the cervicomedullary junction further enhances anterior exposure (Fig. 2-10).

Following resection of the lesion, meticulous dural closure is performed. Small violations of the mastoid air cells can be sealed with bone wax, whereas larger violations are packed with fat or muscle graft (Fig. 2-11).

Preoperative and intraoperative assessment of stability influences the decision to perform arthrodesis. Generally, if more than 50% of the occipital condyle is resected, arthrodesis is performed.[11]

Transoral Transpharyngeal Approach

The approach provides exposure of anterior lesions in the upper cervical spine, namely, midline lesions involving the caudal clivus and the odontoid process (Fig. 2-12).

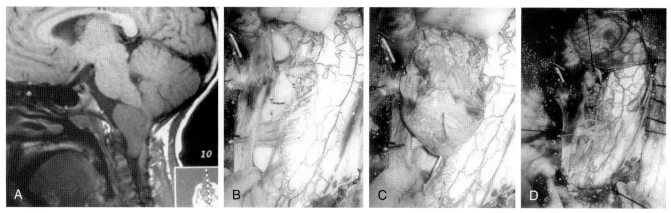

FIGURE 2-11 A, Sagittal T1-weighted magnetic resonance image of a foramen magnum meningioma with compression at the ventral cervicomedullary junction (inset demonstrating mid-sagittal cut). Intraoperative imaging showing the location of the tumor ventral to the cervicomedullary junction (**B**) and after resection (**C**). **D,** The surgical bed after tumor removal.

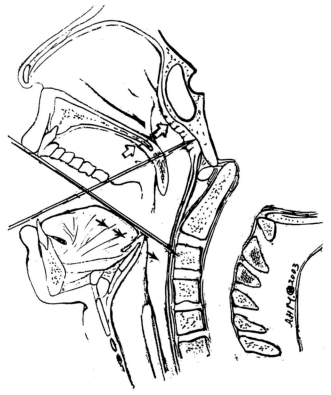

FIGURE 2-12 Illustration demonstrating the extent of exposure achieved with the transoral transpalatopharyngeal approach. (Courtesy of Arnold H. Menezes, MD.)

Preoperative cervical traction (to assess for reducible lesions that would obviate a transoral approach) or intraoperative cervical traction (after the induction of general anesthesia) is applied with an MRI-compatible halo device. Irreducible basilar invagination causing ventral compression is approached through the transoral transpharyngeal route as well.

Reports have described endoscopic approaches to access disorders in this area; however, the authors' preference is the open transoral approach, which allows wide exposure and careful closure. After anterior decompression, almost 97% of patients are supplemented with posterior fusion.[12]

The dreaded complication of this approach is postoperative wound infection. To prevent this complication, the authors have adopted a protocol whereby nasal and pharyngeal cultures are obtained 3 days before the operation, to treat any pathogenic bacteria with antibiotics. In cases of normal flora, preoperative antibiotics are not administrated. All patients perform nystatin and chlorhexidine gluconate gargles three times per day, and mupirocin nasal ointment is used for 2 days before the operation.

The patient's nutritional status is optimized preoperatively. Occasionally, patients who are malnourished because of dysphagia are admitted several days before the operation for aggressive dietary supplementation. Custom-made mouth guards are also created to minimize the risk of oral injury during the operation. Penicillin G is started 2 hours before the beginning of the operation.

Topical oropharyngeal and nasopharyngeal analgesia is used and at times may be supplemented with bilateral superior laryngeal blocks to facilitate fiberoptic intubation with a malleable endotracheal tube. After the endotracheal tube is secured, gauze packing is used to occlude the pharynx to prevent blood leakage into the stomach.

The patient is positioned supine on the operating table with the head resting on a padded Mayfield horseshoe headrest with mild extension. Cervical traction is maintained at 7 pounds in adults and at 4 to 5 pounds in children. The surgical approach has been described in detail elsewhere.[12,13] The custom-made mouth guards are applied, and a Dingman retractor is used to keep the mouth open. The tongue is kept depressed with self-retaining retractors that are attached to the frame of the Dingman retractor.

When the operative procedure takes place at the foramen magnum and above it, the soft palate and at times the hard palate must be split. Conversely, if the operation is limited to the level of the atlas and the axis, the soft palate is elevated by catheters attached to the soft palate through the nasal passages and secured to either side of the soft palate and then withdrawn into the high nasopharynx to allow for exposure. Then 1% lidocaine with 1:200,000 epinephrine is injected into the median raphe of the soft palate.

The microscope is then brought for the operative dissection. The incision starts at the right of the midline at the base of the ovula and continues into the soft palate midline. Stay sutures are applied to hold apart the flaps of the soft palate. When the surgical procedure must proceed through the clivus, or in patients with platybasia, the hard palate is exposed, and the posterior 7 to 10 mm of it is resected, if needed.

The posterior pharyngeal wall is then exposed and is topically anesthetized with 2% cocaine, and the midline raphe is infiltrated with 1% lidocaine and 1:200,000 epinephrine. A midline incision is then made into the posterior pharyngeal median raphe and extends from the middle of the clivus to the upper border of the C3 vertebra. Stay sutures are applied to the reflected pharyngeal wall flaps.

The longus colli and longus capitis muscles are detached from the ventral surfaces of the vertebral bodies and are retracted with self-retaining sutures. The anterior longitudinal ligament is then exposed and coagulated. Subperiosteal dissection using a subperiosteal elevator completes the exposure of the anterior body of the axis, the anterior arch of the atlas, and the caudal anterior clivus. The 20-mm width of the anterior arch of the atlas is then resected, with a high-speed drill with a 4-mm cutting burr and then a diamond attachment. This procedure exposes the caudal odontoid process.

The apical ligament is then resected, and depending on the degree of invagination, the caudal portion of the clivus may be resected. The distal tip of the odontoid process is identified by subperiosteal dissection of the ligamentous tissue from its osseous ventral surface. The bulk of the odontoid process is then resected with a steel cutting burr. Following that, a diamond burr is used to remove the tip and "eggshell" the dorsal wall of the dens to avoid violating the posterior soft tissue. After the posterior tissue plane at the odontoid tip is identified, the odontoid process and the body of the axis are removed in a rostral-to-caudal fashion.

If ligamentous hypertrophy and an inflammatory pannus are encountered, these must be resected. In children, the cruciate ligament and the tectorial membrane should be preserved because these structures allow for new bone formation. If the dura is inadvertently violated, closure can often be challenging. Dural repair can be performed by placing up to three layers of fascia over the rent. The fascia is harvested from the external oblique aponeurosis or the fascia lata. The fascial graft is augmented with a fat pad before closure. Moreover, a lumbar drain is inserted and is kept in place for 7 to 10 days.

Detailed description of intradural dissection through this route is described elsewhere.[14]

At the end of the resection, aerobic and anaerobic cultures are obtained from the depths of the wound. Bacitracin powder combined with microfibrillar collagen is applied to the resection bed. The longus colli and longus capitis muscles are approximated with 3-0 polyglycolic sutures. This is followed by approximating the pharyngeal constrictor muscles and aponeurosis with similar suture in two layers. The soft palate is approximated with interrupted sutures for the nasal mucosa and interrupted mattress sutures for the palatal oral mucosa, along with the muscularis (Fig. 2-13).

Postoperative care is critical. Intravenous fluids and enteral feedings are continued for 5 to 6 days. This regimen is followed by gradually increasing feedings to a regular diet by postoperative day 15. Antibiotics are discontinued after 48 hours, given that the dura is intact and a lumbar drain is not needed. The dorsal fusion is then made.

Patients are kept in a soft collar while they are intubated. After extubation, a custom-fitted occipital-cervical orthosis is used while these patients are mobilized. This is used for 4 to 6 months until osseous fusion is visualized.

Transcervical Extrapharyngeal Approach

Another approach that provides anterior access to the upper cervical spine and avoids the transoral route is the anterior extrapharyngeal approach.[15] The same steps with regard to anesthesia induction and intubation are followed. The incision extends from the mastoid process to 2 cm below the angle of the mandible and proceeds toward the midline at the level of the hyoid bone. At the level of the omohyoid muscle, the incision is extended over the sternocleidomastoid muscle, thus achieving a T-shaped incision (Fig. 2-14).

The subcutaneous tissue is dissected, and then the platysma muscle is undermined. The lower facial nerve division is identified and retracted. The dissection is kept in the fascial plane medial to the sternocleidomastoid muscle and the carotid sheath. The submandibular gland is then retracted; if that is not possible, it can be resected after ligation of the salivary duct. This is done to prevent fistula formation.

The posterior belly of the digastric muscle is then identified and is sectioned at its tendinous insertion after it is tagged with a suture for subsequent approximation. Next, the stylohyoid muscle is identified and divided to allow for medial retraction of the laryngopharynx. The hypoglossal nerve runs between the external and internal carotid arteries and must be carefully mobilized superiorly. The prevertebral fascia is then accessed and incised, to expose the longus colli muscles (Fig. 2-15). Subperiosteal dissection of these muscles exposes the atlas and the clivus. The steps of anterior bony decompression are similar to those described for the transoral approach.

After decompression, bone autograft harvested from the iliac crest or a fibular or rib strut is placed between the caudal clivus and the vertebra. Closure is done by approximating the longus colli muscles. The digastric muscle is reapproximated at the level of its tendinous insertion with 2-0 Nurolon suture. This is followed by approximating the platysma muscle, the subcutaneous tissue, and then the skin. Patients are usually immobilized in a cervical collar postoperatively until posterior fusion is accomplished.

The transoral approach is more popular than the anterior extrapharyngeal approach for several reasons. The anterior extrapharyngeal approach requires more extensive dissection, has a lateral orientation in approaching midline pathologic processes, and is associated with an increased risk of injury of the hypoglossal nerve.

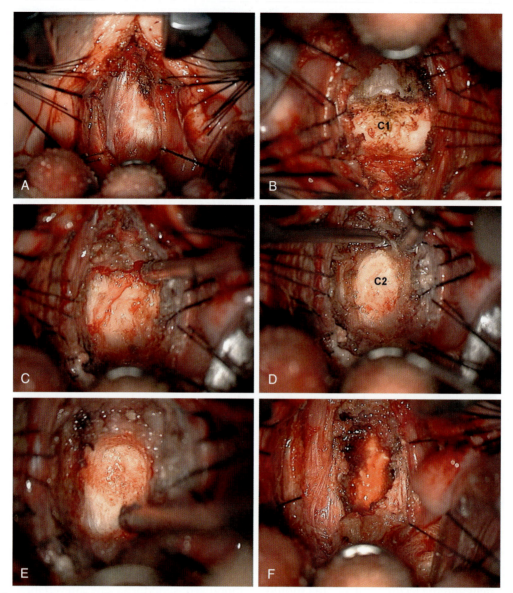

FIGURE 2-13   The transoral transpalatopharyngeal approach in a 12-year-old patient with Down syndrome and a history of a suboccipital decompression who presented with quadriparesis secondary to basilar invagination. After the soft palate and pharyngeal muscle and mucosa are incised (**A**), the anterior arch of C1 and the body of C2 are exposed (**B**). The anterior arch of C1 is resected (**C**), exposing the dens of C2 (**D**). The dens is then resected with the use of curettage and an electric or pneumatic drill (**E**), thus achieving decompression (**F**).

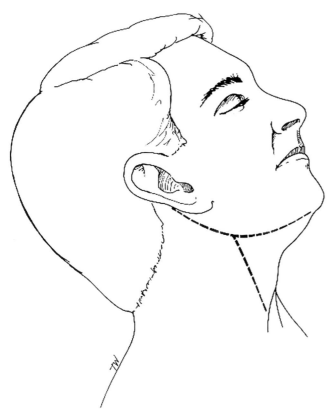

FIGURE 2-14   Illustration depicting the type of incision made for a high cervical extrapharyngeal approach to the upper cervical spine. (Courtesy of Arnold H. Menezes, MD.)

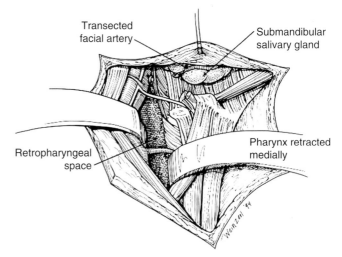

FIGURE 2-15   Diagram illustrating exposure for the high cervical extrapharyngeal route to the upper cervical spine. The posterior belly of the digastric muscle and the stylohyoid muscles are divided to help with retraction of the laryngopharynx. (Courtesy of Arnold H. Menezes, MD.)

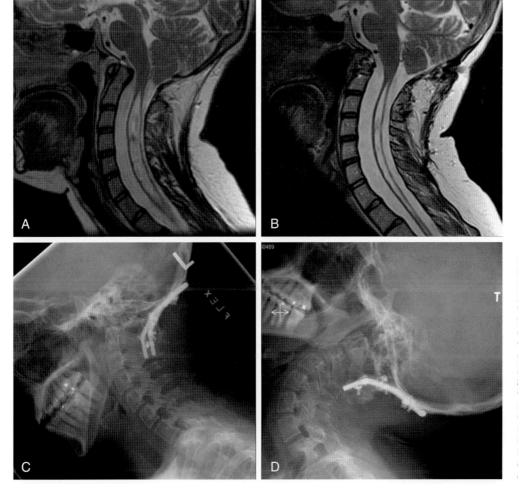

FIGURE 2-16   **A,** Preoperative sagittal T2-weighted magnetic resonance imaging (MRI) of the craniocervical junction showing Chiari I malformation with tonsillar ectopia and impaction of the foramen of magnum. The clivus canal angle measured 90 degrees, with basilar invagination and ventral compression of the cervical medullary junction. Note the presence of syringomyelia. **B,** Sagittal T2-weighted MRI of the craniocervical junction 4 years postoperatively showing ventral and dorsal decompression at the cervicomedullary junction with improvement in the size of the syrinx. Dynamic flexion (**C**) and extension (**D**) radiographs obtained 7 years later show evidence of bony fusion, with no instability.

CLINICAL CASE

Clinical presentation and physical examination: A 22-year-old woman who was known to have congenital panhypopituitarism presented for evaluation of headaches that were induced by coughing, sneezing, and straining. She also reported bilateral arm and hand numbness. All symptoms had been progressively worsening over the past 18 months. Her neurologic examination revealed that her cranial nerves II through XII were grossly normal, with the exception of a mildly decreased gag reflex bilaterally. Her deep tendon reflexes were mildly hyperreflexic on all four extremities. Motor and sensory power examination results were normal. Results of the Romberg test were negative. Gait was steady and normal.

Imaging: Magnetic resonance imaging (MRI) of the brain and cervical spine revealed a Chiari I malformation with tonsillar ectopia and impaction of the foramen of magnum. The clivus canal angle was 90 degrees, with basilar invagination and ventral compression of the cervical medullary junction. Moreover, holocord syringomyelia was noted (Fig. 2-16, *A*).

Operation: The patient underwent fiberoptic intubation while she was awake, and a nasogastric feeding tube was placed. She then underwent application of a crown halo for traction and transoral transpalatopharyngeal resection of the anterior atlas arch, the inferior clivus, and the odontoid process with medullary decompression. The patient then was placed in the prone position and underwent posterior fossa dorsal decompression of the foramen magnum, partial C1 laminectomy, and dorsal occiput–C1-C2 fusion with custom-contoured threaded titanium loop instrumentation, calvarial bone grafts, and bone morphogenetic protein.

Postoperative course: The patient was kept intubated and was admitted to the neurosurgical intensive care unit. She was kept intubated for 6 days, and nasogastric tube feedings were initiated. The crown halo was discontinued, and she was placed in a soft collar. Once the patient was transferred to the regular floor, she was fitted with an Aspen Minerva brace and participated in physical therapy. On postoperative day 7, she was started on a clear fluid diet and transitioned gradually to a regular diet. Once caloric intake was adequate, the nasogastric tube was discontinued. The patient was then discharged on postoperative day 17.

On her first 6-week clinic visit, the patient reported improvement of her bilateral upper extremity numbness, and she had a normal gag reflex on examination. At her 3-month visit, the patient was asymptomatic and had returned to regular physical activity. The patient continued to wear the cervical collar for 4 months. MRI of the craniocervical spine obtained 4 years later showed good decompression at the foramen of magnum ventrally and dorsally, with a decrease in the size of the syrinx (Fig. 2-16, *B*). Flexion and extension radiographs obtained 7 years later showed bony fusion, with no dynamic instability at the craniocervical junction (Fig. 2-16, *C* and *D*).

REFERENCES

1. Ahmed R, Traynelis VC, Menezes AH: Fusions at the craniovertebral junction, *Childs Nerv Syst* 24:1209–1224, 2008.
2. Menezes AH: Craniovertebral junction database analysis: incidence, classification, presentation, and treatment algorithms, *Childs Nerv Syst* 24:1101–1108, 2008.
3. Sawin PD, Traynelis VC, Menezes AH: A comparative analysis of fusion rates and donor-site morbidity for autogeneic rib and iliac crest bone grafts in posterior cervical fusions, *J Neurosurg* 88:255–265, 1998.
4. Garrido BJ, Myo GK, Sasso RC: Rigid versus nonrigid occipitocervical fusion: a clinical comparison of short-term outcomes, *J Spinal Disord Tech* 24:20–23, 2011.
5. Lindley TE, Dahdaleh NS, Menezes AH, Abode-Iyamah KO: Complications associated with recombinant human bone morphogenetic protein use in pediatric craniocervical arthrodesis, *J Neurosurg Pediatr* 7:468–474, 2011.
6. Gallie WE: Fractures and dislocations of the cervical spine, *Am J Surg* 46:495–499, 1939.
7. Bertalanffy H, Seeger W: The dorsolateral, suboccipital, transcondylar approach to the lower clivus and anterior portion of the craniocervical junction, *Neurosurgery* 29:815–821, 1991.
8. Menezes AH: Surgical approaches: postoperative care and complications "posterolateral-far lateral transcondylar approach to the ventral foramen magnum and upper cervical spinal canal," *Childs Nerv Syst* 24:1203–1207, 2008.
9. Spetzler RF, Grahm TW: The far-lateral approach to the inferior clivus and the upper cervical region: technical note, *Barrow Neurol Inst Q* 27:197–204, 1990.
10. Karam YR, Menezes AH, Traynelis VC: Posterolateral approaches to the craniovertebral junction, *Neurosurgery* 66:135–140, 2010.
11. Vishteh AG, Crawford NR, Melton MS, et al.: Stability of the craniovertebral junction after unilateral occipital condyle resection: a biomechanical study, *J Neurosurg* 90:91–98, 1999.
12. Menezes AH: Surgical approaches: postoperative care and complications "transoral-transpalatopharyngeal approach to the craniocervical junction," *Childs Nerv Syst* 24:1187–1193, 2008.
13. Menezes AH, Foltz GD: Transoral approach to the ventral craniocervical border, *Oper Tech Neurosurg* 8:150–157, 2005.
14. Menezes AH, Greenlee JDW: Transoral approach. In Harsh G, editor: *Chordomas and chondrosarcomas of the skull base and spine*, New York, 2003, Thieme.
15. McAfee PC, Bohlman HH, Riley LH Jr, et al.: The anterior retropharyngeal approach to the upper part of the cervical spine, *J Bone Joint Surg Am* 69:1371–1383, 1987.

Anterior Surgical Approach to the Cervical Spine*

Melvin D. Helgeson and Todd J. Albert

3

CHAPTER PREVIEW

Chapter Synopsis	The approach to the anterior cervical spine is one of the most common approaches performed in cervical spine surgery. Because of the vital anatomy near the surgical dissection, potential complications from this approach are severe. Therefore, a thorough understanding of the anatomy is crucial to performing this elegant approach safely and expeditiously. This chapter describes and illustrates the approach and provides insight into prevention of complications.
Important Points	A thorough understanding of the anatomy allows for a safe anterior exposure of the cervical spine.
	The surgeon should recognize all potential complications to avoid and prevent them.
Clinical and Surgical Pearls	All patients undergoing cervical revision procedures should be referred to otolaryngology for either direct or indirect laryngoscopy and vocal cord evaluation.
	Preintubation, postintubation, and postpositioning neuromonitoring should be considered when the spinal cord is at risk.
	Below the deep cervical fascia, blunt dissection is the rule.
Clinical and Surgical Pitfalls	Retractors should be kept below the longus colli muscle, and the esophagus and carotid sheath should be protected.
	The crossing vessels should be identified when the surgeon is working in the upper or lower cervical spine, to protect them.
	The surgeon should ensure adequate hemostasis at closure and consider ligation of crossing vessels if needed to sacrifice.

The approach to the anterior cervical spine was first described by Robinson and Smith in 1955 and was then modified by Southwick and Robinson in 1957.[1,2] Since then, the approach has remained very similar, with slight modifications based on increased experience with the procedure. Because of the predictable and successful results, the anterior cervical diskectomy and fusion operation has become one of the most common procedures performed in the United States and around the world. Therefore, most surgeons have experience with the procedure. The purposes of this chapter are to outline the procedure for those who may not be familiar with it and to provide technical tips for those who are seeking to improve their surgical skills.

Preoperative Considerations

History

Although the surgical indications for anterior cervical procedures are discussed in later chapters, the history that is pertinent to the approach is any previous history of anterior neck surgery. Included are previous carotid artery surgery and thyroid surgery because both have also been

---

*The views expressed in this manuscript are those of the authors and do not reflect the official policy of the Department of Army, Department of Defense, or U.S. government. One author is an employee of the U.S. government. This work was prepared as part of official duties, and as such, there is no copyright to be transferred.

reported to damage the innervation of the vocal cords. If patients present with any history of anterior surgery or have any concern about vocal cord paralysis, preoperative direct or indirect laryngoscopy should be performed by an otolaryngologist. Because of adjacent segment degeneration in the cervical spine, vocal cord paralysis is unfortunately not an uncommon occurrence, and preoperative planning is a must. Additional history that is relevant to the approach includes the diagnosis of a carotid bruit or carotid artery stenosis. It is reasonable to approach a side away from the carotid artery stenosis or bruit, out of concern for causing a stroke.[3,4]

Physical Examination

When a patient is evaluated for anterior cervical surgery, the most important aspect of the physical examination is the presence or absence of neck extension with or without pain. This feature guides the options for intubation and intraoperative neck extension. Additional findings that should be considered are previous incisions and their anatomic locations near the planned surgical procedure.

Imaging

Preoperative imaging is important for obtaining the correct diagnosis, but it is also relevant to the approach. The course of the vertebral artery should be thoroughly evaluated on preoperative magnetic resonance imaging, to ensure that this vessel does not have an aberrant course. The vertebral artery can course through the vertebral body or disk or anterior to it instead of maintaining its normal location through the foramen transversarium. If the vertebral artery traverses the anterior aspect of the vertebral body or disk, it is at risk with the approach, and therefore, surgical dissection must proceed with caution. Additionally, if this artery courses through the vertebral body or disk, corpectomy and diskectomy may be contraindicated.

Indications and Contraindications

The relative contraindications to anterior cervical approaches are a previous history of cervical radiation, radical neck dissection or excision, and esophageal surgery. An anterior cervical approach has no absolute contraindications, but any history of the foregoing procedures makes the approach more challenging and higher risk.

Left-Sided Versus Right-Sided Approach

Currently, no conclusive evidence demonstrates improved outcomes or reduced complication rates with either a left-sided or a right-sided cervical approach.[5] Proponents of the left-sided approach argue that the recurrent laryngeal nerve has a more predictable course within the tracheo-esophageal groove and is at less risk, although the evidence in the literature to support this view is limited.[6] Proponents of the right-sided approach state that it is more comfortable for the right-handed surgeon, avoids the thoracic duct, and has less risk to the esophagus (which is slightly more to the left).

Ultimately, no difference exists, and the approach side is surgeon specific unless the patient has any previous history of neck surgery. If a patient had previous neck surgery and the vocal cords are functioning normally (as confirmed by indirect laryngoscopy), then the approach

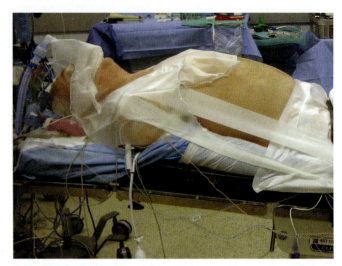

FIGURE 3-1   Positioning with 20 to 30 degrees of reverse Trendelenburg, with the patient's arms tucked and padded, shoulders taped, and neck extended using an inflatable bag.

should be from the contralateral side. Conversely, if the vocal cords are not functioning normally on the side of a previous approach, then the approach should be from the same side as before, to avoid damage to the one remaining normal vocal cord.

Surgical Technique

Anesthesia and Positioning

Communication with anesthesia providers and neuromonitoring personnel is the key to avoiding complications with positioning for anterior cervical surgery. If a patient cannot safely extend the neck without pain or neurologic symptoms preoperatively, then indirect laryngoscopy (i.e., GlideScope or fiberoptic intubation) should be considered. Additionally, if the patient has a history of myelopathy, or if concern about the spinal cord exists, mean arterial pressure requirements (>85 mm Hg) may be indicated. Furthermore, if any concern with neck extension exists, preintubation neuromonitoring baselines values should be obtained. Once total intravenous anesthesia is induced, bite blocks should be placed, and baseline motor-evoked potentials (MEPs) and somatosensory-evoked potentials (SSEPs) should be obtained before intubation. Communication with the anesthesia team to avoid muscle relaxants if possible during intubation allows postintubation monitoring. Only by constant communication with the anesthesia team can this be done expeditiously.

If intubation did not require muscle relaxants, then positioning can be adequately monitored with MEPs and SSEPs. First, the authors place the bed in approximately 20 degrees of reverse Trendelenburg positioning, which allows for venous drainage (Fig. 3-1). If the patient can tolerate neck extension, a small roll can be placed between the scapulae. In the authors' practice, an inflatable pressure bag covered by a gel pad placed behind the scapula allows for more controlled neck extension. Obviously, if the patient's head is lifted from the table with neck extension, too much neck extension has been attempted. Additionally, in patients with significant motion, neck extension may tether the trachea or esophagus to the anterior spine, thus making mobilization of these structures difficult. Therefore, a simple manual check of tracheal mobility can be performed following neck extension.

Gentle caudal traction to the shoulders should be applied using tape. If the surgical procedure is going to extend to the upper cervical spine, minimal traction is required; however, for surgical procedures in the lower cervical spine or in patients with extensive soft tissue, more aggressive traction may be required. After shoulder taping and again after neck extension, neuromonitoring should be checked to ensure that no loss of amplitude in the brachial plexus or spinal cord has occurred.

Surgical Landmarks and Incisions

After gentle neck extension, the anatomic landmarks for surgical incision are as follows: C3, hyoid bone; C4 to C5, thyroid cartilage; and C6, cricoid cartilage. An incision centered on the level of the cricothyroid membrane, an easily palpable structure, is best suited for exposure to C5-C6 disk disorders. Another easily palpable landmark is the carotid (Chassaignac) tubercle, which is the anterior tubercle of the C6 transverse process (the anterior tubercle of C5 may also be prominent). However, some surgeons do not recommend palpation of this structure before incision because of the theoretical risk of massaging the carotid barorecepters (which can consequently slow the heart rate and blood pressure). If a skin crease is present within 1 to 2 cm of the desired location for the skin incision, then use of that skin crease will be more cosmetically appealing. The authors prefer transverse incisions for up to three-level procedures and vertical incisions when approaching four or more levels. The transverse incision should be slightly curved to match the skin crease and rarely needs to extend more than 1 cm past the midline medially or past the border of the sternocleidomastoid (SCM) muscle laterally (Fig. 3-2). If a vertical incision is required, it should be made parallel to the SCM and approximately 1 cm medial to the medial border of the SCM (Fig. 3-3). With the closure of a vertical incision, the surgeon should ensure that "dog ears" at the cephalad aspect of the incision are avoided because they are cosmetically unattractive.

Specific Steps

Step 1: Skin Incision

Sharp dissection is made down to the platysma muscle. The platysma can be minimal in female patients, and at midline it has no muscle fibers, only a thin fascia or fatty layer representing the superficial cervical fascia (Fig. 3-4). Located within this layer near the midline is the anterior jugular vein, which can be sacrificed, although this is rarely needed.

Step 2: Platysma and Deep Cervical Fascia Incision

The platysma can be divided vertically or horizontally. Deep to the platysma is the deep cervical fascia, which covers the strap muscles (infrahyoid) and the SCM

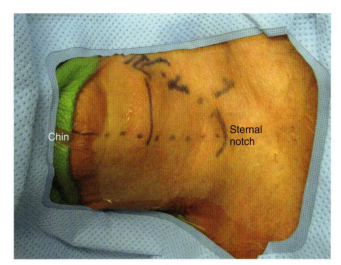

FIGURE 3-2 Skin incision made horizontal and curvilinear from the midline to the border of the sternocleidomastoid (SCM). The midline and border of the SCM are marked with a *dotted line*.

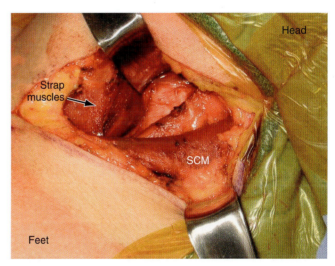

FIGURE 3-3 Vertical skin incision along the border of the sternocleidomastoid (SCM).

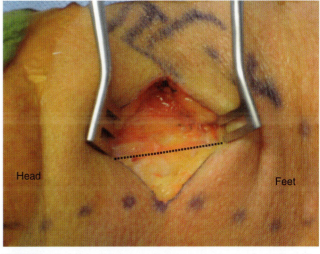

FIGURE 3-4 Minimal platysma with fatty appearance at the midline. The *dotted line* represents the border of the platysma.

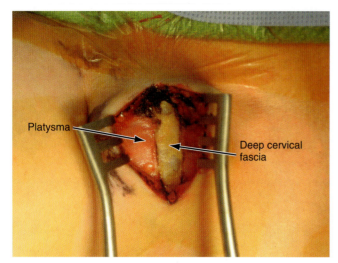

FIGURE 3-5   Division of the platysma layer with the deep cervical fascia immediately behind it.

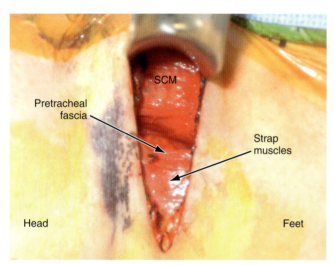

FIGURE 3-6   After the deep cervical fascia has been incised and elevated, the sternocleidomastoid (SCM) and strap muscles can be easily identified.

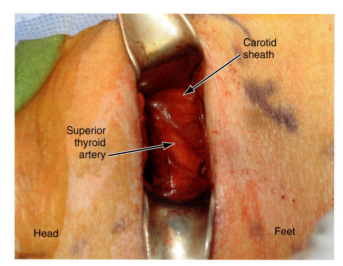

FIGURE 3-7   Within the layer of the pretracheal fascia, the dissection should proceed bluntly with identification of any crossing neurovascular structures. Seen here, in an approach to C3 to C4 crossing from medial to lateral, is the neurovascular bundle containing the superior thyroid artery and superior laryngeal nerve. Care has been taken to avoid damage to these tissues.

(Fig. 3-5). The deep cervical fascia can be incised with the platysma and then elevated away from the SCM and strap muscles. The subplatysmal dissection increases visibility for multiple levels and is important for three-level procedures performed through a transverse incision. Once this layer is developed, the medial border of the SCM and the lateral border of the strap muscles are easily identified (Fig. 3-6).

Step 3: Pretracheal Fascia Incision

The pretracheal fascia is the least resistant of the fascial layers encountered with this approach. It is important to penetrate this layer bluntly, to avoid injury to the thyroid vessels or laryngeal nerves. The easiest manner to pierce this layer is with blunt dissection vertically along the medial border of the SCM by using Metzenbaum scissors in a spreading fashion. Once this layer is pierced, the spine can be palpated and the esophagus and trachea can be mobilized manually with the surgeon's finger. To gain additional access, the omohyoid muscle can be divided

(although this is not necessary for a one-level approach). It is important to stay midline with the dissection to avoid the carotid sheath and therefore, before palpating the spine, palpate the carotid artery to ensure that the dissection is carried medial to it.

Dissection must be done cautiously because several important structures course through this layer (Fig. 3-7). Along the cephalad aspect of the exposure is the superior thyroid artery, which can be sacrificed if necessary, but coursing alongside the artery is the superior laryngeal nerve, which must be spared. The superior laryngeal nerve supplies motor function to the cricothyroid muscle (external branch) and sensation to the posterior larynx (internal branch). Consequently, damage to these branches can cause voice changes or loss of the laryngeal cough reflex, respectively. Additionally, if exposing C2 to C3, the dissection through this plane should start in a more lateral location, thus avoiding the submandibular region, and effort should be made to identify and protect the superior laryngeal nerve. Furthermore, if the caudal aspect of the cervical spine is exposed, the inferior thyroid artery can be seen crossing the plane of dissection. If the superior or inferior thyroid arteries are damaged or must be sacrificed for adequate exposure, they should be ligated with suture instead of bipolar electrocautery, to avoid a postoperative hematoma and damage to the surrounding tissue. If the approach is from the right side in the lower cervical spine, the recurrent laryngeal nerve should be identified and protected.

Step 4: Prevertebral Fascial Incision

By using a lipless retractor to retract the esophagus and trachea, the prevertebral fascia can be exposed (Fig. 3-8). The authors prefer a lipless retractor (i.e., handheld Cloward retractor) when operating are above the prevertebral fascia, to avoid inadvertent injury to the recurrent laryngeal nerve within the tracheoesophageal groove. After the prevertebral fascia is identified, the surgeon's finger can again be used to mobilize the esophagus and trachea. If these structures are not able to be mobilized,

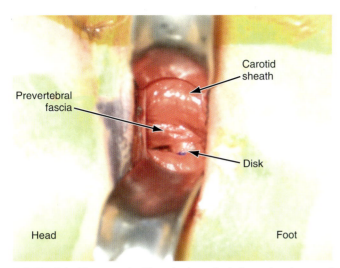

FIGURE 3-8 The pretracheal fascia has been divided, revealing the carotid sheath laterally and the prevertebral fascia deep over the anterior spine.

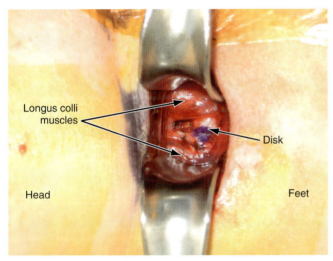

FIGURE 3-9 The prevertebral fascia has been divided and retracted to reveal the longus colli muscles.

the neck may be overextended. Additionally, during a revision surgical procedure (even when exposure is performed from the opposite side), the esophagus is adherent to the prevertebral fascia. The esophagus must slowly be dissected away from the prevertebral fascia by using peanut dissector sponges to avoid injury to the esophagus. The prevertebral fascia can be incised sharply with Metzenbaum scissors, and the longus colli can be identified deep to it (Fig. 3-9).

Step 5: Imaging

The appropriate level is verified by using a marker and a lateral radiograph. A useful landmark in the lower cervical spine is the carotid tubercle, which can be safely palpated after the foregoing dissection. Although the carotid tubercle is at C6, the anterior tubercle of the C5 transverse process can also be prominent. Additionally, when in the upper cervical spine, palpation of the C2 keel can identify the appropriate level. Regardless, an intraoperative radiograph is mandatory.

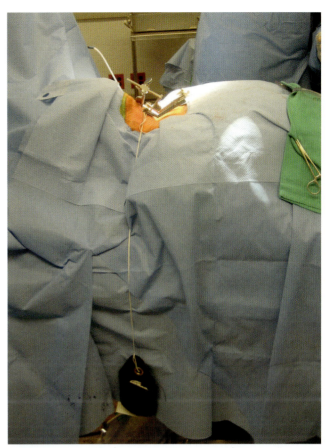

FIGURE 3-10 Self-retaining retractors can be attached to weights (1 to 2 pounds) to keep them in position below the longus colli muscles.

Step 6: Elevation of the Longus Colli Muscles

Staying directly on the bone and disk annulus, elevate the longus colli muscle away from both sides. The sympathetic chain is located along the anterolateral aspect of the longus colli muscle. If possible, avoid transverse cuts in the longus colli, as well as dissection along the anterior aspect of the muscle. After the uncovertebral joints are adequately visualized, the dissection is far enough laterally. Preoperative imaging should be used to verify the absence of an aberrant course to the vertebral artery anteriorly. Finally, at the midpoint of the vertebral body, one should proceed with caution once the vertebral body begins to slope posterolaterally because this is the location where a normal vertebral artery can be injured (above and below the transverse process). After the longus colli muscle has been elevated, self-retaining retractors can be placed, and diskectomy can be performed. Using retractors with teeth and/or attaching weights to the retractors will assist with keeping the retractors under the longus colli (Fig. 3-10). However, if the retractors slide above the muscle, they should be repositioned to prevent damage to the sympathetic chain, esophagus, or carotid vessels.

Step 7: Closure

Although this approach is generally associated with minimal blood loss, a drain can be placed to ensure that a hematoma does not develop over the first night. The authors close the platysma muscle and skin separately,

Nerve Injuries
Hypoglossal Nerve
Superior laryngeal nerve
Recurrent laryngeal nerve
Sympathetic chain
Vagus nerve

Vascular Injuries
Vertebral artery
Carotid artery and internal jugular vein

Esophageal Injury
Trachea Injury
Thoracic Duct Injury

using interrupted sutures. The drain is generally removed on postoperative day 1.

Postoperative Considerations

Postoperatively, patients should be monitored overnight and kept in an upright position of at least 45 degrees. This positioning ensures that any venous drainage or swelling moves caudally and is not problematic. Patients are also encouraged to continue elevation for the first 2 to 3 days at home.

Complications

The complications associated with the anterior cervical approach are discussed in detail in the chapters in Section 8. These complications are listed in Box 3-1.

REFERENCES

1. Robinson RA, Smith G: Anterolateral cervical disk removal and interbody fusion for cervical disk syndrome, *Bull Johns Hopkins Hosp* 96:223–224, 1955.
2. Southwick WO, Robinson RA: Surgical approaches to the vertebral bodies in the cervical and lumbar regions, *J Bone Joint Surg Am* 39:631–644, 1957.
3. Chozick BS, Watson P, Greenblatt SH: Internal carotid artery thrombosis after cervical corpectomy, *Spine (Phila Pa 1976)* 19:2230–2232, 1994.
4. Inamasu J, Guiot BH: Iatrogenic carotid artery injury in neurosurgery, *Neurosurg Rev* 28:239–247, 2005. discussion 248.
5. Beutler WJ, Sweeney CA, Connolly PJ: Recurrent laryngeal nerve injury with anterior cervical spine surgery risk with laterality of surgical approach, *Spine (Phila Pa 1976)* 26:1337–1342, 2001.
6. Jung A, Schramm J: How to reduce recurrent laryngeal nerve palsy in anterior cervical spine surgery: a prospective observational study, *Neurosurgery* 67:10–15, 2010; discussion 15.

Posterior Surgical Approach to the Cervical Spine

4

Brian C. Werner and Isador H. Lieberman

CHAPTER PREVIEW

Chapter Synopsis	The midline posterior approach is the most commonly used approach to the cervical spine. It allows efficient and safe access to the posterior elements of the occipitocervical region and the subaxial cervical spine. It is indicated for a variety of cervical spine procedures, including fusions, decompressions, evacuation of tumors, reduction of facet dislocations and posterior element fractures, and removal of accessible herniated disks.
Important Points	This versatile access is through the midline subperiosteal dissection.
	The surgical technique involves prone positioning, midline incision, and careful superficial and deep dissection to avoid excessive bleeding.
	Potential complications include spinal cord or nerve injury, especially the greater occipital nerve, and vertebral artery or venous plexus injury.
Clinical and Surgical Pearls	Depending on the procedure and the region to be addressed, positioning of the head and neck in flexion and extension must be optimized to gain convenient access and trajectories.
	During the operative setup, the surgeon should check the ability to obtain appropriate images with the fluoroscope and verify appropriate head and neck position.
Clinical and Surgical Pitfalls	Throughout the procedure, the surgeon should continuously identify and verify the appropriate operated levels clinically and radiographically.

The midline posterior approach, which is the most commonly used surgical approach to the cervical spine, allows efficient and safe access to the posterior elements of the occipitocervical junction and the subaxial cervical spine. Although the posterior approach is one of the most elementary approaches in spine surgery, involving a simple midline incision, it is indicated for a variety of cervical spine procedures, including posterior fusion, enlargement of the spinal canal through laminectomy or laminoplasty, excision or debulking of tumors, open treatment of facet dislocations, open reduction of posterior element fractures, decompression of nerve roots, and removal of accessible herniated disks.

Preoperative Considerations

General Principles

A careful history and physical examination, as well as appropriate imaging studies, should be performed preoperatively in all patients. The surgical approach depends on the condition being treated, the specific signs and symptoms, and the patient's expectations. Once surgery is planned for the patient and a posterior approach is chosen, the physical examination should be focused on ensuring that the appropriate landmarks and tactile cues, such as the external occipital protuberance and large C2 and C7 spinous processes, can be palpated. Other less common but important anatomic preoperative considerations include evaluating for unusual anatomy such as an aberrant vertebrobasilar artery, location and condition of preexisting scars in the setting of a revision procedure, and a Klippel-Feil segment or other congenital anomaly that could alter or complicate the surgical approach.

Imaging

An essential step in preoperative preparation is obtaining appropriate imaging studies. Anteroposterior, lateral, and open-mouth plain film radiographs of the cervical spine with full and clear views from C1 to T1 should be standard parts of the diagnostic evaluation. Preoperative computed tomography (CT) scans can help define the bony anatomy and facilitate the preoperative plan. Magnetic resonance imaging (MRI) is almost universally obtained before cervical spine surgery as well because these imaging sequences allow evaluation of the neural structures and disks and provide additional information on potential infections, tumors, or other pathologic processes. A thorough review of all available imaging should be completed when selecting the optimal surgical approach for the patients' disorder.

Indications and Contraindications

A broad range of disorders may be addressed through a posterior approach to the cervical spine. It is easiest to consider the approach in two distinct anatomic regions: the occipitocervical junction (including the occiput to C2) and the subaxial cervical spine (C3 to C7). Although the approach to both regions is similar, the anatomy, function, and associated pathologic features of these two vertebral segments differ. Therefore, it is simpler to discuss these regions separately throughout this chapter. At the occipitocervical junction, both posterior decompressions and posterior fusions can be performed. Various types of decompressions, including that of the skull base, foramen magnum, spinal canal, and nerve roots, can be accomplished through this approach. A posterior approach is indicated for posterior occipitocervical and C1 to C2 fusions for atlantoaxial dissociations, C1 or C2 fractures, transverse cervical ligament disruptions, tumors, or infections. In the subaxial cervical spine, decompression of the canal and nerve roots, including laminectomy, laminoplasty, and keyhole laminoforaminotomy, can be performed through a posterior approach. Posterior fusion procedures for fractures, tumors, or infections can be undertaken through this approach. Additionally, treatment of facet joint dislocations and excision of some herniated disks can also be accomplished through a posterior approach.

If the posterior approach to the cervical spine is the most direct and least invasive access to the pathologic process being treated, this approach has essentially no contraindications. Having said that, many cervical spine disorders are better surgically managed through an anterior approach (see Chapter 3). Thus, it is important to consider the specific pathologic process and to determine the most appropriate and least invasive approach before the surgical procedure.

Surgical Technique

Positioning

Typically, prone positioning is used for the posterior approach to the cervical spine (Fig. 4-1), although some surgeons prefer positioning the patient in a seated position. Preoperatively, the patient's cervical spine should be carefully ranged in flexion and extension to determine a safe range of motion that does not produce symptoms. Additionally, movements of the cervical spine should be minimized as much as possible during intubation, especially for myelopathic patients.

The proper and safest operative head positioning is best achieved with the use of a halo head frame or Mayfield tongs for stabilization (see Fig. 4-1). Head and neck flexion separates the occiput and ring of C1 and also reduces overlap of the laminae and facet joints, thereby facilitating exposure of the occipitocervical region and allowing easier decompression of the subaxial spinal canal. The neck should be returned to a neutral position before any fusion or instrumentation procedures. The arms and shoulders should be placed at the patient's side. Gentle taping of the shoulders to the distal end of the bed can facilitate intraoperative radiographic visualization. Excessive traction on the shoulders should be avoided to minimize the risk of intraoperative brachial plexus traction injury or skin blisters. The caudal scalp should be shaved of hair 1 to 2 cm cephalad of the external occipital protuberance to facilitate draping and palpation of landmarks.

Elevating the head of the operating table to 30 degrees of reverse Trendelenburg positioning can reduce venous epidural bleeding. Knee flexion prevents the patient from sliding inferiorly in this position. All bony prominences and peripheral nerves should be carefully padded to prevent intraoperative neurapraxia. Once satisfactory positioning has been obtained, fluoroscopy should be used for final assessment of cervical spine alignment and positioning before draping.

Hazards

Although the posterior approach to the cervical spine is relatively straightforward, the surgeon should be aware of certain significant hazards. Significant morbidity can result from improper positioning. Hyperextension or hyperflexion while the patient is under anesthesia can contribute to spinal cord injury. Excessive traction on the shoulders can result in brachial plexus injury. Improper padding of bony prominences or peripheral nerves can cause intraoperative decubitus ulcers or neurapraxia. Failure to allow the abdomen to hang free through the table can hamper venous return and also increase required inspiratory pressures.

Anatomic hazards are also present. Neural structures such as the spinal cord and cervical nerve roots, especially the greater occipital nerve (C2), must be properly handled during this approach. Vascular structures such as the vertebral artery (particularly at risk near the C1 ring), transverse sinus, and epidural veins must be properly identified and protected during the surgical approach.

Surgical Landmarks and Incisions

The external occipital protuberance and the spinous processes of C2 and C7 should be identified by palpation and fluoroscopy and marked because they assist in identifying the midline. When approaching the occipitocervical region, the surgeon should make a longitudinal midline incision beginning at the external occipital protuberance and extending distally to at least the level of C3 (approximately 6 to 7 cm) (Fig. 4-2). When the subaxial cervical spine is approached, a similar longitudinal midline incision should be made, beginning at the C2 spinous process and extending distally to at least the C7 spinous process (Fig. 4-3).

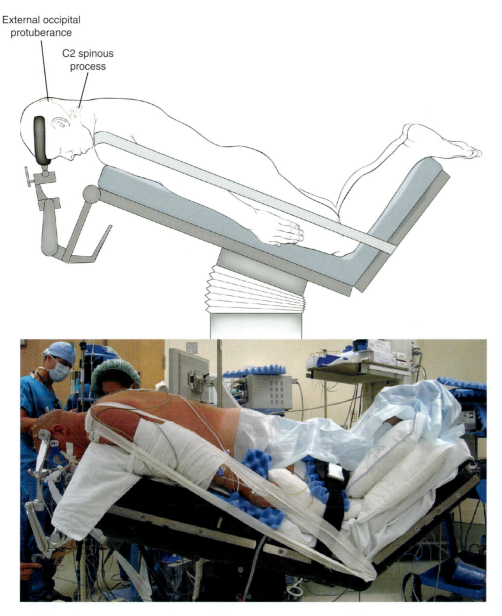

External occipital protuberance

C2 spinous process

FIGURE 4-1 Prone positioning. (From Shen FH: Spine. In Miller MD, Chhabra AB, Hurwitz SR, et al, editors: *Orthopaedic surgical approaches*, Philadelphia, 2008, Saunders.)

Specific Steps

Occipitocervical Region

Incision

See the earlier section on surgical landmarks and incisions.

Superficial Dissection

The incision should be deepened through the median raphe, which is relatively avascular and is seen as a thin white line in the midline. The nuchal ligament is then identified and is incised by electrocautery (Fig. 4-4). The posterior cervical musculature is very vascular, a property that heightens the importance of maintaining the dissection in the avascular median raphe at the midline to reduce bleeding. Intermittent palpation of the spinous processes can assist the surgeon in staying oriented with the midline.

The incision should then be deepened with electrocautery to the external occipital protuberance and down to the posterior tubercle of C1 and the bifid spinous processes of

C2 and C3. The dissection is carried laterally for approximately 2.5 cm on either side of the median occipital crest. Excessive lateral dissection or retraction should be avoided to minimize the risk of injuring the greater occipital nerve. Care should be taken to avoid inadvertently entering the spinal canal through the occipitocervical membrane or the C1 to C2 ligamentum flavum.

Deep Dissection

The occiput is exposed in a subperiosteal fashion down to the foramen magnum. Care must be taken because a group of veins is frequently present at the skull base near the foramen magnum. The surgeon may then proceed with exposure of the C1 ring, which does not have a spinous process and lies deep in the space between the occiput and C2 (Fig. 4-5, *top left*). Subperiosteal elevation with a small Cobb elevator or a fine curet is used to dissect the ligamentum flavum and the tectorial membrane from the posterior arch of C1, with care taken to remain

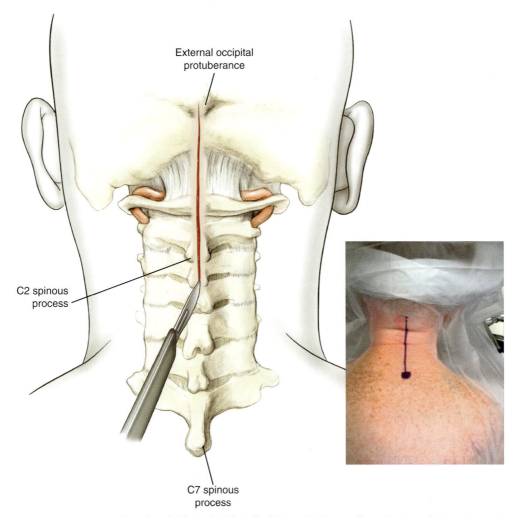

External occipital
protuberance

C2 spinous
process

C7 spinous
process

FIGURE 4-2   Longitudinal midline incision. (From Shen FH: Spine. In Miller MD, Chhabra AB, Hurwitz SR, et al, editors: *Orthopaedic surgical approaches*, Philadelphia, 2008, Saunders.)

within 12 mm from the midline on the posterior aspect of C1 and 8 mm from the midline on the superior aspect of the C1 ring, to avoid injury to the vertebral arteries (Fig. 4-5, *top right* and *bottom*). Preoperative planning should include an assessment of vertebral artery location, and the previously mentioned guidelines should be adjusted in the case of aberrant vertebral artery anatomy.

The large bifid spinous process of C2 is typically palpable and easily identified. It is exposed subperiosteally. The C1-C2 joint should then be identified by following the spinous process of C2 to the lamina and then superiorly to the C1-C2 joint (Fig. 4-6). The C1-C2 joint lies 2 to 3 cm anterior to the facet joint of C2-C3. The greater occipital nerve (C2 nerve) lies posterior to the C1-C2 joint and is typically covered by a venous plexus. Keeping the dissection on the C2 posterior arch avoids injuring this nerve. Preserving the soft tissue attachments on the distal and lateral portions of C2 and C1-C2 facet joint assists in maintaining postoperative subaxial stability.

Exposure of the C1-C2 facet joint is necessary to allow visualization for the placement of C1 lateral screws and C2 pedicle screws. Once the musculature has been dissected and retracted from the posterior aspects of C1 and C2, the lamina of C2 is easily identified. Soft tissue can

then be carefully dissected from the lamina of C2. Continuing this dissection proximally exposes the pars interarticularis of C2, the medial border of the C2 pedicle, and the undersurface of the C1 lateral mass (Fig. 4-7).

Subaxial Cervical Spine

Incision

See the earlier section on surgical landmarks and incisions.

Superficial Dissection

The incision should be deepened through the avascular median raphe, as previously described. Subcutaneous fat and deep cervical fascia should be divided in line with the skin incision, and the nuchal ligament should be identified (Fig. 4-8). Remaining in the midline, using electrocautery, and proceeding with subperiosteal dissection in a caudal-to-cephalad direction all assist in minimizing bleeding. Care should be taken to protect the supraspinous and interspinous ligaments during the initial dissection.

Using subperiosteal dissection, the surgeon should then follow the spinous process out laterally first onto the lamina and then to the lateral mass, thus exposing both these structures (Fig. 4-9). Dissection should stop

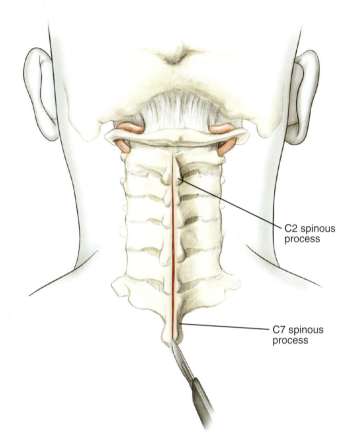

FIGURE 4-3   Longitudinal midline incision. (From Shen FH: Spine. In Miller MD, Chhabra AB, Hurwitz SR, et al, editors: *Orthopaedic surgical approaches,* Philadelphia, 2008, Saunders.)

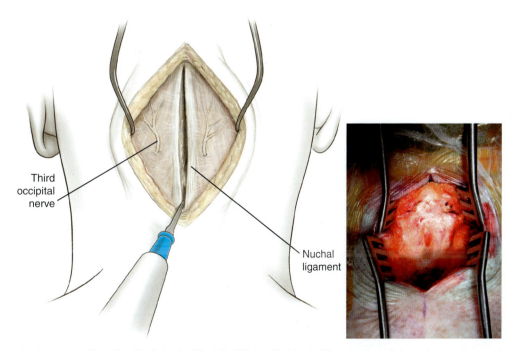

FIGURE 4-4   **Superficial dissection.** (From Shen FH: Spine. In Miller MD, Chhabra AB, Hurwitz SR, et al, editors: *Orthopaedic surgical approaches,* Philadelphia, 2008, Saunders.)

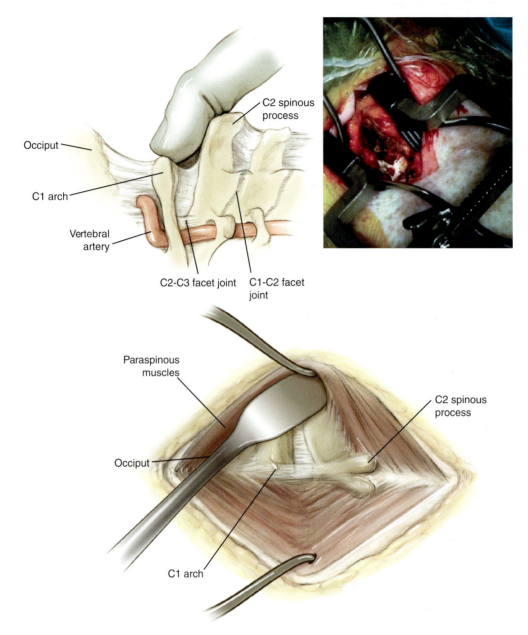

FIGURE 4-5 Deep dissection and exposure of the C1 ring. (From Shen FH: Spine. In Miller MD, Chhabra AB, Hurwitz SR, et al, editors: *Orthopaedic surgical approaches*, Philadelphia, 2008, Saunders.)

at the medial third of the facet joint, and the facet joint capsule should be preserved unless a fusion procedure is planned at that level. If facet fusion or instrumentation is required, then dissection is extended to the lateral border of the lateral mass. The starting point of a lateral mass screw is usually 1 mm medial to the center of the lateral mass, with the trajectory angulated superiorly 15 degrees and laterally approximately 30 degrees.

Deep Dissection

Deeper dissection proceeds by identifying the ligamentum flavum running between the lamina then detaching this ligament from the lamina by using a fine curet. If laminectomy or laminotomy is to be performed, the spinous processes and laminae are typically removed en bloc (Fig. 4-10). The interspinous tissues should first be cauterized to minimize bleeding. Intraoperative lateral radiographs or fluoroscopy should be used to confirm the correct operative levels. Specific surgical procedures are discussed in other chapters.

Postoperative Considerations

The use of deep drains following a posterior approach is based on the surgeon's preference. Most surgeons also place their patients in a cervical collar for a period of time. Once the patient awakens from anesthesia, inpatient hospital stay is recommended, and careful serial neurovascular examinations are essential for detecting any complications. Postoperative anteroposterior and lateral plain film radiographs should be obtained. Advanced imaging such as CT or MRI may be necessary to confirm screw placement, to evaluate decompression if the patient's symptoms have not improved, or to investigate any findings on neurovascular examination that elicit concern for epidural hematoma or nerve root impingement.

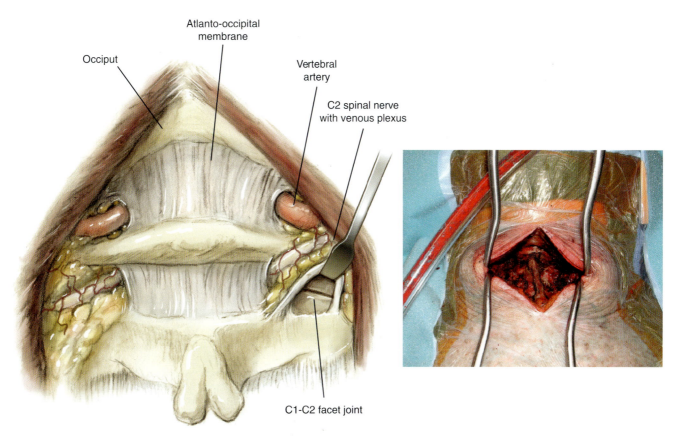

FIGURE 4-6   **Exposure of C2.** (From Shen FH: Spine. In Miller MD, Chhabra AB, Hurwitz SR, et al, editors: *Orthopaedic surgical approaches,* Philadelphia, 2008, Saunders.)

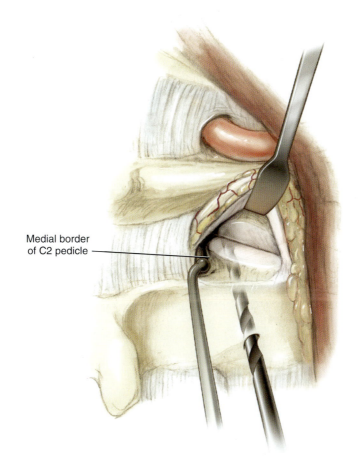

FIGURE 4-7   **Exposure of the C2 facet joint.** (From Shen FH: Spine. In Miller MD, Chhabra AB, Hurwitz SR, et al, editors: *Orthopaedic surgical approaches,* Philadelphia, 2008, Saunders.)

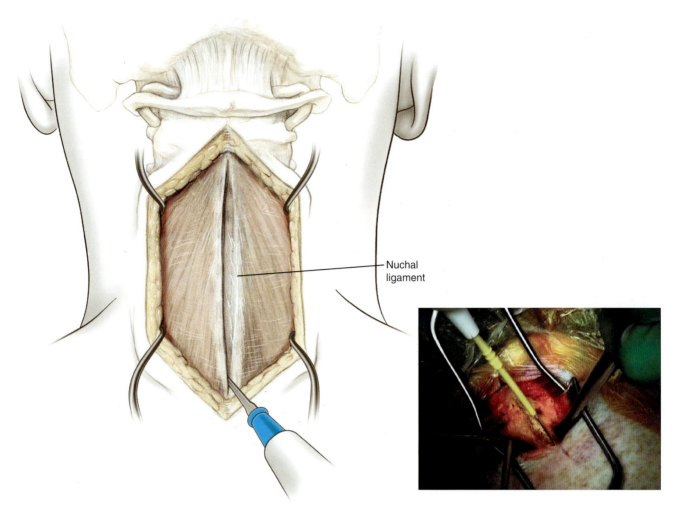

Nuchal
ligament

FIGURE 4-8 **Superficial surgical dissection.** (From Shen FH: Spine. In Miller MD, Chhabra AB, Hurwitz SR, et al, editors: *Orthopaedic surgical approaches,* Philadelphia, 2008, Saunders.)

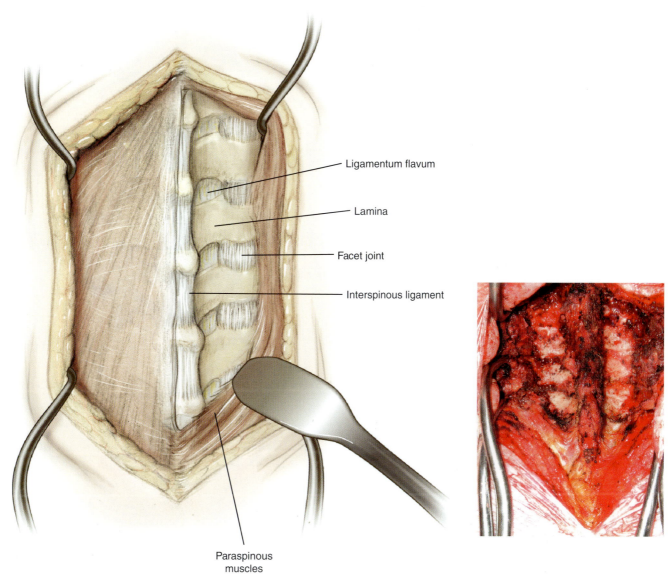

— Ligamentum flavum

— Lamina

— Facet joint

— Interspinous ligament

Paraspinous
muscles

FIGURE 4-9   **Exposure of the lamina and lateral masses.** (From Shen FH: Spine. In Miller MD, Chhabra AB, Hurwitz SR, et al, editors: *Orthopaedic surgical approaches*, Philadelphia, 2008, Saunders.)

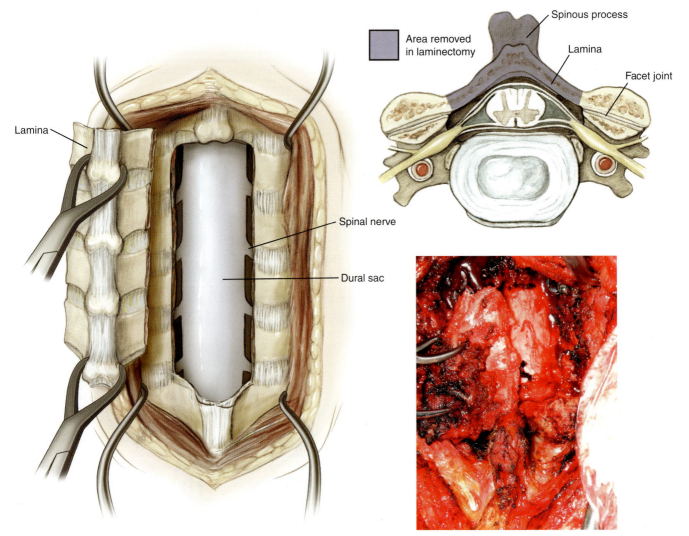

FIGURE 4-10   Deep dissection: laminectomy or laminotomy. (From Shen FH: Spine. In Miller MD, Chhabra AB, Hurwitz SR, et al, editors: *Orthopaedic surgical approaches*, Philadelphia, 2008, Saunders.)

SELECTED READINGS

1. Chesnut R M, Abitbol J J, Garfin S R: Surgical management of cervical radiculopathy: indication, techniques, and results, *Orthop Clin North Am* 23:461–474, 1992.
2. Dvorak M F, Fisher C G, Fehlings M G, et al.: The surgical approach to subaxial cervical spine injuries: an evidence-based algorithm based on the SLIC classification system, *Spine (Phila Pa 1976)* 32:2620–2629, 2007.
3. Ebraheim N A, An H S, Xu R, et al.: The quantitative anatomy of the cervical nerve root groove and the intervertebral foramen, *Spine (Phila Pa 1976)* 21:1619–1623, 1996.
4. Lehman R A Jr, Riew K D: Thorough decompression of the posterior cervical foramen, *Instr Course Lect* 56:301–309, 2007.
5. Martin M D, Bruner H J, Maiman D J: Anatomic and biomechanical considerations of the craniovertebral junction, *Neurosurgery* 66:2–6, 2010.
6. Russell S M, Benjamin V: Posterior surgical approach to the cervical neural foramen for intervertebral disc disease, *Neurosurgery* 54:662–665, 2004; discussion 665–666.
7. Sekhon L H: Posterior cervical decompression and fusion for circumferential spondylotic cervical stenosis: review of 50 consecutive cases, *J Clin Neurosci* 13:23–30, 2006.
8. Xu R, Kang A, Ebraheim N A, Yeasting R A: Anatomic relation between the cervical pedicle and the adjacent neural structures, *Spine (Phila Pa 1976)* 24:451–454, 1999.
9. Yonenobu K, Oda T: Posterior approach to the degenerative cervical spine, *Eur Spine J* 12(Suppl 2):S195–S201, 2003.
10. Zhang J, Tsuzuki N, Hirabayashi S, et al.: Surgical anatomy of the nerves and muscles in the posterior cervical spine: a guide for avoiding inadvertent nerve injuries during the posterior approach, *Spine (Phila Pa 1976)* 28:1379–1384, 2003.

Anterior Approaches and Surgical Considerations for Pathology of the Cervicothoracic Junction

5

Zachary A. Smith, Albert Wong, and Richard G. Fessler

CHAPTER PREVIEW

Chapter Synopsis	Surgical exposure of the anterior cervicothoracic junction poses a unique challenge for spine surgeons. Several distinct features of this region contribute to the difficulty of approach. However, given the complexities and challenges of this region, subsequent modifications have been described. This chapter primarily focuses on two anterior cervicothoracic junction exposure techniques: the supraclavicular approach and the transmanubrial transclavicular approach.
Important Points	The supraclavicular approach is most familiar because it is essentially an oblique extension of the typical anteromedial approach.
	If necessary, the surgical exposure in the supraclavicular approach can be extended by disarticulating the clavicle.
	The recurrent laryngeal nerve is at risk, particularly during the caudal dissection of this approach.
	The thoracic duct lies laterally in the field at the junction of the internal jugular and subclavian veins, and aberrant dissection lateral to the carotid sheath places the thoracic duct at risk for injury.
	The transmanubrial transclavicular approach provides access to the anterior cervicothoracic junction by resecting the medial third of the clavicle and a portion of the manubrium.
	The subclavian vein is at risk for injury during resection of the clavicle.
	Care should be taken to assess for the presence of pleural violation and pneumothorax, which may necessitate placement of a chest tube.

Surgical exposure of the anterior cervicothoracic junction poses a unique challenge for spine surgeons. Several distinct features of this region contribute to the difficulty of approach. First, major anatomic structures can impede surgical access. These structures include the contents of the carotid sheath, the thyroid gland, and osseous structures such as the sternum and clavicle. Furthermore, many of the contents of the thoracic inlet, including the esophagus, trachea, thoracic duct, and essential nerves (i.e., vagus, recurrent laryngeal, phrenic, and sympathetic), must also be safely negotiated during the approach. Finally, in cases of significant disease, anatomic boundaries can be poorly defined, thus contributing to increased difficulty with anterior approaches to the cervicothoracic junction.

The anterior cervical approach was originally described in the 1950s.[1] However, given the complexities and aforementioned challenges of this region, subsequent modifications of this technique were later described. In particular, approaches to the cervicothoracic junction require specific attention. This chapter primarily focuses on two anterior cervicothoracic junction exposure techniques: the supraclavicular approach and the transmanubrial transclavicular approach.

Cervicothoracic Junction: Anatomic Considerations

The cervicothoracic junction can pose multiple challenges given the presence of numerous visceral and vascular structures and the location of this region as a transition zone between two regions of the spine. The cervical spine has a developmentally normal anatomic lordosis and is generally flexible. In contrast, the thoracic spine is kyphotic and generally rigid.

This region has many unique characteristics, such as the ratio of the spinal canal to spinal cord diameter. The spinal canal diameter is the narrowest at the cervicothoracic junction, but the spinal cord in this region is near its widest diameter. Thus, pathologic processes in this region can cause early compressive symptoms. Furthermore, the cervicothoracic junction is a vascular watershed zone. Cervical radicular branches provide blood supply to the lower subaxial cord, whereas thoracic radicular arteries from the aorta provide much of the blood to the spinal cord parenchyma at the level of the cervicothoracic junction (C6 to T2).

Another surgical challenge to the lower neck includes the soft tissue, which traverses vasculature and essential peripheral nerves. The anterolateral region of the neck contains the muscles of the hypopharynx and the carotid sheath (including the carotid artery, jugular vein, and vagus nerve). Deep and medial to the sternocleidomastoid (SCM) muscle are the esophagus and trachea. Ventral to the trachea are the thyroid and parathyroid glands. Injury to any of these vital structures can produce undesired morbidity and contribute to the challenges of the cervicothoracic junction.

Developing a bloodless plane is critical to the surgical approach. Thus, identification of the SCM muscle is critical.[1,2,3,4] This muscle originates from the mastoid process and inserts at the sternum and the clavicle. Just medial and deep to this muscle are the midline structures: strap muscles, trachea, and esophagus. The strap muscles include the sternohyoid, sternothyroid, omohyoid, and thyrohyoid. Between the SCM and strap muscles are multiple neurovascular structures. The right recurrent laryngeal nerve branches from the vagus nerve and curves around the subclavian artery. The left recurrent laryngeal nerve curves underneath the aortic arch and runs superiorly between the trachea and the esophagus in the tracheoesophageal groove more caudally (and is often less aberrant).[2,5,6] Other important structures in this region include the carotid artery, the vagus nerve, and the jugular vein. Within the superior mediastinum, the subclavian artery and vein, the brachiocephalic artery and vein, and the thoracic duct can all be encountered. The thoracic duct is medially bounded by the first thoracic vertebrae and the manubrium and laterally by the first ribs.[3,4,7] The cupula of the lung lies just inferior to the thoracic duct.[3,4,7]

Surgical Techniques

Supraclavicular Approach

The supraclavicular approach to the cervicothoracic junction provides excellent exposure without requiring disruption of the sternum or clavicle. Surgical exposure using this technique is perhaps the most familiar because it is essentially an oblique extension of the typical anteromedial approach. However, this technique can pose specific challenges. This technique is often extremely difficult in patients with short necks, prominent muscular development, or significant kyphosis. Furthermore, this approach can result in a deep operative field and may require an acute angle to place anterior instrumentation.

The authors traditionally use a transverse skin incision that is 2 cm above the clavicle and extends from the midline to the lateral border of the SCM. Like many surgeons, the authors employ a left-sided approach because of the more consistent course of the left recurrent laryngeal nerve.[8] However, a right-sided approach can be used if attention is given to a potentially aberrant course of this nerve.

The initial operative steps are similar to those employed with a traditional anterior cervical approach. Following careful dissection of more superficial structures (including the platysma muscle), the first critical landmark is the SCM muscle. At the anterior border of this muscle, the superficial and deep cervical fascia should be dissected thoroughly, both cranially and caudally. The SCM can be isolated with finger dissection, and its attachment to the sternal and clavicular heads can be identified. Subsequently, the muscular attachments can be transected in a subperiosteal manner and reflected superiorly (Fig. 5-1).

For complete surgical exposure, the authors suggest disarticulation of the clavicle from the manubrium. The free-floating portion of the clavicle can be removed. However, careful attention should be given to the undersurface of this bone fragment because the subclavian vein commonly underlies the clavicular head. In addition, the omohyoid and sternohyoid muscles can also be divided. This technique allows for visualization of the anterior scalene muscle and the phrenic nerve.[9]

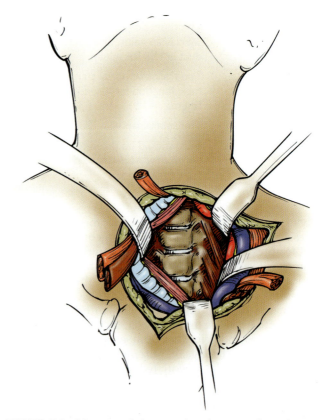

FIGURE 5-1 Schematic of the supraclavicular approach to the anterior cervicothoracic junction. The sternal and clavicular attachments of the sternocleidomastoid, as well as the omohyoid and sternohyoid, have been transected and reflected. (From Fessler RG, Sekhar LN, editors: *Atlas of neurosurgical techniques: spine and peripheral nerves*, New York, 2006, Thieme.)

An equally important surgical landmark, the carotid sheath, should be given attention at this time. Located below the SCM muscle, the carotid artery (and its sheath) should be laterally retracted, and dissection should occur in a plane medial to the carotid artery.[6,10,11] A potential pitfall during dissection of the caudal portion of this plane is injury to the recurrent laryngeal nerve that runs in the groove between the trachea and the esophagus. If attention is not given to this structure, it can be damaged during the approach. Similarly, aggressive surgical dissection of the longus colli muscles laterally can lead to an injury of the sympathetic nerves and plexuses. This injury may potentially result in Horner syndrome.

At the most caudal portions of the exposure, additional structures must be carefully identified and preserved. The thoracic duct is located laterally in the field, at the junction of the internal jugular and subclavian veins. If the dissection is focused medially from the carotid sheath, this structure is rarely injured. In addition, both the subclavian artery and the thyrocervical trunk can be injured with this approach.

When the level of disease is reached, the prevertebral fascia must be incised in the midline to complete the exposure. A bent spinal needle can be used to identify the surgical level with fluoroscopy, followed by development of longus colli "cuffs" to place permanent retractor blades. These muscular cuffs help to protect the midline esophagus and lateral carotid sheath from injury.[5] At this point of the procedure, the surgeon can address spinal column disorders in a fashion to similar to other approaches in the spine. However, because of the narrow opening of the thoracic inlet, wide surgical access is rarely possible. Therefore, if this access is desired, splitting of the manubrium and sternum may be required.

Transmanubrial Transclavicular Approach

The transmanubrial transclavicular approach allows for a direct corridor to the cervicothoracic junction. With this approach, the medial one third of the clavicle and a small percentage of the manubrium are removed. This technique allows excellent exposure of the upper thoracic vertebrae and provides autologous bone grafts during the approach. Depending on the location of the pathologic process, the focus and degree of osseous exposure can be modified as needed. This surgical approach, albeit technically demanding, can be both safe and effective when undertaken by an experienced surgeon.

For the transmanubrial transclavicular approach, the authors typically use a T-shaped incision.[7,4,12,13] This curvilinear incision usually is 2 cm above the clavicle and extends to both sides of the SCM muscle (Fig. 5-2). The incision's vertical portion extends down the midline and just caudal to the manubriosternal junction (halfway down the sternum). Following opening of the skin, subplatysmal flaps are created in a fashion similar to the classic anterior cervical approach. In many circumstances, external jugular veins and a portion of the jugular venous arch require mobilization. However, in some situations, these structures must be sacrificed. Although the senior author's preference is to use a left-sided approach given the decreased variability of the left recurrent laryngeal nerve,[14] either side may be used for exposure.

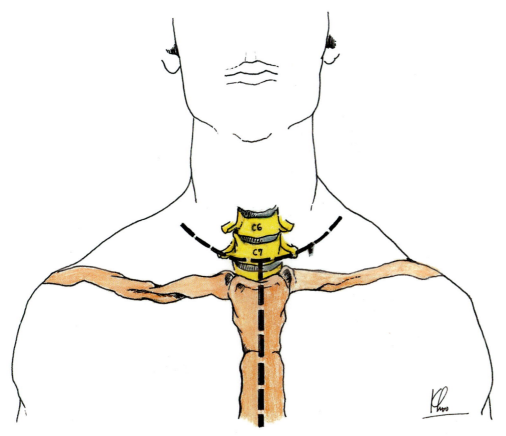

FIGURE 5-2 Incision for the transmanubrial transclavicular approach. (From Fessler RG, Sekhar LN, editors: *Atlas of neurosurgical techniques: spine and peripheral nerves,* New York, 2006, Thieme.)

The focus now shifts to the muscular attachments to the clavicle and manubrium. The two heads of the SCM muscle (sternal and clavicular) are dissected with cautery or with periosteal dissection from their osseous attachments. These muscle attachments are reflected superiorly and laterally. In addition, the sternohyoid and sternothyroid muscles must also be sectioned and elevated. If careful attention is paid to the investments of the deep cervical fascia during elevation of these muscles, injury to their neurovascular bundles is minimal. At this point, the suprasternal space is entered, and subperiosteal dissection can be completed. The soft tissue dissection is carried out to include the medial third of the clavicle and the left two thirds of the manubrium. Finally, the origin of the pectoralis major muscle must be freed from the inferior manubrium and the sternum.

With a high-speed drill, the medial portion of the clavicle is then resected, and the first costal cartilage is also divided. The sternoclavicular joint is disarticulated, and a portion of the clavicle is removed. As mentioned previously during the discussion of the supraclavicular approach, removal of the medial clavicle must be done carefully. Given its location under this bony structure, the subclavian vein can be injured during this step of the procedure. After subperiosteal dissection, the manubrium and medial clavicle can be resected en bloc with an osteotome (Fig. 5-3). These structures can be saved for future bone grafting. As with other approaches, this exposure can now be modified and tailored for each patient's pathologic features.

Conclusions

Both the supraclavicular approach and the transmanubrial approach are closed in similar fashion. After appropriate bone grafting and instrumentation, the area is irrigated copiously with antibiotic-impregnated saline solution. Hemostasis is obtained, and fluoroscopy is used to confirm placement of hardware or bone grafting, or both. The authors typically place a no. 7 Jackson-Pratt drain at the time of closure to prevent postoperative hematoma formation. This drain is kept in place for 2 to 3 days after the operation. Further, if any evidence of pleural violation is noted, a chest tube can be inserted through a separate stab wound. Subcutaneous and skin tissue is closed in a routine fashion, and the choice of a cervical brace is based on the surgeon's preference.

Attention should be given to patients with extensive disease or prolonged surgical procedures. These patients may have significant soft tissue edema, requiring close observation in an intensive care setting in the immediate (24-hour) postoperative period. Judicious evaluation for significant fluid shifts and signs of potential airway edema should be completed before extubation.

Not uncommonly, many patients also have postoperative hoarseness following this procedure. This complication may result from traction on the recurrent laryngeal nerve. In addition, damage to the superior laryngeal nerve can cause difficulty with clearing of the secretions and may promote aspiration. This possibility is further reason to monitor these patients closely after surgery

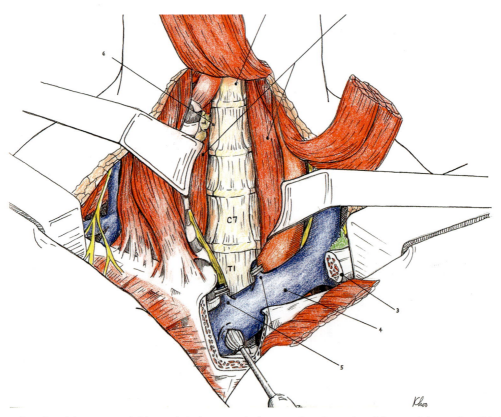

FIGURE 5-3   Deep dissection of the transmanubrial transclavicular approach after resection of a portion of the manubrium and medial clavicle. (From Fessler RG, Sekhar LN, editors: *Atlas of neurosurgical techniques: spine and peripheral nerves,* New York, 2006, Thieme.)

and promote rapid mobilization, pulmonary toilet, and the use of speech therapy. These potential perioperative complications highlight the necessity for careful attention to the details of surgical anatomy. When performed correctly, a successful outcome is attainable with anterior approaches to the cervicothoracic junction.

REFERENCES

1. Cloward R: The anterior approach for removal of ruptured cervical disks. *Journal of neurosurgery* 15:602–617, 1958.
2. Riley LJ: Surgical approaches to the anterior structures of the cervical spine, *Clin Orthop Relat Res* 91:16–20, 1973.
3. Lu J, Ebraheim NA, Nadim Y, et al: Anterior approach to the cervical spine: surgical anatomy. *Orthopedics* 23:841–845, 2000.
4. Cheung KM, Mak KC, Luk KD: Anterior approach to cervical spine. *Spine* 37:E297–302, 2012.
5. Albert T: Relevant cervical anatomy and anterior, middle, and lower cervical exposures. In Albert T, Balderston RA, Northrup BE, editors: *Surgical approaches to the spine*, Philadelphia, 1997, Saunders.
6. Kilburg C, Sullivan HG, Mathiason MA: Effect of approach side during anterior cervical discectomy and fusion on the incidence of recurrent laryngeal nerve injury. *Journal of neurosurgery. Spine* 4:273–277, 2006.
7. Choi S, Samudrala S: Supraclavicular apporach to the cervicothoracic junction. In Fessler RG, Sekhar LN, editors: *Atlas of neurosurgical techniques: spine and peripheral nerves*, New York, 2006, Thieme, pp 306–311.
8. Sundaresan N, DiGiacinto GV: Surgical approaches to the cervicothoracic junction. In Sundaresan N, Schmidek HH, Schiller AL, Rosenthal DI, editors: *Tumors of the spine*, Philadelphia, 1990, Saunders, pp 358–368.
9. McAfee P: Anterior surgical approaches to the lower and upper cervical spine. In Sherk HH, editor: *The cervical spine: an atlas of surgical procedures*, ed 3, Philadelphia, 1994, Lippincott, pp 37–69.
10. Sundaresan N, Shah J, Foley KM, Rosen G: An anterior surgical approach to the upper thoracic vertebrae, *J Neurosurg* 61:686–690, 1984.
11. Pointillart V, Aurouer N, Gangnet N, et al: Anterior approach to the cervicothoracic junction without sternotomy: a report of 37 cases. *Spine* 32:2875–2879, 2007.
12. Khoo L, Samudrala S: Transmanubrial transclavicular approach to the cervicothoracic junction. In Fessler RG, Sekhar LN, editors: *Atlas of neurosurgical techniques: spine and peripheral nerves*, New York, 2006, Thieme. pages 318-325.
13. Tarantino R, Donnarumma P, Marruzzo D, et al: Anterior surgical approaches to the cervicothoracic junction: when to use the manubriotomy? *The spine journal : official journal of the North American Spine Society* 13:1064–1068, 2013.
14. Capener N: The evolution of lateral rhachotomy, *J Bone Joint Surg Br* 36:173–179, 1954.

6

Developmental and Congenital Disorders of the Cervical Spine

Panagiotis Glavas, Lauren A. Tomlinson, and Denis S. Drummond

CHAPTER PREVIEW

Chapter Synopsis	Congenital anomalies of the pediatric cervical spine arise from a failure of normal development occurring early in the embryonic process. Failure to recognize these pathologic processes risks overlooking segmental instability, developing progressive spinal deformity, encroachment on the space available for the spinal cord (SAC), and the risk for myelopathy. This chapter reviews the embryology, biomechanics, and associated developmental and congenital disorders of the cervical spine.
Important Points	Better recognition and management of the congenital spine can be achieved by understanding the embryology and biomechanics of the normal immature cervical spine.
	These issues can include failures in segmentation, chondrification, and ossification, alone or in combination.
	Additional organ system abnormalities can occur in children with congenital spinal deformities.
Clinical and Surgical Pearls	Because the immature spine is largely cartilaginous, recognition and definition of pathologic features can be difficult even for experienced clinicians.
	Magnetic resonance imaging and three-dimensional computed tomography can define bony and cartilaginous anatomy and help assist in identifying any associated encroachment on neurovascular structures. Traction should be used with caution and applied progressively, and neurologic examination should be performed after every incremental increase in weight.
Clinical and Surgical Pitfalls	Relative ligamentous laxity in most children can have adverse effects on spinal stability.
	Facet and condylar development of the atlanto-occipital articulation are relatively shallow compared with the mature spine.
	The relatively larger heads of children can result in higher risks for instability.

Congenital anomalies of the pediatric cervical spine arise from a failure of normal development occurring early in the embryonic process. These anomalies can lead to problems for treating physicians and surgeons. Because the immature spine is largely cartilaginous, recognition and definition of pathologic features can be difficult even for experienced clinicians. Failure to recognize these pathologic processes risks overlooking segmental instability, developing progressive spinal deformity, encroachment on the space available for the spinal cord (SAC), and the risk for myelopathy. To recognize congenital anomalies and best manage these patients, it is helpful to understand the embryology and biomechanics of the normal immature cervical spine. Once these fundamental issues are understood, then anomalous development can be better appreciated.

Embryology

Segmentation

By the end of the fifth week of development, mesodermal cells that surround the notochord segment into epithelial spheres called somites[1] (Fig. 6-1). This process is known as segmentation and produces 42 to 44 pairs of somites. The somites develop in a craniocaudal fashion, and each somite has three parts: the sclerotome, the dermatome, and the myotome. The sclerotomes are responsible for

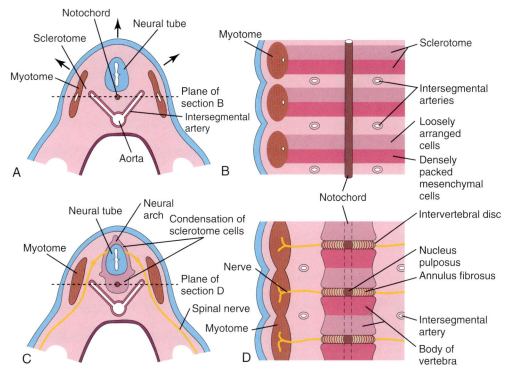

FIGURE 6-1 **A** to **D,** Segmentation produces 42 to 44 pairs of somites. The cells within the somites are arranged such that the cranial half are loosely packed and the caudal half are densely packed. The cranial half becomes the disk space and the annulus fibrosus, whereas the caudal half becomes the vertebral body. (From Moore KL, Persaud TVN, Torschia MG: *The developing human,* ed 9, Philadelphia, 2013, Saunders.)

the formation of the vertebrae, whereas the dermatomes and myotomes are responsible for the formation of the overlying dermis and muscles, respectively.[1]

The paired aggregation of cells within the somites is patterned so that the cells in the caudal half are densely packed and the cells in the cranial half are loosely packed (see Fig. 6-1). Separation or segmentation of the stacked somites occurs through the loosely packed cells in the cranial half of each somite. The cranial half becomes the disk space and the annulus fibrosus, whereas the caudal, tightly packed half of the somite becomes the vertebral body. Finally, the notochord slowly regresses to become the nucleus pulposus within the annulus fibrosus.[1]

For one complete vertebra to form properly, a tight interaction between a pair of somites is necessary. Failure of the proper segmentation process may result in congenital abnormalities. Two families of regulatory genes have been implicated in the control of the processes of somitogenesis and segmentation: *Pax* and *Hox*.[2] The *Pax* family of genes contributes to the development of the central nervous system and also controls the establishment of boundaries for each sclerotome. The *Hox* family of genes regulates the sequential craniocaudal development of the midline axial structures. Mutations in these genes may contribute to the development of congenital anomalies and are a topic of ongoing investigation.[2]

Chondrification and Ossification

During the sixth week of development, chondrification occurs and ultimately leads to ossification of relevant structures and regression of the notochord.[1] Defects in these two processes, which are controlled by signals

from the notochord, can lead to congenital abnormalities.[1] The vertebrae of the lower cervical spine (C3 to C7) have a similar pattern of development. Each vertebra has three primary ossification centers: one on either side of the neural arch and one in the vertebral centrum.[1] The ossification centers are separated anteriorly by the neurocentral synchondroses, which lie parallel to each other on either side of the centrum (Fig. 6-2). To develop normal vertebral growth, it is important for the neurocentral synchondroses to have paired growth that is symmetric and equal. Asymmetric growth leads to deformity. Normally, the synchondroses close between 6 and 8 years of age, at which time the spinal canal diameters have reached adult size. Premature closure of the neurocentral synchondroses may lead to reduced spinal cord diameters with an increased risk of spinal stenosis and deformity.[3,4]

Additional organ systems are derived from the same primitive areas of the mesoderm. Any process that can affect the normal development of the mesoderm can lead to spinal defects, as well as anomalies in other areas.[1] The estimated incidence of additional abnormalities in children with congenital spinal anomalies is up to 60%.[5] The genitourinary system is most commonly associated with congenital spine abnormalities.[1]

Upper Cervical Spine

The development of the occipitoatlantoaxial complex is a unique variation of the foregoing process (Fig. 6-3).

Atlas

Cells from the fourth occipital somite, also called the proatlas, combine with cells from the first cervical

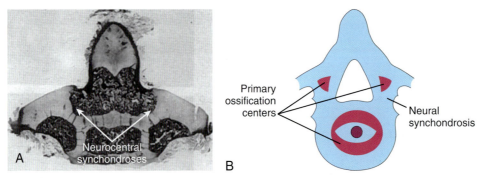

FIGURE 6-2   A, Neurocentral synchondroses of the atlas. **B,** Ossification centers and neurocentral synchondroses of a subaxial vertebra. (**A,** From Ganey TM, Ogden JA: Development and maturation of the axial skeleton. In Weinstein SL, editor: *The pediatric spine*, ed 2, Philadelphia, 2001, Lippincott Williams & Wilkins; **B,** adapted from Moore KL, Persaud TVN, Torschia MG: *The developing human*, ed 9, Philadelphia, 2013, Saunders.)

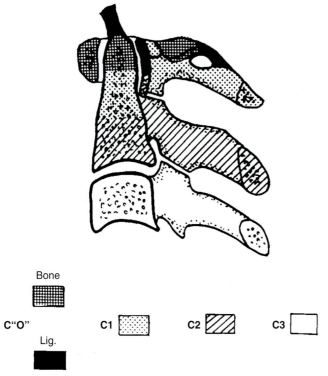

FIGURE 6-3   Development of the atlantoaxial spine. *Lig.*, Ligament. (From Sherk HH: Developmental anatomy of the normal cervical spine. In Clarke CR, editor: *The cervical spine*, ed 4, Philadelphia, 2005, Lippincott Williams & Wilkins, pp 37–45.)

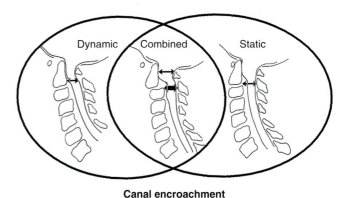

Canal encroachment

FIGURE 6-4   Types of encroachments on the spinal cord. (From Hosalkar HS, Sankar WN, Wills B, et al: Congenital osseous anomalies of the upper cervical spine. *J Bone Joint Surg Am* 90:337–348, 2008.)

Axis

Cells from the first and second somites contribute to formation of the axis (C2). The migration of cells that form the centrum of the proatlas also aids formation of the odontoid or dens and the supporting ligaments (see Fig. 6-3). Failure of this process may cause odontoid aplasia or hypoplasia. Finally, the basilar synchondrosis of the dens is a weak spot that can become the site of failure in the event of injury; this sequence of events is believed to be the cause of os odontoideum (OO).[7]

Biomechanics of the Immature Cervical Spine with Congenital Osseous Anomalies

Spinal biomechanics of the normal cervical spine in children differs significantly from that of healthy adults.[8] First, the relative ligamentous laxity in most children can have an adverse effect on stability of the facet joints, as well as on the competence of both the atlanto-occipital and the atlantoaxial joints. Second, the facet joints and the condylar development of the atlanto-occipital articulation are relatively shallow compared with those in the mature spine. Third, the relatively larger heads of children subject the immature spine to increased acceleration-deceleration forces and a higher risk of instability.

somite to form the atlas.[6] During the segmentation period, failure to segment or separate can occur, leading to synostosis between the atlas and the occiput. This condition is known as occipitalization of the atlas (Fig. 6-4). Another developmental failure can occur in the condylar joints. The result is a loss of the normal rounded shape of the joints, thus causing a loss of the required smooth motion with flexion and extension and leading to relative instability. In addition, cells from the first and second somites that contribute to the atlas centrum descend to form part of the odontoid process or dens. The caudal migration of cells from the centrum of the proatlas results in a central space and the ring shape of the atlas.

Table 6-1   Classification of Congenital Osseous Anomalies of the Cervical Spine with Associated Conditions

Classification	Anomalies	Associated Conditions[2,6,7,10,12,13]
1. Congenital	Occipitalization	KFS, Goldenhar syndrome, 22q11.2 deletion, Morquio syndrome, basilar invagination, atlas defects, os odontoideum, occipital vertebra, syringomyelia
	Condylar hypoplasia	Down syndrome, Goldenhar syndrome, skeletal dysplasias
	Atlas defects	Down syndrome, Goldenhar syndrome, Morquio syndrome
	Proatlas segmentation failure	Chiari type I malformation
	Basilar invagination	Chiari type I malformation, KFS, syringomyelia, syringobulbia, atlas defects, hydrocephalus
2. Developmental	Os odontoideum	Skeletal dysplasia, Down syndrome, KFS, Larsen syndrome, occipitalization
	Ossiculum terminale persistens	Down syndrome

KFS, Klippel-Feil syndrome.
Adapted from Menezes AH: Craniocervical developmental anatomy and its implications. *Childs Nerv Syst* 24:1109–1122, 2008.

With the addition of congenital anomalies, the risk of cervical instability is considerably greater. For example, in patients with vertebral fusion, excess motion can develop, and vertebral translation may occur at the adjacent motion segment. This translation of a vertebra can result in dynamic encroachment on the SAC and an increased risk for developing spinal cord injury[9] (see Fig. 6-4). An example of this is observed in a patient with occipitalization of the atlas combined with congenital fusion of C2 and C3. This situation leaves the atlantoaxial joint as the only motion segment in the upper cervical spine and increases the risk of encroachment on the SAC. This type of phenomenon is also observed in Klippel-Feil syndrome (KFS), in which a single mobile disk space exists between two fusion masses.

Another type of encroachment is static.[9] This disorder occurs when, for example, an intraspinal mass, such as protrusion of the dens in basilar invagination (BI) or the Chiari type I malformation, encroaches on the SAC. A combination of static and dynamic encroachment may also exist. Thus, encroachment and instability are the underlying mechanisms that can ultimately lead to neurologic signs and symptoms in the setting of congenital osseous anomalies.[9]

Congenital Osseous Anomalies of the Cervical Spine

Menezes provided a practical classification of craniocervical anomalies.[6] He divided these anomalies into a congenital group and a developmental group, with abnormal embryology and abnormalities that develop later in childhood (Table 6-1). The two groups are not mutually exclusive because some abnormalities may be present at birth but more frequently develop as the patient matures.

Occipitalization of the Atlas

Assimilation of the atlas to the occiput, or occipitalization, is defined as partial or complete congenital fusion of the atlas to the occiput[10] (Fig. 6-5). It results from failure of segmentation of the fourth occipital and first cervical sclerotomes.[6] This fusion may be partial, complete, unilateral, or bilateral. It can occur in conjunction with many other abnormalities and syndromes such as KFS, BI, spina

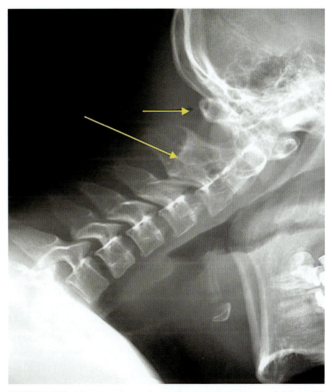

FIGURE 6-5 Flexion radiograph showing occipitalization and C2 to C3 fusion (*arrows*) in a patient with Klippel-Feil syndrome. This combination of anomalies produces excessive stress at the C1 to C2 motion segment and may lead to instability. (From Hosalkar HS, Sankar WN, Wills B, et al: Congenital osseous anomalies of the upper cervical spine. *J Bone Joint Surg Am* 90:337–348, 2008.)

bifida of the atlas, 22q11.2 deletion syndrome, occipital vertebrae, and Morquio syndrome[6,10] (see Table 6-1).

The spectrum of clinical findings can range from asymptomatic to pain and stiffness of the neck to neurologic deficits. Findings can resemble those associated with KFS and include a low hairline, short neck, and decreased cervical mobility. Gholve and associates reported on a series of 30 children with occipitalization.[10] The most frequent presenting symptoms were pain and stiffness in the neck. Myelopathy was observed in 5 of the 30 patients.[10]

Because of the occipitoatlantal fusion, increased mobility of the C1 to C2 segment is often observed. This can lead to atlantoaxial instability (defined as an atlantodental interval [ADI] greater than 4 mm on lateral flexion-extension radiographic films), as noted in up to 57% of the patients studied by Gholve and colleagues.[10] Of these patients, almost half had additional fusion of the C2 to C3 segment.[10] Therefore, occipitalization in conjunction with a fusion at C2 to C3 increases the risk that a patient will develop atlantoaxial instability. A thorough neurologic and radiologic evaluation of the cervical spine, with close attention to additional cervical spine anomalies, is important in the presence of instability. Families of affected children should be advised of potential signs of spinal cord compression and myelopathy. Patients should seek regular follow-up into adulthood.[10]

Usually, occipitalization in the absence of neurologic symptoms does not require any treatment. However, when associated malformations such as BI or C1 to C2 instability are present, surgical intervention may be indicated to prevent the progression of neurologic signs and symptoms. This intervention can consist of a combination of surgical decompression and posterior stabilization.

Atlas Defects

Malformations of the atlas are rare and result from segmentation failure.[11] Numerous malformations have been described, including aplasia, hypoplasia, and median clefts of the posterior or anterior arches.[2] The most common malformation is a cleft of the posterior arch, with a reported prevalence of 4%.[2] This is important clinically when the patient has associated instability and when a posterior approach to the upper cervical spine is planned. Connective tissue diseases resulting in ligamentous laxity, such as Down syndrome, are associated with clefts or spina bifida of the anterior and posterior arch of the atlas[2] (see Table 6-1). Abnormal movements during the chondrification period are believed to be the cause of spina bifida of the C1 arches.[12]

Usually, defects of the arches of C1 are asymptomatic except when they are associated with syndromes. Persistence of a bifid anterior and posterior arch has also been reported in Morquio, Down, and Goldenhar syndromes. The clinical presentation of patients with atlas defects in a series by Menezes consisted of torticollis and plagiocephaly.[6]

The ring of C1 should be complete by 3 years of age.[6] Persistence of the bifid arch past 3 years of age in addition to ligamentous laxity can lead to instability. Menezes reported on 20 infants with a bifid anterior or posterior arch or absent anterior or posterior arches.[6] Sixty percent of these patients reformed their anterior arch and stabilized the craniocervical junction with a custom-built cervical brace.[6] If the malformation is detected early enough, a bracing trial until approximately 3 years of age is indicated.[6] In the setting of continued abnormal movement in the patient with a syndrome and ligamentous laxity, it is thought that the ring will not form and can lead to neurologic deficits. In such cases, fusion is recommended.[6] Similarly, the authors' experience suggests that upper cervical fusion is warranted in the child who is more than 3 years old and who has signs of instability.

Proatlas Segmentation Failure

Proatlas segmentation failures result in anomalies of the last occipital sclerotome. These rare anomalies may be mistaken for atlas or odontoid anomalies.[13] Menezes and Fenoy reviewed 72 patients identified as having proatlas segmentation abnormalities from a large database of 5200 patients with symptomatic craniovertebral junction abnormalities.[13] These abnormalities are located around the foramen magnum and were associated with Chiari type I malformations in 33% of cases (see Table 6-1). Other abnormalities included a central bony mass from the clivus or the medial aspects of the occipital condyle in 61%, anterolateral and lateral compression in 37%, and dorsal compression in 17%.[13]

In the series of Menezes and Fenoy, 90% of these patients presented between the first and second decades. Seventy-two percent of the patients had motor dysfunction, as manifested by weakness of the upper extremities, quadriparesis, and hemiparesis. Vertebrobasilar insufficiency was seen in 25% of the patients.[13]

Magnetic resonance imaging (MRI) and three-dimensional computed tomography (CT) scans are best suited to evaluate encroachment on the neurovascular structures and to guide treatment. For example, anterior and anterolateral protrusions are best addressed from a transpalatopharyngeal approach, whereas dorsal compression is relieved through a posterolateral approach. As imaging techniques and an understanding of the embryologic development of the craniovertebral junction continue to evolve, new insight into segmentation failures of the proatlas will be acquired and will lead to novel treatments.

Basilar Invagination

BI consists of occipital hypoplasia and upward protrusion of the dens into the foramen magnum.[2] True congenital BI is associated with other occipitoatlantal malformations, including failure of closure of the atlas ring (anterior or posterior, or both), KFS, Chiari type I malformation, and syringomyelia[2,14] (see Table 6-1).

Normally, the dens progressively descends relative to the foramen magnum. This may be a result of the growth and development of the occipital condyles. When this descent is incomplete, BI can occur.[2]

BI is defined radiologically as a protrusion of the dens into the foramen magnum.[2] Craniometric lines (McGregor, Chamberlain, and McRae) on the lateral radiograph are used to determine whether BI is present. However, these lines rely on landmarks that are difficult to visualize in the immature spine. Advanced imaging such as with CT or MRI is recommended to diagnose BI when the condition is suspected based on plain films (Fig. 6-6).

Goel and colleagues evaluated 190 patients with BI. The series was divided into 2 groups: group 1 consisted of 88 patients with no associated Chiari malformation, and group 2 consisted of 102 patients with an associated Chiari malformation.[15] Of the 88 patients in group 1, weakness and neck pain were the most common presenting symptoms (100% and 59%, respectively). Localizing signs included short neck (41%), low hairline (48%), webbed neck (47%), torticollis (69%), and restricted neck movements (59%).[15]

A trial of presurgical traction can be used to assess the reducibility of the BI.[14] Caution should be used whenever traction is applied: weights should increase progressively, and neurologic examination should be performed after every incremental increase of weight. If the BI is reducible, then surgical stabilization from a posterior-only approach can be used.[14] If the dens is not reducible, transoral decompression followed by posterior occipitocervical stabilization is performed.[14]

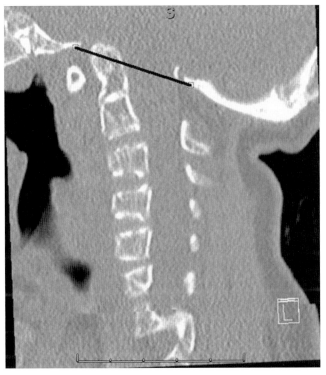

FIGURE 6-6 Basilar invagination. Note the protrusion of the dens into the foramen magnum.

Os Odontoideum

OO can be defined as a separate ossicle of variable size with smooth, rounded cortical margins that lies in place of the odontoid process and leaves a clear space between it and the hypoplastic odontoid process[2] (Fig. 6-7). Therefore, OO should not be considered an isolated odontoid process, but rather a unique ossicle cranial to a foreshortened odontoid process. Moreover, it should not be confused with ossiculum terminale, which refers to nonunion at the apex of the dens and does not lead to atlantoaxial instability. The two anatomic types of OO are orthotopic and dystopic.[16] In orthotopic OO, the ossicle is in a normal position relative to the dens and moves in unison with the anterior arch of the atlas. In the dystopic form, the ossicle is displaced cranially and may fuse with the clivus.

The pathogenesis of OO has been extensively debated. Two theories have been proposed: congenital (embryologic) or acquired (traumatic). In support of the congenital theory are a report of familial OO[17] and another case report of identical twins with OO and partial fusion of the posterior elements of C2 and C3.[18] The congenital theory supposes a congenital failure of fusion between the base of the dens and the body of the axis. This would create a gap at the level of the neurocentral synchondrosis. Anatomically, however, the gap is rarely seen at this level. Instead, the gap is more rostral at the anatomic base of the dens. Moreover, this area of the dens has been shown to have a 55% reduction of bone mass when compared with the rest of the dens and axis body. In addition, cortical thickness at the base of the dens is 35% less than in the rest of the dens.[19] Therefore, the current prevailing theory is acquired (traumatic),[6,7] in which OO results from an early and chronic fracture of the dens. OO is frequently

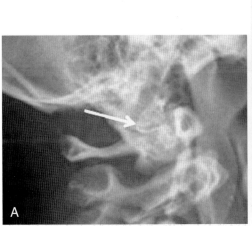

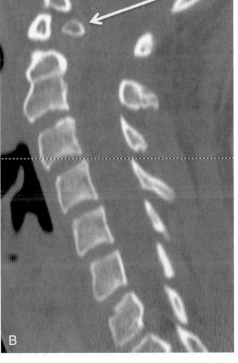

FIGURE 6-7 Radiograph (**A**) and computed tomography (CT) scan (**B**) of an os odontoideum. A fortuitous finding of os odontoideum in a patient presenting with neck pain following a low-velocity motor vehicle accident. *Arrows* indicate the location of the os odontoideum on the radiograph and CT scan, respectively.

encountered in patients with congenital syndromes such Down syndrome, KFS, and Morquio syndrome[7] (see Table 6-1). Although one can argue that this finding supports the congenital theory, another explanation could be that the abnormal and excessive movements in the cervical spine of these individuals can produce a stress fracture at the weak anatomic base of the dens, thus leading to OO with atlantoaxial instability.[7]

The range of symptoms associated with OO is wide.[7] Patients may report the following: (1) no symptoms, with the diagnosis been made incidentally; (2) local mechanical irritation manifested as pain and torticollis; (3) progressive myelopathy; and (4) transient neurologic symptoms related to vertebral artery compression.

As in other anomalies of the craniovertebral junction, the goals of treatment are to relieve the compression on the neurovascular structures and to provide stability to the cervical spine. Arvin and co-workers recommended that asymptomatic patients with an incidental finding of OO and no atlantoaxial instability should have a yearly clinical and radiologic examination with flexion-extension radiographs. In addition, MRI should be performed every 5 years to assess for the appearance of myelomalacia. Counseling regarding avoidance of contact sports should be offered.[7]

In the presence of instability, most patients can be managed by a posterior stabilization technique; the most successful rate of fusion has been demonstrated with transarticular screw fixation of C1 and C2.[2] Anterior decompression followed by posterior stabilization may be necessary in patients who present with fixed OO, typically seen in the dystopic type. Finally, extension of the fusion to the occiput may be indicated in patients who have OO in the presence of BI or with an absent posterior arch of the atlas.

Ossiculum Terminale Persistens

By the age of 8 to 10 years, a secondary ossification center develops within the proximal dens epiphysis. This is termed the ossiculum terminale, and it fuses with the rest of the dens by the age of 10 to 13 years.[20] Occasionally, this fusion does not occur; it is then called an ossiculum terminale persistens. The main clinical significance of this condition lies in the fact that it should not be confused with OO, which is much larger. Otherwise, ossiculum terminale persistens is a benign variation of normal with no associated atlantoaxial instability.

Klippel-Feil Syndrome

KFS was first described by French neurologist Maurice Klippel and his intern André Feil in their original report in 1912.[21] They reported in a 46-year-old patient what has become known as the classic triad of KFS: decreased movement in the affected area, a short neck, and a low hairline. This classic triad is found in less than 50% of patients with KFS.[22] In addition, many other abnormalities associated with KFS have been described, including brainstem malformations, scoliosis, webbing of the neck, spina bifida, Sprengel deformity, deafness, and cardiovascular and renal abnormalities (Table 6-2). This multitude of associations relates to the proximity of the cervical somites to other regions of the developing embryo. Thus,

KFS describes a heterogeneous group of patients unified by the presence of fusions of some or the entire cervical spine.

The final common pathway that leads to KFS results from a failure of segmentation of the cervical spine during embryogenesis. Several genes are under investigation for their possible role in the development of KFS.[22] For example, the *HOX* family of genes plays an important role in the specification and identity of vertebrae. In the murine model, inactivation of *Hoxd3* causes occipitalization of the atlas. In addition, the *Pax* family of genes plays an important role in somite segmentation. Further study is necessary to determine whether these genes play a role in the development of KFS.

KFS can be classified into three categories.[1] Type I KFS manifests with numerous cervical fusions, type II manifests with fusion of one or two vertebrae and other abnormalities of the cervical spine, and type III manifests with fusion of cervical vertebrae and thoracic or lumbar vertebrae. The incidence is approximately 1 in 42,000 live births.[1] Sixty percent of patients have scoliosis, with the more severe curves appearing in type I KFS. Thirty-five percent of patients have associated urinary abnormalities, and 30% have a hearing impairment.

The presenting signs and symptoms of patients with KFS are related to pain and decreased range of motion of the cervical spine and typically occur during the second or third decades of life. More extensive fusions tend to cause patients to present earlier, perhaps because of the cosmetic deformity.[22] In other patients, the discovery of cervical synostoses can be incidental when radiographs are ordered for other reasons. Regardless of the initial presentation, once cervical spine fusion is discovered, meticulous examination of the radiographs is warranted to evaluate the extent of the fusion and determine whether any adjacent instability exists. This may be difficult to evaluate in the pediatric spine because pseudosubluxation of C2 on C3 or C3 on C4 may be normal in children less than 8 years old. Advanced imaging can provide additional information. MRI (including dynamic flexion-extension MRI) can evaluate the SAC and assess for the presence of intraspinal abnormalities, such as tethered spinal cord and syringomyelia. In addition, because of the numerous nonspinal abnormalities present in KFS, thorough examination of the patient is warranted, including

Table 6-2 Common Abnormalities Associated with Klippel-Feil Syndrome

Anomaly	Percentage of Patients
Congenital scoliosis	>50
Rib abnormalities*	33
Deafness	30
Genitourinary abnormalities	25-35
Sprengel deformity	20-30
Synkinesia	15-20
Cervical ribs	12-15
Cardiovascular abnormalities	4-29

*Excluding cervical ribs.

From Tracy MR, Dormans JP, Kusumi K: Klippel-Feil syndrome: clinical features and current understanding of etiology. *Clin Orthop Relat Res* (424):183–190, 2004.

neurologic, cardiac, renal, and audiologic evaluations. Any abnormalities noted should be addressed by the concerned specialties. Although the gastrointestinal, respiratory, and integumentary systems are less frequently involved, the clinician should be prepared to perform a workup as needed.[22]

The degree of symptom severity from the fused segments can vary from asymptomatic to decreased mobility to more serious complications, including stenosis, hypermobility, and instability, which occur infrequently. Three specific patterns of cervical fusion can result in a high risk of instability[22]: fusion of C2 and C3 with occipitocervical synostosis (see Fig. 6-4), extensive fusion over several segments with occipitocervical synostosis, and two fused segments separated by a normal joint space. This condition may lead to altered biomechanics and neurologic sequelae typically during the second or third decade of life.

Periodic radiographic evaluation of the cervical spine is warranted in the child to rule out progressive instability. In a study by Pizzutillo and associates, the investigators concluded that patients at the highest risk of developing neurologic deficits were individuals with BI, iniencephaly, or hypermobility of the upper cervical spine.[23] In these patients, annual clinical and radiographic examinations are warranted. In addition, Auerbach and colleagues demonstrated that patients with KFS have smaller spinal cords when compared with age-matched controls.[24] These investigators postulated that the abnormal motion that occurs at segments adjacent to the fusions may lead to degenerative changes and ultimately to stenosis later in life. Hypermobility of the lower cervical spine did not correlate with neurologic deficits, but it did correlate with degenerative disk disease.[23]

Most patients with stable fusions do not develop cervical symptoms. Theiss and co-workers reported on the long-term follow-up of 32 patients with congenital scoliosis and KFS.[25] Seven patients developed cervical symptoms, and 2 patients required surgery at the 10-year follow-up. If symptoms do arise, treatment is indicated and may include conservative management in the form of activity modification and bracing. In patients with progressive instability and neurologic compromise, surgical stabilization with or without decompression of the affected cervical region is indicated. In the occipitocervical region, arthrodesis is accomplished through a posterior approach. Numerous techniques have been adapted from the adult literature for the pediatric population. One technique developed specifically for the pediatric patient was reported by Dormans and associates[26] (Fig. 6-8). This procedure involves a corticocancellous iliac crest graft that is positioned and secured to the occipitocervical region with wires that are passed through burr holes in the occiput. A halo ring and vest are usually added as an adjunct to the arthrodesis.

Similarly, many techniques have been described for arthrodesis of the atlantoaxial and subaxial cervical spine. In children, the favored procedures for atlantoaxial and subaxial arthrodesis involve sublaminar fixation unless the posterior elements are incompetent or the SAC is decreased. In these cases, lateral mass, transpedicular, or transarticular screw-plate fixation is an alternative.

In summary, patients with KFS display failure of segmentation of at least one level in the cervical spine. Although the exact pathogenesis of KFS remains to be elucidated, an interplay between genetic and environmental factors may cause damage to the developing embryo. The classic clinical picture of a short neck, low hairline, and decreased cervical motion is seen in 50% of patients; most patients present only with decreased range of motion and pain. Other systems may also be affected, and a general examination is warranted. Radiographs provide some information, but more sophisticated imagery such as dynamic flexion-extension MRI helps determine whether instability or stenosis with myelopathy is present. Instability is more likely to occur in patients with fusion of C2 and C3 with occipitocervical synostosis, extensive fusion over several segments with occipitocervical synostosis, and two fused segments separated by a normal joint space. Although uncommon, instability of the upper cervical spine is an indication for surgical stabilization. In addition, cervical stenosis superimposed on an intrinsically small spinal cord may lead to neurologic symptoms typically in the second to third decade. In such cases, decompression and stabilization of the spine are indicated.

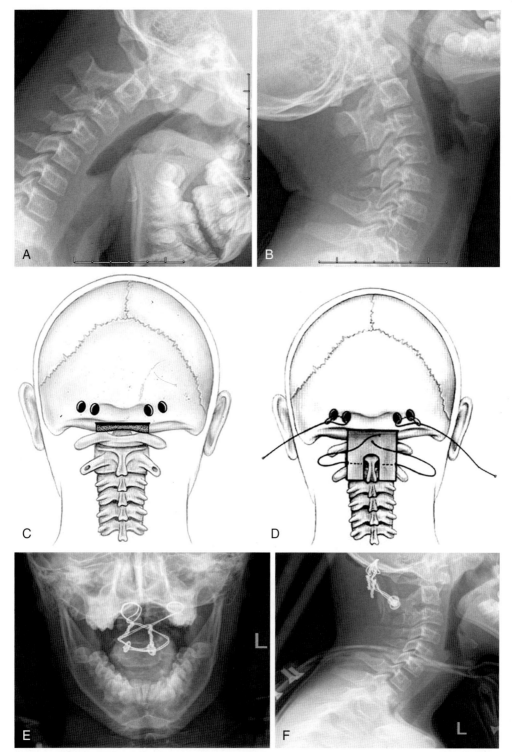

FIGURE 6-8 Flexion (**A**) and extension (**B**) radiographs of a patient with Down syndrome that demonstrate gross atlantoaxial instability. Illustrations of the authors' preferred surgical technique (**C** to **D**) for occipito-C2 arthrodesis. Postoperative radiographs, both anteroposterior (**E**) and lateral (**F**) of the same patient following occiput-C2 arthrodesis. (Courtesy John M. Flynn, MD.)

REFERENCES

1. Kaplan KM, Spivak JM, Bendo JA: Embryology of the spine and associated congenital abnormalities, *Spine J* 5:564–576, 2005.
2. Dàvid KM, Crockard A: Congenital malformations of the base of the skull, atlas, and dens. In Clarke CR, editor: *The cervical spine*, ed 4, Philadelphia, 2005, Lippincott Williams & Wilkins, pp 415–427.
3. Kabins MB: Congenital and developmental spinal stenosis. In Weinstein SL, editor: *The pediatric spine*, ed 2, Philadelphia, 2001, Lippincott Williams & Wilkins, pp 203–218.
4. Mik G, Drummond DS, Hosalkar HS, et al.: Diminished spinal cord size associated with congenital scoliosis of the thoracic spine, *J Bone Joint Surg Am* 91:1698–1704, 2009.
5. Jaskwhich D, Ali RM, Patel TC, Green DW: Congenital scoliosis, *Curr Opin Pediatr* 12:61–66, 2000.
6. Menezes AH: Craniocervical developmental anatomy and its implications, *Childs Nerv Syst* 24:1109–1122, 2008.
7. Arvin B, Fournier-Gosselin MP, Fehlings MG: Os odontoideum: etiology and surgical management, *Neurosurgery* 66(Suppl):22–31, 2010.
8. Dormans JP: Evaluation of children with suspected cervical spine injury, *J Bone Joint Surg Am* 84:124–132, 2002.
9. Hosalkar HS, Sankar WN, Wills BP, et al.: Congenital osseous anomalies of the upper cervical spine, *J Bone Joint Surg Am* 90:337–348, 2008.
10. Gholve PA, Hosalkar HS, Ricchetti ET, et al.: Occipitalization of the atlas in children: morphologic classification, associations, and clinical relevance, *J Bone Joint Surg Am* 89:571–578, 2007.
11. Pasku D, Katonis P, Karantanas A, Hadjipavlou A: Congenital posterior atlas defect associated with anterior rachischisis and early cervical degenerative disc disease: a case study and review of the literature, *Acta Orthop Belg* 73:282–285, 2007.
12. David KM, McLachlan JC, Aiton JF, et al.: Cartilaginous development of the human craniovertebral junction as visualised by a new three-dimensional computer reconstruction technique, *J Anat* 192:269–277, 1998.
13. Menezes AH, Fenoy KA: Remnants of occipital vertebrae: proatlas segmentation abnormalities, *Neurosurgery* 64:945–953, 2009. discussion 954.
14. Smith JS, Shaffrey CI, Abel MF, Menezes AH: Basilar invagination, *Neurosurgery* 66(Suppl):39–47, 2010.
15. Goel A, Bhatjiwale M, Desai K: Basilar invagination: a study based on 190 surgically treated patients, *J Neurosurg* 88:962–968, 1998.
16. Hadley MN: Os odontoideum, *Neurosurgery* 50(Suppl):S148–S155, 2002.
17. Morgan MK, Onofrio BM, Bender CE: Familial os odontoideum: case report, *J Neurosurg* 70:636–639, 1989.
18. Kirlew KA, Hathout GM, Reiter SD, Gold RH: Os odontoideum in identical twins: perspectives on etiology, *Skeletal Radiol* 22:525–527, 1993.
19. Amling M, Posl M, Wening VJ, et al.: Structural heterogeneity within the axis: the main cause in the etiology of dens fractures. A histomorphometric analysis of 37 normal and osteoporotic autopsy cases, *J Neurosurg* 83:330–335, 1995.
20. Ogden JA, Murphy MJ, Southwick WO, Ogden DA: Radiology of postnatal skeletal development. XIII. C1-C2 interrelationships, *Skeletal Radiol* 15:433–438, 1986.
21. Klippel M, Feil A: The classic: a case of absence of cervical vertebrae with the thoracic cage rising to the base of the cranium (cervical thoracic cage), *Clin Orthop Relat Res* (109)3–8, 1975.
22. Tracy MR, Dormans JP, Kusumi K: Klippel-Feil syndrome: clinical features and current understanding of etiology, *Clin Orthop Relat Res* (424)183–190, 2004.
23. Pizzutillo PD, Woods M, Nicholson L, MacEwen GD: Risk factors in Klippel-Feil syndrome, *Spine (Phila Pa 1976)* 19:2110–2116, 1994.
24. Auerbach JD, Hosalkar HS, Kusuma SK, et al.: Spinal cord dimensions in children with Klippel-Feil syndrome: a controlled, blinded radiographic analysis with implications for neurologic outcomes, *Spine (Phila Pa 1976)* 33:1366–1371, 2008.
25. Theiss SM, Smith MD, Winter RB: The long-term follow-up of patients with Klippel-Feil syndrome and congenital scoliosis, *Spine (Phila Pa 1976)* 22:1219–1222, 1997.
26. Dormans JP, Drummond DS, Sutton LN, et al.: Occipitocervical arthrodesis in children: a new technique and analysis of results, *J Bone Joint Surg Am* 77:1234–1240, 1995.

7

Biomechanics of the Cervical Spine

Fernando Techy and Edward C. Benzel

CHAPTER PREVIEW

Chapter Synopsis   The determination of spine stability is a controversial topic and continues to evolve. Understanding the anatomy and the biomechanical principles is fundamental to the performance of successful cervical spine surgery. The clinician must possess broad knowledge of the properties and characteristics of the implants available in spine reconstructions. The goals of this chapter are to introduce the basic biomechanical principles of the intact and diseased cervical spine, to define the most accurate parameters regarding the definition of spine stability, and to assist in crafting the optimal strategy for management of the unstable spine.

Important Points   Radiographic instability of the occipitoatlantal junction should be considered when the patient has more than 2 mm of translation or 5 degrees of rotation between the occiput and C1.

Radiographic instability is seen between C1 and C2 when the atlantodens interval (ADI) is greater than 3 mm in adults and 5 mm in children.

An ADI greater than 5 mm indicates that the transverse ligament is ruptured.

An ADI greater than 9 mm indicates that both the transverse and alar ligaments are incompetent. More than 50% of rotation between C1 and C2 is also considered a radiographic sign of instability.

Subaxial spine injuries with greater than 3.3 mm of displacement at the disk level or greater than 3.8 degrees of rotation are considered unstable.

Subaxial spine injuries with increased angulation greater than 30 degrees are considered unstable.

Resection of more than 50% of bilateral cervical facets results in instability.

Adding a dorsal tension band wire to the transarticular C1-C2 construct biomechanically increases flexion-extension stability.

Minimal complications and high fusion rates have been reported when using intralaminar screws for constructs at C2 and C7.

Unplated grafts are loaded in flexion and unloaded in extension.

The addition of an anterior cervical plate acts as a tension band and results in reversal of spinal biomechanics with graft loading in neck extension and unloading in flexion.

The determination of spine stability and instability is a challenge. It depends on the definition of the anatomic elements involved and the determination of the extent to which they are injured. The study of the biomechanics of the spine encompasses many controversial topics and continues to evolve. The goals of this chapter are to introduce the basic biomechanical principles of the intact and diseased cervical spine, to define the most accurate parameters regarding the definition of spine stability, and, through biomechanical scientific evidence, to assist treating physicians in crafting the optimal strategy for management of the unstable spine.

Spine Biomechanics

More important than biomechanical instability itself is the definition of clinical instability. In their classic biomechanical textbook, White and Panjabi introduced the most widely accepted definition of clinical spine instability: "Clinical instability is the loss of the ability of the spine, under physiologic loads to maintain relationships between vertebrae in such a way that there is neither initial or subsequent damage to the spinal cord or nerve roots, and in addition, there is neither development of incapacitating deformity nor severe pain."[1] Spine instability may be caused by trauma leading to bony or ligamentous injury, by infection, by tumor, or by iatrogenic resection of the spinal elements. Multiple in vitro and in vivo studies have been performed with the goal of defining the stability of the spine segment in question, and the results of these studies aid in treatment decisions.

Upper Cervical Spine Stability: Principles and Biomechanical Evidence

Unique bone and ligamentous anatomica features form the elements responsible for the stability of the upper cervical spine. Heller and colleagues tested the isolated biomechanical properties of the transverse ligament of C1 by simulating an anteroposterior shear injury mechanism.[2] Eleven specimens failed in the midsubstance of the ligament, and 2 failed by bony avulsion. The mean load to failure was 692 N (range, 220 to 1590 N), and the mean displacement to failure was 6.7 mm (2 to 14 mm). These investigators concluded that anteroposterior translation of the C1 transverse ligament in relation to the C2 dens is essential for its fracture, and the rate of loading affects the type of injury (the greater the rate, the more probable it is a ligamentous injury, as opposed to a fracture). When the transverse ligament-dens complex fails, either by midsubstance tear or by dens fracture, the greatest increase in instability is in flexion and extension (42% or 22 degrees), followed by lateral bending (24% or 8 degrees), and least in axial rotation (5% or 5 degrees).[3]

The alar ligaments have been extensively studied, and although the involved mechanics is more complex, the alar ligaments have been shown mainly to limit axial rotation. Their transection increases contralateral axial rotation by approximately 15%; as in the transverse ligament, alar ligament rupture is rate dependent. In one report, these ligaments failed at 13.6 Nm at 4 degrees per second and at 27.9 Nm at 100 degrees per second.[4] Radiographically, occipitoatlantal instability should be considered when the patient has more than 2 mm of translation or 5 degrees of rotation between the occiput and C1. Significant variability exists from patient to patient, and patients with rheumatoid arthritis perhaps should be assessed by more lenient parameters. Radiographic instability is seen between C1 and C2 when the atlantodens interval (ADI) is greater than 3 mm in adults and 5 mm in children. When the ADI is greater than 5 mm, the transverse ligament is considered ruptured, and when the ADI is greater than 9 mm, both the transverse and alar ligaments are deemed incompetent. More than 50% of rotation between C1 and C2 is also considered a radiographic sign of instability.[5]

Subaxial Cervical Spine Stability: Principles and Biomechanical Evidence

For many years, multiple clinical and biomechanical studies have been performed to understand the factors responsible for subaxial cervical spine stability. In 1978, Panjabi and associates axially loaded cadaveric cervical spines in increments of 5 kg until failure of the specimens.[6] Ventral and dorsal soft tissue injuries were created. Ventral injuries with greater than 3.3 mm displacement at the disk level or greater than 3.8 degrees of rotation were considered unstable. Similarly, dorsal injuries resulting in 27 mm of interspinous space widening or an increase in angulation greater than 30 degrees with the axial loading were considered unstable.

The laminae and spinous processes serve as insertion points for such important dorsal stabilizers as the supraspinous and interspinous ligaments and the ligamentum flavum. Clinical studies showed that resection of these elements causes cervical spine instability in children and adults.[7,8] In a cadaveric study, Goel and co-workers reported a 10% increase in the flexion-extension motion after multilevel cervical spine laminectomy.[9] In another in vitro study, no instability was observed after multilevel laminoplasty, whereas a significant increase in motion in all planes was observed after multilevel laminectomy with 25% bilateral facetectomy.[10]

In a clinical series, instrumentation was not performed after multilevel cervical laminectomy for resection of intramedullary tumors. The investigators wanted to avoid implant-related imaging interference on postoperative magnetic resonance imaging, to accurately monitor progression of disease more accurately. Cervical deformity developed in 52% of patients and cervical instability in 36%. Sixteen percent had moderate to severe disabling neck pain. Laminectomy of C2 was associated with cervical instability ($P = 0.02$). Old age at the time of surgery correlated with cervical deformity ($P = 0.05$), and multiple surgical procedures were associated with greater disability related to neck pain ($P = 0.01$). The investigators ultimately concluded that only 12% of patients will develop clinical instability, and all will need postoperative magnetic resonance imaging. These investigators recommended that stabilization should be performed only in patients who develop instability.[7]

The cervical facet joint and its capsule provide significant contribution to the stability of the cervical spine. In cadaveric studies, Zdeblick and associates showed that resection of more than 50% of bilateral cervical facets,[11] or more than 50% of the bilateral cervical facet joint capsule,[12] results in instability. In a finite element modeling (FEM) study, Voo and colleagues confirmed that instability, indeed, begins to develop after resection of more than 50% of both joints at the same level.[13] An evaluation of unilateral facetectomy showed that even resection of 75% or 100% of one facet joint was more stable than resection of 50% of both joints, in flexion and extension. Unilateral complete cervical facetectomy and 75% facet resection were more unstable than bilateral 50% facet resection in lateral bending and axial rotation. Unilateral 50% facetectomy was more stable than bilateral 50% facetectomy in all planes of range of motion. A cadaveric study assessed bilateral and unilateral complete cervical facetectomy. Furthermore, Cuisick and co-workers found that bilateral facetectomy reduced the stability of the joint in 53% of specimens and that unilateral facetectomy resulted in stability reduction of 32%.[14]

Even though ventral diskectomy without fusion was performed for many years, ultimately it was determined that the anterior elements also play a role in spine stability. Therefore, fusing the segment after complete anterior diskectomy became the gold standard of treatment. After C5-C6 diskectomy, Shulte and associates noticed an increase in the range of motion between segments (66% in flexion, 69% in extension, 41% for lateral bending, and 40% for axial rotation).[15]

Biomechanics of Cervical Spine Instrumentation

Dens Screw Fixation

Odontoid fixation of a dens fracture was first described in the early 1980s.[16,17] Initially, the use of two screws was advocated, with the theoretical advantage of increased stability and rotation resistance properties. However, because of the difficulty of placing two screws in such a small space and the findings of subsequent studies that showed no difference in biomechanical stability or fusion rate when using one or two screws,[18] the current standard of practice is to use one screw only for the fixation of dens fractures.

Dorsal C1 and C2 Instrumentation

Initially, dorsal fixation of C1 and C2 was accomplished with dorsal wiring techniques.[19-22] More rigid modern constructs improved biomechanical stability and have achieved fusion rates that approach 100%. Biomechanically, transarticular C1-C2 screws using the Magerl technique have shown a 10-fold increased rotational stiffness over dorsal wiring techniques, with similar lateral bending stiffness.[19,22] C1 lateral mass and C2 pars constructs have been shown to have superior biomechanical stability characteristics in lateral bending and axial rotation when compared with dorsal wiring techniques. This same study also found no difference in stability between C1 lateral mass and C2 pars fixation when using the technique popularized by Harms and Magerl transarticular screws.[21] Adding a dorsal tension band (wires) to the transarticular C1-C2 construct has been shown to increase flexion-extension stability biomechanically,[20] thus making this combination construct a popular choice among clinicians when transarticular screws are used.

Dorsal Instrumentation of the Subaxial Cervical Spine

Wire constructs for stabilizing the subaxial cervical spine have been used for many years. In a biomechanical study, Cuisick and colleagues showed that either facet-lamina wiring or interfacet wiring can partially restore (20% of the intact joint strength) the stability of unilateral or bilateral complete facet joint resection.[14] Currently, one of the most popular techniques among spine surgeons for dorsal cervical instrumentation is the use of lateral mass screws. This relatively simple technique has a low complication rate and is associated with excellent results overall. Biomechanically, the fixation strength of lateral mass screws is strongest at C4, and it becomes progressively weaker toward either end of the cervical spine (C2 and C7).[23] In addition, bone quality has been consistently shown to be worse at the lateral mass of C7 when compared with the other cervical levels.[23] The lateral mass fixation at C2 and C7 is often hindered by lack of high-quality or sizable bone mass. At these two levels, other fixation techniques are usually used. Biomechanically, pedicle screws are superior to lateral mass fixation in any level of the cervical spine. Pedicle screws have demonstrated a significantly lower rate of loosening at the bone-screw interface, greater strength after fatigue testing, and greater pull-out strength when compared with lateral mass screws.[24] Their placement is, however, technically demanding and not free of complications. Cervical pedicle screw insertion has been considered too risky and maybe unnecessary, except at the C2 and C7 levels.

Intralaminar Screw Fixation for the Upper and Lower Cervical Spine

The use of intralaminar (also known as translaminar) screws for the fixation of C2, C7, T1, and T2 has become increasingly popular. Minimal complications and high fusion rates have been reported when using intralaminar screws for constructs at C2 and C7.[25] Intralaminar screws from C3 to C6 are not recommended because the laminar thickness of these segments is usually less than 3.0 mm, too small to accept a 3.5- or 4.0-mm screw safely.[26] C2 intralaminar screw fixation has been shown to be biomechanically equivalent to more traditional C2 screw fixation techniques while decreasing the risk of the vertebral artery injury[27,28] (Fig. 7-1). Moreover, this type of intralaminar screw fixation has also been used as an alternative technique for patients with intact dorsal elements who require fixation in the upper thoracic spine and C7 vertebra, where pedicle screw insertion is possible but not risk free, and the lateral mass bone quality and size are not optimal.[29,30]

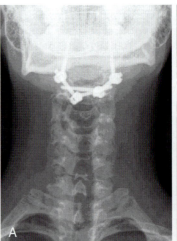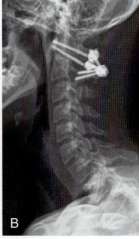

FIGURE 7-1 This 22-year-old man had a painful C2 odontoid nonunion after a fracture managed in a collar. He was then treated with C1-C2 fusion with posterior instrumentation, after which the neck pain resolved. Anteroposterior (**A**) and lateral (**B**) plain radiographs illustrate the C1 lateral mass with C2 intralaminar screw fixation. The C2 intralaminar fixation provides strength equivalent to that obtained by other screw fixation techniques at C2. It also obviates the risk of injury to the nerve root, vertebral artery, or sympathetic ganglia. (Case courtesy Gordon Bell, MD, Center for Spine Health, Cleveland Clinic, Cleveland, Ohio.)

Biomechanically, intralaminar screws in T1 and T2 were only slightly less stable than pedicle screws in long cervicothoracic constructs in one report (in the cervical portion, lateral mass screws from C4 to C6 were used).[31]

Anterior Instrumentation of the Cervical Spine

The fusion rate after anterior cervical diskectomy and fusion (ACDF) increased once surgeons began using rigid plates to enhance stability. Excessive motion is known to impede fusion, but the absolute elimination of motion can retard bone growth (stress shielding).[32,33] Rigid plate fixation for ACDF provides a clear advantage in terms of stability augmentation and improved fusion rates.[34,35] However, it is also associated with a biomechanical drawback regarding the reduction of load sharing through the bone graft. Therefore, a reduction of the stresses applied to bone and the resultant elimination of micromotion at the graft–end plate interface have an adverse effect on bone healing.

The more rigid the plate, the greater is the unloading effect on the bone graft. In a cadaveric C5 corpectomy study, rigid plates bore 23% of the load, as opposed to 9% in dynamic plates. The difference was statistically significant.[33] Other biomechanical studies demonstrated that rigid plates bear even more load when the graft initially subsides; thus, they theoretically function as distraction devices that can further interfere with the fusion.[32,33] To address concerns related to excessive plate stability and the stress shielding of bone healing, dynamic plates were developed. When considering their use, one must weigh all the aforementioned theory and information. Currently, investigators have determined that more stability than simply graft insertion is optimal for spinal fusion in ACDF, and absolute stability may cause stress shielding and interfere with bone healing because of a lack of bone formation stimulated by micromotion. The optimal stability for fusion to occur lies somewhere in between these parameters.

The reconstruction of multilevel corpectomies is biomechanically much more complex than is plate fixation for ACDF. Stand-alone anterior plating for the stabilization of long strut-graft constructs has been associated with unfavorable biomechanics. Many clinical series reported high complication rates of graft dislodgement and construct failure.[36,37]

One study showed that, under fatigue loading (1000 cycles), three-level corpectomy constructs significantly lose their initial stability, whereas one-level constructs remain stable.[38] DiAngelo and co-workers demonstrated that the addition of a rigid plate to a multilevel corpectomy reconstructed with a long strut graft may paradoxically reverse load transfer through the graft.[39] Normally, the unplated graft would be loaded in flexion and unloaded in neck extension. The plate acts as a tension band placed ventral to the spine. The graft then becomes loaded during neck extension and unloaded in flexion. The forces created within this construct can be sufficient to overcome the strength of the end plates and may lead to its failure. Therefore, when multilevel corpectomies are reconstructed, strong consideration

should be given to supplemental dorsal fixation or to a more stable, hybrid corpectomy-ACDF construct, if possible (Fig. 7-2).

An anterior cervical plate functions as an anterior cantilever fixation device. A cantilever is a beam supported on only one end, similar to a flagpole bolted to a wall or, in the case of spine instrumentation, a screw connected to a plate. Fixed moment arm cantilever beam constructs are those in which the screws are rigidly secured to the plate, thus not permitting toggling of the screws. Hence, no screw toggling occurs, to accommodate subsidence. These are the most stable of constructs. Therefore, they are the most prone to complications associated with attempts at achieving excessive stability (i.e., stress shielding).[32,33]

Nonfixed moment arm cantilever beam systems are those in which the screws are not locked into the plate. Screw toggling can take place and accommodates subsidence to a moderate degree. These constructs are not as rigid as the fixed variant. True dynamic implants permit axial implant subsidence. Mechanisms include implant shortening and slotted holes for screws.

All cervical implants, and in fact all implants in general, exhibit varying responses to different loading conditions. Under axial loading, ventral implants resist compression and, as such, act as distraction devices (as do interbody spacers) (Fig. 7-3, *A*). If an extension moment is applied to the spine, an anterior implant resists segmental extension and thus functions as a compression device (tension band principle) (Fig. 7-3, *B*). The same happens to dorsal implants with neck flexion.

An implant can resist three-point bending forces, without an intervening fixation anchor (e.g., screw), if the spine comes in contact with the longitudinal member (e.g., plate) (Fig 7-3, *C*). Anterior plates are extremely effective in resisting axial loads and spine extension. They are not as effective in controlling flexion. Supplemental dorsal fixation may be needed to preserve stability, especially with highly unstable long anterior constructs.[40]

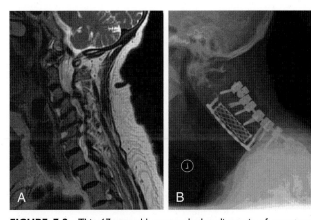

FIGURE 7-2 This 67-year-old woman had a diagnosis of symptomatic progressive cervical myelopathy secondary to fixed cervical deformity and multilevel stenosis. Posterior fixation should be strongly considered in such patients to supplement multilevel anterior corpectomy reconstructions. Preoperative magnetic resonance imaging (**A**) and postoperative plain radiographs (**B**) of this patient with multilevel stenosis. (Case courtesy Richard Lim, MD, Advocate Christ Medical Center. Oak Lawn, Ill.)

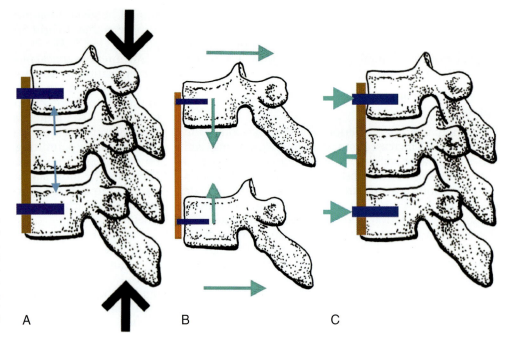

FIGURE 7-3   A, Like an interbody spacer, an anterior plate and screw system functions as a distraction device during the application of axial loads. **B,** With an anterior plate, cervical spine extension results in compression of an interbody strut. **C,** An anterior implant can resist three-point fixation forces if the midportion of the implant contacts bone.

A   B   C

Conclusions

Understanding the anatomy and the biomechanical principles associated with spine instability and spine stabilization is fundamental to the performance of successful cervical spine surgery. The clinician must possess broad knowledge of the properties and characteristics of the implants available in spine reconstructions. Construct failure rarely results from intrinsic implant failure. The surgeon's inability to understand the relevant biomechanical concepts is the most common cause of suboptimal surgical technique and outcomes.

REFERENCES

1. White AA, Panjabi MM: *Clinical biomechanics of the spine,* ed 2, Philadelphia, 1990, Lippincott.
2. Heller JG, Amrani J, Hutton WC: Transverse ligament failure: a biomechanical study, *J Spinal Disord* 6:162–165, 1993.
3. Oda T, Panjabi MM, Crisco JJ 3rd, Oxland TR: Multidirectional instabilities of experimental burst fractures of the atlas, *Spine (Phila Pa 1976)* 17:1285–1290, 1992.
4. Panjabi MM, Yue JJ, Dvorak J, et al.: Cervical spine kinematics and clinical instability. In Clark CR, editor: *The cervical spine,* ed 4, Philadelphia, 2005, Lippincott Williams & Wilkins.
5. Maak TG, Grauer JN: The contemporary treatment of odontoid injuries, *Spine (Phila Pa 1976)* 31(Suppl):S53–S60, 2006.
6. Panjabi MM, White AA, Keller D, et al.: Stability of the cervical spine under tension, *J Biomech* 11:189–197, 1978.
7. Asthagiri AR, Mehta GU, Butman JA, et al.: Long-term stability after multilevel cervical laminectomy for spinal cord tumor resection in von Hippel-Lindau disease, *J Neurosurg Spine* 14:444–452, 2011.
8. Bell DF, Walker JL, O'Connor G, Tibshirani R: Spinal deformity after multilevel cervical laminectomy in children, *Spine (Phila Pa 1976)* 19:406–411, 1994.
9. Goel VK, Clark CR, Harris KG, et al.: Kinematics of the cervical spine: effects of multiple total laminectomy and facet wiring, *J Orthop Res* 6:611–619, 1988.
10. Nowinski GP, Visarius H, Nolte LP, et al.: A biomechanical comparison of cervical laminaplasty and cervical laminectomy with progressive facetectomy, *Spine (Phila Pa 1976)* 18:1995–2004, 1993.
11. Zdeblick TA, Abitbol JJ, Kunz DN: Cervical stability after sequential capsule resection, *Spine (Phila Pa 1976)* 18:2005–2008, 1993.
12. Zdeblick TA, Zou D, Warden KE, et al.: Cervical stability after foraminotomy: a biomechanical in vitro analysis, *J Bone Joint Surg Am* 74:22–27, 1992.
13. Voo LM, Kumaresan S, Yoganandan N, et al.: Finite element analysis of cervical facetectomy, *Spine (Phila Pa 1976)* 22:964–969, 1997.
14. Cuisick JF, Yoganandan N, Pintar F, et al.: Biomechanics of cervical spine facetectomy and fixation techniques, *Spine (Phila Pa 1976)* 13:808–812, 1988.
15. Schulte KR, Clark CR, Goel VK: Kinematics of the cervical spine following discectomy and stabilization, *Spine (Phila Pa 1976)* 14:1116–1121, 1989.
16. Bohler J: Anterior stabilization for acute fractures and nonunions of the dens, *J Bone Joint Surg Am* 64:18–27, 1982.
17. Nakanishi T: Internal fixation of the odontoid fracture, *J Orthop Trauma Surg* 23:399–406, 1980.
18. Sasso R, Doherty BJ, Crawford MJ, Heggeness MH: Biomechanics of odontoid fracture fixation: comparison of the one- and two-screw technique, *Spine (Phila Pa 1976)* 18:1950–1953, 1993.
19. Grob D, Crisco JJ 3rd, Panjabi MM, et al.: Biomechanical evaluation of four different posterior atlantoaxial fixation techniques, *Spine (Phila Pa 1976)* 17:480–490, 1992.
20. Henriques T, Cunningham BW, Olerud C, et al.: Biomechanical comparison of five different atlantoaxial posterior fixation techniques, *Spine (Phila Pa 1976)* 25:2877–2883, 2000.
21. Melcher RP, Puttlitz CM, Kleinstueck FS, et al.: Biomechanical testing of posterior atlantoaxial fixation techniques, *Spine (Phila Pa 1976)* 27:2435–2440, 2002.
22. Montesano PX, Juach EC, Anderson PA, et al.: Biomechanics of cervical spine internal fixation, *Spine (Phila Pa 1976)* 16(Suppl):S10–S16, 1991.
23. Heller JG, Estes BT, Zaouali M, Diop A: Biomechanical study of screws in the lateral masses: variables affecting pull-out resistance, *J Bone Joint Surg Am* 78:1315–1321, 1996.
24. Johnston TL, Karaikovic EE, Lautenschlager EP, Marcu D: Cervical pedicle screws vs. lateral mass screws: uniplanar fatigue analysis and residual pullout strengths, *Spine J* 6:667–672, 2006.
25. Hong JT, Yi JS, Kim JT, et al.: Clinical and radiologic outcome of laminar screw at C2 and C7 for posterior instrumentation: review of 25 cases and comparison of C2 and C7 intralaminar screw fixation, *Surg Neurol* 73:112–118, 2010.

26. Nakanishi K, Tanaka M, Sugimoto Y, et al.: Application of laminar screws to posterior fusion of cervical spine: measurement of the cervical vertebral arch diameter with a navigation system, *Spine (Phila Pa 1976)* 33:620–623, 2008.
27. Cassinelli E H, Lee M, Skalak A, et al.: Anatomic considerations for the placement of C2 laminar screws, *Spine (Phila Pa 1976)* 31:2767–2771, 2006.
28. Gorek J, Acaroglu E, Berven S, et al.: Constructs incorporating intralaminar C2 screws provide rigid stability for atlantoaxial fixation, *Spine (Phila Pa 1976)* 30:1513–1518, 2005.
29. Kretzer R M, Sciubba D M, Bagley C A, et al.: Translaminar screw fixation in the upper thoracic spine, *J Neurosurg Spine* 5:527–533, 2006.
30. Xing-guo L, Yun H, Yan Z, et al.: Applied anatomy of the lower cervical pedicle screw insertion, *Chin J Traumatol* 10:299–305, 2007.
31. McGirt M J, Sutter E G, Xu R, et al.: Biomechanical comparison of translaminar screw versus pedicle screws at T1 and T2 in long subaxial cervical constructs, *Neurosurgery* 65:167–172, 2009.
32. Brodke D S, Gollogly S, Alexander Mohr R, et al.: Dynamic cervical plates: biomechanical evaluation of load sharing and stiffness, *Spine (Phila Pa 1976)* 26:1324–1329, 2001.
33. Reidy D, Finkelstein J, Nagpurkar A, et al.: Cervical spine loading characteristics in a cadaveric C5 corpectomy model using a static and dynamic plate, *J Spinal Disord Tech* 17:117–122, 2004.
34. Kaiser M G, Haid RW Jr, Subach B R, et al.: Anterior cervical plating enhances arthrodesis after discectomy and fusion with cortical allograft, *Neurosurgery* 50:229–236, 2002. discussion 236–238.
35. Xie JC, Hurlbert R J: Discectomy versus discectomy with fusion versus discectomy with fusion and instrumentation: a prospective randomized study, *Neurosurgery* 61:107–116, 2007. discussion 116–117.
36. Riew K D, Sethi N S, Devney J, et al.: Complications of buttress plate stabilization of cervical corpectomy, *Spine (Phila Pa 1976)* 24:2404–2410, 1999.
37. Vaccaro A R, Falatyn S P, Scuderi GJ, et al.: Early failure of long segment anterior cervical plate fixation, *J Spinal Disord* 11:410–415, 1998.
38. Isomi T, Panjabi M M, Wang J L, et al.: Stabilizing potential of anterior cervical plates in multilevel corpectomies, *Spine (Phila Pa 1976)* 24:2219–2223, 1999.
39. DiAngelo DJ, Foley KT, Vossel K A, et al.: Anterior cervical plating reverses load transfer through multilevel strut grafts, *Spine (Phila Pa 1976)* 25:783–795, 2000.
40. Benzel E: *Ventral subaxial spine constructs in biomechanics of spine stabilization*, New York, 2001, Thieme. pp 239–253.

8 Evaluation of the Cervical Spine

Christopher K. Kepler and D. Greg Anderson

CHAPTER PREVIEW

Chapter Synopsis   This chapter describes a methodical approach to the patient with suspected cervical spine disease. Characteristic aspects of the history and physical examination are discussed and warning flags for musculoskeletal and neurologic diseases which mimic spinal disease are discussed. Relevant diagnostic tests are described. The chapter concludes with a brief discussion of disability and workers' compensation assessments and how these evaluations differ from a standard patient evaluation.

Important Points   Careful selection of patients is critical and relies heavily on the history and physical examination.

Developing a knowledge of the characteristic natural history and symptomatology of myelopathy, radiculopathy, and axial neck pain is important as these clinical entities have some shared features.

Different types of musculoskeletal, psychiatric, and neurologic disease states can mimic cervical spine disease and must be distinguished by clinical history and physical examination.

Electrodiagnostic testing may help make or confirm the diagnoses and are a valuable adjunct to clinical judgment.

Achieving a successful outcome after spinal surgery relies as heavily on careful selection of appropriate operative indications as it does on the technical aspects of the operative procedure. Degenerative changes within the spine are ubiquitous in asymptomatic individuals.[1] Therefore, the history and physical examination make up the key components of establishing a diagnosis. Imaging studies are confirmatory but can be interpreted only in light of knowledge gained from a careful history and physical examination.

Interpreting a patient's symptoms and establishing a diagnosis are skills that can be honed with knowledge of the natural history of common and uncommon disease entities and a careful physical examination. Fortunately, diseases of the cervical spine generally manifest with reproducible physical findings that offer substantial clues to the underlying diagnosis. Imaging modalities and laboratory tests provide useful confirmatory data to substantiate and quantify the clinical impression gained from the history and physical examination.

History

The diagnostic process begins with the taking of a thorough medical history. The history of the condition, as obtained from the patient, is the most important portion of the diagnostic process. It is not possible to evaluate findings on the physical examination or imaging studies accurately without knowledge gained from the history. Thus, this portion of the workup should come first in sequence and should provide early clinical impressions about the probable diagnosis. These impressions are then confirmed or refuted, based on the physical examination, imaging studies, and any other ancillary medical tests. During the history, the physician must understand the presenting symptoms in terms of location, character, onset, severity, exacerbating and alleviating factors, neurologic deficits, prior treatments and their effects, and the course of the symptoms since onset. The physician must also understand the medical history of the patient including health, medications, prior surgical interventions, habits, and family history.

Natural History of Common Cervical Conditions

When formulating a diagnostic impression, the physician must understand the natural history of common cervical conditions. Cervical radiculopathy generally manifests with pain along a dermatomal distribution as the primary symptom and may be associated with sensory or motor complaints related to the involved nerve root. Patients commonly complain of associated sharp parascapular pain. The onset of cervical radiculopathy may be insidious or acute. It may be associated with a particular inciting event, or the disorder may manifest with an acute-on-chronic history of rapid worsening of symptoms that were already present in a less severe form. Although the symptoms may regress spontaneously, they have the potential to erupt again in an unpredictable fashion. Cervical radiculopathy is relatively common and is the most frequent indication for cervical spinal surgery.

Myelopathy, conversely, typically manifests with a slowly progressive process that may be subtle enough initially that the patient may not be aware of early neurologic deficits or may believe that the symptoms are simply part of aging. Common complaints include a loss of fine dexterity in hand function (inability to fasten buttons), nondermatomal finger numbness, changes in balance, urgency with bladder control, and increasing muscle atrophy (particularly involving the hand intrinsics).[2] Myelopathy may be painless or may be associated with symptoms of neck or arm pain, depending on the specific neural tissues involved. As the disease progresses, the neurologic symptoms generally worsen, although this occurs classically in a slow, stepwise fashion with long periods of stability between changes in neurologic functioning.[3] Rarely, a patient may have a more rapid neurologic decline, particularly in the setting of trauma.

Axial neck pain is relatively common, although the severity of the condition varies widely. In most cases, the symptoms are self-limited.[4] The symptoms are usually described as having a deep, aching character and are located along the posterior neck. The pain may be described as radiating across the shoulders (along the trapezius muscle distribution) or to the posterior occipital region (where it may be associated with occipital region headaches). The symptoms often wax and wane in severity and may be aggravated by repetitive function, prolonged positions, or an awkward sleeping position.

Symptoms

Radiculopathy usually manifests with classic, well-defined symptoms of nerve root irritation secondary to compression in the neural foramen (Table 8-1). Arm pain is the classic symptom and is generally more severe than neck pain (which may or may not be an associated symptom). Patients often note that the pain is worse with neck flexion, extension, or rotation. They may report relief

when abducting the ipsilateral arm and placing their hand behind their head (shoulder abduction relief sign). Although nerve roots have stereotypic patterns of associated motor, sensory, and reflex functions, the examiner must keep in mind that overlap between adjacent root distributions is common. Although pain is usually the predominant symptom, discrete neurologic symptoms may be noted. In some cases, the pain may subside, leaving the affected individual with residual persistent numbness or weakness, or both. The surgeon should be aware of the possibility of a less classic presentation of radicular pain such as isolated parascapular pain or atypical chest pain. For patients presenting with atypical symptoms, the physician must be careful to characterize the symptoms fully, to rule out potential disease in an alternative organ system (e.g., cardiac angina).

Myelopathy has a wide variety of presenting symptoms and is classically associated with hand or finger numbness, increasing clumsiness or difficulty holding objects with one or both hands, and a shuffling and unsteady gait. Patients may complain of difficulty walking at night when they have fewer visual clues or may note problems navigating uneven terrain. Generally, the changes in coordination and weakness are symmetric, although this is not always the case. Patients may also complain of aching pain in the neck and upper back or radicular pain radiating to the arms. Myeloradiculopathy is relatively common and may have the clinical features of both conditions. Although complete bladder or bowel incontinence is rare, more subtle symptoms of urgency are seen more commonly.

Axial neck pain, by definition, consists of pain without associated pain down the extremity or neurologic findings. The pain is usually described as deep seated, along the posterior aspect of the neck and upper shoulders. Patients with axial neck symptoms may complain of associated posterior headaches or constitutional symptoms. The physician must distinguish axial neck pain from radicular pain related to the upper cervical radiculopathy, which is less likely to have a waxing-waning course and is generally localized to one side. Additionally, radicular pain is generally affected by maneuvers that narrow or widen the neural foramina.

Warning Signs of Mimetics of Cervical Spine Disorders

Because many nonspinal sources of pain and disability can have a presentation similar to that of cervical spine disease, the spinal surgeon must always be attentive for features of the patient's history that suggest an alternative diagnosis. Other musculoskeletal disorders that can masquerade as cervical spine disease include shoulder disorders, especially rotator cuff disease, which may manifest with shoulder pain radiating to the upper arm and is not relieved by shoulder elevation. Suprascapular nerve entrapment can cause aching shoulder or periscapular pain that may be noted on physical examination to be associated with atrophy of either the supraspinatus or infraspinatus muscles and confirmed by electromyography (EMG). Peripheral nerve entrapment commonly creates sensory deficits (with or without associated pain) that may be similar in distribution to patterns of

Table 8-1 Stereotypic Nerve Root Functions			
Nerve Root	**Sensory Distribution**	**Motor Distribution**	**Skeletal Reflex**
C5	Lateral arm	Deltoid, biceps	Biceps
C6	Thumb and index finger	Biceps, wrist extensors	Brachioradialis
C7	Middle finger	Triceps, wrist flexors	Triceps
C8	Small finger	Hand intrinsics	None

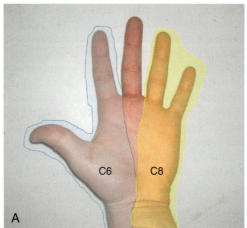
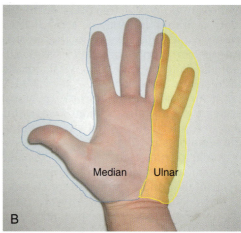

FIGURE 8-1 Photograph demonstrating the distributions of C6 and C8 (**A**) and the median and ulnar nerves (**B**), compression of which can easily be confused for nerve root level compression.

radiculopathy. In particular, carpal tunnel syndrome (similar to C6 radiculopathy) and cubital tunnel syndrome (C8 radiculopathy) should be considered and ruled out when patterns of sensory disturbance suggest their inclusion in the differential diagnosis (Fig. 8-1). Again, EMG can be helpful in excluding these conditions.

The presenting complaints and symptoms of fibromyalgia overlap with those of cervical spine disease, but several notable differences may be identified to distinguish between these two entities. Whereas diffuse pain around the shoulder girdle and neck is common in fibromyalgia, this generalized condition also commonly involves pain in the lower back, buttocks, and lower limbs (Fig. 8-2). Additionally, nearly all patients with fibromyalgia have some degree of sleep disturbance and complain of chronic fatigue or tiredness, symptoms that are not common in the presentation of cervical spine disorders.[5]

Thoracic outlet syndrome is rare but manifests with symptoms that mimic radiculopathy, most commonly in the C8 distribution. In contrast to cervical spine disease, the pain in thoracic outlet syndrome is often centered around the thoracic outlet and may be accompanied by arm swelling or discoloration that worsens with lifting or carrying heavy objects. Brachial plexopathy and Parsonage-Turner syndrome (brachial plexus neuritis) both manifest with symptoms referable to the brachial plexus and can affect the distributions of any nerve root in the brachial plexus (C5 to T1). Brachial plexopathy may be preceded by a specific traumatic event, so patients should be specifically questioned about injury to the neck or shoulders. Parsonage-Turner syndrome (acute brachial plexitis) has a characteristic presentation that typically begins with shoulder pain in the C5 distribution that is exacerbated by shoulder motion. As the pain begins to subside, the patient develops weakness involving any or all of the C5 to C8 distributions; this weakness may vary in severity by level. Although both brachial plexopathy and Parsonage-Turner syndrome are most often unilateral, Parsonage-Turner syndrome is bilateral in a third of cases.

Several neurologic diseases can be confused with cervical spine disorders. Amyotrophic lateral sclerosis (ALS) often manifests with weakness, atrophy, and loss of coordination. Distinguishing features include an absence

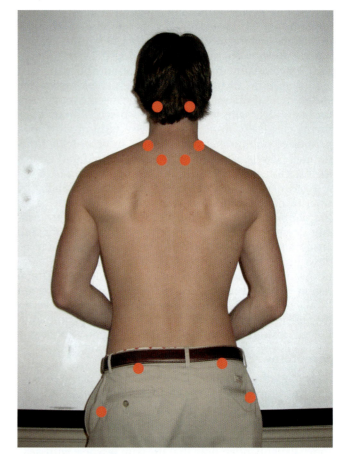

FIGURE 8-2 The *red circles* represent "trigger points" that are commonly tender in patients with fibromyalgia.

of pain or sensory changes and the presence of grossly visible muscle fasciculation (classically of the tongue). Transverse myelitis, as its name suggests, affects an entire segment of the spinal cord at once, so symptoms are bilateral. Associated neurologic deficits in transverse myelitis can be profound, progress more rapidly than in degenerative cervical conditions (ranging from several hours to several weeks), and may be preceded by back or neck pain.[6] Multiple sclerosis (MS) can manifest in a wide variety of ways, and it may have a slow or rapid

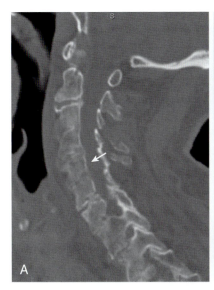
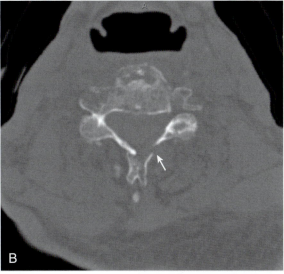

FIGURE 8-3 Sagittal (**A**) and axial (**B**) images from a computed tomography scan of a patient with ankylosing spondylitis. This patient presented with complaints of neck pain after a near fall in which he managed to grab hold of a railing, thus preventing a fall. Despite the lack of direct trauma, C5 body and lamina fractures occurred (*arrows* in **A** and **B**), and the patient developed a progressing neurologic deficit requiring decompression and fusion resulting from an expanding hematoma within the spinal canal.

clinical course. In MS, the symptoms may demonstrate a relapsing-remitting pattern. Because of the susceptibility of the entire central nervous system to MS, symptoms vary widely, and patients with MS may have seemingly unrelated symptoms such as visual abnormalities or cranial nerve findings.

For patients presenting with axial pain, the physician should consider the potential of neoplastic involvement (most commonly metastatic disease) or spinal infection in the differential diagnosis. Therefore, symptoms of fevers, chills, night sweats, weight loss, or anorexia should be sought. In addition, symptoms or night or rest pains that are worse than activity-related pain may suggest these entities. A Pancoast tumor is a type of apical lung cancer that can erode into the superior chest and causes an uncommon but stereotypic array of symptoms related to the lower brachial plexus or the sympathetic chain.

Spinal surgeons should identify previous cervical or shoulder trauma in the patient's history. Occult spinal column trauma is a particular concern with patients with a prior history of ankylosing spondylitis or diffuse idiopathic skeletal hyperostosis (DISH) because even minor trauma can result in fractures with catastrophic neurologic consequences in this population (Fig. 8-3). Patients with rheumatoid arthritis should be questioned not only about current symptoms, which often include myelopathy secondary to neural element compression from the rheumatoid pannus, but also about general disease activity and any disease-modifying agents that may result in immune suppression if surgery is planned.

Physical Examination

General Examination

The physical examination begins before any contact with the patient, by observing the positioning of the neck and the patient's active range of cervical motion and inquiring whether any particular position acutely exacerbates symptoms.[7] The Spurling' maneuver is performed by gently extending and rotating the patient's head to the painful side

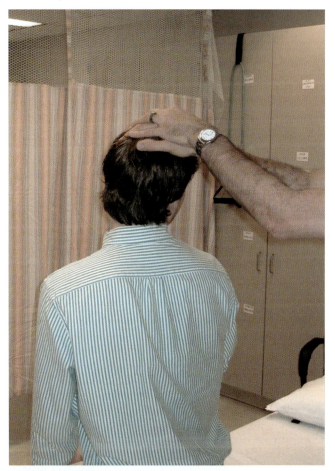

FIGURE 8-4 Photograph demonstrating the Spurling maneuver. Axial pressure is applied with the neck in an extended position with rotation to the side of suspected nerve root compression.

while applying axial compression (Fig. 8-4). This maneuver decreases the neural foraminal area and stretches the nerve roots, thereby exacerbating any radicular symptoms. Evaluating the range of motion in the shoulders, elbows, and wrists is important for those patients with upper extremity

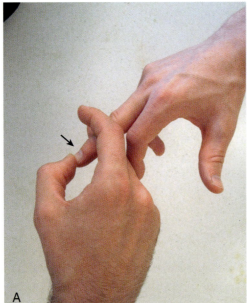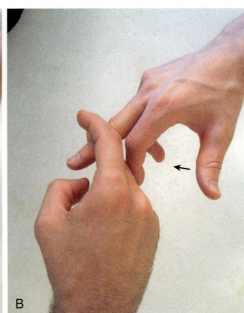

FIGURE 8-5 Photographs demonstrating the Hoffmann test. **A,** The nail of the middle finger is flicked in a dorsal-to-volar direction while the middle phalanx is stabilized. **B,** Reflexive flexion of the interphalangeal joint of the thumb suggests cervical myelopathy.

symptoms. The upper extremities should also be examined for evidence of muscle atrophy, which may suggest the distribution of a compressive peripheral or central lesion. Next, the examination should progress to palpation of the neck and periscapular muscles to elicit local tenderness, asymmetry, or muscle spasm in regions. Lymph nodes in the axilla and anterior neck should be palpated because findings may suggest disseminated cancer or regional infection. Appropriate care should be taken in the examination of patients with suspected trauma, especially those with ankylosing spondylitis or DISH, and of patients with rheumatoid arthritis, who may have cervical spine instability.

In the cervical spine, the C5 to C8 nerve roots have a motor component that should be tested using formal strength testing (see Table 8-1). Strength is important to document, and testing ideally includes multiple muscles with shared innervation to distinguish root-level weakness from weakness related to peripheral compression. The examiner should evaluate muscle tone and note involuntary movement such as fasciculations or tremors. Patients with suggestive symptoms referable to the upper extremity should be examined specifically for common musculoskeletal afflictions, such as rotator cuff dysfunction, medial epicondylitis, or carpal tunnel syndromes.

Similarly, upper extremity dermatomes should be examined for sensory disturbances (see Table 8-1). Patients who present with complaints of altered upper extremity or neck sensation can be examined in greater detail, if necessary, by using multiple sensory modalities (pinprick, vibration). Dermatomal innervation is usually partially redundant, a property that may mask the sensory component of some lesions.

Every patient should undergo evaluation of muscle stretch reflexes. Lower motor neuron lesions result in the loss or attenuation of reflexes, whereas upper motor neuron lesions result in exaggeration of reflexes. Cervical nerve roots C5, C6, and C7 have well-defined associated muscle tendon reflexes (see Table 8-1). When reflexes are graded, any proximal or distal propagation of the reflex

that suggests myelopathy should be noted. Lower extremity skeletal reflexes should also be tested because they are likely to show hyperactivity in patients with myelopathy or other upper motor neuron disorders.

Special Tests Associated with Myelopathy

Several special tests evaluate for the presence of myelopathy by testing for loss of coordination or the onset of pathologic reflexes that accompany compression of the cervical spinal cord. Patients should undergo a gait evaluation, both during normal, unaltered gait and during tandem gait, to highlight any subclinical balance problems indicative of myelopathy. An upper extremity test for loss of motor coordination can be performed by evaluating a patient's ability to perform repetitive tasks rapidly, such as opening and clenching the fist, which a person without myelopathy should be able to perform at least 20 times in 10 seconds. Similarly, patients with myelopathy may have difficulty with the Romberg test as a result of diminished proprioception. Pathologic reflexes present in myopathic patients include the inverted radial reflex, in which testing of the brachioradialis reflex elicits little, if any, wrist extension and instead results in finger flexion. The Hoffmann sign occurs when flicking or tapping the terminal phalanx of the middle or ring finger elicits reflexive flexion of the thumb interphalangeal joint (Fig. 8-5). Finally, although it is not specific to myelopathy, the Lhermitte sign (barber chair sign) occurs when an electric sensation occurs in the upper extremities on maximal neck flexion and suggests compression of the dorsal columns of the cervical spinal cord. Although this condition does occur in myelopathy, it also occurs in several cervical spine disease mimetics including MS and transverse myelitis.

Several aspects of the physical examination may allow surgeons to distinguish among clinical entities with similar presentations. The presence of multiple nondermatomal areas of tenderness around the buttocks, hip, lower back, and legs, along with a consistent history, is diagnostic for fibromyalgia (see Fig. 8-2). Although potential peripheral nerve entrapment sites in the upper extremity are numerous, the spinal surgeon should be familiar with provocative tests for the most common conditions, including carpal tunnel syndrome and ulnar nerve compression at the elbow. Patients suspected of having thoracic outlet syndrome should have blood pressures taken in both arms. The Adson maneuver (diminution of the radial pulse with ipsilateral head rotation is diagnostic), radial pulse palpation during arm abduction with or without head rotation, and auscultation of the supraclavicular and infraclavicular regions for the presence of a bruit related to vascular compression may be helpful in such cases.

Imaging

Cervical spine imaging is covered in detail in Chapters 9 and 10. Prospective studies established that degenerative changes in the cervical spine are common in asymptomatic individuals; disk degeneration was found on magnetic resonance imaging in nearly 60% and foraminal narrowing in 20% of individuals who were more than 40 years old.[1] This high prevalence of degenerative changes in patients without symptoms cautions against the use of advanced imaging studies as a stand-alone diagnostic technique (Fig. 8-6). Early computed tomography or magnetic resonance imaging, or both, should be obtained when concern exists for trauma or tumor and when patients present with a progressive neurologic deficit or severe symptoms. Patients who do not present with these concerns are best treated with a short course of conservative care before advance imaging studies are obtained.

Diagnostic and Therapeutic Tests

Neurophysiologic testing is a critical diagnostic tool for the spinal surgeon when evaluating patients with focal upper extremity symptoms. EMG is the gold standard test to distinguish between spinal disease and compressive neuropathies of the upper extremity.[8] Denervation of muscle by compressive neuropathy either proximally at the nerve root level or distally in the upper extremity results in muscle activity in the absence of neural stimuli as the process of nerve stimulation of voluntary muscle firing becomes uncoupled. The location of muscle denervation and the muscles affected provide insight into the anatomic location of compression to help distinguish between nerve root compression (which affects every muscle innervated by the affected roots) and peripheral nerve compression (which affects only muscles distal to compression). EMG may be useful in the diagnosis of MS and ALS, as well as other degenerative neurologic diseases that demonstrate characteristic EMG patterns.

Diagnostic injections and blocks may help the spinal surgeon to distinguish among potential pain generators. Epidural steroid injections are commonly used for both diagnostic and therapeutic purposes and can be delivered under fluoroscopic guidance by either interlaminar or transforaminal techniques (Fig. 8-7). Although some investigators have questioned the efficacy of this treatment modality, the use of epidural steroid injections may provide relief for some patients with isolated

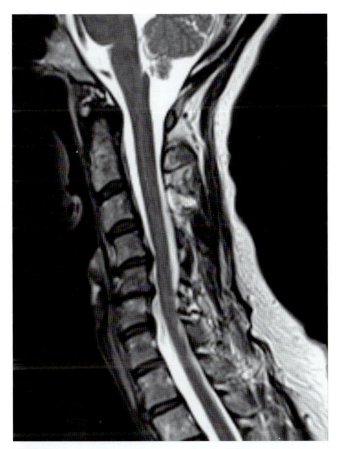

FIGURE 8-6 Sagittal magnetic resonance imaging (MRI) scan from a patient presenting to the emergency department who complained of neck soreness immediately following a car accident and who had no prior history of neck pain or radicular symptoms. The MRI scan was negative for acute traumatic injury but demonstrates signs of asymptomatic disk degeneration with disk protrusions at C4-C5 and C5-C6.

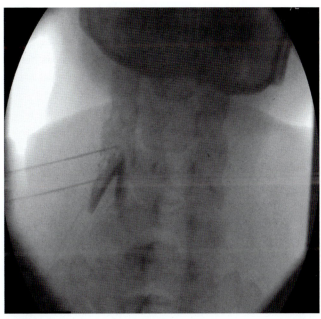

FIGURE 8-7 Fluoroscopic image demonstrating a transforaminal epidural steroid injection.

radicular symptoms and generally has a favorable complication profile, although symptom relief is variable and often temporary. Similarly, facet blocks are used by some physicians to help identify a source of pain in patients with neck pain when axial symptoms are the principal complaint.

Finally, diskography of the cervical spine has been used by some physicians, but this technique is controversial in terms of its utility, efficacy, and risks. Advocates of diskography use this technique in patients with severe axial neck pain when imaging demonstrates either multiple degenerative levels or only mild degenerative changes that do not adequately explain the symptoms. The role and efficacy of surgical intervention in this patient population are controversial because outcomes tend to be suboptimal.

Laboratory Testing

Other than routine preoperative laboratory tests, blood tests may be useful to the spinal surgeon in the evaluation of patients with suspected infection (complete blood count, erythrocyte sedimentation rate, C-reactive protein) or blood dyscrasia (complete blood count). Although it is outside the scope of practice of a spinal surgeon, patients suspected of having MS may be referred for a spinal tap and analysis of cerebrospinal fluid immunoglobulins.

Wide Differential Diagnosis

The surgeon should consider a wide differential diagnosis early in the evaluation of a new patient. As described earlier, various disparate nonspinal diseases can mimic spinal disease, especially myelopathy. Patients who present with a constellation of seemingly unrelated symptoms or symptoms that are not adequately explained by known anatomic distributions should alert the examiner to widen the differential diagnosis. In these types of conditions, it may be useful to refer the patient for additional evaluation by a qualified neurologist or other specialist, to assist in establishing the optimal diagnosis before embarking on a treatment plan.

Disability Evaluation

Although chronic pain resulting from cervical spine disease is less common than chronic low back pain, it similarly is responsible for a disproportionate amount of the direct treatment costs and indirect costs associated with work absenteeism and chronic disability compared with other conditions. Because of the high rates of disability associated with chronic neck pain, spinal surgeons may be asked to perform evaluations related to disability and workers' compensation claims. Whereas many elements of the history, examination, and consideration of diagnostic and imaging modalities are the same as in a standard examination of the cervical spine, the goals are different. In addition to diagnosing the source of pain or neurologic deficit, the disability examiner must also evaluate the capacity of the patient to work in an occupation or in an alternate job with decreased physical demands and determine when a patient has reached maximal improvement after a course of treatment. Limitations in the ability of a patient to perform a given job may be related to pain, weakness, or the risk of progressive disability or injury if the patient continues to work. Although portions of this evaluation are objective, the spinal surgeon must use reasonable judgment about the severity of pain and the patient's ability to work. In determining whether the symptoms constitute a true organic disability, Waddell signs can help to distinguish findings of inorganic disease.[9] These criteria use five examination techniques that should distinguish between organic and nonorganic spine pain: (1) excessive tenderness, (2) simulated movement that inappropriately causes pain, (3) distraction techniques, (4) atypical regional symptoms, and (5) overreaction. In addition to determining the ability of a patient to work, the disability examination often is charged with determining whether a specific injury at work could conceivably have resulted in the anatomic derangement and related degree of disability.

Spinal surgeons treating patients who receive disability or workers' compensation benefits must be aware of the challenges implicit in treating this difficult population. Although the specific reason is unclear, numerous studies evaluating outcomes after both surgical and nonsurgical treatment of patients receiving workers' compensation or disability benefits have consistently demonstrated significantly inferior results in this population.[10] Therefore, surgeons must factor the work injury process into the decision-making process and appropriately counsel the patient regarding the likelihood of a successful intervention when surgery is considered.

REFERENCES

1. Boden SD, McCowin PR, Davis DO, et al.: Abnormal magnetic-resonance scans of the cervical spine in asymptomatic subjects: a prospective investigation, *J Bone Joint Surg Am* 72:1178–1184, 1990.
2. Dvorak J, Sutter M, Herdmann J: Cervical myelopathy: clinical and neurophysiological evaluation, *Eur Spine J* 12(Suppl 2):S181–S187, 2003.
3. Lees F, Turner JW: Natural history and prognosis of cervical spondylosis, *Br Med J* 2:1607–1610, 1963.
4. Devereaux M: Neck pain, *Med Clin North Am* 93:273–284, 2009. vii.
5. Hawkins RA: Fibromyalgia: a clinical update, *J Am Osteopath Assoc* 113:680–689, 2013.
6. Frohman EM, Wingerchuk DM: Clinical practice: transverse myelitis, *N Engl J Med* 363:564–572, 2010.
7. Rao RD, Currier BL, Albert TJ, et al.: Degenerative cervical spondylosis: clinical syndromes, pathogenesis, and management, *J Bone Joint Surg Am* 89:1360–1378, 2007.
8. Hakimi K, Spanier D: Electrodiagnosis of cervical radiculopathy, *Phys Med Rehabil Clin N Am* 24:1–12, 2013.
9. Waddell G, McCulloch JA, Kummel E, Venner RM: Nonorganic physical signs in low-back pain, *Spine (Phila Pa 1976)* 5:117–125, 1980.
10. Anderson PA, Subach BR, Riew KD: Predictors of outcome after anterior cervical diskectomy and fusion: a multivariate analysis, *Spine (Phila Pa 1976)* 34:161–166, 2009.

Radiographic and Computed Tomography Evaluation of the Cervical Spine

9

John P. Malloy, Ashvin Kumar Dewan, and A. Jay Khanna

CHAPTER PREVIEW

Chapter Synopsis Conventional radiographs and computed tomography (CT) imaging are integral parts of the evaluation of a patient with suspected cervical spine abnormalities. The treating clinician must have a thorough understanding of the role of the imaging studies available, the radiographic views that should be obtained, and the ability to differentiate normal from abnormal findings. This chapter discusses the conventional radiographic views most commonly used in the cervical spine and their key roles in evaluating for cervical spine disease. It also reviews the benefits of obtaining multiplanar CT imaging and describes when this imaging technique should be used to evaluate patients with known or suspected spinal disorders.

Important Points Conventional radiographs and CT images play major roles in the evaluation of patients with known or suspected cervical spine abnormalities.

The lateral view of the cervical spine provides most of the information the clinician obtains from conventional radiographic images.

A systematic approach to the interpretation of radiographic studies is important to ensuring that adequate views are obtained and all structures are appropriately visualized.

The cervical spine is often divided into separate regions: the occipitocervical junction, the atlantoaxial region, and the subaxial region. The unique anatomy of the individual regions leads to characteristic radiographic findings and appearances. The anteroposterior, oblique, dynamic, odontoid, and swimmer's views all offer specific advantages to complete a thorough evaluation of particular cervical spinal abnormalities.

CT allows for multiplanar image reconstruction, which improves overall visualization and detail in imaging of the cervical spine.

Although both conventional radiographs and CT images allow for evaluation of the cervical spine, clinicians should know when magnetic resonance imaging is the optimal modality for a particular diagnosis or clinical situation.

The evaluation of a patient with a suspected spinal abnormality always begins with a thorough history and physical examination. The next most important tool in the spine surgeon's armamentarium is the ability to evaluate imaging studies accurately. Imaging begins with conventional radiographs and often progresses to advanced planar imaging studies such as computed tomography (CT) and magnetic resonance imaging (MRI) (see Chapter 10). In the context of correlating clinical findings, the ability to order and interpret radiographic studies appropriately leads to more accurate diagnosis and treatment. This chapter focuses on the individual radiographic views that aid the clinician in the evaluation of the cervical spine. A discussion of the indications for CT-based evaluation of the cervical spine is also included.

Conventional Radiographic Evaluation

Conventional radiographs are commonly obtained to (1) diagnose (e.g., fracture from trauma), (2) localize the level or levels of abnormality, (3) observe and follow the progression of disease (e.g., tumor, infection, or degenerative or inflammatory conditions such as rheumatoid arthritis or diffuse idiopathic skeletal hyperostosis), (4) observe and follow the progression of deformity (e.g., kyphosis, scoliosis), (5) plan the levels and extent of surgery preoperatively, and (6) follow-up operative procedures.

An understanding of the information that can be obtained from individual radiographic views is necessary to ensure that appropriate studies are initially ordered. Next, the clinician must develop a systematic approach to radiographic studies. This approach should begin by ensuring that the image is of the correct patient and that it adequately visualizes the anatomic structures to be evaluated and allows for assessment of spinal alignment.

Lateral View

The lateral cervical spine radiograph provides most of the information for the evaluation of patients with cervical spine disorders or suspected cervical spine abnormalities.

For a cervical spine lateral radiograph to be considered adequate, the clinician must be able to visualize the area from the occiput to the superior end plate of T1 (Fig. 9-1). The overall spinal alignment should be noted in terms of lordosis, straightening, or kyphosis. Normal vertebral bodies are symmetric and rectangular. The margins of the vertebral body should be visually traced to rule out fracture or an osteolytic process, such as tumor. Disk space height should also be evaluated; a loss of disk space height may indicate degenerative disk disease or chronic infectious conditions. A loss of disk space height with nonbridging, nonmarginal osteophytes or syndesmophytes is a classic finding in patients with degenerative spinal disease.

Harris and associates[1,2] described five lines for the evaluation of the cervical spine on the lateral radiograph: (1) the anterior vertebral body line, (2) the posterior vertebral body line, (3) the spinolaminar line, (4) the spinous process line, and (5) the soft tissue line. These lines should be evaluated carefully in every patient. Disruption of one of these lines, even if subtle, should prompt the examiner to scrutinize that area further for abnormality. For example, spondylolisthesis, or displacement of one vertebral body over another, as classified by Wiltse and colleagues[3] and graded by Meyerding,[4] results in disruption of these radiographic lines and indicates abnormality with the potential for instability. These findings should be interpreted according to the clinical situation. For example, after acute trauma to the cervical spine, such a finding may warrant immediate immobilization or surgical stabilization (Fig. 9-2). In contrast, in the setting of chronic degenerative or rheumatologic disease, this finding would prompt further clinical or radiographic evaluation, such as flexion and extension views, as described later.

In addition to osseous structures, soft tissue shadows can be appreciated on lateral radiographs. In particular, the shadow anterior to the vertebral bodies representing the retropharyngeal soft tissues should be evaluated. According to some clinicians, the shadow should be less than 5 mm at the C3 level (Fig. 9-3), and it should be less than 22 mm at the C6 level.[5] However, other clinicians have found this measurement to be unreliable.[6,7] A larger

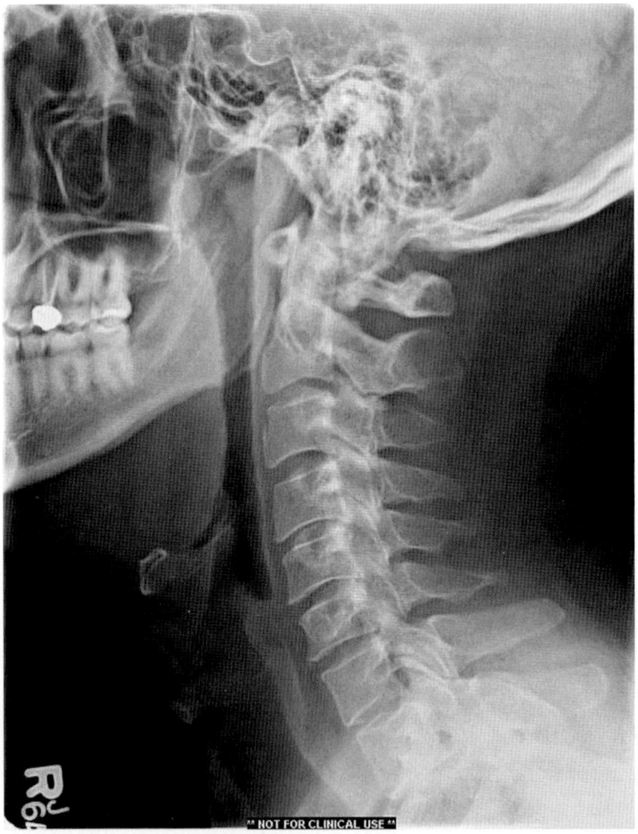

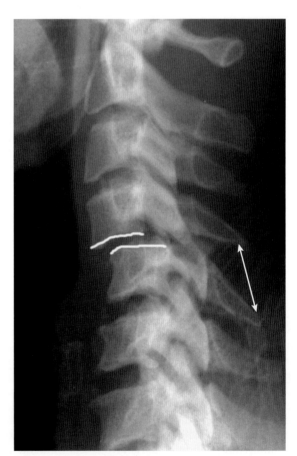

FIGURE 9-2 Spondylolisthesis. Lateral radiograph of the cervical spine showing disruption of the spinal lines, widening of the spinous processes (*arrow*), and anterolisthesis of C4 on C5. The degree of listhesis can be measured as a percentage of the displacement of the inferior end plate of the superior vertebral body over the superior end plate of the inferior vertebral body (end plates highlighted with *lines*).

FIGURE 9-1 Lateral radiograph of the cervical spine. The entire cervical spine, including the occipitocervical junction and the cervicothoracic junction, are well visualized, and the five spinal lines (anterior vertebral body line, posterior vertebral body line, spinolaminar line, spinous process line, and soft tissue shadow line) are well maintained.

soft tissue shadow may be the result of edema related to a fracture, an infection in a patient with a retropharyngeal abscess, or a retropharyngeal hematoma in a patient who recently underwent an anterior cervical spinal procedure.

Occipitocervical Junction

The occipitocervical junction can be a particularly challenging region to evaluate on conventional radiographs because of the overlap of anatomic landmarks. Radiographic lines and parameters have been described to aid in evaluating the relationship of the base of the occiput with C1 and C2 for disassociation, basilar invagination, and cranial settling.[8] The Harris "rule of twelves"[1,2] is one such relationship with which the spine surgeon should be familiar, especially in the setting of major occipitocervical trauma. The dens-basion interval, measured as the distance from the basion to the tip of the odontoid process, should be less than 12 mm. Similarly, the basion-axial interval, the distance from a vertical line drawn along the posterior aspect of the dens (termed the posterior axial line) to the basion, should be less than 12 mm. A distance of more than 12 mm for either interval indicates atlanto-occipital dissociation. Additional radiographic lines and parameters can aid in the evaluation

of the occipitocervical junction (Fig. 9-4 and Table 9-1). The reliable use of these lines and parameters largely depends on the ability to visualize their corresponding landmarks. CT and MRI have aided substantially in the accurate evaluation of these parameters in this region and have widely replaced conventional radiographs for definitive evaluation.

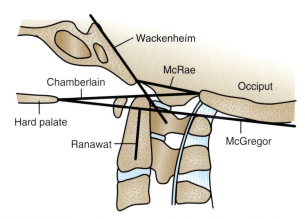

FIGURE 9-4   Lines and measurements for the evaluation of basilar invagination. (Redrawn from Zebala LP, Buchowski JM, Daftary AR, et al: The cervical spine. In Khanna AJ, editor: *MRI for orthopaedic surgeons,* New York, 2010, Thieme, pp 229-268.)

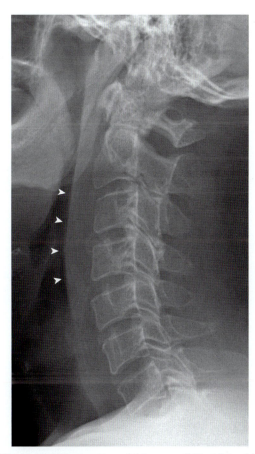

FIGURE 9-3   This 35-year-old man fell from a scaffold, with forcible extension of the neck, and sustained an extension-distraction injury with incomplete spinal cord injury. This lateral conventional radiograph shows substantial edema in the anterior soft tissues (*arrowheads*). (From Khanna AJ, Kwon BK: Subaxial cervical spine injuries. In Rao RD, Smuck M, editors: *Orthopaedic knowledge update: spine 4,* ed 4, Rosemont, Ill, 2012, American Academy of Orthopaedic Surgeons, pp 221–233.)

Table 9-1   Occipitocervical Junction: Anatomic Relationships, and Lines for Use with Magnetic Resonance Imaging, Computed Tomography, and Conventional Radiographs

Eponym	Parameters	Pathologic Features
Wackenheim clivus baseline	Tangent drawn along the superior surface of the clivus	Dens should be below the line.
Clivus canal angle	Angle formed between Wackenheim line and the posterior vertebral body line	Normal ranges are 180 degrees in extension to 150 degrees in flexion. An angle of <150 degrees is considered abnormal.
Chamberlain line	Between the hard palate and the opisthion	Protrusion of the dens >3 mm above this line is considered abnormal.
McRae line	Basion to the opisthion	Protrusion of the dens above this line is abnormal.
McGregor line	From the hard palate to the most caudal point on the midline occipital curve	Odontoid process rising >4.5 mm above this line is considered abnormal.
Ranawat criterion	Distance between the center of the pedicle of C2 and the transverse axis of C1	Measurement of <15 mm in males and <13 mm in females is abnormal.
Welcher basal angle	Tangent to the clivus as it intersects a tangent to the sphenoid bone	The normal range is 125 to 143 degrees. Platybasia exists when the basal angle is >143 degrees.

From Zebala LP, Buchowski JM, Daftary AR, et al: The cervical spine. In Khanna AJ, editor: *MRI for orthopaedic surgeons,* New York, 2010, Thieme, pp 229–268.

Atlantoaxial Region

After the occipitocervical junction, the next region that is evaluated on the lateral cervical spine radiograph is the atlantoaxial junction, which includes the anterior arch of C1, the odontoid process, and the posterior arch of C1. Relationships that should be evaluated in this area include the anterior atlantodens interval and the posterior atlantodens interval. The uses of these intervals have been described primarily in the evaluation of patients with rheumatoid arthritis.[9-11] The anterior atlantodens interval should measure less than 3 mm in adults and less than 3.5 mm in children less than 10 years old. A posterior atlantodens interval of less than 14 mm is considered a relative indication for surgery in a patient with rheumatoid arthritis.[9]

In the trauma setting, the atlantoaxial region should be evaluated in conjunction with the open-mouth view (see details later) for hangman's fractures, Jefferson or burst fractures, and odontoid fractures (see Chapter 17 for details on the classification and treatment of these fractures). A more thorough evaluation of these fractures can be performed with CT and MRI.

Subaxial Region

The third region of the cervical spine that is evaluated on conventional radiographs is the subaxial cervical spine (C3 to C7). Along with the five lines described earlier, several other specific parameters should be evaluated in this area. One such parameter is the Pavlov or Torg ratio, which can be evaluated in patients with suspected or known congenital cervical spinal stenosis. A ratio of less than 0.8 (ratio of the anteroposterior [AP] canal diameter to the AP vertebral body diameter) suggests the presence of congenital cervical spinal stenosis.[12,13] One study described the use of this ratio to limit return to play or participation in contact sports for athletes.[14] The space available for the spinal cord is another similar parameter and can be used to define the degree of stenosis in the subaxial cervical spine. The degree or amount of stenosis is defined as absolute when the space available for the spinal cord is less than 10 mm, and it is defined as relative when the space measures 11 to 13 mm.[15-18]

The subaxial cervical spine is the primary location where facet subluxations or dislocations may be noted. In the setting of the unilateral facet fracture or subluxation, the degree of spondylolisthesis is typically between 0% and 25%, whereas in bilateral facet dislocation (or "jumped facets"), the degree of subluxation is 50% or greater. An additional radiographic finding in patients with bilateral jumped facets is the sail sign or bow tie sign.

Other fractures with classic radiographic appearances seen in the subaxial cervical spine region include compression fractures, burst fractures, teardrop fractures, quadrangular fractures, and clay-shoveler's fractures.[19] Denis[20,21] described the spine as divisible into three columns: anterior, middle, and posterior. Evaluation of the three columns on the lateral radiograph aids in identifying these fractures. For example, a loss of anterior vertebral body height in comparison with maintained posterior vertebral body height signifies an anterior column injury or compression fracture. Involvement of the posterior vertebral body or middle column indicates a two-column injury or burst fracture. Teardrop and quadrangular fractures are associated with interspinous process widening, thereby indicating posterior column disruption or a three-column injury. A clay-shoveler's fracture results from an avulsion of the spinous process secondary to hyperflexion.

Anteroposterior View

On the AP cervical spine radiograph (Fig. 9-5), the coronal alignment should be evaluated. In the normal cervical spine, the AP radiograph shows the spinous processes in the midline, symmetric uncovertebral joints (joints of Luschka), bilateral lateral masses with undisrupted and undulating lateral cortical margins, vertebral bodies of equal height, and parallel disk spaces. On the AP view, the presence of the first rib serves as a marker to help localize the C7-T1 articulation. In general, the AP cervical spine view does not provide as much information as the lateral view for patients with cervical degenerative and traumatic abnormalities.

Oblique Views

Oblique cervical radiographs allow for the evaluation of the pedicle, facet joints, and neural foramina and for the presence of foraminal osteophytes. Before the more widespread availability of CT and MRI, oblique radiographs were more frequently used to evaluate patients for foraminal stenosis. The direction, or side of the patient, to which the spinous process points on an oblique radiograph indicates the side of the foramina visualized (Fig. 9-6).

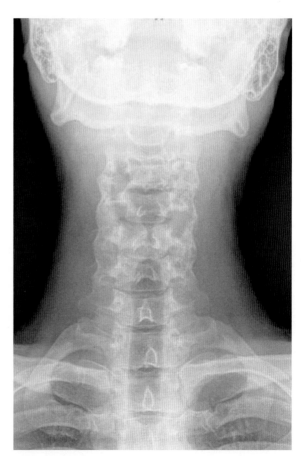

FIGURE 9-5 Anteroposterior radiograph of the cervical spine showing normal anatomy.

Dynamic Views

Flexion and extension cervical spine radiographs allow for the dynamic evaluation of cervical spine alignment for instability or dynamic spondylolisthesis.[22] For example, as part of the preoperative evaluation for a surgical procedure requiring intubation of a patient with rheumatoid arthritis, flexion and extension lateral radiographs are important, to assess for subclinical instability. Changes in the anterior atlantodens interval on flexion and extension views indicate atlantoaxial instability and could be missed on a static lateral radiograph (Fig. 9-7).

After arthrodesis, flexion and extension radiographs can be used to evaluate for the presence or absence of fusion, as evidenced by movement of the spinous processes of more than 1 to 2 mm or a change in angulation of the vertebral bodies of more than 4 degrees.[23,24] Additional pathologic radiographic findings in the postoperative patient include lucency around the screws or at the graft-vertebrae junction, indicating pseudarthrosis, or, conversely, the presence of the sentinel sign, indicating fusion.[25] Although flexion and extension radiographs are more feasible to obtain and follow clinically for postoperative follow-up, CT is more accurate and should be obtained in the clinical setting for the postoperative evaluation of the patient with suspected pseudarthrosis.[26-28]

Finally, with more recent developments in motion-preservation technologies, these dynamic radiographs have become useful for evaluating maintenance of range of motion after procedures such as total disk replacement.[29-31]

Odontoid or Open-Mouth View

The open-mouth or odontoid view can also be used to evaluate the C1-C2 articulation in the AP plane (Fig. 9-8). This view allows for evaluation of odontoid process or dens fractures in an orthogonal plane and also for evaluation of C1 burst fractures (Jefferson burst fracture). With

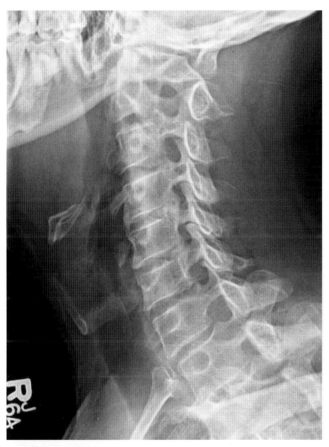

FIGURE 9-6   Oblique radiograph of the cervical spine. The spinous processes point to the patient's left; thus, the left neural foramina are the ones visualized. Foraminal stenosis secondary to osteophyte formation is well visualized at the C4-C5 and C5-C6 foramina.

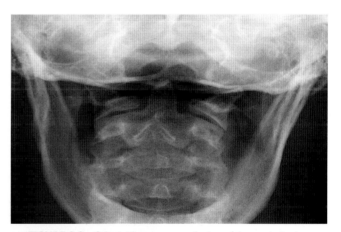

FIGURE 9-8   Odontoid or open-mouth view of the cervical spine.

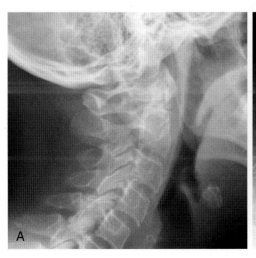
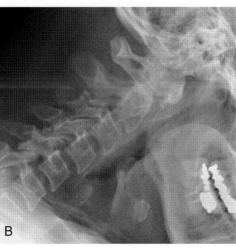

FIGURE 9-7   The cervical spine of a patient with rheumatoid arthritis. **A,** Lateral view. The anterior atlantodens interval is normal. **B,** Flexion lateral view shows widening of the anterior atlantodens secondary to atlantoaxial instability.

such fractures, the clinician or radiologist measures the amount of overhang of C1 lateral masses bilaterally. If the degree of the lateral mass overhang (beyond the lateral margins of C2) is greater than 6.9 mm when both sides are combined, disruption of the transverse ligament should be suspected in addition to the burst fracture.[32] This finding may be a relative indication for surgical intervention or for close clinical follow-up.

Swimmer's View

The swimmer's view can be used to help evaluate the cervicothoracic junction.[33] This view is indicated in patients whose conventional lateral radiographs provide poor visualization of C7 to T1 (Fig. 9-9). The cervicothoracic junction is often poorly visualized because of the mass effect created by the shoulders obscuring visualization of the spine. One option to aid in visualization is to have an individual wearing a lead

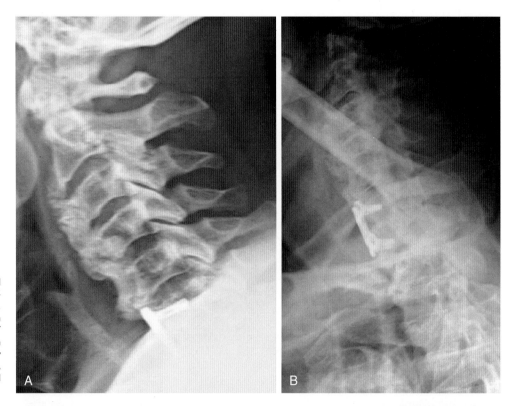

FIGURE 9-9 This 45-year-old man underwent anterior cervical diskectomy and arthrodesis at C6 to C7. **A,** Postoperative lateral radiograph of the cervical spine. The C6-C7 surgical level with instrumentation is poorly visualized and obscured by the mass effect of the shoulders. **B,** Swimmer's view provides improved visualization of C6 and C7.

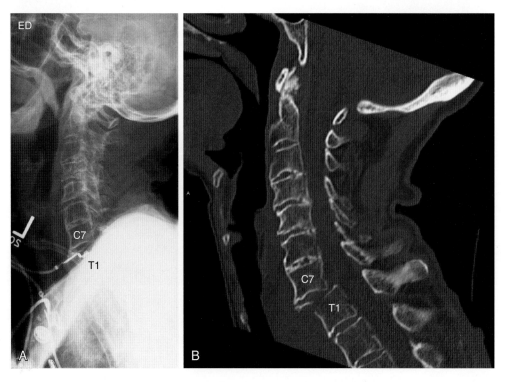

FIGURE 9-10 This 67-year-old woman presented to the emergency department with severe neck pain without neurologic compromise after a ground-level fall. **A,** A conventional lateral cervical radiograph. **B,** A computed tomography scan with sagittal reconstruction shows a C7-T1 fracture-subluxation that initially was not well visualized on conventional radiographs.

gown pull down on a patient's arms to bring the shoulder below the level of C7 to T1. Alternatively, having the patient raise one arm overhead while maintaining the contralateral arm at the side, in the motion of a swimmer, may allow for improved visualization of the cervicothoracic junction. With greater availability of CT scanning, conventional radiographs are often replaced by CT in the poorly visualized regions such as the cervicothoracic junction.

Computed Tomography Evaluation

CT images use high-resolution conventional radiographs transmitted through multiple planes. Through the use of computer software algorithms, images can be reconstructed in any plane, as opposed to the single-plane projection obtained with conventional radiographs.

In the cervical spine, this technique is quite useful for the evaluation of areas with substantial osseous overlap. In the occipitocervical junction, for example, conventional radiography is challenging because the osseous elements of the cranium overlap with those of the C1 and C2 vertebrae and thus obstruct detailed visualization. Similarly, conventional radiographic imaging of the cervicothoracic junction is also challenging because the shoulders and structures of the thorax overlap with those of the lower cervical spine (Fig. 9-10, *A*). For these regions, CT facilitates assessment of the anatomic relationships between adjacent cervical segments and patency of the spinal canal (Fig. 9-10, *B*). CT imaging also facilitates the detection of cervical spine fractures, evaluation of fusion, and evaluation of instrumentation (Fig. 9-11). For patients in whom MRI is contraindicated, CT in conjunction with intrathecal injection of contrast material can be used to produce a myelogram.

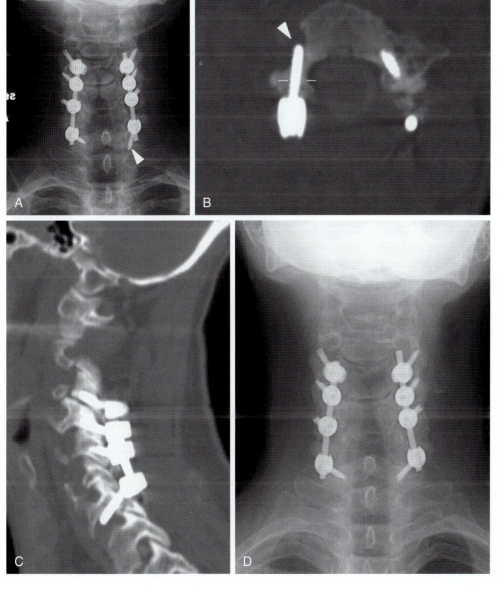

FIGURE 9-11 This 63-year-old woman with progressive myelopathy underwent C3-C7 laminectomy and fusion with placement of bilateral lateral mass screws at C3, C4, and C5 and pedicle screw fixation at C7. Postoperatively, the myelopathy gradually improved, but the patient developed new left-side arm pain radiating into the hand and fingers. **A,** A postoperative anteroposterior radiograph shows subtle asymmetry of the left C7 pedicle screw (*arrowhead*). Axial (**B**) and sagittal (**C**) computed tomography myelograms confirm a lateral-medial breach of the left C7 pedicle screw (*arrowhead* in **B**). **D,** Persistent arm and hand symptoms resulted in subsequent repositioning of the screw and resolution of the symptoms.

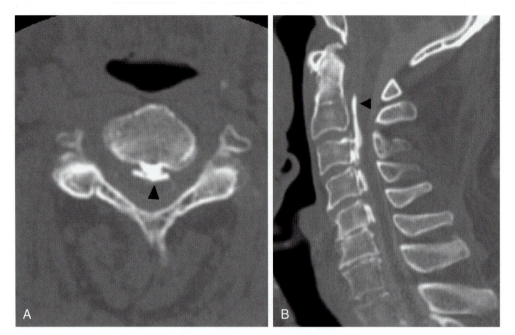

FIGURE 9-12 This patient had ossification of the posterior longitudinal ligament, which can result in a variety of shapes. **A,** In this axial computed tomography (CT) scan, the *arrowhead* indicates a more classic mushroom-shaped ossification. **B,** A sagittal CT scan shows the cephalad (*arrowhead*) extension of the ossification in this patient.

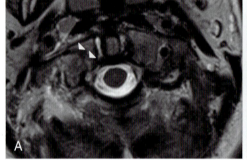
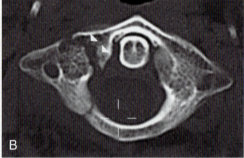

FIGURE 9-13 A C1 anterior and posterior ring fracture results in a minimally displaced C1 lateral mass fracture. **A,** A T2-weighted axial magnetic resonance imaging (MRI) sequence. **B,** An axial computed tomography (CT) scan. Although the fracture (*arrowheads* in **A** and **B**) can be visualized on the MRI sequence, it is better characterized on the CT scan.

In the setting of trauma, cervical spine instability, tumor, or infection, CT assessment can be indispensable. On conventional radiographs, nondisplaced fractures and more subtle osseous abnormalities can be overlooked or missed, especially in the presence of conditions such as ankylosing spondylitis or ossification of the posterior longitudinal ligament (Fig. 9-12). Such fractures and abnormalities can be detected much more readily with CT imaging. Consequently, many trauma centers are beginning to substitute CT imaging for cervical spine conventional radiographs in the initial evaluation of patients with known or suspected cervical spine trauma (Fig. 9-13).

Another advantage of CT imaging is the better visualization it provides of osseous detail and morphology after cervical spine fusion surgery. Evaluating bony arthrodesis can be difficult on conventional radiographs, but CT imaging readily shows bony growth between two osseous structures. For example, with anterior cervical interbody fusions, radiographs may show a persistent lucency at the vertebral body–allograft interface; the integrity of the fusion is difficult to assess on the conventional radiograph. On CT, however, localized areas of bone joining the two vertebral bodies and suggesting union are much easier to discern. Furthermore, CT avoids the metallic artifact seen on MRI that may complicate the interpretation of regions in the cervical spine in proximity to implanted instrumentation. CT can accurately evaluate hardware positioning relative to important neurovascular structures.

Finally, the use of pacemakers or other implantable devices such as spinal cord stimulators often contraindicates the use of MRI. In such patients, similarly formatted sagittal, coronal, and axial CT images can be obtained after the administration of intrathecal contrast material. Although the soft tissue detail supplied is not equivalent to that provided by MRI, the osseous detail is superior, and the resulting myelogram can help visualize compression of neural structures in the cervical spine.

Conclusions

Correct interpretation of radiographic studies requires knowledge of the anatomy, spinal alignment, and specific parameters unique to a particular view. A thorough understanding of the various radiographic views enables the clinician to order the appropriate view, evaluate its adequacy, and accurately diagnose and treat patients with cervical spine disorders.

CT of the cervical spine offers unique benefits in comparison with conventional radiographs and MRI in the evaluation of the occipitocervical and cervicothoracic junctions, fusions in patients with previous arthrodesis procedures, the position of implanted instrumentation, and patients in whom MRI is contraindicated. Any clinician dealing with cervical spinal abnormalities must be aware of the indications for and benefits of CT to ensure its timely and appropriate use.

REFERENCES

1. Harris JH Jr, Carson GC, Wagner LK: Radiologic diagnosis of traumatic occipitovertebral dissociation: 1. Normal occipitovertebral relationships on lateral radiographs of supine subjects, *AJR Am J Roentgenol* 162:881–886, 1994.
2. Harris JH Jr, Carson GC, Wagner LK, Kerr N: Radiologic diagnosis of traumatic occipitovertebral dissociation: 2. Comparison of three methods of detecting occipitovertebral relationships on lateral radiographs of supine subjects, *AJR Am J Roentgenol* 162:887–892, 1994.
3. Wiltse LL, Newman PH, Macnab I: Classification of spondylolisis and spondylolisthesis, *Clin Orthop Relat Res* (117)23–29, 1976.
4. Meyerding HW: Spondylolisthesis, *Surg Gynecol Obstet* 54:371–377, 1932.
5. Weir DC: Roentgenographic signs of cervical injury, *Clin Orthop Relat Res* (109)9–17, 1975.
6. DeBehnke DJ, Havel CJ: Utility of prevertebral soft tissue measurements in identifying patients with cervical spine fractures, *Ann Emerg Med* 24:1119–1124, 1994.
7. Herr CH, Ball PA, Sargent SK, Quinton HB: Sensitivity of prevertebral soft tissue measurement of C3 for detection of cervical spine fractures and dislocations, *Am J Emerg Med* 16:346–349, 1998.
8. Riew KD, Hilibrand AS, Palumbo MA, et al.: Diagnosing basilar invagination in the rheumatoid patient: the reliability of radiographic criteria, *J Bone Joint Surg Am* 83:194–200, 2001.
9. Boden SD, Dodge LD, Bohlman HH, Rechtine GR: Rheumatoid arthritis of the cervical spine: a long-term analysis with predictors of paralysis and recovery, *J Bone Joint Surg Am* 75:1282–1297, 1993.
10. Castro S, Verstraete K, Mielants H, et al.: Cervical spine involvement in rheumatoid arthritis: a clinical, neurological and radiological evaluation, *Clin Exp Rheumatol* 12:369–374, 1994.
11. Collins DN, Barnes CL, FitzRandolph RL: Cervical spine instability in rheumatoid patients having total hip or knee arthroplasty, *Clin Orthop Relat Res* (272)127–135, 1991.
12. Torg JS: Cervical spinal stenosis with cord neurapraxia and transient quadriplegia, *Clin Sports Med* 9:279–296, 1990.
13. Torg JS, Pavlov H, Genuario SE, et al.: Neurapraxia of the cervical spinal cord with transient quadriplegia, *J Bone Joint Surg Am* 68:1354–1370, 1986.
14. Torg JS, Corcoran TA, Thibault LE, et al.: Cervical cord neurapraxia: classification, pathomechanics, morbidity, and management guidelines, *J Neurosurg* 87:843–850, 1997.
15. Arnold JG Jr: The clinical manifestations of spondylochondrosis (spondylosis) of the cervical spine, *Ann Surg* 141:872–889, 1955.
16. Murone I: The importance of the sagittal diameters of the cervical spinal canal in relation to spondylosis and myelopathy, *J Bone Joint Surg Br* 56:30–36, 1974.
17. Penning L: Some aspects of plain radiography of the cervical spine in chronic myelopathy, *Neurology* 12:513–519, 1962.
18. Wolf BS, Khilnani M, Malis L: The sagittal diameter of the bony cervical spinal canal and its significance in cervical spondylosis, *J Mt Sinai Hosp N Y* 23:283–292, 1956.
19. Khanna AJ, Kwon BK: Subaxial cervical spine injuries. In Rao RD, Smuck M, editors: *Orthopaedic knowledge update: spine 4*, ed 4, Rosemont, Ill, 2012, American Academy of Orthopaedic Surgeons, pp 221–233.
20. Denis F: The three column spine and its significance in the classification of acute thoracolumbar spinal injuries, *Spine (Phila Pa 1976)* 8:817–831, 1983.
21. Denis F: Spinal instability as defined by the three-column spine concept in acute spinal trauma, *Clin Orthop Relat Res* (189)65–76, 1984.
22. Wang JC, Hatch JD, Sandhu HS, Delamarter RB: Cervical flexion and extension radiographs in acutely injured patients, *Clin Orthop Relat Res* (365)111–116, 1999.
23. Cannada LK, Scherping SC, Yoo JU, et al.: Pseudoarthrosis of the cervical spine: a comparison of radiographic diagnostic measures, *Spine (Phila Pa 1976)* 28:46–51, 2003.
24. Hilibrand AS, Dina TS: The use of diagnostic imaging to assess spinal arthrodesis, *Orthop Clin North Am* 29:591–601, 1998.
25. Epstein NE, Silvergleide RS: Documenting fusion following anterior cervical surgery: a comparison of roentgenogram versus two-dimensional computed tomographic findings, *J Spinal Disord Tech* 16:243–247, 2003.
26. Carreon LY, Glassman SD, Djurasovic M: Reliability and agreement between fine-cut CT scans and plain radiography in the evaluation of posterolateral fusions, *Spine J* 7:39–43, 2007.
27. Epstein NE: Evaluation and treatment of clinical instability associated with pseudoarthrosis after anterior cervical surgery for ossification of the posterior longitudinal ligament, *Surg Neurol* 49:246–252, 1998.
28. Ploumis A, Mehbod A, Garvey T, et al.: Prospective assessment of cervical fusion status: plain radiographs versus CT-scan, *Acta Orthop Belg* 72:342–346, 2006.
29. Duggal N, Bertagnoli R, Rabin D, et al.: ProDisc-C: an in vivo kinematic study, *J Spinal Disord Tech* 24:334–339, 2011.
30. Kim SW, Limson MA, Kim SB, et al.: Comparison of radiographic changes after ACDF versus Bryan disc arthroplasty in single and bi-level cases, *Eur Spine J* 18:218–231, 2009.
31. Sasso RC, Best NM, Metcalf NH, Anderson PA: Motion analysis of bryan cervical disc arthroplasty versus anterior discectomy and fusion: results from a prospective, randomized, multicenter, clinical trial, *J Spinal Disord Tech* 21:393–399, 2008.
32. Spence KF Jr, Decker S, Sell KW: Bursting atlantal fracture associated with rupture of the transverse ligament, *J Bone Joint Surg Am* 52:543–549, 1970.
33. Rethnam U, Yesupalan RSU, Bastawrous SS: The swimmer's view: does it really show what it is supposed to show? A retrospective study, *BMC Med Imaging* 8:2, 2008.

10 Magnetic Resonance Imaging of the Cervical Spine

Ashvin Kumar Dewan, John P. Malloy, and A. Jay Khanna

CHAPTER PREVIEW

Chapter Synopsis	Magnetic resonance imaging (MRI) is instrumental in evaluation of symptomatic cervical spine degeneration and guidance of surgical treatment. In the setting of trauma, MRI can help define unexplained neurologic injuries, assess for soft tissue damage, and exclude cervical spine injury. It has also become extremely beneficial in the diagnosis and management of spinal infection and inflammatory conditions of the spine and in the differential diagnosis of spinal tumors. The emphasis of this chapter is the utility of MRI in the diagnosis of different pathologic processes of the cervical spine.
Important Points	Spinal anatomy is challenging; therefore, gaining an understanding of normal spinal anatomy is vital before one can recognize subtleties of pathologic processes.
	Systematic evaluation and review of MRI images greatly enhance the interpretation of the images and reduce the risk of missing pathologic features.
	MRI abnormalities do not always correlate with symptomatic degenerative lesions. Sixty percent of asymptomatic patients who are more than 40 years old can have MRI evidence of cervical degenerative disorders.
	Correlation of the patient's history and examination with imaging findings is vital.
	Although MRI is the imaging modality of choice for soft tissue lesions, it is only half as sensitive for osseous injuries.
	Gadolinium-enhanced MRI can be helpful in the diagnosis and management of recurrent disk herniations, spinal infections, and tumors.
	Techniques such as magnetic resonance angiography continue to evolve and can provide noninvasive means of assessing vascular injury and integrity in the cervical spine.

Magnetic resonance imaging (MRI) is a very useful tool for assessing the cervical spine because it provides high-resolution multiplanar images of both osseous and soft tissue structures.[1,2] The specifics of MRI image acquisition and physics are discussed in detail elsewhere.[1] The emphasis of this chapter is the utility of MRI in the diagnosis of different pathologic processes of the cervical spine.

Pulse Sequences

Although the specifics of MRI procurement are discussed in detail elsewhere,[1,2] the clinician should be able to identify the basic pulse sequences and be aware of the roles they play in imaging the cervical spine. Imaging protocols of the cervical spine vary by institution, but standard MRI sequences of the cervical spine include the following: sagittal T1-weighted spin-echo (SE), sagittal T2-weighted fast SE, axial gradient-echo, and axial T2-weighted fast SE.

T1-weighted images are best used to evaluate anatomy, fracture lines, and other osseous details.[3] T2-weighted images are excellent for evaluating spinal cord parenchyma for lesions and edema. T2-weighted images are sensitive to pathologic changes in tissue, including any cellular process that increases the local water content.[4] Gadolinium contrast–enhanced T1-weighted images are useful for assessing neoplasms, infections, and the postoperative spine. Fat-suppressed T2-weighted fast SE and short tau inversion recovery images accentuate fluid and edema and make abnormalities more conspicuous by eliminating the signal of fat. Gradient-echo images help detect degenerative changes, including osteophytes and neural foraminal narrowing.[3] The susceptibility of gradient-echo sequences to magnetic artifact make it ideal for detecting areas of hemorrhage, such as those from trauma, or vascular malformations.[5]

Steps in Cervical Spine Image Interpretation*

The complex anatomy of the cervical spine can be difficult to evaluate. A systematic approach to imaging can greatly enhance the interpretation of the images. The following algorithm, proposed by Khanna and associates,[3] is one approach to the interpretation of MRI of the cervical spine:

1. Determine the pulse sequence for all images.
2. Locate the T2-weighted midsagittal image. Evaluate all normal structures.
3. Serially evaluate all parasagittal images in each direction toward the facet joints and neural foramina. Use the coronal localizer to confirm right-left orientation.
4. Repeat steps 2 and 3 for other pulse sequences (usually T1 and occasionally gradient-echo and postgadolinium T1).
5. Locate the odontoid process on the T2-weighted axial images. Serially evaluate all images from the odontoid toward the first thoracic vertebra (determined by the presence of ribs). Use the intervertebral disks and sagittal localizer to confirm levels. Repeat this process for other pulse sequences.
6. Correlate the MRI findings with the clinical history to arrive at the most likely differential diagnosis.

Normal Anatomy†

Before one can recognize the subtleties of pathologic processes, it is important to gain an appreciation of normal anatomy. When evaluating a cervical MRI scan, close attention should be paid to the following structures‡:

- Spinal column and vertebral bodies: alignment, vertebral body fracture, posterior element fracture, edema, degenerative change
- Ligaments: anterior longitudinal ligament, posterior longitudinal ligament, interspinous ligaments, edema or rupture
- Spinal cord: edema, hemorrhage, compression, syrinx
- Epidural space: hematoma, disk herniation, osseous fragment
- Vascular: vertebral artery

Sagittal Images

Following the approach outlined previously, and starting with midsagittal image of the T2-weighted sequence, the full profile of the odontoid, most vertebral bodies, and the spinal cord can be appreciated in patients without scoliosis. The facet joints and neural foramina are assessed next on parasagittal images. The dorsal and ventral nerve

roots can be visualized within the neural foramina. The nerve roots show intermediate signal intensity and are surrounded by high-signal-intensity fat on T1-weighted images (Fig. 10-1).[3] While panning lateral to the midsagittal plane, the clinician can evaluate end plate and osteophyte anatomy and the margins of the anterior and posterior longitudinal ligaments.[3]

Healthy intervertebral disks show intermediate signal intensity on T1-weighted images and high signal intensity on T2-weighted, gradient-echo, and T2-weighted images. For vertebral bodies, the normal fatty marrow shows bright signal intensity on T1-weighted images. A lordotic curvature of the cervical spine is expected, with tapering of the spinal canal diameter initially from the first to the third cervical vertebrae and a constant diameter thereafter (Fig. 10-2). The entry site of basivertebral veins can often be seen at the midposterior portions of the vertebral bodies. The short cervical pedicles are seen on the parasagittal images (Fig. 10-3).

Cerebrospinal fluid is seen as low signal intensity on T1-weighted images and as high signal intensity on T2-weighted images. Spinal cord sagittal T2-weighted images provide a myelographic effect that allows evaluation of spinal cord morphology and evaluation for extrinsic compression. The spinal cord usually has a homogeneous signal without intrinsic abnormality.[3] Ligaments show low signal intensity on all sequences. Ligaments that are important to identify in the review of sagittal images include the transverse ligament, ligamentum flavum, and anterior and posterior longitudinal ligaments. The transverse ligament lies posterior to the odontoid process. The ligamentum flavum starts superiorly as a hypointense band just posterior to the dura and descends to the posterior aspect of the spinal canal. The anterior and posterior longitudinal ligaments typically adhere to the vertebral column.[3]

Axial Images

Accurate identification of the vertebral level is always challenging on axial MRI scans. Most modern MRI studies provide a sagittal localizer, but in its absence, the level can be determined by identifying the odontoid process and numbering each vertebral body from that level. The difference in intervertebral disk and vertebral body signal facilitates distinction between vertebral levels. At each vertebral level, the spinal canal morphology, the traversing spinal cord, and associated roots should be scrutinized.[3]

Coronal Images

Although almost all spinal structures can be examined with sagittal and axial images alone, coronal plane images should be reviewed to confirm normal anatomy. In addition, coronal plane images add an indispensable perspective when evaluating pathologic features in the presence of coronal plane deformities such as scoliosis, particularly with regard to the morphology of the neural foramen, lateral recesses, and facet joints.

Cervical Spine Disorders

Degenerative Disk Disease

Degenerative abnormality can affect multiple areas of the cervical spine, including intervertebral disks, facet joints,

*Adapted from Khanna AJ, Carbone JJ, Kebaish KM, et al: Magnetic resonance imaging of the cervical spine: current techniques and spectrum of disease. *J Bone Joint Surg Am*; 84:70–80, 2002.
†Adapted from Khanna AJ, Carbone JJ, Kebaish KM, et al: Magnetic resonance imaging of the cervical spine: current techniques and spectrum of disease. *J Bone Joint Surg Am*; 84:70–80, 2002.
‡Adapted from Takhtani D, Melhem ER: MR imaging in cervical spine trauma. *Magn Reson Imaging Clin N Am*; 8:615–634, 2000.

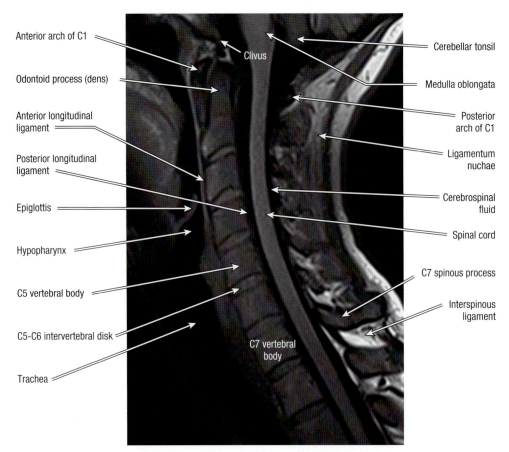

Anterior arch of C1

Odontoid process (dens)

Anterior longitudinal ligament

Posterior longitudinal ligament

Epiglottis

Hypopharynx

C5 vertebral body

C5-C6 intervertebral disk

Trachea

Clivus

C7 vertebral body

Cerebellar tonsil

Medulla oblongata

Posterior arch of C1

Ligamentum nuchae

Cerebrospinal fluid

Spinal cord

C7 spinous process

Interspinous ligament

FIGURE 10-1   Sagittal T1-weighted magnetic resonance image of the cervical spine shows the cervical spinal cord, cerebrospinal fluid, anterior and posterior longitudinal ligaments, and anterior and posterior elements of the cervical spine and intervertebral disks. (From Dunleavy JD, Khanna AJ, Carrino JA: Normal MRI anatomy of the musculoskeletal system. In Khanna AJ, editor: *MRI for orthopaedic surgeons,* New York, 2010, Thieme, pp 17–76.)

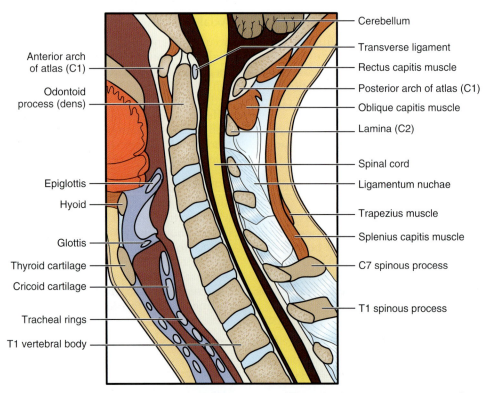

Anterior arch of atlas (C1)

Odontoid process (dens)

Epiglottis

Hyoid

Glottis

Thyroid cartilage

Cricoid cartilage

Tracheal rings

T1 vertebral body

Cerebellum

Transverse ligament

Rectus capitis muscle

Posterior arch of atlas (C1)

Oblique capitis muscle

Lamina (C2)

Spinal cord

Ligamentum nuchae

Trapezius muscle

Splenius capitis muscle

C7 spinous process

T1 spinous process

FIGURE 10-2   Artist's sketch shows the normal cervical spine anatomy seen on a sagittal T1-weighted magnetic resonance image. (Redrawn from Dunleavy JD, Khanna AJ, Carrino JA: Normal MRI anatomy of the musculoskeletal system. In Khanna AJ, editor: *MRI for orthopaedic surgeons,* New York, 2010, Thieme, pp 17–76.)

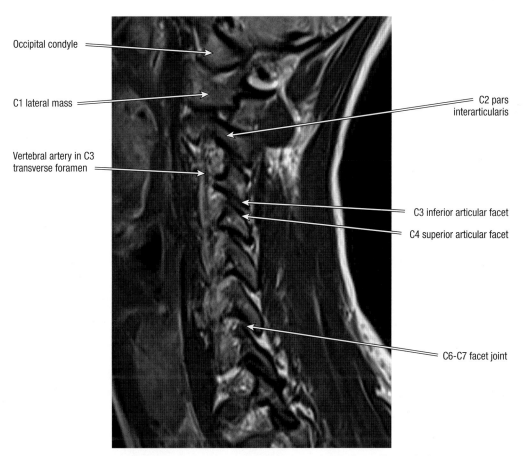

Occipital condyle

C1 lateral mass

Vertebral artery in C3
transverse foramen

C2 pars
interarticularis

C3 inferior articular facet

C4 superior articular facet

C6-C7 facet joint

FIGURE 10-3 A sagittal T2-weighted paramidline magnetic resonance image of the cervical spine shows the vertebral artery in its long axis coursing through the transverse foramina of the cervical spine. The facet joints are most easily evaluated in the parasagittal plane, as shown here. (From Dunleavy JD, Khanna AJ, Carrino JA: Normal MRI anatomy of the musculoskeletal system. In Khanna AJ, editor: *MRI for orthopaedic surgeons,* New York, 2010, Thieme, pp 17–76.)

uncovertebral joints of Luschka, ligaments, and para-vertebral musculature.[5] MRI is considered the preferred initial advanced imaging modality for the evaluation of symptomatic cervical spine degeneration, with a reported sensitivity and specificity of 91% each for the detection of cervical degenerative changes.[6,7] Despite this high sensitivity and specificity, however, MRI abnormalities do not always correlate with symptomatic degenerative lesions.[8] Boden and associates[9] reported that almost 60% of asymptomatic patients who were more than 40 years old had cervical spine degenerative disk disease on MRI. Therefore, correlating a patient's history and physical examination with imaging findings is of paramount importance.

The structural composition of the intervertebral disk changes with age: the water content of the nucleus pulposus and annulus fibrosis decreases from approximately 90% in the first year of life to 70% to 75% in the eighth decade.[10-12] Disk desiccation results in bulging of the annulus fibrosus and concomitant loss of disk height; the result is increased stress transfer to the facet and uncovertebral joints that propagates osteocartilaginous hypertrophy and osteophyte formation.[7] On MRI, a normal intervertebral disk has intermediate signal intensity on T1-weighted images and high signal intensity on T2-weighted images, whereas disk desiccation is seen as low signal intensity on T1-weighted and T2-weighted images (Fig. 10-4).[6,7] Degeneration and desiccation of the

annulus fibrosus can result in annular tears. Tears manifest as areas of high signal intensity within the annulus on T2-weighted sequences (Fig. 10-5).[6,7] A weakened annulus fibrosus may lead to a spectrum of intervertebral disk abnormality based on the extent of annulus bulging and disk herniation (Table 10-1). Findings of degenerative disk disease on MRI should always be correlated with cervical radiographs.

Disk herniation resulting from degenerative disease can impinge on structures in the spinal canal. The size of the disk abnormality is less important than the degree of the mass effect on neighboring neural structures. The direction and location of herniation (i.e., central, para-central [left-right], foraminal, or far lateral) should be noted and carefully correlated with the patient's history and examination.

In addition to being evaluated for the level, direction, and configuration of disk displacement, the MRI should also be scrutinized for the presence or absence of areas of calcium deposition, anterior or posterior osteophyte formation, and vertebral end plate changes.[6,7] These findings should be correlated with lateral and oblique cervical spine radiographs.

Cervical stenosis secondary to disk displacement must be distinguished from ossification of the posterior longitudinal ligament because treatment algorithms for each condition are distinct. Stenosis secondary to disk

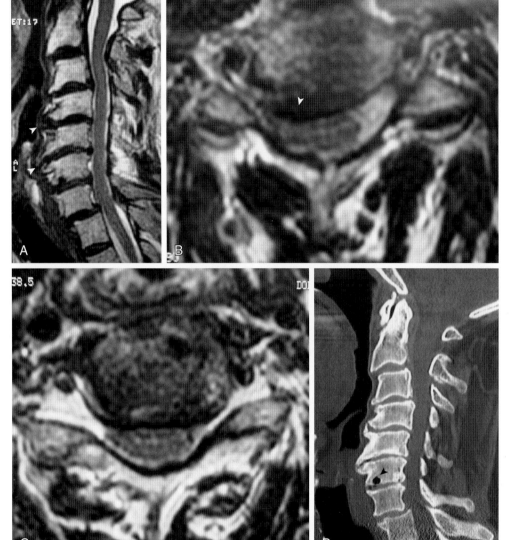

FIGURE 10-4 Multilevel degenerative disk disease. **A,** A sagittal T2-weighted image shows multilevel degenerative disk disease as evidenced loss of the normal high signal intensity within the disks. Note the degenerative spondylolisthesis at C2 to C3, C3 to C4 (subtle), and C7 to T1 and the multilevel anterior osteophyte formation (*arrowheads*). A loss of the normal cervical lordosis is also noted. **B,** An axial T2-weighted magnetic resonance image at the C3-C4 level shows a right paracentral disk bulge (*arrow*) resulting in moderate stenosis with asymmetric cord compression. **C,** An axial T2-weighted magnetic resonance image at the C5-C6 level shows moderate central stenosis. **D,** A sagittal reconstructed computed tomography image also shows multilevel degenerative disk disease and provides improved osseous detail that complements the information seen on the images. Note the subchondral cyst at the inferior end plate of C6 (*arrowhead*) and the multilevel anterior osteophyte formation. (From Zebala LP, Buchowski JM, Daftary AR, et al: The cervical spine. In Khanna AJ, editor: *MRI for orthopaedic surgeons*, New York, 2010, Thieme, pp 229–268.)

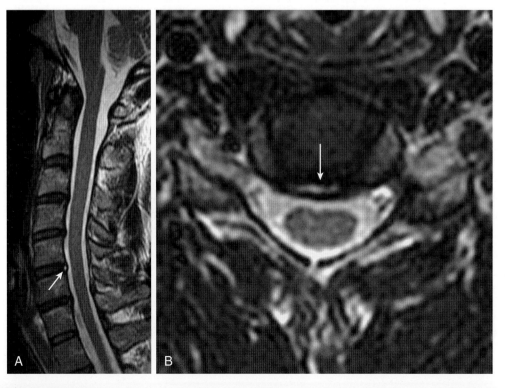

FIGURE 10-5 Annular tear. Sagittal (**A**) and axial (**B**) T2-weighted magnetic resonance images show a high-intensity zone in the posterior annulus at C5-C6. This finding is compatible with an annular tear that may be responsible for the patient's diskogenic neck pain. (From Zebala LP, Buchowski JM, Daftary AR, et al: The cervical spine. In Khanna AJ, editor: *MRI for orthopaedic surgeons*, New York, 2010, Thieme, pp 229–268.)

abnormality is seen only posterior to the vertebral disk (in the absence of extrusion with migration) (Fig. 10-6). In contrast, stenosis in patients with ossification of the posterior longitudinal ligament is shown on MRI along the course of the posterior longitudinal ligament, not just posterior to the disk (Fig. 10-7). In patients with suspected ossification of the posterior longitudinal ligament, computed tomography (CT) imaging provides optimal visualization of calcification in the ligament and helps confirm this diagnosis.

Spinal Stenosis

General Description

Spinal stenosis can have congenital or acquired causes (Table 10-2). On MRI, central canal stenosis is characterized by focal or concentric compression of the thecal sac that is best seen on sagittal and axial T2-weighted images. The cerebrospinal fluid around the spinal cord produces a bright signal anterior and posterior to the cord on midsagittal images and circumferentially around the spinal cord on axial images. Parasagittal images allow for visualization of lateral recess and foraminal stenosis. The degree of central spinal canal stenosis can range from mild encroachment on the ventral subarachnoid space to severe compression and flattening of the spinal cord with myelomalacia. MRI findings may correspond to the severity and duration of the compression.[6] Acute spinal cord compression can produce spinal cord edema with high-signal areas on T2-weighted images. Progressive compression may trigger spinal cord atrophy (Fig. 10-8), cystic degeneration, and syrinx formation.[6]

Several objective measures of cervical spinal stenosis have been proposed. Relative stenosis and absolute stenosis of the spinal canal are defined as an anteroposterior canal diameter of less than 13 mm and 10 mm, respectively.[5] The Torg or Pavlov ratio is calculated by dividing the anteroposterior spinal canal diameter by the anteroposterior vertebral body diameter; a ratio of less than 0.8 is defined as stenotic.[13]

Occipitocervical Stenosis

Occipitocervical stenosis can occur secondary to developmental processes such as Arnold-Chiari malformation, congenital C1 and C2 dysplasias, or diseases such as rheumatoid arthritis (RA), Down syndrome, or tumors.[5] Relationships of the occipitocervical junction were originally defined using landmarks on conventional radiography (see Table 9-1). Many of these relationships have been extrapolated for use with MRI and are helpful for quantifying degree of basilar invagination and cranial settling.

Unique to MRI are the capabilities to visualize erosion of the dens or presence of a pannus and to measure the cervicomedullary angle. The cervicomedullary angle is a measurement of the angle created between the long axis of the brainstem and the spinal cord. A normal

Table 10-1 Intervertebral Disk Pathology	
Disk Pathology	**Magnetic Resonance Imaging Findings**
Bulge	Symmetric extension of annulus beyond the confines of adjacent end plates
Protrusion	Focal area of disk material that extends beyond vertebral margin but remains contained within the outer annular fibers
Extrusion	Herniation of nucleus pulposus beyond the confines of the annulus with disk attached to the remainder of nucleus pulposus by a narrow pedicle
Sequestration	Portion of disk fragment entirely separated from the parent disk

Modified from Khanna AJ, Carbone JJ, Kebaish KM, et al: Magnetic resonance imaging of the cervical spine. *J Bone Joint Surg Am* 84:70–80, 2002.

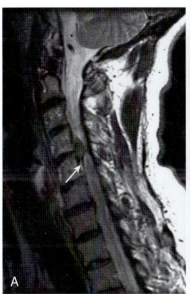 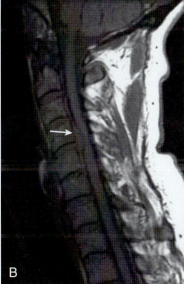 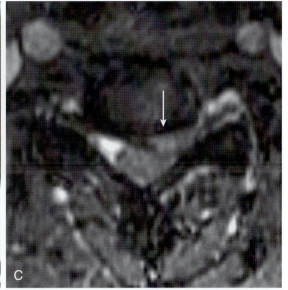

FIGURE 10-6 Cervical disk extrusion. **A,** A sagittal T2-weighted magnetic resonance image shows a large disk extrusion at the C4-C5 level (*arrow*) that has migrated proximally, tenting the posterior longitudinal ligament. **B,** A sagittal T1-weighted magnetic resonance image shows the disk extrusion at the C4-C5 level (*arrow*) that is isointense to the intervertebral disk. **C,** An axial T2-weighted magnetic resonance image shows a left paracentral disk extrusion (*arrow*) that produces severe foraminal stenosis and deformity on the left side of the spinal cord. (From Zebala LP, Buchowski JM, Daftary AR, et al: The cervical spine. In Khanna AJ, editor: *MRI for orthopaedic surgeons*, New York, 2010, Thieme, pp 229–268.)

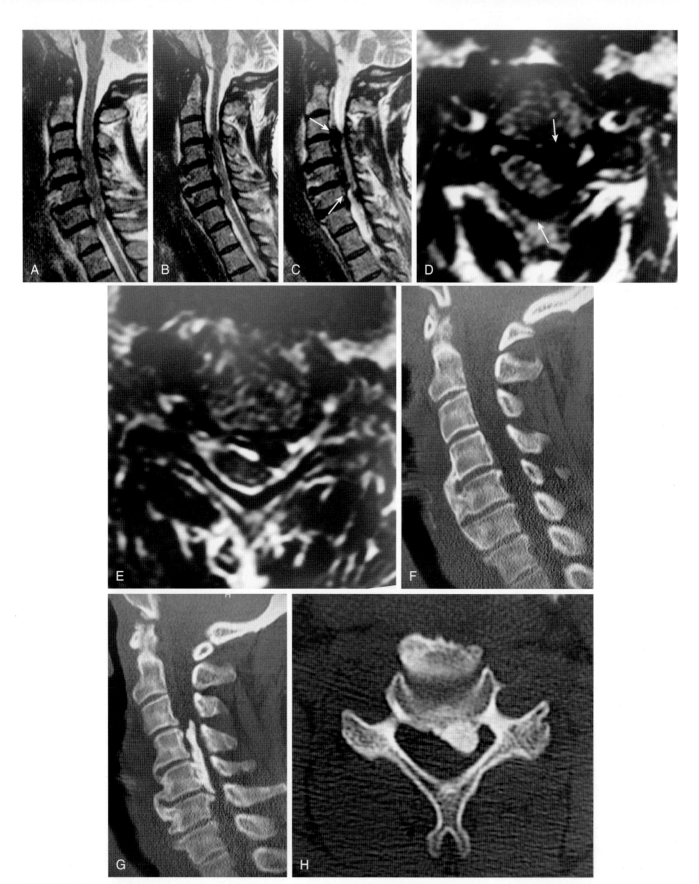

FIGURE 10-7 Ossification of the posterior longitudinal ligament. **A,** Midline sagittal T2-weighted magnetic resonance imaging (MRI) study shows multilevel degenerative disk disease and moderate stenosis from C3 and C4 to C6 and C7. The stenosis appears to be centered at the level of the disk spaces on this midline image. **B,** A parasagittal T2-weighted MRI study obtained a few millimeters lateral to the midline suggests that the posterior longitudinal ligament is thickened and that the stenosis is present at the level of the vertebral bodies and disks from C3 to C7. **C,** A parasagittal T2-weighted MRI study obtained farther from the midline shows that the posterior longitudinal ligament is markedly hypertrophied and nearly fills the spinal canal (*between arrows*). **D,** An axial T2-weighted MRI study shows severe left paracentral stenosis secondary to what appears to be a disk protrusion (*upper arrow*) but is actually a focal region of ossification of the posterior longitudinal ligament at the level of the C4 vertebral body. (The *lower arrow* is a pointer from the computer workstation and should be ignored.) **E,** An axial T2-weighted MRI study at the level of the C4-C5 disk shows similar findings. **F,** A sagittal reconstructed computed tomography (CT) image shows anterior osteophyte formation but no substantial spinal canal stenosis. **G,** A parasagittal reconstructed CT image (obtained at the same level as **C**) shows ossification of the posterior longitudinal ligament extending from C3 and C4 to C5 and C6. **H,** An axial CT image (obtained at the same level as **D**) shows that what appears to be a disk protrusion on MRI is actually a focal region of **ossification.** (From Zebala LP, Buchowski JM, Daftary AR, et al: The cervical spine. In Khanna AJ, editor: *MRI for orthopaedic surgeons,* New York, 2010, Thieme, pp 229–268.)

measurement ranges between 135 and 175 degrees. An angle of less than 135 degrees has been shown to have 100% correlation with neurologic symptoms.[14]

Chiari Malformations

Chiari malformations are associated with herniation of cerebellar tonsils through the foramen magnum with resultant

Table 10-2	Acquired and Congenital Factors Associated with Spinal Stenosis
Type	**Factor**
Acquired	Intervertebral disk disease
	Uncovertebral joint hypertrophy
	Facet joint hypertrophy
	Ligamentous (ligamentum flavum hypertrophy or ossification, ossification of the posterior longitudinal ligament, diffuse idiopathic skeletal hyperostosis)
	Spondylosis
	Metabolic conditions
	Postinflammatory status
	Spondylolisthesis
	Postoperative status
	Neoplastic disorders
Congenital	Idiopathic condition with short pedicles
	Skeletal growth disorders
	Down syndrome
	Achondroplasia
	Mucopolysaccharidosis
	Scoliosis

From Zebala LP, Buchowski JM, Daftary AR, et al: The cervical spine. In Khanna AJ, editor: *MRI for orthopaedic surgeons*, New York, 2010, Thieme, pp 229–268.

occipitocervical stenosis. Patients with advanced lesions that produce symptoms may benefit from suboccipital decompression. Three types of Chiari malformations have been described.[15,16] Type I is defined as a defect in the cerebellum with a downward displacement of the tonsils greater than 5 mm below the plane of the foramen magnum.[17,18] Type II involves herniation of the inferior cerebellar vermis, fourth ventricle, and medulla. Type III involves herniation of the hindbrain into a high cervical encephalocele.[5]

Rheumatoid Arthritis

RA is a systemic inflammatory disease of synovial joints that can produce occipitocervical stenosis (see the discussions of other RA MRI findings later and in Chapter 27). In the cervical spine, RA produces MRI-detectable erosions of C1 lateral masses, occipital condyles, and facets of C2. Consequently, as RA progresses, cranial settling occurs, and the odontoid process migrates rostrally; unlike with other disease entities, however, as cranial settling advances, the C1 arch migrates with the skull base caudally.[19] Two commonly cited studies reported on the use of MRI to measure the space available for the spinal cord as a technique for predicting recovery after cervical stabilization for patients with RA and atlantoaxial instability.[20,21] The investigators noted that a spinal cord space or space available for the cord of more than 14 mm on MRI was associated with better clinical outcomes and prognosis than was a space of less than 10 mm.

Trauma

Although the cervical spine is injured in only 2% to 3% of blunt trauma accidents,[1] the potential for catastrophic

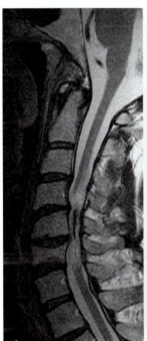
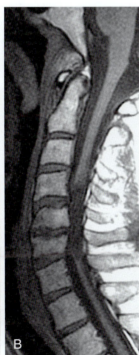
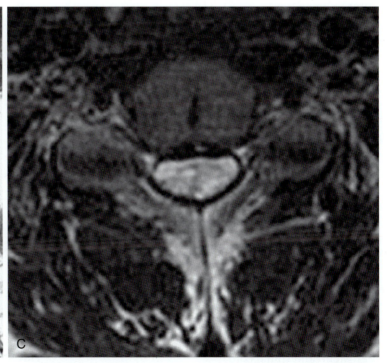

FIGURE 10-8 Spinal cord atrophy. **A,** A sagittal T2-weighted magnetic resonance image shows moderate to severe stenosis at C4 to C6 with resultant atrophy of the spinal cord at the level of C5 and regions of spinal cord edema proximal and distal to the region of atrophy. **B,** A sagittal T1-weighted magnetic resonance image shows a segment of low signal intensity within the spinal cord from C4 to C7. **C,** An axial T2-weighted magnetic resonance image at the level of C4 to C5 shows atrophy of the spinal cord and indistinct margins between the spinal cord and the surrounding cerebrospinal fluid. (From Zebala LP, Buchowski JM, Daftary AR, et al: The cervical spine. In Khanna AJ, editor: *MRI for orthopaedic surgeons*, New York, 2010, Thieme, pp 229–268.)

injury makes prompt identification paramount. However, MRI is not the initial examination of choice for cervical spine trauma; it is indicated specifically when neurologic deficit, vascular injury, or soft tissue injury is suspected.[22]

Currently, MRI is the most sensitive imaging technique for *soft tissue injuries* of the cervical spine.[22,23] Saltzherr and colleagues[22] reviewed several studies and reported that MRI is approximately half as sensitive as CT for osseous injuries. Consequently, MRI alone is not sufficient to clear the cervical spine, and it should be used as an adjunct to CT under the appropriate circumstances. MRI should be reserved for patients with unexplained neurologic symptoms and for the evaluation of extensive soft tissue injuries.

In high-risk patients (i.e., unconscious, sedated, intoxicated, or noncooperative patients or those with distracting injury), in whom an adequate neurologic examination is compromised, MRI can be considered when a CT scan shows injury.[22] In the setting of a normal CT scan in this patient population, clinicians may elect to use MRI, but its utility is debatable. No general consensus exists on the incidence and relevance of pure ligamentous injuries of the cervical spine. For example, Saltzherr and co-workers[22] reviewed the literature and reported an incidence of 0.04% to 0.6% of unstable ligamentous injuries without osseous defects. Another study, a retrospective review of 366 patients with normal CT scans, found that subsequent MRI detected no new unstable or other soft tissue injuries that required more than symptomatic treatment.[24] Conversely, an MRI scan that does not disclose anything abnormal can conclusively exclude cervical spine injury in a high-risk patient who has sustained blunt trauma.[23]

Therefore, MRI findings must be interpreted in conjunction with other available imaging modalities, including radiography and CT.

Blunt Trauma

Cervical spine injuries resulting from blunt trauma can be classified by location or mechanism.

Classification by Location

The occipitocervical junction, suboccipital cervical spine (C1-C2), and vertebral artery have unique injury patterns that deserve special mention. Injuries to the subaxial cervical spine (C3 to C7) are easier to characterize according to mechanism (see later).

Occipitocervical Junction Injuries. Atlanto-occipital dissociation is a devastating injury involving any separation of the atlanto-occipital articulation.[25-28] The primary injury is to the ligaments that provide structural support to the cervicocranial junction. MRI is the best modality for detecting injury to the cervicocranial ligaments (e.g., transverse, apical, cruciate, atlanto-occipital membrane and capsular ligaments, tectorial membrane), brainstem, and spinal cord.[29-31]

Suboccipital Cervical Spine (C1 and C2) Injuries. Axial load to the occipitocervical junction at the atlas may result in a Jefferson burst fracture seen on radiographs or CT scans and possible injury to the transverse ligament.[5] The axial T2-weighted images should be scrutinized for increased signal and regions of discontinuity representing injury along the course of the transverse ligament. According to Spence and associates,[32] a combined overhang of the lateral masses of C1 over C2 of 6.9 mm or more is associated with transverse ligament rupture and indicates an unstable burst fracture.

C2 is the most commonly fractured cervical spine level.[33] Once a fracture has been characterized by radiographs or CT scans, MRI can provide insight into the age of the fracture (acute versus chronic) to help guide treatment (Fig. 10-9). The sagittal and axial T2-weighted images can determine the extent of neural compression from a displaced fracture or underlying degenerative changes.[5]

The relationship of the axis and atlas is clearly visible with MRI. Specifically, the integrity of the transverse ligament and the condition of spinal cord can be evaluated, along with the approximate size of the anterior atlantodens interval.[31] This measurement is more frequently evaluated on flexion and extension lateral cervical spine radiographs.

Vertebral Artery Injury. Vertebral artery injury is associated with 11% of blunt cervical trauma,[34] and it

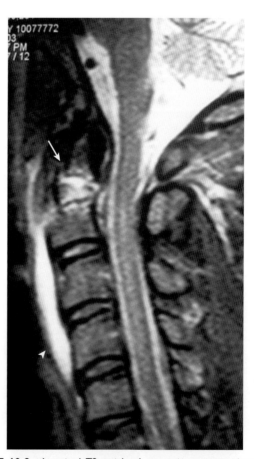

FIGURE 10-9 A sagittal T2-weighted magnetic resonance image of a type II odontoid fracture shows edema at the fracture site (*arrow*), indicating an acute or subacute fracture. Note the prevertebral edema or hematoma (*arrowhead*). (From Zebala LP, Buchowski JM, Daftary AR, et al: The cervical spine. In Khanna AJ, editor: *MRI for orthopaedic surgeons*, New York, 2010, Thieme, pp 229–268.)

usually results from cervical spine fractures extending into the transverse foramen or from unilateral or bilateral facet dislocations.[30,35] Magnetic resonance angiography may be used to assess vertebral artery patency in the setting of these injuries. Bowen and associates[36] described a signal void on axial T2-weighted images and bright signal on gradient-echo images created by flowing blood. The types of vertebral artery injuries are thrombosis, dissection, and transection. According to Zebala and colleagues,[5] "MR angiography shows vertebral artery thrombosis as the absence of flow-related enhancement on images in the expected course of the vertebral artery; dissections as a tapering of the vessel; and transections as a focal discontinuity of the vessel" (Fig. 10-10).

Classification by Mechanism

The classification of traumatic cervical spine injury according to mechanism can be simplified into three categories: hyperflexion, hyperextension, and axial loading.

Hyperflexion. Hyperflexion injuries produce compression of the anterior elements of the spinal column and reciprocal distraction of the posterior elements. The severity of flexion-compression injuries anteriorly ranges from minor impaction of the anterosuperior end plate (Fig. 10-11) to severe quadrangular vertebral body fractures with end plate compression producing kyphosis. Flexion-distraction forces posteriorly can lead to facet subluxations, dislocations, or fracture-dislocations that are associated with a spectrum of osteoligamentous abnormalities. Unlike conventional radiographs and CT scans, MRI can detect spinal cord compression from retrolisthesis, as well as posterior element compromise in the setting of circumferential soft tissue disruption. MRI can assess the integrity of the posterior musculature, interspinous ligaments, ligamentum flavum, and facet capsules that are often compromised with flexion-distraction injuries.[37] Facet joint injuries and capsule tears are best seen on parasagittal or axial images that

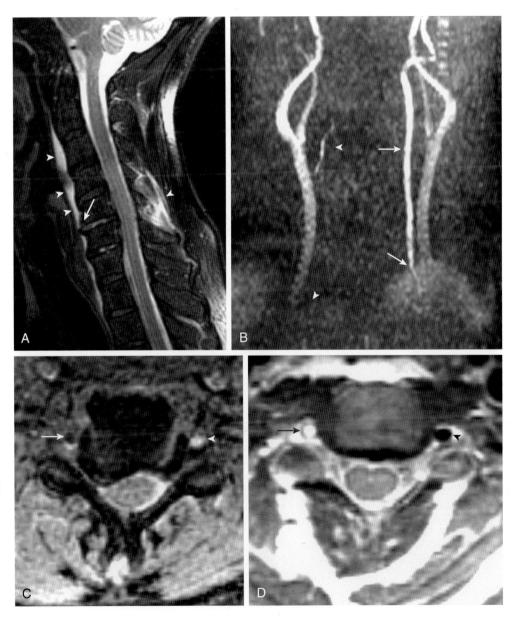

FIGURE 10-10 Vertebral artery injury after unilateral interfacetal dislocation at C5 to C6 without spinal cord injury. **A,** A sagittal T2-weighted magnetic resonance image shows an injured disk at C5-C6 with increased signal intensity in the disk and probably avulsion of the anterior longitudinal ligament (*arrow*). Prevertebral edema (*small arrowheads*) and edema in the posterior paraspinal musculature (*single arrowhead*) are present. **B,** A magnetic resonance image (anterior view) from a two-dimensional time-of-flight acquisition shows absence of signal intensity in the expected course of the right vertebral artery (*arrowheads*). Note the course of the normal course of the left vertebral artery (*arrows*). **C,** An axial magnetic resonance image from a three-dimensional gradient-echo acquisition shows an oval area of low signal intensity in the right foramen transversarium (*arrow*) corresponding to a thrombus in the right vertebral artery. Note the normal flow-related enhancement in the left foramen transversarium (*arrowhead*). **D,** An axial fast spin-echo magnetic resonance image obtained at a similar level to that in **C** shows a high-signal-intensity thrombus (*arrow*) in the right foramen transversarium, indicative of a thrombosed vertebral artery. Note the normal flow void of the left vertebral artery in the left foramen transversarium (*arrowhead*). (From Torina PJ, Flanders AE, Carrino JA, et al: Incidence of vertebral artery thrombosis in cervical spine trauma: correlation with severity of spinal cord injury. *AJNR Am J Neuroradiol* 26:2645–2651, 2005.)

show surrounding increased signal on T2-weighted images secondary to edema.[1,10,30,31] Injury to posterior elements is easiest to detect as areas of hyperintensity on fat-suppressed T2-weighted or short tau inversion recovery images (Fig. 10-12).

The role of MRI in the acute setting for patients with bilateral cervical facet dislocations without neurologic compromise is controversial[24,37,38] (Fig. 10-13). Some clinicians advocate obtaining an MRI scan before attempting closed reduction or surgery to rule out the possibility of extruded disk that could theoretically displace into the spinal canal with manipulation (Fig. 10-14). Other clinicians attempt with closed reduction while monitoring the patient's neurologic examination and then proceed with surgical stabilization.[24,37,38]

Hyperextension. Cervical spine hyperextension injuries (typically produced by rear-impact motor vehicle collisions or direct facial injuries that create distraction across the anterior elements and compression posteriorly) result in the posterior translation or rotation of a vertebral body in the sagittal plane.[31,39,40] Findings on MRI can include anterior longitudinal ligament tears, intervertebral disk avulsion from an adjacent vertebrae, and horizontal intervertebral disk rupture (Fig. 10-15).[10,30,31,39,40] Additional findings that may suggest an unstable hyperextension injury include prevertebral hematoma, disk space widening, posterior ligament complex edema, and a herniated disk.[39] In the elderly patient with preexisting narrowing of the spinal canal from posterior vertebral osteophytes, spinal cord injury may occur with posterior infolding of the ligamentum flavum alone, and without vertebral fracture or ligamentous injury.

Intervertebral disk abnormality, such as acute annular tears and disk herniation secondary to hyperextension injury, can be detected by MRI. However, multiple investigators have shown that annular tears can be seen in asymptomatic individuals,[9,41,42] so distinguishing between acute tears and preexisting chronic tears can be challenging. Intervertebral disk separation from an adjacent vertebral body may be seen as a horizontal hyperintense T2-weighted signal.[10,30,31] Subtle fractures, such as end plate fractures, are best visualized with MRI because it can detect osseous edema and hemorrhage.[10,30,31]

In the absence of neurologic findings, whiplash injuries often have no associated injury on imaging studies, and MRI has limited benefit.[1,43] However, in patients with a fused spine secondary to ankylosing spondylitis or diffuse idiopathic skeletal hyperostosis, MRI may reveal subtle fractures, instability, or neurologic compromise.[44]

Axial Load. Axial loads are transmitted through the occipital condyles and into the spine; this process can cause burst fractures of the subaxial cervical spine. MRI findings include lateral mass displacement on coronal images, atlantodental interval increase on sagittal images, and transverse ligament disruption on axial images.[31] Although pure axial forces do not injure the posterior spinal elements, a degree of flexion during

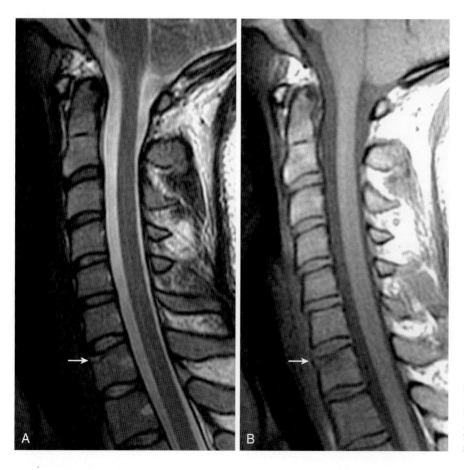

FIGURE 10-11 C7 vertebral compression fracture. Sagittal T2-weighted (**A**) and T1-weighted (**B**) magnetic resonance images show the fracture (*arrow* on each) with minimal loss of height. (From Zebala LP, Buchowski JM, Daftary AR, et al: The cervical spine. In Khanna AJ, editor: *MRI for orthopaedic surgeons*, New York, 2010, Thieme, pp 229–268.)

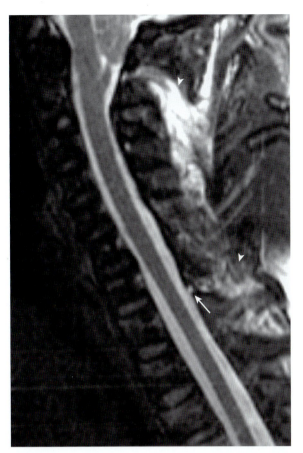

FIGURE 10-12   A sagittal short tau inversion recovery image shows edema in the supraspinous ligament region (*arrowhead*) and interspinous region at C6 to C7 and C7 to T1, with a small, focal region of increased T2-weighted signal in the ligamentum flavum at the level of C7 to T1 (*arrow*) compatible with a partial tear. (From Zebala LP, Buchowski JM, Daftary AR, et al: The cervical spine. In Khanna AJ, editor: *MRI for orthopaedic surgeons,* New York, 2010, Thieme, pp 229–268.)

the traumatic event can introduce injury to the posterior spinal elements.[40] The clinician must scrutinize the fat-suppressed T2-weighted images for evidence of posterior ligamentous and osseous injury that may alter treatment. With burst fractures, it is important to assess axial images for any violation of the spinal canal and for evidence of retropulsion from a compromised posterior vertebral wall.[5]

Penetrating Trauma

Penetrating injuries of the cervical spine can be divided into two broad categories: ballistic injuries and impaling or stabbing injuries. Ballistic mechanisms can injure the spine by direct penetration, displacement into the spinal canal of bone fragments that compress the spinal cord, or blast effect. In this setting, the myelographic effect of cerebrospinal fluid on T2-weighted MRI scans is useful for assessing the degree of bone fragment displacement and compression into the spinal cord in the spinal canal. Intramedullary signal on T2-weighted images can represent edema from the blast effect of an acute ballistics insult, but radiographs and CT scans are better at characterizing osseous injuries produced by penetrating projectiles. Imaging spinal ballistics injuries with MRI is controversial because of the theoretical risk that embedded mobile ferrous gunshot or missile fragments in proximity to the spinal cord could migrate during image acquisition.[45,46]

Impaling or stabbing injuries generally produce primarily soft tissue damage. The osseous architecture of the spine usually protects the spinal cord, thus deflecting the impaling object into the paraspinal tissues. MRI is useful for assessing the specific location and extent of soft tissue damage, particularly on T2-weighted sequences, which show edema and inflammation after an acute impaling injury.

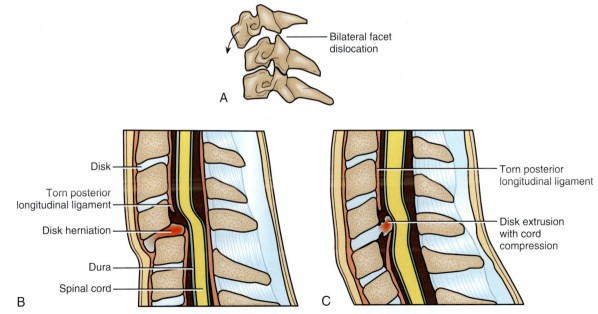

FIGURE 10-13   Artist's sketches illustrating the pathologic processes in bilateral facet dislocation. **A,** A lateral view of osseous structures shows that the facets are perched and that additional translation will lead to complete dislocation. **B,** A lateral view before reduction shows approximately 50% translation of the superior vertebral body relative to the inferior vertebral body and displacement of the intervertebral disk. **C,** A lateral view after reduction shows that the intervertebral disk has displaced into the spinal canal and compressed the spinal cord during the reduction maneuver. (Redrawn from Zebala LP, Buchowski JM, Daftary AR, et al: The cervical spine. In Khanna AJ, editor: *MRI for orthopaedic surgeons,* New York, 2010, Thieme, pp 229–268.)

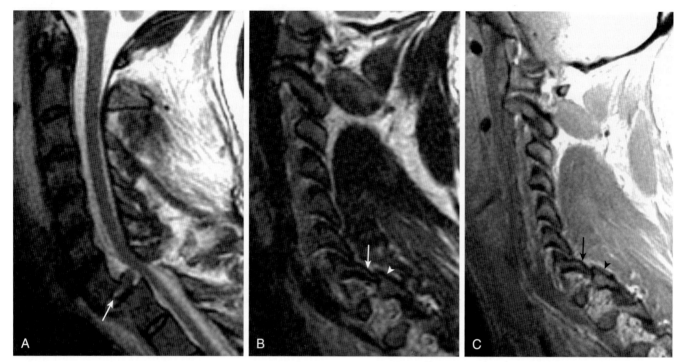

FIGURE 10-14   Bilateral cervical facet dislocation. **A,** A sagittal T2-weighted magnetic resonance image shows anterior translation of C7 over T1 with an associated disk extrusion (*arrow*) and spinal cord compression. Parasagittal T2-weighted (**B**) and gradient-echo (**C**) magnetic resonance images showing the inferior articular process of C7 (*arrow*) displaced anterior to the superior articular process of T1 (*arrowhead*). (From Zebala LP, Buchowski JM, Daftary AR, et al: The cervical spine. In Khanna AJ, editor: *MRI for orthopaedic surgeons,* New York, 2010, Thieme, pp 229–268.)

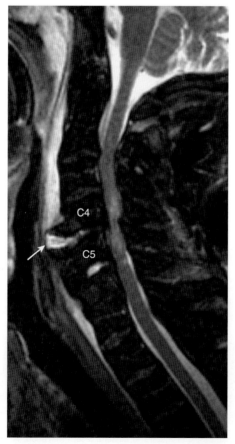

FIGURE 10-15   A sagittal short tau inversion recovery image shows an intervertebral disk rupture at C4-C5 (*arrow*) in a patient who sustained a hyperextension injury to the cervical spine. Note the associated prevertebral hematoma and the severe stenosis with associated spinal cord signal change. (From Zebala LP, Buchowski JM, Daftary AR, et al: The cervical spine. In Khanna AJ, editor: *MRI for orthopaedic surgeons,* New York, 2010, Thieme, pp 229–268.)

Infectious Conditions

MRI is the imaging modality of choice for the diagnosis and evaluation of spinal infections and for monitoring treatment response.[47]

Cervical Vertebral Osteomyelitis and Diskitis

MRI has been described as having a sensitivity of 96%, a specificity of 93%, and accuracy of 94% for the diagnosis of vertebral osteomyelitis,[48] and it is reported to be more sensitive than radiographs or CT and more specific than nuclear scintigraphy for this diagnosis.[47] According to Zebala and co-workers,[5] infectious spondylitis is indicated by the following MRI findings: "low T1-weighted signal with or without high T2-weighted signal; increased T2-weighted signal within the intervertebral disc; contrast enhancement in the disc, subchondral marrow, and epidural space; erosion of end plates; epidural fluid collections; paraspinous soft tissue abnormalities; and posterior element involvement" (Fig. 10-16). Isolated diskitis is common in the pediatric population, but in adults, with their differing patterns of vascularity, bacteria cannot access the disk as readily, and infection is usually limited to vertebral body metaphysis and end plates. In adult vertebral infections, bacteria affect intervertebral disk destruction through bacterial proteolytic enzyme infiltration from adjacent vertebral end plates.

The nonspecific features of infection can be difficult to distinguish from other spinal processes such as neoplasm. However, the epicenter of infectious abnormality of the spine tends to be the intervertebral disk, whereas neoplastic processes tend to originate within the vertebral body, and edema usually does not cross the adjacent intervertebral disks. As infection advances, it erodes the vertebral end plates, and disk height loss or collapse occurs. Moreover, gadolinium enhancement of the disk is evident in diskitis, and edema of adjacent vertebral subchondral bone suggests chronic infection.[10,47,49]

Some spinal infections such as tuberculosis have distinct features. With *Mycobacterium tuberculosis* infection, disk destruction is less severe compared with that seen in other infections.[47] Tuberculous spondylodiskitis is a slow-growing process that results in the collapse of the vertebral body, and telescoping of one vertebral body disk into an adjacent level may be seen. Contiguous subligamentous spread of tuberculosis is often observed.[5]

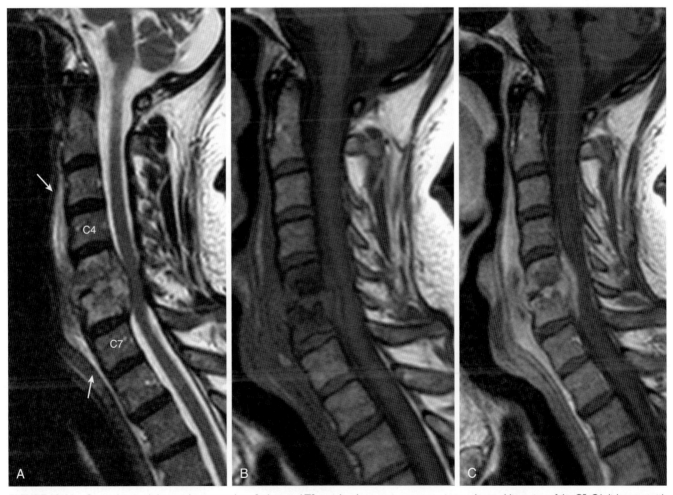

FIGURE 10-16   Cervical spine diskitis and osteomyelitis. **A,** A sagittal T2-weighted magnetic resonance image shows obliteration of the C5-C6 disk space with associated edema in the C5 and C6 vertebral bodies and an associated epidural component, which produces moderate spinal stenosis in a patient with infectious symptoms and findings. Note the prevertebral edema and soft tissue fullness (between *arrows*). Pregadolinium (**B**) and postgadolinium (**C**) T1-weighted magnetic resonance images show enhancement at the disk space, in the vertebral body's epidural component, and in the prevertebral space. (From Zebala LP, Buchowski JM, Daftary AR, et al: The cervical spine. In Khanna AJ, editor: *MRI for orthopaedic surgeons*, New York, 2010, Thieme, pp 229–268.)

Gadolinium-enhanced MRI is essential for monitoring the efficacy of treatment for spinal infection.[50] Regression of T2-weighted signal hyperintensity suggests resolution of the infection.[49] The sequelae of infection can include scar development, osteophytic bridging, or fusion.[49]

Infection in the postoperative patient is more difficult to determine with MRI. Signs of disk enhancement can occur in an uninfected disk in the postoperative setting and are therefore unreliable markers of infection. Consequently, MRI should be scrutinized for other findings of infection such as subchondral bone and marrow enhancement after contrast administration.[47] Bone graft usually has a high T2-weighted signal during the first postoperative year. With vascularization and fusion of the graft, the signal gradually declines.[47] According to Ruiz and associates,[47] an enhancing mass adjacent to the graft or graft dislodgement is concerning for potential infection.

Epidural Abscess

MRI is the diagnostic study of choice for the diagnosis of an epidural abscess.[10,47,49] A spinal epidural abscess is a collection of purulent infectious material that forms outside the dura mater, often immediately adjacent to vertebral osteomyelitis.[47] Most commonly, the C4 to C7 levels are involved.[47] Gadolinium-enhanced, fat-suppressed, T1-weighted images provide anatomic detail of location and extension of abscess and highlight any associated vertebral infections.[47] The gadolinium enhancement pattern varies from a thin peripheral pattern representing a collection of liquefied pus to a homogeneous pattern seen with phlegmon. T2-weighted images are scrutinized for associated spinal cord compression.

Intradural Infection

Intradural infections include subdural abscesses, leptomeningitis, and myelitis. Subdural abscesses are seen on gadolinium-enhanced MRI as peripheral enhancing intradural-extramedullary abscesses next to a compressed spinal cord. Associated T2-weighted images show a relative increase in signal intensity of the spinal cord, secondary to compression or myelitis, compared with the adjacent normal parenchyma. In patients with severe compression, a T2-weighted image can distinguish an epidural from an intradural abscess. Leptomeningeal infections affect the meninges or the peripheral covering of the spinal cord, and gadolinium-enhanced MRI can show abnormal meningeal enhancement on the surface of the cord or roots.[51] Myelitis directly involves the spinal cord. Early spinal cord infection shows increased T2-weighted signal and poor enhancement with gadolinium.[47,49] With progression of the infection, cavitation (seen as areas of low signal intensity on T2-weighted images and high signal intensity on T2-weighted images) can develop. Furthermore, myelitis generates edema and a concomitant increase in the size of the spinal cord.

Other Pathologic Conditions

Intrinsic Inflammatory Myelopathies

Although surgeons typically do not treat intrinsic inflammatory myelopathies, they should be able to differentiate them from myelopathy secondary to extrinsic compression. Multiple sclerosis can produce plaques in the spinal cord that usually span one or two vertebral levels, occupying less than half the spinal cord diameter, usually along the periphery.[52] MRI characteristics include increased signal on T2-weighted images, decreased signal on T1-weighted images, patchy spinal cord enhancement with gadolinium enhancement, and spinal cord swelling or atrophy with larger plaques (Fig. 10-17).[52] Acute transverse myelopathy is a monophasic, acute inflammatory condition of the entire spinal cord, and the MRI findings are variable. MRI may show areas of hyperintensity of various lengths and widths on T2-weighted images and usually involving three or four spinal segments.[53] Subacute necrotizing myelopathy is a rare progressive myelopathy that occurs in elderly persons. It is often attributed to spinal dural arteriovenous fistula, and it produces venous congestion, ischemia, and infarction of the spinal cord. MRI typically reveals a long segment of fusiform spinal cord swelling and edema with peripheral contrast enhancement.[54] Patients with acquired immunodeficiency syndrome commonly have human immunodeficiency virus myelitis and vacuolar myelopathy; T2-weighted MRI images of such patients reveal spinal cord atrophy and symmetric hyperintense focal lesions in the dorsal and lateral columns, but no cord swelling or enhancement.[55] Viral, bacterial, parasitic, and granulomatous diseases produce variable MRI findings, including spinal cord swelling, cord edema, rim-enhancing lesions, and nerve enhancement or clumping or both, depending on the offending organism.[54] Metabolic conditions, such as vitamin B_{12} deficiency or nitrous oxide poisoning, can be complicated by subacute combined degeneration, which can cause increased signal on MRI in the dorsal and lateral columns on T2-weighted images along with demyelination, gliosis, and axonal loss.[54] Finally, radiation myelopathy is a progressive process produced by spinal cord necrosis, demyelination, and gliosis; the corresponding MRI findings are spinal cord swelling, edema, and contrast enhancement.[56]

Arthritides

MRI provides specific findings that facilitate the selection of one or two entities from the differential diagnoses of arthritides that affect the spine, including RA, ankylosing spondylitis, juvenile RA, psoriatic arthritis, amyloidosis, gout, and calcium pyrophosphate deposition disease.[57] By itself, MRI is not diagnostic of any particular arthritides.

RA is the most common inflammatory arthropathy, and the cervical spine is the most common area of RA spinal involvement.[57] Juvenile RA is the most common connective tissue disorder in children.[57] MRI is useful for the evaluation of the craniocervical junction and for the assessment of atlantoaxial and subaxial subluxation, basilar invagination, and spinal cord compression in RA and juvenile RA (Fig. 10-18).[57,58] MRI depicts the extent of periodontoid pannus formation (and atlantoaxial instability), associated odontoid process fractures, nodular fibrosis, and perivertebral erosions.[57] The space-occupying effect of the periodontoid pannus can be visualized clearly on MRI, well before conventional radiographic signs become evident. MRI is considered highly specific for RA and may clarify the diagnosis in otherwise

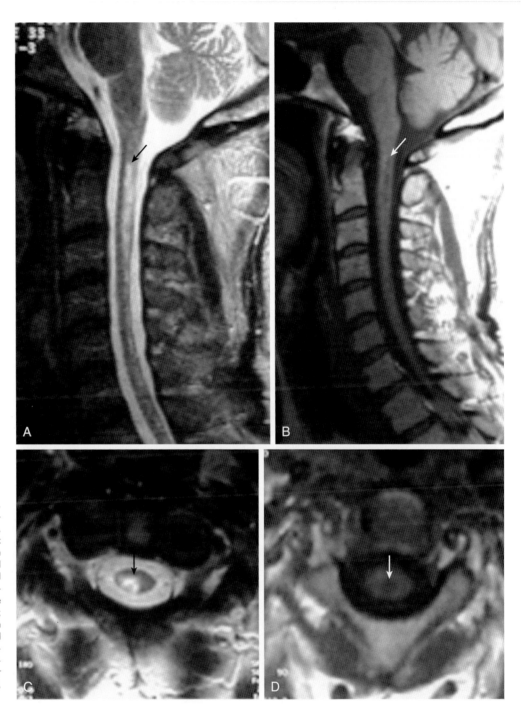

FIGURE 10-17 Multiple sclerosis. Sagittal T2-weighted (**A**), sagittal T1-weighted (**B**), axial T2-weighted (**C**), and axial T1-weighted (**D**) magnetic resonance images show a focal region of increased (**A** and **C**) and decreased (**B** and **D**) signal within the spinal cord (*arrow* on each). In the appropriate clinical setting, these findings are compatible with multiple sclerosis; the diagnosis can be confirmed with lumbar puncture and cerebrospinal fluid analysis. (From Zebala LP, Buchowski JM, Daftary AR, et al: The cervical spine. In Khanna AJ, editor: *MRI for orthopaedic surgeons*, New York, 2010, Thieme, pp 229–268.)

nonspecific cases.[59] Rheumatoid diskitis that manifests as increased T2-weighted and decreased T1-weighted signal in the disk may also be noted. In addition, facet joint involvement (inflammation, edema, and fusion) may be detected on MRI. The cervicomedullary angle can be measured on MRI by drawing a line along the anterior aspect of the cervical spinal cord and the medulla. This angle normally is between 135 and 175 degrees. With progressive craniocervical disease in RA, the brainstem angulates ventrally over the displaced odontoid process, thus leading to increased obliquity of the cervicomedullary angle. One study reported a 100% correlation between a cervicomedullary angle of less than 135 degrees and neurologic

signs of cervicomedullary compression, myelopathy, or C2 radiculopathy.[14]

The use of flexion-extension MRI for evaluating patients with RA, and specifically those with instability at the occipitocervical junction and suboccipital cervical spine, is controversial (Fig. 10-19).[57,60,61] A theoretical advantage is the ability to identify, when the patient is in the neutral position, potentially clinically significant dynamic spinal cord compression before static compression is apparent. One study suggested that a spinal cord diameter in cervical flexion of less than 6 mm is a risk factor for neurologic deficit.[60] However, a theoretical risk of sudden death exists as a result of prolonged cervical

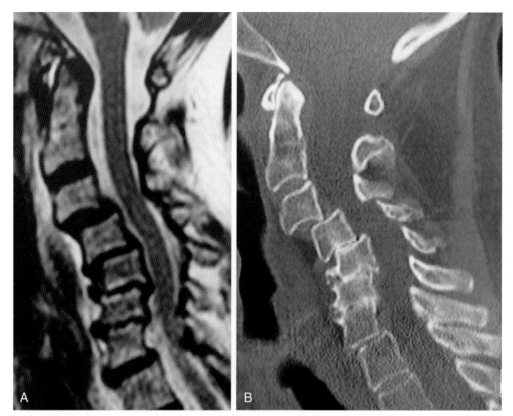

FIGURE 10-18 Subaxial subluxation in rheumatoid arthritis. Sagittal T2-weighted magnetic resonance **(A)** and sagittal reconstructed computed tomography **(B)** images show multilevel subaxial subluxation and degenerative disk disease. Specifically, spondylolisthesis is noted at C3 to C4 and C4 to C5 and retrolisthesis at C5 to C6. Note the improved osseous detail provided by the computed tomography image. (From Zebala LP, Buchowski JM, Daftary AR, et al: The cervical spine. In Khanna AJ, editor: *MRI for orthopaedic surgeons,* New York, 2010, Thieme, pp 229–268.)

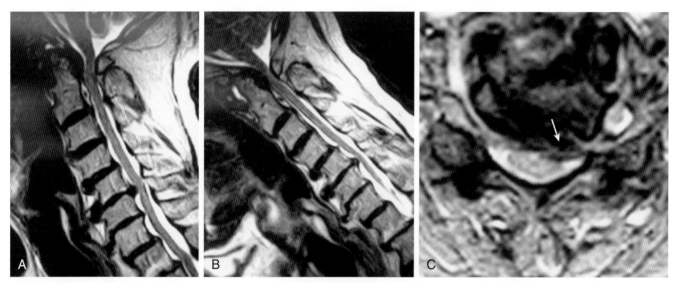

FIGURE 10-19 Occipitocervical stenosis. **A,** A sagittal T2-weighted magnetic resonance image obtained with the patient in neutral position shows moderate stenosis at the occipitocervical junction and at the level of C5 to C6. Multilevel degenerative disk disease is also seen. **B,** A sagittal T2-weighted magnetic resonance image in flexion shows exacerbation of the occipitocervical stenosis to severe. **C,** An axial T2-weighted magnetic resonance image at the level of C5 to C6 shows moderate stenosis at this level from degenerative changes and a left paracentral disk protrusion (*arrow*). (From Zebala LP, Buchowski JM, Daftary AR, et al: The cervical spine. In Khanna AJ, editor: *MRI for orthopaedic surgeons,* New York, 2010, Thieme, pp 229–268.)

flexion in a patient with severe instability; therefore, the recommendation for routine dynamic MRI in these patients may change.[58]

Psoriatic arthritis may manifest with cervical spine disease before skin lesions. MRI findings may reveal disk space narrowing and erosions of the apophyseal joints, vertebral end plates, and spinous processes.[5] On MRI, the atlantoaxial damage in patients with psoriatic arthritis is indistinguishable from that in patients with RA.[57]

MRI is useful for the evaluation of the early development of ankylosing spondylitis. MRI can detect acute nondisplaced fractures of the ankylosed spine (often missed on radiographs), pseudarthrosis, advanced degenerative changes, vertebral body subluxations, epidural hematoma, spinal cord compression, and deformity.[57]

Amyloidosis is characterized by extracellular deposition of insoluble fibrillar proteins throughout the body.[57] The dialysis-associated form, β_2-microglobulin, can cause destructive spondyloarthropathy of the cervical spine.[62] Findings in amyloid arthritis can mimic those of degenerative change. On MRI, amyloid deposits exhibit low signal intensity and have variable enhancement patterns with gadolinium.[57]

Gout rarely involves the spine. Gouty tophi on MRI are of intermediate signal intensity on T1-weighted images and of variable intensity on T2-weighted sequences. Calcium pyrophosphate dihydrate deposition disease occasionally involves the spine, with deposition in the intervertebral disks or ligaments. Relative to brain tissue, calcium pyrophosphate dihydrate deposition appears as an isointense or hypointense signal on T1-weighted images, has mixed signal intensity on T2-weighted images, and shows marked peripheral enhancement with gadolinium.[57] Sometimes calcification can surround the dens, which produces a characteristic "crowned dens" sign.[5]

Tumors

MRI is an effective technique for imaging spinal tumors. Through clinical history, physical examination, and MRI findings, a reasonable differential diagnosis of the tumor can be established.[3] MRI provides unparalleled soft tissue detail, assesses the extent of spinal cord compression, and reveals tissue characteristics of the tumor (e.g., vascularity, density, vascular perfusion, extent of marrow involvement). Spinal tumors are categorized by anatomic location as extradural, intradural-extramedullary, and intramedullary.[63] When a tumor is suspected, the entire spine should be screened for skip lesions, multiple primary sites, or a syrinx.[5] Contrast enhancement is beneficial for increasing the detection of most intramedullary and intradural-extramedullary tumors.[3] However, gadolinium enhancement may obscure the contrast between metastatic lesions and normal bone marrow if fat suppression is not applied.[64] With the exception of osseous tumors, in which gradient-echo imaging can reveal areas of calcification or hemorrhage, gradient-echo images have limited utility in imaging spinal cord tumors.[64]

Conclusions

Understanding the MRI features of certain pathologic processes and integrating that knowledge with other imaging modalities and clinical information can be challenging. Nonetheless, cervical spine MRI has revolutionized the spinal surgeon's ability to diagnose and treat cervical spine disease. T1-weighted images are best for anatomic detail. T2-weighted images, in particular fat-suppressed images, are excellent for identifying disease. MRI has been instrumental in evaluation of symptomatic cervical spine degeneration and guidance of surgical treatment.

Symptomatic disk herniation and spinal stenosis with spinal cord impingement can be readily identified. In the setting of trauma, MRI is reserved for unexplained neurologic injuries and extensive soft tissue damage and for excluding cervical spine injury in the high-risk trauma patient. Infectious conditions such as vertebral osteomyelitis and epidural abscess are readily diagnosed by MRI. Many arthritides such as RA have unique MRI features that aid in treatment and characterization of the disease. Finally, MRI is important in the differential diagnosis of spinal tumors.

REFERENCES

1. Kaiser J A, Holland B A: Imaging of the cervical spine, *Spine (Phila Pa 1976)* 23:2701–2712, 1998.
2. Lejay H, Holland B A: Technical advances in musculoskeletal imaging. In Stoller DW, editor: *Magnetic resonance imaging in orthopaedics and sports medicine*, ed 3, Baltimore, 2007, Lippincott Williams & Wilkins, pp 1–28.
3. Khanna A J, Carbone J J, Kebaish K M, et al.: Magnetic resonance imaging of the cervical spine: current techniques and spectrum of disease, *J Bone Joint Surg Am* 84:70–80, 2002.
4. Laiho K, Soini I, Kauppi M: Magnetic resonance imaging of the rheumatic cervical spine, *J Bone Joint Surg Am* 85:2482, 2003. author reply 2483.
5. Zebala L P, Buchowski J M, Daftary A R, et al.: The cervical spine. In Khanna A J, editor: *MRI for orthopaedic surgeons*, New York, 2010, Thieme, pp 229–268.
6. Boutin R D, Steinbach L S, Finnesey K: MR imaging of degenerative diseases in the cervical spine, *Magn Reson Imaging Clin N Am* 8:471–489, 2000.
7. Uhlenbrock D: Degenerative disorders of the spine. In Uhlenbrock D, editor: *MR imaging of the spine and spinal cord*, New York, 2004, Thieme, pp 159–268.
8. Matsumoto M, Fujimura Y, Suzuki N, et al.: MRI of cervical intervertebral discs in asymptomatic subjects, *J Bone Joint Surg Br* 80:19–24, 1998.
9. Boden S D, Davis D O, Dina T S, et al.: Abnormal magnetic-resonance scans of the lumbar spine in asymptomatic subjects: a prospective investigation, *J Bone Joint Surg Am* 72:403–408, 1990.
10. Boden S D, Lee R R, Herzog R J: Magnetic resonance imaging of the spine. In Frymoyer JW, editor: *The adult spine: principles and practice*, ed 2, Philadelphia, 1997, Lippincott-Raven, pp 563–629.
11. Boos N, Weissbach S, Rohrbach H, et al.: Classification of age-related changes in lumbar intervertebral discs: 2002 Volvo Award in basic science, *Spine (Phila Pa 1976)* 27:2631–2644, 2002.
12. Mercer S, Bogduk N: The ligaments and annulus fibrosus of human adult cervical intervertebral discs, *Spine (Phila Pa 1976)* 24:619–626, 1999. discussion 627–628.
13. Pavlov H, Torg J S, Robie B, Jahre C: Cervical spinal stenosis: determination with vertebral body ratio method, *Radiology* 164:771–775, 1987.
14. Bundschuh C, Modic M T, Kearney F, et al.: Rheumatoid arthritis of the cervical spine: surface-coil MR imaging, *AJR Am J Roentgenol* 151:181–187, 1988.
15. Batzdorf U: Pathogenesis and development theories. In Anson J A, Benzel E C, Awad I A, editors: *Syringomyelia and the Chiari malformations*, Park Ridge, Ill, 1997, American Association of Neurological Surgeons, pp 35–40.
16. Schenk M, Ruggieri P M: Imaging of syringomyelia and the Chiari malformations. In Anson J A, Benzel E C, Awad I A, editors: *Syringomyelia and the Chiari malformations*, Park Ridge, Ill, 1997, American Association of Neurological Surgeons, pp 41–56.
17. Aboulezz A O, Sartor K, Geyer C A, Gado M H: Position of cerebellar tonsils in the normal population and in patients with Chiari malformation: a quantitative approach with MR imaging, *J Comput Assist Tomogr* 9:1033–1036, 1985.
18. Barkovich A J, Wippold F J, Sherman J L, Citrin C M: Significance of cerebellar tonsillar position on MR, *AJNR Am J Neuroradiol* 7:795–799, 1986.
19. Smoker W R K: MR imaging of the craniovertebral junction, *Magn Reson Imaging Clin N Am* 8:635–650, 2000.

20. Boden S D: Rheumatoid arthritis of the cervical spine: surgical decision making based on predictors of paralysis and recovery, *Spine (Phila Pa 1976)* 19:2275–2280, 1994.

21. Boden S D, Dodge L D, Bohlman H H, Rechtine G R: Rheumatoid arthritis of the cervical spine: a long-term analysis with predictors of paralysis and recovery, *J Bone Joint Surg Am* 75:1282–1297, 1993.

22. Saltzherr T P, Fung Kon Jin P H, Beenen L F, et al.: Diagnostic imaging of cervical spine injuries following blunt trauma: a review of the literature and practical guideline, *Injury* 40:795–800, 2009.

23. Muchow R D, Resnick D K, Abdel M P, et al.: Magnetic resonance imaging (MRI) in the clearance of the cervical spine in blunt trauma: a meta-analysis, *J Trauma* 64:179–189, 2008.

24. Lee J Y, Nassr A, Eck J C, Vaccaro A R: Controversies in the treatment of cervical spine dislocations, *Spine J* 9:418–423, 2009.

25. Adams V I: Neck injuries: I. Occipitoatlantal dislocation: a pathologic study of twelve traffic fatalities, *J Forensic Sci* 37:556–564, 1992.

26. Adams V I: Neck injuries: III. Ligamentous injuries of the craniocervical articulation without occipito-atlantal or atlanto-axial facet dislocation: a pathologic study of 21 traffic fatalities, *J Forensic Sci* 38:1097–1104, 1993.

27. Ahuja A, Glasauer F E, Alker G J Jr, Klein D M: Radiology in survivors of traumatic atlanto-occipital dislocation, *Surg Neurol* 41:112–118, 1994.

28. Alker G J Jr, Oh Y S, Leslie E V: High cervical spine and craniocervical junction injuries in fatal traffic accidents: a radiological study, *Orthop Clin North Am* 9:1003–1010, 1978.

29. Goldberg A L, Baron B, Daffner R H: Atlantooccipital dislocation: MR demonstration of cord damage, *J Comput Assist Tomogr* 15:174–175, 1991.

30. Mirvis S E: Use of MRI in acute spinal trauma. In Uhlenbrock D, editor: *MR imaging of the spine and spinal cord*, New York, 2004, Thieme, pp 437–465.

31. Takhtani D, Melhem E R: MR imaging in cervical spine trauma, *Magn Reson Imaging Clin N Am* 8:615–634, 2000.

32. Spence K F Jr, Decker S, Sell K W: Bursting atlantal fracture associated with rupture of the transverse ligament, *J Bone Joint Surg Am* 52:543–549, 1970.

33. Goldberg W, Mueller C, Panacek E, et al.: Distribution and patterns of blunt traumatic cervical spine injury, *Ann Emerg Med* 38:17–21, 2001.

34. Hadley M N: Management of vertebral artery injuries after nonpenetrating cervical trauma, *Neurosurgery* 50:S173–S178, 2002.

35. Kathol M H: Cervical spine trauma: what is new? *Radiol Clin North Am* 35:507–532, 1997.

36. Bowen B C, Pattany P M: Contrast-enhanced MR angiography of spinal vessels, *Magn Reson Imaging Clin N Am* 8:597–613, 2000.

37. Vaccaro A R, Madigan L, Schweitzer M E, et al.: Magnetic resonance imaging analysis of soft tissue disruption after flexion-distraction injuries of the subaxial cervical spine, *Spine (Phila Pa 1976)* 26:1866–1872, 2001.

38. Hart R A: Cervical facet dislocation: when is magnetic resonance imaging indicated? *Spine (Phila Pa 1976)* 27:116–117, 2002.

39. Davis S J, Teresi L M, Bradley W G Jr, et al.: Cervical spine hyperextension injuries: MR findings, *Radiology* 180:245–251, 1991.

40. Kwon B K, Vaccaro A R, Grauer J N, et al.: Subaxial cervical spine trauma, *J Am Acad Orthop Surg* 14:78–89, 2006.

41. Quencer R M: The abnormal annulus fibrosus: can we infer the acuteness of an annular injury? *AJNR Am J Neuroradiol* 23:1069, 2002.

42. Stadnik T W, Lee R R, Coen H L, et al.: Annular tears and disk herniation: prevalence and contrast enhancement on MR images in the absence of low back pain or sciatica, *Radiology* 206:49–55, 1998.

43. Ronnen H R, de Korte P J, Brink P R G, et al.: Acute whiplash injury: is there a role for MR imaging? A prospective study of 100 patients, *Radiology* 201:93–96, 1996.

44. Kwon B K, Hilibrand A S: Management of cervical fractures in patients with diffuse idiopathic skeletal hyperostosis, *Curr Opin Orthop* 14:187–192, 2003.

45. Silberstein M, Tress B M, Hennessy O: Delayed neurologic deterioration in the patient with spinal trauma: role of MR imaging, *AJNR Am J Neuroradiol* 13:1373–1381, 1992.

46. Dewan A K, Khanna A J: Penetrating injuries to the spine. In Anderson D G, Vaccaro A R, editors: *Decision making in spinal care*, ed 2, New York, 2012, Thieme, pp 567–574.

47. Ruiz A, Post M J, Sklar E M, Holz A: MR imaging of infections of the cervical spine, *Magn Reson Imaging Clin N Am* 8:561–580, 2000.

48. Modic M T, Feiglin D H, Piraino D W, et al.: Vertebral osteomyelitis: assessment using MR, *Radiology* 157:157–166, 1985.

49. Uhlenbrock D, Henkes H, Weber W, et al.: Inflammatory disorders of the spine and spinal canal. In Uhlenbrock D, editor: *MR imaging of the spine and spinal cord*, New York, 2004, Thieme, pp 357–435.

50. DiGiorgio M L, Sklar E M L: Donovan Post M J: Role of MR in determining the efficacy of medical therapy in spine infections, *Radiology* 189:193, 1997.

51. Murphy K J, Brunberg J A, Quint D J, Kazanjian P H: Spinal cord infection: myelitis and abscess formation, *AJNR Am J Neuroradiol* 19:341–348, 1998.

52. Tartaglino L M, Friedman D P, Flanders A E, et al.: Multiple sclerosis in the spinal cord: MR appearance and correlation with clinical parameters, *Radiology* 195:725–732, 1995.

53. Choi K H, Lee K S, Chung S O, et al.: Idiopathic transverse myelitis: MR characteristics, *AJNR Am J Neuroradiol* 17:1151–1160, 1996.

54. Finelli D A, Ross J S: MR imaging of intrinsic inflammatory myelopathies, *Magn Reson Imaging Clin N Am* 8:541–560, 2000.

55. Chong J, Di Rocco A, Tagliati M, et al.: MR findings in AIDS-associated myelopathy, *AJNR Am J Neuroradiol* 20:1412–1416, 1999.

56. Wang P Y, Shen W C, Jan J S: Serial MRI changes in radiation myelopathy, *Neuroradiology* 37:374–377, 1995.

57. Janssen H, Weissman B N, Aliabadi P, Zamani A A: MR imaging of arthritides of the cervical spine, *Magn Reson Imaging Clin N Am* 8:491–512, 2000.

58. Kim D H, Hilibrand A S: Rheumatoid arthritis in the cervical spine, *J Am Acad Orthop Surg* 13:463–474, 2005.

59. Hopkins J S: Lower cervical rheumatoid subluxation with tetraplegia, *J Bone Joint Surg Br* 49:46–51, 1967.

60. Dvorak J, Grob D, Baumgartner H, et al.: Functional evaluation of the spinal cord by magnetic resonance imaging in patients with rheumatoid arthritis and instability of upper cervical spine, *Spine (Phila Pa 1976)* 14:1057–1064, 1989.

61. Reijnierse M, Breedveld F C, Kroon H M, et al.: Are magnetic resonance flexion views useful in evaluating the cervical spine of patients with rheumatoid arthritis? *Skeletal Radiol* 29:85–89, 2000.

62. Brzeski M, Fox J G, Boulton-Jones J M, Capell H A: Vertebral body collapse due to primary amyloidosis, *J Rheumatol* 17:1701–1703, 1990.

63. Lee R R: MR imaging of intradural tumors of the cervical spine, *Magn Reson Imaging Clin N Am* 8:529–539, 2000.

64. Keogh C, Bergin D, Brennan D, Eustace S: MR imaging of bone tumors of the cervical spine, *Magn Reson Imaging Clin N Am* 8:513–527, 2000.

Neurophysiologic Monitoring of the Cervical Spine

11

Faisal R. Jahangiri

CHAPTER PREVIEW

Chapter Synopsis

This chapter discusses the application of various intraoperative neurophysiologic monitoring (IONM) techniques (also known as modalities) during cervical spine surgery, namely, somatosensory-evoked potentials (SSEPs), transcranial electrical motor-evoked potentials (TCeMEPs), direct epidural potentials, spontaneous electromyography (sEMG), triggered electromyography (tEMG), and train of four (TOF). Each modality is briefly discussed separately and in terms of technical and anesthetic considerations, to provide better understanding of how best to use IONM during anterior and posterior cervical spine surgery.

Important Points

Benefits of IONM:
Improved patient care
Reduced patient neurologic deficits
Reduced surgical morbidity and mortality

Secondary benefits:
Effects of improved surgical guidance
Allowance of a more aggressive surgical approach by identification and monitoring of structures
Identification of physiologically important changes such as blood flow changes: brain ischemia, spinal ischemia, and peripheral ischemia
Identification of anesthetic effects such as burst suppression

Goals of IONM:
Identification of significant changes in spinal function
Intervention and prevention of permanent neurologic damage

Intraoperative neurophysiologic monitoring (IONM) is the application of a variety of electrophysiologic monitoring procedures during surgery to allow early warning and avoidance of injury to nervous system structures. Cervical spine surgery involves a wide variety of surgical procedures that place the spinal cord, nerve roots, and blood vessels at risk. IONM during cervical spine surgery has become common to evaluate spinal cord function. This chapter discusses the application of various IONM techniques (also known as modalities) during cervical spine surgery (Box 11-1), namely, somatosensory-evoked potentials (SSEPs), transcranial electrical motor-evoked potentials (TCeMEPs), direct epidural potentials (D waves), spontaneous electromyography (sEMG), triggered electromyography (tEMG), and train of four (TOF). Each modality is briefly discussed separately and in terms of technical and anesthetic considerations, to provide better understanding of how best to use IONM during surgical procedures of the cervical spine.

IONM plays a key role in minimizing the postoperative deficits during the various types of surgical procedures (neurosurgery, orthopedic, vascular). Dorsal (sensory) and ventral (motor) pathways can be monitored by IONM during cervical spine surgical procedures with real-time feedback to the surgeons.[1]

Modalities are specific types of neurophysiologic tests that can be used for testing and evaluating specific neurologic and functional pathways during different types of surgical procedures. Ascending somatosensory pathways (dorsal columns) and descending motor pathways (ventral columns) are monitored and protected by using various modalities such as SSEPs, TCeMEPs, D waves, and EMG. Multimodality IONM, in general, can prevent or lower the risk of devastating neurologic deficits in a wide variety of situations that place neural structures at risk.[2] Although these modalities all have advantages and disadvantages, they are, in combination, effective means for providing patient protection.

Somatosensory-Evoked Potentials

SSEPs have been used as monitoring tools during surgical procedures since the 1960s. SSEPs are the most widely

- Somatosensory-evoked potentials (SSEPs)
- Transcranial electrical motor-evoked potentials (TCeMEPs)
- Epidural direct waves (D waves)
- Spontaneous electromyography (sEMG)
- Triggered electromyography (tEMG)
- Train of four (TOF)

Table 11-1 Somatosensory-Evoked Potential Setup

Stimulus Parameters

Pulse	Electric monopolar rectangular
Duration	100-300 µsec
Intensity	30-40 mA
Stimulation rate	
Median	2-8/sec
Tibial	2-10/sec
Sweep	
Median	40 msec
Tibial	60 msec
Averages	500-2000
Band-pass	
Cortical	1-30 to 250-3000 Hz
Spinal	100-200 to 1000-3000 Hz
Peripheral	100-200 to 1000-3000 Hz

Recording Parameters: aEEG Guidelines

Median and Ulnar		Posterior Tibial	
−	+	−	+
CPc	CPi	CPi	FPz
CPi	Ref	CPz	FPz
C5s	Ref	FPz	C5s
EPi	Ref	TI2S	Ref
		PFd	PFp

used monitoring modality and are routinely used during brain, spinal, and peripheral surgical procedures. SSEPs are optimal for protection of the patient's ascending sensory spinal pathways (dorsal column) during high-risk surgical procedures.[3] These ascending dorsal column pathways mediate stereognosis, proprioception, tactile discrimination, vibration sensation, and form recognition.[4]

Upper and lower extremity SSEP monitoring is usually performed during all surgical procedures of the cervical spine. Median nerve (C5 to T1 roots) and ulnar nerve (C8 to T1 roots) SSEPs are frequently performed in the upper extremities, whereas in the lower extremities, posterior tibial nerve (L4 to S2) and peroneal nerve (L4 to S1) SSEPs are typically performed. SSEPs are generated by a low-intensity (≈25 mA) electrical stimulation of peripheral nerves in the hands and feet (Table 11-1). Recordings made at multiple locations along the sensory pathway (brachial plexus and popliteal fossa, brainstem, and somatosensory cortex) can determine the anatomic and functional integrity at different locations as the signal travels from the periphery to the cortex. SSEPs are also useful in detection of mechanical and ischemic changes in the peripheral nerves, posterior spinal cord, and cerebral cortex.[5]

Electrical stimulation of nerves in upper and lower extremities produces major positive and negative deflections as signals travel along the somatosensory pathway. The negative potential (N20) is recorded from the somatosensory cortex at the scalp corresponding to upper extremity stimulation (median and ulnar nerves). Conversely, a positive potential (P37) is recorded from the somatosensory cortex at the scalp corresponding to lower extremity stimulation (posterior tibial and peroneal nerves) (Fig. 11-1).

Adequacy of stimulation, peripheral limb perfusion, and peripheral nerve compression can be monitored by a peripheral response recorded at the level of

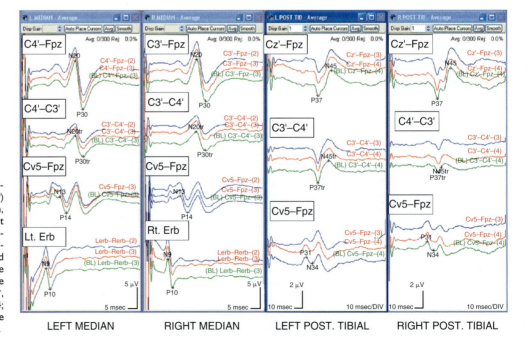

FIGURE 11-1 From *left to right*, Somatosensory-evoked potential (SSEP) data showing left median, right median, left posterior (post.) tibial, and right posterior (post.) tibial nerve SSEP responses. Cortical responses are C4'-Fpz, C3'-Fpz, Cz'-Fpz, C3'-C4', and C4'-C3'. Subcortical responses are CV5-Fpz. Peripheral responses are Erb (brachial plexus point (Erb). *C3'*, Placed at CP3; *C4'*, placed at CP4; *Cz'*, placed at CPz; *Cv5*, placed at the fifth cervical spine; *Lt.*, left; *Rt.*, right.

LEFT MEDIAN RIGHT MEDIAN LEFT POST. TIBIAL RIGHT POST. TIBIAL

the brachial plexus (for the upper extremities) or the popliteal fossa (for the lower extremities). In SSEPs, peripheral and subcortical responses are less sensitive to anesthesia and are frequently used to differentiate SSEP monitoring changes resulting from anesthesia and surgical manipulation. The SSEP responses are transmitted by the fasciculus cuneatus (upper extremity) and the fasciculus gracilis (lower extremity). Therefore, the spinothalamic pathways for pain and temperature are not covered by SSEP monitoring. SSEP uses three orders of neurons. First order neurons carry the signal from the stimulation site, enter the spinal cord through the dorsal root entry zone (DREZ), and travel upward in the dorsal columns forming the fasciculus cuneatus (upper extremity) and the fasciculus gracilis (lower extremity). These fibers make the first synapse with the second order neurons at the nucleus cuneatus (upper extremity) and the nucleus gracilis (lower extremity) in the lower medulla. This is followed by decussation at the medial lemniscus and the making of another synapse, with third order neurons in the thalamus. The third order neurons travel to the somatosensory cortex and terminate in the postcentral or somatosensory gyrus.

Usually, any changes of 50% or more in amplitude or 10% or more in latency of SSEP responses are considered significant and must be reported to the surgeon. Such changes should prompt a search for an intervention to reverse the procedure to reduce the risk of permanent damage.

Advantages

Sensory pathways can be monitored continuously by SSEPs intraoperatively without interrupting the surgical procedure. SSEPs are very effective in monitoring the dorsal column pathways. This monitoring decreases the risk of any mechanical and ischemic changes to the dorsal column pathways, brainstem, brain, and peripheral nerves.[6]

Disadvantages

Averaging of 200 to 300 signals is needed to perform SSEP monitoring in patients under anesthesia, to cancel out unwanted signals such as noise, electroencephalography, and EMG. This signal averaging requires approximately 2 to 3 minutes for each trace. The scope of SSEP monitoring is also limited in assessing spinal cord function, because SSEPs do not detect changes in descending motor pathways. However, in a few reported cases, SSEP responses were not changed but TCeMEP responses were lost. Multiple perisurgical factors affect SSEP responses such as anesthesia, blood pressure, ischemia, and temperature. Therefore, SSEP responses should be monitored only by personnel trained in IONM.

Transcranial Electrical Motor-Evoked Potentials

Since their discovery in the 1980s, TCeMEPs have emerged as extremely useful tools for activation and monitoring of the corticospinal tracts. Many research studies have proven that the evaluation of functional integrity of the descending corticospinal tracts by TCeMEPs during high-risk neurosurgical and orthopedic procedures makes a significant difference in the motor outcome of patients.[7,8]

TCeMEPs assess in real time the function of motor pathways in the spinal cord and reduce the risk of paralysis. They also help in detecting ischemic changes in the motor cortex, spinal cord, and peripheral motor nerves. Since 2000, further research has refined the use of TCeMEP techniques during high-risk spinal procedures. The Stagnara wake-up test was the only way to assess the functional integrity of the motor pathways during spine operations before the introduction of TCeMEP monitoring. The Stagnara wake-up test involved waking patients up during surgical procedures and asking them to move their feet. This technique can be difficult in noncompliant patients (e.g., language issues, hearing impairment) and can also delay the surgical procedure. Although patients do not feel any pain and have no memory of the test postoperatively, this method does not give continuous feedback to the surgeon during critical surgical steps, and the surgeon must stop the procedure to perform the test.

When the Stagnara wake-up test result is positive and the patient cannot move one or both feet, the period between incurring the injury and performing the test may be prolonged. Because of this potential delay between the injury and the test, a risk exists of missing the critical period during which an intervention may have been performed to reverse the neurologic insult.

In the past, SSEPs comprised the only modality performed during spine procedures. The assumption was that any damage to the spinal cord would affect both ascending sensory and descending motor pathways in the spinal cord. In some reported cases, no change in SSEP data was noted, and the patient woke up with motor deficits. TCeMEPs are very sensitive in predicting postoperative motor deficits as compared with SSEPs. This difference may be related to the disparate blood supplies to the ventral and dorsal spinal cord.[9] The blood supply for dorsal columns that supply SSEPs is through the posterior spinal artery. However, the anterior spinal artery is the major source of perfusion to the anterior and lateral corticospinal tracts. If the anterior spinal artery is compressed, it may result in loss of TCeMEP responses while leaving SSEPs unaffected. Intraoperative loss of muscle MEPs indicates some postoperative impairment of voluntary motor control with a specificity of approximately 90% and a sensitivity of 100%.

During spinal surgical procedure, an anode and a cathode are placed on the patient's scalp. Multipulse electrical anodal stimulation transcranially through these electrodes transcranially results in activation of upper motor neurons. The signals are transmitted to lower motor neurons at anterior horn cells in the spinal cord that synapse with distal muscle fibers through the neuromuscular junction, with resulting compound muscle action potentials (Fig. 11-2). The downward volley can be recorded over the spinal cord by placing an epidural electrode. These responses are generated by direct activation (direct or D waves) and indirect activation (indirect or I waves).

For TCeMEP stimulation, electrodes are placed at the C3 and C4 position or the C1 and C2 position.

The recording electrodes are placed in all four extremities. Multiple stimulation and recording sites should be selected especially in patients in whom TCeMEPs are difficult to elicit, such as patients with myelopathy. Increasing the stimulation intensity results in spatial summation, whereas increasing the number of stimulation trains results in temporal summation. The stimulation rate is set between 200 and 500 Hz (Table 11-2). The latency of responses in upper extremity muscles is earlier than in lower extremity muscles. TCeMEP responses are very sensitive to neuromuscular blocking agents and are somewhat sensitive to inhalational anesthetic agents and infused agents. Appropriate anesthetic technique must be used for adequate monitoring. The alarm criteria for TCeMEP consist of various factors, including all or none response, changes in signal morphology, changes in stimulation intensity, and changes in amplitude.

Advantages

TCeMEP monitoring has multiple advantages during high-risk cervical spine procedures. TCeMEPs assess the function of voluntary motor pathways (corticospinal and motor tracts) of the spinal cord in real time and reduce the risk of paralysis. The pyramidal motor pathways can be evaluated in real time by TCeMEP monitoring. TCeMEPs record corticospinal tract information, thus allowing the neurophysiologist to evaluate the functional integrity of the descending motor tracts during high-risk portions of the procedure.[10] TCeMEPs also help in detecting ischemic changes in the motor cortex, spinal cord, and peripheral motor nerves.

Disadvantages

TCeMEPs have some disadvantages, too. They are affected by a high level of anesthesia and by muscle relaxants. The ideal recommended anesthetic technique is total intravenous anesthesia (TIVA) without any muscle relaxants when TCeMEP monitoring is performed.

Another disadvantage of TCeMEP monitoring is that it is not very sensitive to damage to the nerve roots in the lumbosacral area. TCeMEP monitoring is also limited by its contraindication in patients with cochlear implants and deep brain stimulator implants. Any patient with a history of seizures also has a higher risk of a seizure episode related to transcranial stimulation. The benefits of TCeMEP monitoring must be weighed against all these limitations and contraindications. Even though this technique is generally safe, tongue laceration from forced contraction of the facial muscles is the most common complication reported. Tongue lacerations can easily be avoided by placing bite blocks before applying any motor stimulation.

Table 11-2 Transcranial Electrical Motor-Evoked Potential Setup

Stimulus Parameters	
Pulse	Electric monopolar rectangular
Duration	50 μsec
Intensity	100-1000 V
Interstimulus interval (ISI)	1.1-9.0
Trains	1-9
Averages	1

Recording Parameters	
Low cut	10 Hz
High cut	3000-10,000 Hz
Sweep	10 msec/Div
Gain	100 μV/Div
Reject	Off
Upper extremity	Delt, FCU, BR, APB, ADM
Lower extremity	Quads, TA, MG, AH, EHB

ADM, Abductor digiti minimi; *AH,* abductor hallucis; *APB,* abductor pollicis brevis; *BR,* brachioradialis; *Delt,* deltoid; *EHB,* extensor hallucis brevis; *FCU,* flexor carpi ulnaris; *MG,* medial gastrocnemius; *Quads,* quadriceps; *TA,* tibialis anterior.

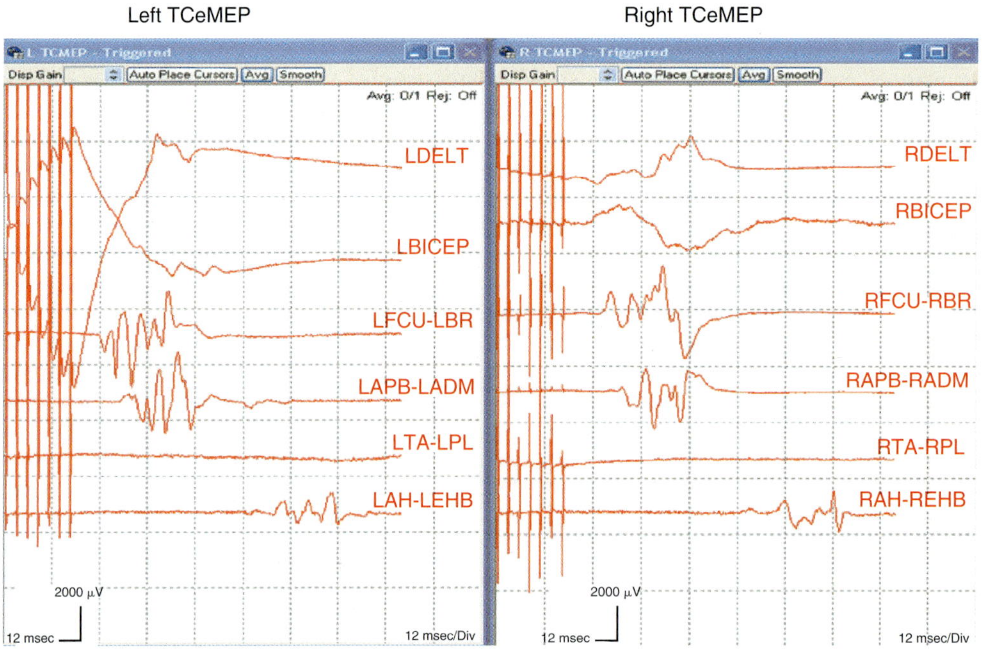

FIGURE 11-2 Transcranial electrical motor-evoked potentials (TCeMEPs). *Left,* Responses from muscles of the left (L) upper and lower extremity muscles. *Right,* Responses from muscles of the right (R) upper and lower extremity muscles. *AH,* Abductor hallucis; *APB,* abductor pollicis brevis; *ADM,* abductor digiti minimi; *BR,* brachioradialis; *BICEP,* biceps brachii; *DELT,* deltoid; *EHB,* extensor hallucis brevis; *FCU,* flexor carpi ulnaris; *PL,* peroneus longus; *TA,* tibialis anterior.

Epidural Potentials (Direct or D Waves and Indirect or I Waves)

An epidural electrode is placed in the epidural space for recording MEPs directly from the spinal cord generated in response to single pulse stimulation (Table 11-3). Direct and indirect activation of upper motor neurons results in transmission of a volley in the spinal cord. By placing an electrode in the epidural space over the cervical spinal cord, these responses can be recorded as single D waves and multiple I waves.[8] D waves are produced by direct activation of the upper motor neurons, whereas indirect activation of upper motor neurons through multiple interneurons produces multiple I waves (Fig. 11-3). Anesthetics have minimal effect on D waves, but they abolish I waves. Epidural recordings are recommended for all patients with intramedullary spinal cord tumors.[11] The advantage of epidural recording is that surgeons do not have to stop the procedure for monitoring, and recordings can be done without any patient movement during tumor resection (Table 11-4). Another benefit is that anesthetic inhalational agents and neuromuscular blocking agents have minimal effects on the recordings.

Spontaneous Electromyography

EMG is a modality used during surgical procedures for the evaluation and recording of muscle activity produced by nerve root irritation. Intraoperatively, sEMG activity is used to monitor the muscles of the corresponding nerve roots at risk. During cervical spine procedures, recording subdermal needle electrodes are placed bilaterally in muscles of the upper extremity, depending on the level of structures at risk. A pair of electrodes is placed in each muscle to be root specific.[12] sEMG monitors spontaneous activity without using any nerve root stimulation. Intraoperatively, sEMG is very sensitive to any injury, and any stretching, pulling, heating, or compression of the nerve root during the procedure will result in abnormal sEMG activity (Fig. 11-4). The various types of abnormal activities resulting from nerve root irritation are spikes, bursts, trains, and neurotonic discharges. The source of nerve root or nerve irritation can be mechanical, electrical, or thermal. Any baseline EMG activity, such as fasciculation or fibrillation potentials, means that the corresponding nerve root irritation was present preoperatively.

In contrast to clinical EMG testing, intraoperative EMG monitoring is focused on identifying any type of abnormal activity in any muscle supplied by the nerve roots at risk. Monitoring is focused only on the presence or absence and type of EMG activity. The latency and amplitude of abnormal EMG findings are not important. Prolonged neurotonic discharges are considered to represent a type of more serious nerve injury. The muscles

Table 11-3 Epidural and D-Wave Setup

Stimulus Parameters: FDA Guidelines	
Pulse	Electric monopolar rectangular
Duration	50 μsec
Intensity	100-400 V
Interstimulus interval (ISI)	1.1-9.0
Trains	1
Averages	1
Recording Parameters	
Low cut	10 Hz
High cut	3000-10,000 Hz
Sweep	1-3 msec/Div
Gain	100 μV/Div
Reject	Off
Epidural electrodes	

FDA, Food and Drug Administration.

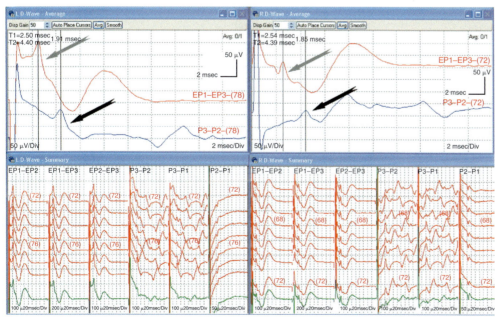

Left D Waves   Right D Waves

FIGURE 11-3 Epidural or D-wave responses. The *upper level (gray arrows)* displays D-wave responses above the surgical site (early latency). The *upper level (black arrow)* also displays D-wave responses below the surgical site (delayed latency). The *lower level* displays stack view summary of epidural responses for left and right cortical stimulation.

monitored during cervical spine operations may include the trapezius, deltoid, biceps brachii, flexor carpi ulnaris, brachioradialis, abductor pollicis brevis, and abductor digiti minimi, depending on the nerve root at risk (Table 11-5). The C5 nerve root may be at higher risk of injury during cervical spine procedures; thus, monitoring of at least two muscles may minimize C5 nerve root damage.[13] The deltoid and biceps brachii muscles can typically be used to monitor the C5 nerve root.

sEMG for vocal monitoring has also been used during anterior cervical fusion surgery to prevent any damage to the recurrent laryngeal nerve. This nerve is usually monitored by intubating the patient with a specially designed endotracheal tube with two electrodes embedded bilaterally. The electrode wires are insulated, except for a few centimeters of length, which are in direct contact with the false vocal cords. Any irritation of the recurrent laryngeal nerve results in activation of the false vocal cord muscles that can be seen on sEMG monitoring.

Advantages

Monitoring of sEMG takes place in real time and gives immediate feedback to the surgeon. This immediacy allows the surgeon to act accordingly and remove any nerve traction or reverse the procedure that is causing abnormal EMG activity.

Disadvantages

Muscle relaxants cannot be used during sEMG monitoring. A small dose of muscle relaxant can be given only for intubation. Any relaxant suppresses muscle activity and makes accurate monitoring impossible. In addition, if damage is already done to the nerve root, sEMG will not provide any real-time feedback. Occasionally, sEMG monitoring is interrupted by various artifacts caused by electrocautery devices, electrocardiography, and drills, for example.

Triggered Electromyography (Direct Nerve and Pedicle Screw Stimulation)

Neurophysiologic monitoring during cervical spine lateral mass or pedicle screw placement has become more common. tEMG can be used to help determine whether screws have breached the pedicle wall and pose a risk to the exiting nerve root at that level (Fig. 11-5). The bone surrounding the pedicle screw acts as an insulator requiring a high current to stimulate the adjacent nerve roots. The

Table 11-4	D-Wave Alarm Criteria	
D-Wave Response	**TCeMEP Response**	**Motor Status**
No change	Present	Intact
30%-50% decrease	Unilateral or bilateral loss	Temporary postoperative motor deficit
>50% decrease	Unilateral or bilateral loss	Long-term postoperative motor deficit
Lost	Lost	Permanent deficit

Data from Deletis V: Intraoperative neurophysiological monitoring. In McLone D, editor: *Pediatric neurosurgery: surgery of the developing nervous system*, ed 3, Philadelphia, 1999, Saunders, pp 1204-1213.
TCeMEP, Transcranial electrical motor-evoked potential.

Table 11-5	Muscles Used for Monitoring Cervical Nerve Roots	
Root	**Muscle**	**Nerve**
C3, C4	Trapezius	CN XI
C5, C6	Deltoid	Axillary
C5, C6	Biceps brachii	Musculocutaneous
(C5), C6, C7	Brachioradialis	Radial
(C7), C8	Flexor carpi ulnaris	Ulnar
(C8), T1	Abductor pollicis brevis	Median
C8, (T1)	Abductor digiti minimi	Ulnar

CN, Cranial nerve.

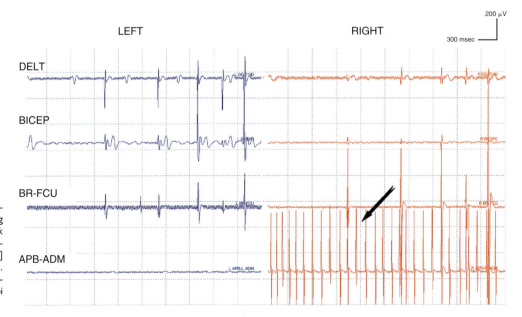

FIGURE 11-4 Spontaneous electromyography (sEMG) view showing abnormal train EMG activity (*black arrow*) mostly in the right hand muscles (abductor pollicis brevis [APB] and abductor digiti minimi [ADM]). *BICEP,* Biceps brachii; *BR,* brachioradialis; *DELT,* deltoid; *FCU,* flexor carpi ulnaris.

screw is stimulated directly with a monopolar probe. The subdermal needle electrodes are placed in corresponding muscle groups to record compound muscle action potentials, which are time locked to the stimulation. The stimulation thresholds are decreased in the presence of a pedicle wall breach. A study by Djurasovis and associates showed that a threshold of less than 10 mA suggests a malpositioned lateral mass or pedicle screw with 100% predictive value.[14] A threshold of 15 mA or higher suggests, with 99% positive predictive value accuracy, that the screw was within the lateral mass or pedicle. False-negative responses to pedicle screw stimulation can be recorded for various reasons. The most common causes of false-negative responses are muscle relaxants, previous damage to nerve roots, and current spread from shunting in any fluid (blood, saline, cerebrospinal fluid).

Direct nerve stimulation can be done by tEMG. If the patient has preexisting nerve root damage, the threshold of the nerve to electrical stimulation will be increased, thus resulting in false-negative findings. The level of muscle relaxant must be monitored by TOF testing from a muscle more distal to the surgical site.

Train of Four

TOF monitoring is performed in conjunction with TCeMEP and EMG monitoring. Patients who receive neuromuscular blocking agents are evaluated intraoperatively with peripheral nerve stimulation and TOF monitoring. The posterior tibial nerve in the foot is typically used for stimulation by recording responses from the abductor hallucis and extensor hallucis brevis muscles. Ulnar nerve stimulation is another option, by recording TOF responses from the abductor digiti minimi muscles. A peripheral nerve is stimulated at the rate of 2 Hz for 2 seconds, with a total of four stimulations (Table 11-6). The presence of responses to all four stimulations means blockade of less than 5% of these muscles. Three twitches correspond to a 75% blockade, two twitches correspond to an 85% blockade, and one twitch corresponds to a 95% blockade. The absence of twitches corresponds to a 100% muscle blockade. To perform appropriate intraoperative monitoring, at least three out of four twitches must be present, if not all four out of four (Fig. 11-6).

Anesthesia and Neurophysiologic Monitoring

Most anesthetic agents have significant effects on evoked potentials by increasing the latency and decreasing the amplitude of cortical SSEP responses. The effect of anesthesia on evoked responses varies from one patient to another, depending on various preoperative factors. These factors include the patient's age, any history of alcohol abuse or abuse, neurologic abnormalities, vascular deficiencies, a history of stroke, and diabetes mellitus. The anesthetic effects are always present bilaterally. Every neural generator on the pathways is affected differently by anesthesia.

Table 11-6 Train of Four Setup

Stimulus Parameters	
Setup mode	TOF
Pulse	Electric monopolar rectangular
Duration	200 μsec
Intensity	10-50 mA
Stimulation rate	2 Hz
Train	2
Nerves	Median or posterior tibial
Recording Parameters	
Low cut	10 Hz
High cut	3000-10,000 Hz
Sweep	20 msec/Div
Gain	100 μV/Div
Muscles	APB/ADM or AH/EHB

ADM, Abductor digiti minimi; *AH,* abductor hallucis; *APB,* abductor pollicis brevis; *EHB,* extensor hallucis brevis; *TOF,* train of four.

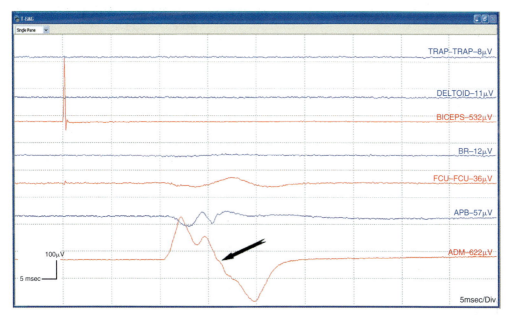

FIGURE 11-5 Triggered electromyography (T-EMG) view showing a response from the abductor digiti minimi (ADM) muscle (*black arrow*) after direct cervical nerve root stimulation. *APB,* Abductor pollicis brevis; *BICEPS,* biceps brachii; *BR,* brachioradialis; *FCU,* flexor carpi ulnaris; *TRAP,* trapezius.

Cortical SSEP responses are most strongly affected by anesthesia. The effect starts from later cortical peaks and moves toward earlier cortical peaks. Anesthesia usually affects the evoked responses by blocking the synaptic transmission of responses. Therefore, when more synapses are involved in response generation, the effect of anesthesia is greater. Therefore, the cortical SSEP potentials are more sensitive to anesthesia as compared with the subcortical and peripheral nerve potentials. The exceptions to this rule are two drugs, etomidate and ketamine, which increase the amplitude of cortical SSEP responses.[5]

Because halogenated agents take a few minutes to cause anesthetic effects, the changes in evoked potentials are always later than the changes in gas concentration. All the halogenated gases including nitrous oxide (N_2O), isoflurane, sevoflurane, and desflurane cause potent suppression of cortical SSEP and all TCeMEP responses. In contrast, the intravenous agents have a much milder effect on SSEP and TCeMEP responses as compared with gas agents. The bolus administration of these agents should be avoided because it may decrease SSEP and TCeMEP responses. Other drugs such as barbiturates, benzodiazepines (midazolam, diazepam), and neuromuscular blocking agents (succinylcholine, vecuronium, rocuronium, and pancuronium) have minimal effects on SSEP if they are given in a steady infusion.

A constant TIVA infusion should be given that ideally causes the least suppression and yields steady potentials. This protocol has proven highly effective in optimizing both SSEP and MEP amplitudes. A combination of propofol with a narcotic agent, such as sufentanil, fentanyl, or remifentanil, without any muscle relaxant can be used for the TIVA infusion for monitoring SSEPs, TCeMEPs, and EMG during cervical spine operations.[1] Short-acting neuromuscular blockade should be used only initially, for intubation. Subsequent neuromuscular blockade levels should be monitored with TOF by stimulating the left posterior tibial nerve and recording from the corresponding abductor hallucis and extensor hallucis brevis muscles. A train of four out of four twitches should be maintained for the entire duration of the procedure.

Positioning-Related Injuries

The use of IONM to assess brachial plexus function in the upper extremities during spine surgery is becoming more accepted as a valid and useful technique to minimize intraoperative positioning-related nerve injuries. This view is supported by the literature indicating that brachial plexopathy can occur from improper arm or shoulder positioning. Additional pressure is applied to the brachial plexus when the arms are tucked and pulled down, thereby stretching the brachial plexus. The American Society of Anesthesiology reported that male patients are at higher risk for position-related nerve injuries.[15] Obesity, preexisting spinal cord disease, and diabetes mellitus are among other patient-related characteristics reported to carry a greater risk for position-related injury. The current recommendation is to use ulnar nerve SSEPs and upper extremity TCeMEPs to monitor for positioning-related brachial plexus injuries. If the ulnar SSEPs or TCeMEPs of the upper extremity muscles change, the surgeon and the anesthesiologist should be notified immediately, to reposition the affected arm until the SSEP or TCeMEP signals are returned to baseline values, to avoid any long-term damage.

Effect of Hypotension

Hypotension can affect SSEP and TCeMEP signals globally. Ischemia results in a delayed time course. Within the spinal cord, the gray matter is most sensitive to ischemia; loss of synaptic activity occurs in 1 to 2 minutes, whereas conduction is delayed in the sensory and motor

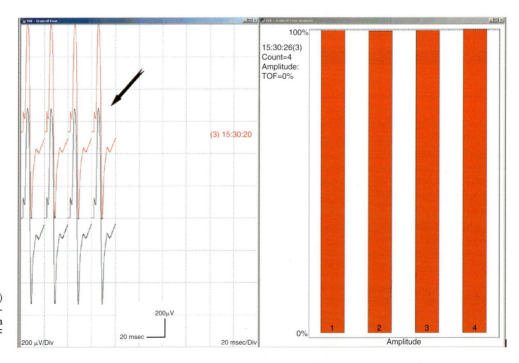

FIGURE 11-6 Train of four (TOF) data showing all four twitches present (*black arrow*). *Left,* TOF data showing all four twitches. *Right,* TOF data in a histogram view.

white matter tracts and shows alteration in different time. Decreased cerebral blood flow from the average of 50 mL/minute/100 g to less than 25 mL/minute/100 g causes signal changes. SSEPs are affected at 20 mL/minute/100 g and are lost between 13 and 18 mL/minute/100 g. Regional hypoperfusion caused by poor positioning, tourniquets, or vascular interruption can also be detected.

Mean arterial pressure (MAP) should be continuously monitored during the surgical procedure. Any significant decrease in MAP results in a decrease or loss of SSEP or TCeMEP responses, or both. This situation is more important in patients with a history of hypertension. The anesthesiologist and the surgeon should be notified immediately to elevate the MAP to the baseline level to avoid permanent damage to the spinal cord or cerebral cortex.

Effect of Hypothermia

Hypothermia alters latency and amplitude primarily by decreasing synaptic function, mostly on the postsynaptic membrane. Thus, changes are more prominent at the cephalic end of long neural tracts or where multiple synapses are involved. Local hypothermia can be caused by cold irrigation fluids, and whole-body hypothermia can result from cold intravenous fluids. Hypothermia of the limbs results in delay of the latency of peripheral responses with normal interpeak intervals.

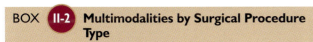

BOX **11-2**   **Multimodalities by Surgical Procedure Type**

Anterior Cervical Procedures
- SSEPs
- sEMG
- TCeMEPs

Posterior Cervical Procedures
- SSEPs
- sEMG
- tEMG
- TCeMEPs

Occiput-C2 Fusion
- SSEPs
- TCeMEPs

Extramedullary Spinal Cord Tumor
- SSEPs
- sEMG
- tEMG
- TCeMEPs

Intramedullary Spinal Cord Tumor
- SSEPs
- sEMG
- tEMG
- TCeMEPs
- D waves

Spinal Arteriovenous Malformation and Vascular Procedures
- SSEPs
- TCeMEPs

D waves, Direct waves; *sEMG*, spontaneous electromyography; *SSEPs*, somatosensory-evoked potentials; *TCeMEPs*, transcranial electrical motor-evoked potentials; *tEMG*, triggered electromyography.

Real-Time Monitoring

On-site or continuous real-time oversight of the monitoring neurophysiologist or a technologist in the operating room by a trained neurologist provides supervision by a highly trained physician regardless of location. It also gives a second expert opinion when intraoperative data have changed during a critical surgical step.

Multimodality Monitoring

Multimodality neurophysiologic monitoring can reduce the risk of neurologic injury during cervical spine procedures.[16] The modalities available for neuromonitoring of the cervical spine surgeries include SSEPs, TCeMEPs, D waves, sEMG, and tEMG. Each modality has its advantages and disadvantages, but if used in combination, these techniques can be very sensitive in preventing postoperative neurologic deficits, which can be devastating to the patient (Box 11-2).[17]

REFERENCES

1. Bose B, Sestokas AK, Schwartz DM: Neurophysiological monitoring of spinal cord function during instrumented anterior cervical fusion, *Spine J* 4:202–207, 2004.
2. Eager M, Shimer A, Jahangiri F, et al: Intraoperative neuromonitoring: lessons learned from 32 case events in 2095 spine surgeries, Eurospine 2010, Vienna, Austria (E-poster): http://eposter.eurospine.org/cm_data/eposter/64.pdf (Accessed 18.02.14).
3. Nuwer MR, Dawson EG, Carlson LG, et al.: Somatosensory evoked potential spinal cord monitoring reduces neurologic deficits after scoliosis surgery: results of a large multicenter survey, *Electroencephalogr Clin Neurophysiol* 96:6–11, 1995.
4. Khan MH, Smith PN, Balzer JR, et al.: Intraoperative somatosensory evoked potential monitoring during cervical spine corpectomy surgery: experience with 508 cases, *Spine (Phila Pa 1976)* 31:E105–E113, 2006.
5. Jahangiri FR: *Surgical neurophysiology: a reference guide to intraoperative neurophysiological monitoring (IONM)*, ed 2, Charleston, SC, 2012, CreateSpace.
6. Jahangiri FR, Crowley RW, Persyn JJ, et al.: Predicting surgical outcome using somatosensory evoked potentials and transcranial electric motor evoked potentials in a cervical-medullary junction hemangioblastoma, *Am J Electroneurodiagnostic Technol* 50:101–110, 2010.
7. Deletis V, Sala F: Intraoperative neurophysiological monitoring of the spinal cord during spinal cord and spine surgery: a review focus on the corticospinal tracts, *Clin Neurophysiol* 119:248–264, 2008.
8. Kothbauer KF, Deletis V, Epstein FJ: Motor-evoked potential monitoring for intramedullary spinal cord tumor surgery: correlation of clinical and neurophysiological data in a series of 100 consecutive procedures, *Neurosurg Focus* 4:e1, 1998.
9. Macdonald DB: Intraoperative motor evoked potential monitoring: overview and update, *J Clin Monit Comput* 20:347–377, 2006.
10. Hilibrand AS, Schwartz DM, Sethuraman V, et al.: Comparison of transcranial electric motor and somatosensory evoked potential monitoring during cervical spine surgery, *J Bone Joint Surg Am* 86:1248–1253, 2004.
11. Deletis V: Intraoperative neurophysiological monitoring. In McLone D, editor: *Pediatric neurosurgery: surgery of the developing nervous system*, ed 3, Philadelphia, 1999, Saunders, pp 1204–1213.
12. Gunnarsson T, Krassioukov AV, Sarjeant R, Fehlings MG: Real-time continuous intraoperative electromyographic and somatosensory evoked potential recordings in spinal surgery: correlation of clinical and electrophysiologic findings in a prospective, consecutive series of 213 cases, *Spine (Phila Pa 1976)* 29:677–684, 2004.

13. Fan D, Schwartz DM, Vaccaro AR, et al.: Intraoperative neurophysiologic detection of iatrogenic C5 nerve root injury during laminectomy for cervical compression myelopathy, *Spine (Phila Pa 1976)* 27:2499–2502, 2002.
14. Djurasovic M, Dimar JR 2nd, Glassman SD, et al.: A prospective analysis of intraoperative electromyographic monitoring of posterior cervical screw fixation, *J Spinal Disord Tech* 18:515–518, 2005.
15. Schwartz DM, Sestokas AK, Hilibrand AS, et al.: Neurophysiological identification of position-induced neurologic injury during anterior cervical spine surgery, *J Clin Monit Comput* 20:437–444, 2006.
16. Kelleher MO, Tan G, Sarjeant R, Fehlings MG: Predictive value of intraoperative neurophysiological monitoring during cervical spine surgery: a prospective analysis of 1055 consecutive patients, *J Neurosurg Spine* 8:215–221, 2008.
17. Pajewski TN, Arlet V, Phillips LH: Current approach on spinal cord monitoring: the point of view of the neurologist, the anesthesiologist and the spine surgeon, *Eur Spine J* 16(Suppl 2):S115–S129, 2007.

SECTION 2

Degenerative Conditions

Cervical Degenerative Disk Disease

12

Jason Pui Yin Cheung, Jaro Karppinen, Jani Takatalo, Hai-Qiang Wang, Francis H. Shen, and Dino Samartzis

CHAPTER PREVIEW

Chapter Synopsis

Cervical disk degeneration becomes more prevalent with increasing age and can affect both male and female patients equally. Genes associated with disk degeneration include those coding for collagen I and IX, vitamin D receptor, and matrix metalloproteinase-3. Disk degeneration begins with a loss of water content in the nucleus pulposus that leads to an increased loss of proteoglycan and altered collagen content. A cascade of changes in the disk follows and causes mechanical incompetence for load transmission. Eventually, the disk fails and collapses, causing annular tears and protrusion of disk material into the spinal canal. Further collapse compromises the facet joints posteriorly. Pain is the main concern for patients with cervical disk degeneration. Pain can be caused by annular ruptures, irritation of nerve roots by protruded disk material, and facet joint instability. Treatment is focused on relieving pain, improving function, and preventing recurrence. Nonoperative management includes rest, medication (e.g., steroids and muscle relaxants), physical therapy, manipulation, and injections. Operative treatment is reserved for patients with intractable pain and neurologic compression unresponsive to nonoperative therapy. Surgical intervention entails decompression for neurologic deficit and fusion and instrumentation for avoiding instability and correcting deformity.

Important Points

The etiology of cervical disk degeneration is multifactorial.

The degenerative process in the cervical spine is similar to that in the lumbar spine.

At present, only genes coding for collagen I and IX, metalloproteinase-3, and vitamin D receptor are found to be associated with cervical disk degeneration.

The most common symptom of cervical disk degeneration is pain, which can be caused by irritation to the outer annular nerve endings, nerve root compression, and compromised facet joints.

Treatment options are decompression for neurologic compromise, fusion to prevent instability, and instrumentation to correct deformity or maintain stability.

Clinical Pearls

Education about the disease is of utmost importance.

Nonoperative treatment includes rest, medical and physical therapy, manipulation, and injections.

Decompression options for disk disorders include a direct approach (anterior) and an indirect approach (posterior).

Both options of anterior and posterior surgical procedures have similar fusion and complication rates.

The main risks encountered in anterior surgery are associated with surgical neck dissection and include injury to the recurrent laryngeal nerve, trachea, and esophagus.

Cervical disk arthroplasty is a popular and promising procedure, but long-term clinical results are lacking; however, current findings show equivalency to single-level anterior cervical diskectomy and fusion with plating.

The first account of the description of cervical degenerative disk disease (DDD) appeared in 1911.[1] Since then, most published studies on cervical DDD have been related to spinal surgery. Although DDD is common in the cervical spine, it manifests later than in the lumbar spine.[2] The quantity of water decreases in the nucleus pulposus as a person ages, and this loss reduces the cushioning effect of the disk. This change further decreases the dynamic function of the disk by directing more mechanical forces to the zygapophyseal joints and reducing the height of the intervertebral space. Not all the degenerative changes are seen on magnetic resonance imaging (MRI), but they can be noted histologically.[3] In addition to the disk, the cartilage end plates of the vertebrae are degenerated, causing blood vessels to grow into the disk and thereby triggering disk ossification.[4] Cervical disk disease encompasses a spectrum of disorders, ranging from diskogenic neck pain to myelopathy. Degenerative disease of the cervical spine can manifest with a variety of clinical signs and symptoms. Nonoperative treatment is the cornerstone of management in the majority of cases. Operative treatment is indicated in patients with neural compression and spinal instability. This chapter presents an overview of cervical DDD.

Epidemiology

Cervical DDD is an age-related phenomenon, as it is in the lumbar spine.[2,5-8] Disk degeneration is a natural aging phenomenon, and its prevalence increases with age whether symptoms are present or not.[2,5-11] In an MRI study, Boden and associates showed that the disk was degenerated or narrowed at one level or more in 25% of subjects who were less than 40 years old and in almost 60% of subjects who were more than 40 years old.[5] Lehto and colleagues, in another MRI study, showed that abnormalities were found in 62% of subjects who were more than 40 years old, whereas no abnormalities were found in subjects who were less than 30 years old.[2] Among asymptomatic Japanese study subjects, 20% of participants in their 20s and almost 90% of participants who were more than 60 years old had cervical disk degeneration.[7] The most commonly involved disk level in patients who were more than 30 years old was C5-C6.[2,12] A study by Lawrence and co-workers similarly showed that the C5-C6 and C6-C7 disks were most often degenerated, and the prevalence of cervical disk degeneration increased with age.[13] No differences were found among male and female study subjects. Matsumoto and associates reported that cervical disks were degenerated in 17% and 12% of asymptomatic men and women in their twenties, respectively.[7] In subjects more than 60 years old, the prevalence rose to 86% in men and 89% in women. Moderate to severe cervical degeneration was associated with a past episode or repeated episodes of pain in the neck-shoulder-brachial region. Moderate to severe cervical disk degeneration was associated significantly with lumbar degeneration in both sexes.[13] Although disk degeneration is common in the cervical spine, it appears to begin later in the cervical spine than in the lumbar region.[2]

Pathophysiology

The intervertebral disk is the largest avascular tissue in the human body.[14] Disk nutrition derives from diffusion across the cartilaginous end plates. The intervertebral disk consists of the central nucleus pulposus and the peripherally encircling annulus fibrosus. These structures are important shock absorbers of the spine to body motion. The nucleus pulposus is a remnant of the notochord and consists of the loose network of collagen fibers in a gelatinous fluid that is composed of 85% to 90% water in a young individual. The rest of the matrix is composed of 25% to 35% collagen and 60% to 65% proteoglycans. Aging causes the water content of the nucleus pulposus to decrease, thus resulting in a relative increase of proteoglycan and collagen. The annulus fibrosus is predominantly composed of water (60% to 70%) and, to a lesser degree, collagen (20% to 30%). Unlike in the nucleus pulposus, however, the water content of the annulus fibrosus does not change with age.[15]

Biochemical changes of the spinal unit begin in the nucleus pulposus. With aging, the nucleus pulposus begins to desiccate and loses its mechanical competence.[16] Effective load transmission is no longer possible when this occurs because the normal nucleus pulposus is similar to a contained fluid.[17] Axial loads to the spine are converted to tensile strain on annular fibers and are then transmitted to the vertebral end plates. With continuous loading, creep occurs in the nucleus pulposus. Eventually, the gel structure degenerates. The collagen content of the disk increases while glycoprotein content decreases after the second decade of life.[16] The loss of glycoproteins decreases imbibition pressure. In its relaxed state, the degenerated disk imbibes fluid.

Loading, genetics, and local autocrine factors all influence the rate and degree of disk degeneration. The significant effect of axial loading is evidenced by the high rates of disk degeneration in the lordotic area of the spine.[18] When static compressive stress exceeds the pressure in the disk, water is forced out, thus causing altered intradiskal stress distribution and resulting in a number of harmful, dose-dependent responses.[17] These include apoptosis of the nuclear cells, loss of cellularity, down-regulation of the collagen II and aggrecan gene expression, and increasingly disorganized annulus fibrosis. Cells of the intervertebral disk are metabolically active and are capable of responding to biochemical stimuli. These autocrine factors function as local cellular signals that affect disk degeneration.

The percentage of matrix metalloproteinase-3 (MMP-3)–positive cells correlates with the degree of degeneration on MRI and osteophyte size.[19] Degenerated disks exhibit MMP-3 but no metalloproteinase tissue inhibitor. Disk degeneration is suggested to be caused by an imbalance of MMP-3 and tissue inhibitor of metalloproteinase-1. Cathepsins and other proteolytic enzymes can separate disks from vertebral bodies, thereby affecting the rate of disk degeneration.[20]

The mature annulus fibrosus contains degenerated cells and necrotic debris. Collagen types I and II predominate in the disk. Type I collagen is suited to withstand tensile-type loading and is located in the annulus fibrosus. Type II collagen can sustain tensile loads and is found in the nucleus pulposus. The proteoglycan content of the disk decreases with age. The normal disk contains enzymes active against type II collagen, whereas in the prolapsed disk, the enzyme systems are active against type I collagen.[21] The prolapsed disk contains elastin-degrading enzymes, which are not found in the normal disk. Elastic fibers are located in the annulus fibrosus at the interface of the disk and the vertebral body. The increased presence of elastin- and type I collagen–degrading enzymes in the annulus fibrosus is likely one mechanism for disk herniation. The histologic changes in disk degeneration are seen in adjacent cartilaginous end plates, where neovascularization, capillary wall thickening, and calcification are found.[22,23]

The normal functions of the annulus fibrosus are to contain the nucleus pulposus and to convert compressive stress to tangential stress. When the nucleus pulposus fails to maintain hydration, strain changes occur at the nucleus-annulus interface. The mechanical effectiveness of the disk decreases with decreasing states of hydration.[24] The disk is no longer able to generate increased intradiskal pressures and is therefore unable to distribute force effectively. The central annular lamellae buckle under constant compressive loading. The disk collapses and causes external concentric bands of annulus fibrosus to bulge outward.

Increased annular stress leads to fibrillation and tearing of annular fibers. In younger patients, disk material prolapses through tears in the annulus fibrosus and causes nerve root or spinal cord impingement. The soft disk herniation causes nerve dysfunction both directly and through vascular compromise of radicular feeder arteries. The exiting nerve root is most commonly affected by disk protrusion. Acute disk herniation and annular degeneration and protrusion are part of a continuum of degeneration that leads to advanced spondylosis. Disk collapse translates into excess motion in the zygapophyseal (facet) joints posteriorly and increased strain in the supporting ligaments.[25] With loss of disk height, the facets begin to override, and uncovertebral joints come into contact, thus forming osteophytes. Decreasing facet competence and increased segmental motion hasten the rate of disk degeneration.[24] Ten years after the disk begins to degenerate, the mechanical competence of the motion segment becomes evident, with facet and uncovertebral joint degeneration.[26] True disk protrusion or a hard disk (osteophytes) can also compress the nerve root and lead to radiculopathy. With continued degeneration, osteophytes along with other pathologic processes, such as disk protrusion or ossification of the posterior longitudinal ligament (OPLL), may compress the central spinal canal. Spinal cord function is affected by vascular insufficiency, and direct mechanical pressure on the neural elements results from central spinal canal stenosis, which may lead to cervical myelopathy.

Risk Factors

DDD has several possible mechanisms, such as decreased proteoglycan and water content,[9] inflammation induced by cytokines such as interleukin-1[27] and tumor necrosis factor-α,[28] genetics,[29] smoking,[30] occupational load,[31-33] atherosclerosis,[34] and history of surgery.[35] However, a longitudinal study could not support all suggested DDD theories such as smoking. In addition, the role of body mass index, gender, sports, and alcohol consumption is not certain in the development of DDD of the cervical spine.[8] Smoking was not found to be related to cervical DDD on lateral plain radiographs in a cross-sectional case-control study.[36] No increased risk for herniation was found for sedentary jobs or jobs requiring twisting of the neck,[37] and no increased risk was noted for any sport including weightlifting.[38] In fact, sport activity has been suggested to be protective of the cervical spine. Hence, causal factors for DDD have not been fully established.

Genetics

Hereditary factors could affect disk degeneration through several mechanisms, such as an influence on the size and shape of spinal structures that affect the mechanical properties of the spine and its vulnerability to external forces. Biologic processes associated with the synthesis and breakdown of structural and biochemical constituents of the disk could be partly genetically predetermined, thus leading to vulnerability to accelerated degenerative changes in some persons. The identification of specific genetic influences may eventually provide key insights into underlying mechanisms.[39] Furthermore, for specific genes and some environmental factors, gene-gene interactions and gene-environment interactions may exist.

Another factor that must be considered is age. A particular gene may possibly be associated with DDD only at a certain age. Some genes have been associated with disk degeneration in human beings, including genes coding for collagen type I (*COL1A1*),[40,41] collagen type IX (*COL9A2* and *COL9A3*),[42-47] collagen type XI (*COL11A2*),[47] interleukin-1,[48,49] aggrecan,[50-52] vitamin D receptor (VDR),[53-57] MMP-3,[58] and cartilage intermediate-layer protein (CILP).[59] At present, only an association of the *COL1A1*, *COL9A2*, MMP-3, and VDR genes with DDD has been verified in different ethnic populations. The annulus fibrosus consists mainly of collagen type I, and the nucleus pulposus contains approximately 50% proteoglycans, mainly aggrecan, and 20% collagen type II. Both contain small amounts of collagen types IX and XI. Studies based on a mouse model indicated that mutations in collagen type IX and aggrecan can cause age-related disk degeneration and herniation.[52,60] Collagen types IX and XI are attractive candidates for lumbar disk degeneration because they serve as minor components in both the annulus fibrosus and the nucleus pulposus[9]; however, their roles in the cervical spine warrant further investigation. Nonetheless, various genetic studies have noted concomitant cervical and lumbar degenerative changes, findings suggesting that these two regions share common risk factors.[61-64]

Collagen Type I

The collagen type I α1 gene (*COL1A1*; chromosomal location, 17q21.3-q22) encodes a part of type I collagen, which is the major protein in bone and in the outer layer of the annulus fibrosus.[62] Pluijm and colleagues evaluated 517 older Dutch individuals (65 to 85 years old) and showed that people with the TT genotype had a higher risk of DDD than did those with the GG and GT genotypes (odds ration [OR], 3.6; 95% confidence interval

[CI], 1.3 to 10).[40] The frequencies of the GG, GT, and TT genotypes were 66%, 30%, and 4% in men, and 70%, 27%, and 3% in women, respectively.

Collagen Type IX

A subsequent study of Finnish families revealed that family members who carry the Trp2 allele have a greater degree of degeneration in the vertebral disk and end plate.[45] Jim and co-workers found that the Trp2 allele was present in 20% of the population and was associated with a fourfold increase in the risk of developing annular tears at age 30 to 39 years and a 2.4-fold increase in the risk of developing DDD and end plate herniations at age 40 to 49 years.[43] Affected Trp2 individuals had more severe degeneration. The Trp3 allele was absent from the southern Chinese population. This study demonstrated that the association between this gene and DDD was age dependent because it was more prevalent in some age groups than in others.

Trp2 was common in the Japanese population, but no association with DDD was found.[65] However, the researchers found an association of a *COL9A2*-specific haplotype with DDD ($P = 0.025$; permutation test); this association was more significant in patients with severe DDD ($P = 0.011$).[65] In another Japanese study of 84 patients (mean age, 43.4 years) who underwent lumbar diskectomy, 21.4% had the Trp2 allele, and no patients had the Trp3 allele.[66] Patients with the Trp2 allele who were less than 40 years old showed more severe disk degeneration at the surgical level than did those without the Trp2 allele (OR, 6.00; $P = 0.043$). In contrast, patients 40 years old or older did not show a significant association between disk degeneration and collagen type IX genotype.

Collagen Type XI, Matrix Metalloproteinase-3, Vitamin D Receptor, and Cartilage Intermediate-Layer Protein

In a study of 164 Finnish men (40 to 45 years old), Solovieva and associates found that the carriers of the *COL11A2* (chromosomal location 6p21.3) minor allele had an increased risk of disk bulges (OR, 2.1; 95% CI, 1.0-4.2) compared with noncarriers.[47] MMP-3 (stromelysin-1) is a potent proteoglycan-degrading enzyme that has an important role in the degeneration of intervertebral disks.[67] Gene polymorphisms of the VDR are thought to contribute to disorders such as osteoporosis, osteoarthritis, and DDD.[54,55,57,68-70] Furthermore, Seki and colleagues concluded that the extracellular matrix protein CILP regulates transforming growth factor-β signaling and that this regulation plays a crucial role in the etiology and pathogenesis of DDD.[59]

Symptoms and Natural Course of Disease

Pain Generator

In the lumbar spine, disk degeneration is associated with low back symptoms.[71-75] Studies indicate that a higher degree of lumbar disk degeneration is related to a higher likelihood of symptoms; moreover, the presence of moderate disk degeneration or degenerative changes at multiple levels increases the likelihood of pain.[72,74] A tissue or structure can generate pain only if it is innervated. Pain generators of the spine have been studied mostly in the lumbar region, but the physiology of nociception in cervical disks is identical to that in lumbar disks. The intervertebral disk is innervated mainly by the sinuvertebral nerve, although it receives direct branches in its posterolateral aspect from the ramus communicans or the ventral ramus.[76] In a normal lumbar disk, nerve endings can be found in the periphery of the outer annulus fibrosus and central end plate but not in the inner annulus fibrosus or nucleus pulposus.[77] The facet joints, the posterior synovial joints, are compromised with advancing disk degeneration.[78] Disk degeneration with reduction of disk height is considered to be the initiating event that leads to secondary deterioration of the posterior elements, such as in the facet joints, most of the time.

Diskographic studies have shown that only annular ruptures, which extend to the outer annulus fibrosus, as expected on the basis of histologic studies on innervation, produce pain.[79] In the lumbar spine, pain among young subjects is more likely to be diskogenic, whereas in older subjects the probability of pain related to the facet joint increases.[80] Although diskography is regarded as the gold standard in the diagnosis of diskogenic pain, this procedure is invasive and may enhance progression of disk degeneration, as noted in the lumbar spine.[81]

Neck Pain

Most cases of cervical DDD can be diagnosed by history and physical examination alone, but patients with concerning signs (red flags) should be screened with neurologic examination for signs of radiculopathy and myelopathy.[82] Cervical disk disease typically manifests with axial neck pain and loss of range of motion of the cervical spine. Headaches have been reported by 2.5% of patients,[83] and 71% of patients experience unilateral or bilateral shoulder pain.[84] The burden and determinants of neck pain in the general population were estimated in a best evidence synthesis of the published literature; the 12-month prevalence of any neck pain ranged between 30% and 50%, and activity-limiting pain ranged between 1.7% and 11.5%.[85] Neck pain was more prevalent among women, and prevalence peaked in middle age. In the state of North Carolina, the prevalence of chronic neck pain was 2.2% among noninstitutionalized individuals, and it was also more common in middle age and among women.[86] In Finland, the prevalence of physician-diagnosed chronic neck syndrome was 5.5% among male patients and 7.3% among female patients, and the highest prevalence was in older age groups.[87]

Risk factors for neck pain include genetics, poor psychological health, and smoking,[85] whereas higher education decreases the risk of chronic neck pain.[87] Disk degeneration was not identified as a risk factor of chronic neck pain.[85] In one retrospective study of patients with chronic neck pain, the most common tissue sources of neck pain were the facet joints (55% of those with completed investigations), followed by diskogenic pain (16%) and lateral atlantoaxial pain (9%).[88] Most episodes of neck and arm pain resolve spontaneously. Underlying cervical degeneration likely increases the time course of healing for minor neck strains. Patients with neck pain usually have difficulty with persistent static positioning (sitting, writing, computer use, driving) and with upper extremity activities (reaching, pushing over the shoulder).

Radiculopathy

Occipital pain, pain in the mastoid-maxillary area, and pain in the supraorbital area can also occur. Interscapular and upper brachial dermatomal pain radiation is also common.[89] Radicular syndromes may result from a wide variety of pathologic conditions. A Rochester, Minnesota, study looked at patients from 13 to 91 years of age and found that the mean age for onset of radicular complaints was similar for men (48.2 years) and women (47.7 years).[90] The most common causes are posterolateral soft disk herniations and spondylotic osteophytes at the neural foramen, with resulting unilateral radiculopathy.

Neurologic problems include specific nerve root signs of weakness, atrophy, decreased deep tendon reflexes, paresthesias, or hypesthesias. The largest intersegmental flexion-extension motion occurs between C4 and C5 and, in particular, between C5 and C6.[91,92] Thus, the C5-C6 interspace exhibits the earliest and greatest degree of degeneration, and the C6 root is the most commonly affected by disk protrusion.[93] Henderson and co-workers showed that 98.7% of 846 cases of cervical radiculopathy occurred at C5-C6 or C6-C7.[94] These patients complain of radiating pain down the biceps into the radial forearm. Other complaints include weakness of the wrist extensors, biceps, and triceps. Diminution of the brachioradialis reflex may also be noted. More than half of these patients have a normal dermatomal pattern of pain and paresthesia.[94] Herniations more commonly cause reflex loss, cervical muscle spasm, restricted motion, a positive Spurling sign, and pain or motor deficit in a single dermatomal or myotomal distribution.[95] Radicular pain from soft disk protrusion may be intensified with a Valsalva maneuver, rotation and flexion of the head toward the side of symptoms, and axial compression of the skull. Abduction of the shoulder often eases radicular pain.

The spinal nerve root, which consists of secondary motor neurons, has a capacity for recovery. Radiculopathies tend to improve with time. For approximately half of patients with cervical radiculopathy, symptoms resolve after 6 to 12 weeks. Only 10% to 15% of patients have residual impairment.[96] However, the evidence supporting nonoperative management is not strong, and studies have reported contrasting findings. Gore and associates showed that 79% of patients treated nonoperatively improved or were asymptomatic at follow-up; however, one third of these patients still rated their pain as moderate to severe.[97] Another series showed that symptoms persisted in more than 50% of patients treated nonoperatively.[98]

Myelopathy

Cervical spondylotic myelopathy arises from cervical spondylosis, OPLL, or soft disk herniation. The average age of patients is reported to be in the middle to late 50s.[99-101] Myelopathy usually has a less favorable natural history. Symptoms evolve slowly and insidiously, but some patients experience periods of stability interspersed with episodes of deterioration. In 44 patients, Lees and Turner showed that symptoms and disability were rapidly progressive in only 5% of cases.[98] In 20% of these

patients, symptoms were slowly progressive. Duration of symptoms ranges from several months to several years before patients require surgery.[99,101]

Large central disks can cause myelopathy and usually require decompression. This disorder usually causes problems with the posterior column function of the upper extremities. Patients describe sensory complaints such as numbness or tingling in the hands. These symptoms start in the fingertips, and the usual feeling is described as being gloved.[102] Thus, the symptoms do not follow a dermatomal distribution that suggests radicular symptoms unless specific nerve roots are involved. Patients have difficulty in fine motor function, such as writing. Hyperreflexia is commonly found in patients with a positive Hoffmann sign, reverse supinator and scapulohumeral reflexes, Babinski reflex, and ankle clonus. Gait deterioration usually follows the severity of the disease and is generally attributable to spasticity rather than weakness. Stiff-knee gait is the usual description for these gait patterns. Patients may require walking aids or even a wheelchair if the condition is severe. Other severe symptoms include sphincter and sexual dysfunction. Soft disk herniation usually produces radicular symptoms along with myelopathy, and pure myelopathy is seen in fewer than 10% of patients.[103] Symptoms usually progress more rapidly than in spondylosis or OPLL.

Vertebral Artery Compression

Vertebral artery compression and vertebrobasilar insufficiency have also been described as caused by degenerative disorders of the cervical spine.[84] Symptoms include headaches, dizziness, vertigo, tinnitus, visual symptoms, facial pain, or numbness. More severe compressions can cause transient ischemic attacks. External compression is rare, however, and these vessels are usually compressed by osteophytes or unstable vertebral elements rather than by herniations.[104]

Imaging

Radiographic changes exhibit a linear increase with age. In the mid-20s, the prevalence of disk degeneration is 10%, and it increases through the age of 65 years, when it approaches 95%.[13] By the sixth decade, more than three fourths of individuals have degenerative changes but may nevertheless be asymptomatic. Lawrence and colleagues found radiographic changes in more than 90% of their patients who were more than 65 years old, but the peak prevalence of pain was only 9%.[13] In another study, 25% of asymptomatic patients in their fifth decade, as opposed to 75% of patients in their seventh decade, demonstrated cervical degeneration.[105] The clinical implications are not clear. Brain and co-workers found no consistent association between radiographs and symptoms.[30] Gore and associates followed 205 patients with neck complaints and failed to identify a relationship between the degree of spinal degeneration and the patients' symptoms.[97] An MRI study of the cervical spine in 497 asymptomatic volunteers between 1993 and 1996 found that the incidence of degenerative changes in the cervical spine on MRI increased with age.[7] For example, a decrease in the signal intensity of the intervertebral disks was observed in 17% and 12% of the disks in men and women, respectively, in their 20s, whereas a decrease was observed in 86% and 89% of the disks in men and women, respectively, after 60 years of age.[8] In general, the quantity of water decreases in the nucleus pulposus as Keep it "as" person ages, and the disk becomes a dry, crumbly, grayish-white, or dark brown mass.[4] This condition can be seen in T2-weighted MRI images as lost signal intensity,[106] as well as decrement of intervertebral space.[107]

Although MRI is widely considered the gold standard for the diagnosis and assessment of cervical DDD, important information can also be gathered from plain radiographs and computed tomography (CT) scans. On plain radiographs, cervical DDD can be diagnosed on the basis of narrowed disk spaces and osteophyte formation. Dynamic scans are also useful to assess the integrity of the cervical disk and the severity of degeneration leading to instability of spinal segments (Fig. 12-1). Findings noted on dynamic scans can drive the decision about whether fusion is required to stabilize the spine. CT scans are useful to distinguish between soft and hard disk disorders (Fig.

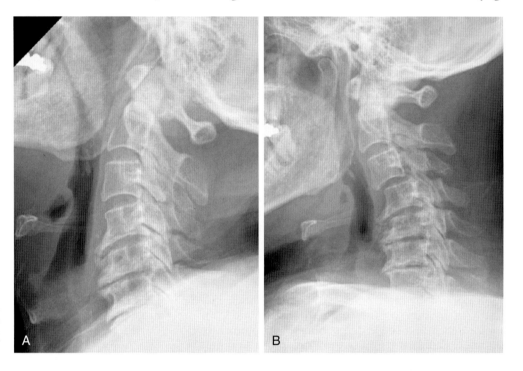

FIGURE 12-1   Flexion (**A**) and extension (**B**) dynamic lateral radiographs of the cervical spine showing multiple levels of degeneration. Note the osteophytes at C4-C5, C5-C6, and C6-C7 and the instability at C3-C4.

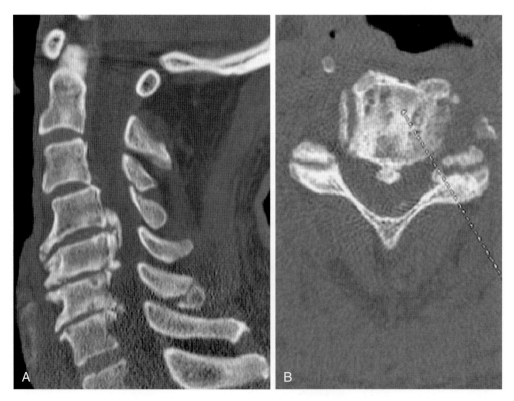

FIGURE 12-2   A, Sagittal computed tomography (CT) scan showing cervical degenerative disk disease with osteophyte formation C4-C5, C5-C6, and C6-C7. **B,** Axial CT scan of C4-C5 shows a posterior osteophyte with spinal canal compromise.

12-2). CT can also assess the severity of involvement and the location of osteophyte formation, as well as establish the diagnosis of OPLL or ossified yellow ligament.

Disk spaces on MRI have moderately high signal intensity in the inner region and are surrounded by a rim of low signal intensity that represents the annulus fibrosus. Herniation that is central or paracentral can be recognized on sagittal images by an area of medium-intensity signal posterior to the disk space. On gradient-echo or T1-weighted sequences, disk material has a higher signal than the dense cortical bone of a ridge. Disk protrusion or herniation can be adequately assessed on MRI scans (Fig. 12-3). Further evidence of myelopathy can be observed by hyperintensity or enhancement of the spinal cord at the level of the compression, thus indicating spinal cord damage. This is important for the diagnosis and location of the lesion for surgical planning.

The main advantage of sagittal T1-weighted MRI sequences is that they allow differentiation of disk disease from osteophytes. A herniated disk has intermediate signal intensity and is continuous with normal disk tissue. The central portion of osteophytes has higher signal intensity than does disk tissue, and most osteophytes have a dark outline representing cortical bone and periosteum. A calcified osteophyte has homogeneous low signal intensity and can be recognized as a bony spur.

Modic changes (MCs) are vertebral end plate and bone marrow signal changes that are visible only on MRI and are shown in the lumbar spine to relate to low back pain.[108] MCs are claimed to represent a specific phenotype of symptomatic lumbar DDD.[109] The prevalence of MCs in the cervical spine has been evaluated only among patients with neck pain.[110,111] In an MRI study by Mann and colleagues of patients who were more than 50 years old, the occurrence of MCs was most common at C5-C6 and C6-C7 (almost 5% for both), and MCs colocalized typically with disk herniations.[110] Currently, no studies exist on the association of cervical MCs and neck pain in a controlled cohort setting.

Management

Nonoperative Treatment

Education about the disease is the first goal of treatment for cervical DDD. Other goals of treatment are to relieve pain, improve function, and prevent recurrence. Chronic cervical disease may entail psychological modifiers that may adversely affect outcomes. Treatment modalities for radiculopathy include rest, medications, physical therapy, manipulation, injections, and patient education. Patients with cervical radiculopathy should not be immobilized for more than 2 days, to maximize their rehabilitation potential. Pharmacologic agents provide symptomatic relief. These include steroids, nonsteroidal anti-inflammatory drugs, and muscle relaxants.[112] Steroids should be used only for short-term initial management because these drugs have a multitude of undesirable side effects. Nonsteroidal

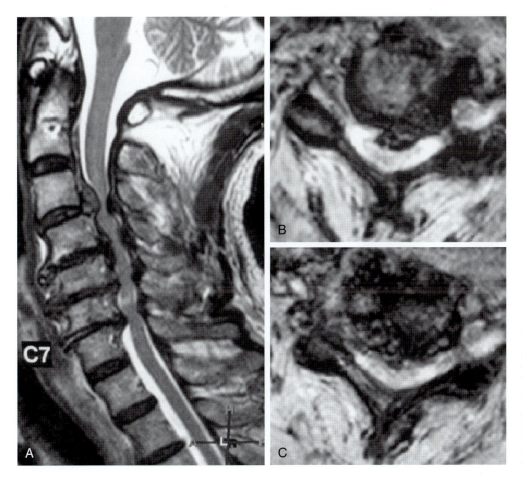

FIGURE 12-3 A, Sagittal magnetic resonance imaging showing cervical spondylotic myelopathy caused by disk protrusions at C3-C4, C4-C5, C5-C6, and C6-C7 with a hypertrophic ligamentum flavum at the same levels. Spinal cord myelomalacic changes are seen posterior to the C6 body. Axial scans of C4-C5 (**B**) and C5-C6 (**C**) show spinal canal compromise by the disk protrusion and compression of the spinal cord.

anti-inflammatory drugs are commonly used. They interfere with prostaglandin synthesis, thus inhibiting the inflammatory cascade of the condition. Muscle relaxants can provide relief for patients with muscle spasms. Drugs with sedative effects should be avoided. Manipulation and mobilization of the neck may provide short-term and intermediate-term relief for neck pain.[113] In patients with intractable pain, a cervical collar or cervical traction may be recommended. It is unclear whether traction is effective, and no evidence indicates that the degree of disk prolapse would be reduced with its use.[114]

Physical therapy includes passive and active modalities, and they should be initiated within the first 3 to 5 days of treatment.[115] Passive modalities include heat, cryotherapy, mechanical traction, ultrasound, massage, and use of a soft cervical collar.[115] Heat therapy is thought to reduce pain at trigger points,[116] as well as reducing muscle spasms.[117] Deep heat by ultrasound can also improve radicular pain and myelopathy to some degree. Cryotherapy can decrease muscle guarding and reduce inflammation.[118,119] Cervical traction can distract joints and relieve pressure off nerve roots and disks, improve epidural blood flow, and reduce inflammation, pain, and muscle spasms. Massage can provide mechanical stimulation to increase circulation and promote muscle relaxation.[120] However, these modalities have no evidence to verify their effectiveness. Active modalities include isometric exercises, aerobic conditioning, range-of-motion exercises, and dynamic muscle training. Isometric exercises allow strengthening of paravertebral muscles without invoking the spinal motion that may cause pain. Aerobic conditioning and range-of-motion exercises with dynamic strength training should be enforced for maintenance of overall health. In the latest *Cochrane Review* by Kay and co-workers,[121] no strong support was found for neck stretching and strengthening exercises in chronic neck pain and for neck endurance training in patients with acute cervicogenic headaches. In addition, evidence supporting neck proprioceptive training for headaches in the short term was minimal. At present, no evidence supports upper extremity strengthening or endurance and extensibility exercises for neck pain.

That myelopathy consists of a nonlinear decline in function is generally accepted.[122] Some patients experience a plateau in symptoms, but spontaneous improvement is rarely encountered. Other patients may have rapid decline instead. Currently, no predictor for the natural course of myelopathy exists because clinical and imaging findings do not correlate with the neurologic condition.[123] Therapeutic modalities are adjunctive to surgery. Physical therapy can assist rehabilitation, as well as endurance and pain control. Cervical collars can increase support during initial phase of treatment.

Operative Treatment

Most symptomatic cervical DDD responds to nonoperative management, but surgical treatment is indicated for patients with intractable pain, severe or progressive neurologic deficits, myelopathy, nonprogressive but disabling motor deficit, and failure to respond to nonoperative therapy.[124-132] Removing a cervical disk solely for neck pain is not indicated. Surgery includes nerve root injections or decompression surgical procedures with or without fusion and instrumentation. Nerve root injections can be diagnostic as well as palliative; however, they have serious complications.[133,134] Trigger point treatments are not proven for long-term effectiveness. Many techniques are used to decompress the cervical spine, including diskectomy, corpectomy, laminoforaminotomy, laminectomy, and laminoplasty. Arm pain may respond better than neck pain to surgical intervention. In the Rochester, Minnesota, series, 26% of patients with cervical radiculopathy underwent surgical intervention.[90] In the United States, the number of orthopedic surgeons performing spine surgery has increased.[135] At the same time, the absolute number of diskectomy-fusions has increased by 67% per year, with a marked increase in the use of allografts and interbody devices and significant regional variation.

Many options are available for decompression of disk disorders. The direct approach to removal of disk compression requires an anterior approach. The standard technique consists of anterior cervical diskectomy and fusion.[124-132,136,137] In general, anterior approaches are recommended for patients with normal to kyphotic alignment because laminectomy in these patients can cause further kyphosis as a result of destabilization of the spine.[138,139] Anterior decompression and fusion require removal of the compressive and degenerative structures with fusion of the segments adjacent to the decompression (Fig. 12-4). Overall, the extent of the operation can range from removal of one disk to removal of several disks, partial vertebrectomy, and strut graft fusion. Corpectomy and strut grafting are required for longer lengths of decompression. Occasionally, an anterior cervical plate can be placed for better stability and earlier mobilization. In a study of 1015 patients undergoing anterior cervical diskectomy and fusion, the fusion rate was reported to be up to 94.5%.[140] Studies by Samartzis and associates noted high fusion rates with single-level fusion with or without plate fixation,[122,125-128,137] but the risk of nonunion increased as the levels of fusion also increased. However, proper patient selection and meticulous operative technique have been advocated as key factors to successful fusion in any situation. Most studies have shown major improvements in symptoms among the majority of patients.[141-143] The most common cause of recurrent symptoms or deterioration of initially favorable results is adjacent level degeneration to the fusion.[142,143] The risk of major neurologic complication is quite rare. Flynn and colleagues found an incidence of 0.01% for major neurologic complications after anterior cervical diskectomy and fusion.[144] Other complications are caused by soft tissue dissection in the anterior approach, as well as by grafting and plating. These complications include recurrent laryngeal nerve palsy causing hoarseness, esophageal and tracheal injury and perforation, graft dislodgement and subsidence, and bone graft donor site morbidity.

Indirect decompression entails a posterior approach to the spinal cord. The posterior elements are decompressed to allow the spinal cord to float away from the anterior compressing disk. Laminectomy, laminectomy with fusion with or without instrumentation (Fig. 12-5),

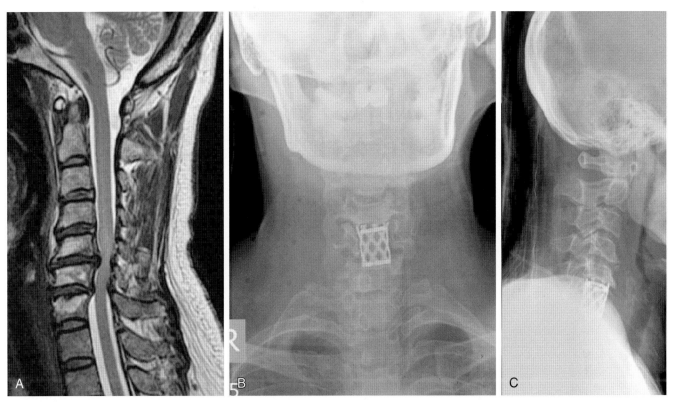

FIGURE 12-4   A, Sagittal magnetic resonance imaging scan showing C5-C6 disk protrusion with spinal cord compression and myelomalacic changes at the corresponding level. C6-C7 was also stenotic, and thus, C6 corpectomy and C5 to C7 anterior spinal fusion with cage insertion were performed, as evidenced in the postoperative anteroposterior (**B**) and lateral (**C**) radiographs.

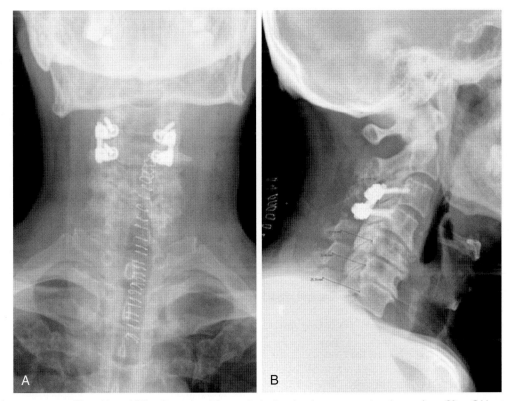

FIGURE 12-5   Anteroposterior (**A**) and lateral (**B**) radiographs of the cervical spine showing postoperative changes from C3 to C4 laminectomy and instrumented fusion.

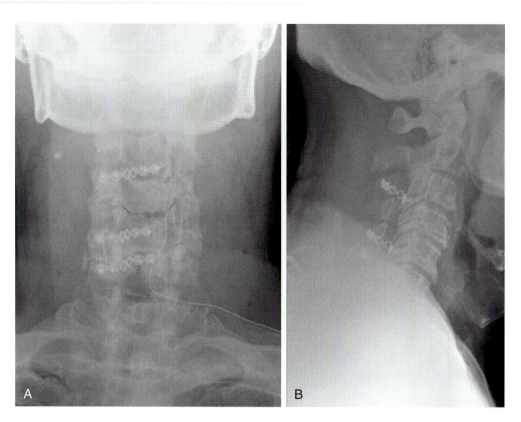

FIGURE 12-6 Anteroposterior (**A**) and lateral (**B**) radiographs of the cervical spine showing postoperative changes from C3 to C6 laminoplasty, with the hinges kept open by miniplates at C3, C5, and C6.

and laminoplasty (Fig. 12-6) are the common options. The diameter of the spinal canal is increased after the procedure, and the potential for further stenosis is decreased. Direct decompression of the nerve roots by foraminotomy is also possible in patients with radiculopathy. Posterior approaches are more often indicated for patients with lordotic or neutral alignment of the cervical spine. Posterior approaches can also tackle multiple levels of compression and cases of congenital stenosis. Involved segments usually include C3 through C6 or C7. C2 posterior muscle attachments are usually preserved to avoid postoperative neck pain and progressive kyphosis. Laminectomy generally is accompanied by fusion and instrumentation to increase stability and to restore or maintain lordosis. Up to 70% to 80% of patients have satisfactory results with laminectomy.[98] Expansive open-door laminoplasty, as described by Hirabayashi and co-workers,[145] was noted to have good results in 66% of patients.[146] Complications include paralysis, hematoma, postoperative C5 palsy, dural injury, and postlaminectomy kyphosis and neck pain (25%).

Cervical disk arthroplasty is a newer method that has growing popularity, although no long-term results are currently available to verify its use. Current evidence shows no difference between arthroplasty and fusion in terms of revision rate up to 2 years of follow-up.[147] Only two studies demonstrated a marginal but clinically questionable benefit of disk replacement over fusion for the end point "overall success."[148,149] However, the end point of "overall success" was not adequately defined in these studies. Huppert and associates found, at 2 years of follow-up, that revision surgery was required in 2.3% of patients who underwent single-level arthroplasty and in 3.6% of patients who underwent multilevel arthroplasty.[150]

Conclusions

The etiology of cervical DDD remains incompletely understood. Numerous studies have attempted to elaborate on the various risk factors associated with cervical DDD, but additional well-controlled, large-scale, and multiethnic studies are needed to delineate the true degree of risk of various factors. Various imaging techniques exist to assess the degree of cervical DDD, with indications and strengths for each. In the majority of cases, cervical disk degeneration is asymptomatic, but symptomatic conditions can be managed nonoperatively. Operatively, the numerous approaches and indications largely depend on the location and extent of the pathologic process, cervical alignment, comorbidities, and the surgeon's preference. Overall, outcomes stemming from the surgical treatment of cervical DDD have been promising.

REFERENCES

1. Bailey P, Casamajor L: Osteoarthritis of the spine as a cause of compression of the spinal cord and its roots, *J Nerv Ment Dis* 38:588–609, 1911.
2. Lehto IJ, Tertti MO, Komu ME, et al.: Age-related MRI changes at 0.1 T in cervical discs in asymptomatic subjects, *Neuroradiology* 36:49–53, 1994.
3. Christe A, Laubli R, Guzman R, et al.: Degeneration of the cervical disc: histology compared with radiography and magnetic resonance imaging, *Neuroradiology* 47:721–729, 2005.
4. Prescher A: Anatomy and pathology of the aging spine, *Eur J Radiol* 27:181–195, 1998.
5. Boden SD, McCowin PR, Davis DO, et al.: Abnormal magnetic-resonance scans of the cervical spine in asymptomatic subjects: a prospective investigation, *J Bone Surg Am* 72:1178–1184, 1990.
6. Gore DR: Roentgenographic findings in the cervical spine in asymptomatic persons: a ten-year follow-up, *Spine (Phila Pa 1976)* 26:2463–2466, 2001.

7. Matsumoto M, Fujimura Y, Suzuki N, et al.: MRI of cervical intervertebral discs in asymptomatic subjects, *J Bone Surg Br* 80:19–24, 1998.

8. Okada E, Matsumoto M, Ichihara D, et al.: Aging of the cervical spine in healthy volunteers: a 10-year longitudinal magnetic resonance imaging study, *Spine (Phila Pa 1976)* 34:706–712, 2009.

9. Buckwalter JA: Aging and degeneration of the human intervertebral disc, *Spine (Phila Pa 1976)* 20:1307–1314, 1995.

10. Gore DR, Sepic SB, Gardner GM: Roentgenographic findings of the cervical spine in asymptomatic people, *Spine (Phila Pa 1976)* 11:521–524, 1986.

11. Wiesel SW, Tsourmas N, Feffer HL, et al.: A study of computer-assisted tomography. I. The incidence of positive CAT scans in an asymptomatic group of patients, *Spine (Phila Pa 1976)* 9:549–551, 1984.

12. Laimi K, Erkintalo M, Metsahonkala L, et al.: Adolescent disc degeneration: no headache association, *Cephalalgia* 27:14–21, 2007.

13. Lawrence JS: Disc degeneration: its frequency and relationship to symptoms, *Ann Rheum Dis* 28:121–138, 1969.

14. Urban JP, Holm S, Maroudas A, Nachemson A: Nutrition of the intervertebral disk: an in vivo study of solute transport, *Clin Orthop Relat Res* (129)101–114, 1977.

15. Sedowofia KA, Tomlinson IW, Weiss JB, et al.: Collagenolytic enzyme systems in human intervertebral disc: their control, mechanism, and their possible role in the initiation of biomechanical failure, *Spine (Phila Pa 1976)* 7:213–222, 1982.

16. Hendry NG: The hydration of the nucleus pulposus and its relation to intervertebral disc derangement, *J Bone Surg Br* 40: 132–144, 1958.

17. Lotz JC, Colliou OK, Chin JR, et al.: Compression-induced degeneration of the intervertebral disc: an in vivo mouse model and finite-element study, *Spine (Phila Pa 1976)* 23:2493–2506, 1998.

18. Lindblom K: Intervertebral-disc degeneration considered as a pressure atrophy, *J Bone Surg Am* 39:933–945, 1957.

19. Kanemoto M, Hukuda S, Komiya Y, et al.: Immunohistochemical study of matrix metalloproteinase-3 and tissue inhibitor of metalloproteinase-1 human intervertebral discs, *Spine (Phila Pa 1976)* 21:1–8, 1996.

20. Ariga K, Yonenobu K, Nakase T, et al.: Localization of cathepsins D, K, and L in degenerated human intervertebral discs, *Spine (Phila Pa 1976)* 26:2666–2672, 2001.

21. Ng SC, Weiss JB, Quennel R, Jayson MI: Abnormal connective tissue degrading enzyme patterns in prolapsed intervertebral discs, *Spine (Phila Pa 1976)* 11:695–701, 1986.

22. Oda J, Tanaka H, Tsuzuki N: Intervertebral disc changes with aging of human cervical vertebra: from the neonate to the eighties, *Spine (Phila Pa 1976)* 13:1205–1211, 1988.

23. Weidner N, Rice DT: Intervertebral disk material: criteria for determining probable prolapse, *Hum Pathol* 19:406–410, 1988.

24. Hunt WE: Cervical spondylosis: natural history and rare indications for surgical decompression, *Clin Neurosurg* 27:466–480, 1980.

25. Lestini WF, Wiesel SW: The pathogenesis of cervical spondylosis, *Clin Orthop Relat Res (239)*69–93, 1989.

26. Holt S, Yates PO: Cervical spondylosis and nerve root lesions: incidence at routine necropsy, *J Bone Surg Br* 48:407–423, 1966.

27. Le Maitre CL, Freemont AJ, Hoyland JA: The role of interleukin-1 in the pathogenesis of human intervertebral disc degeneration, *Arthritis Res Ther* 7:R732–R745, 2005.

28. Weiler C, Nerlich AG, Bachmeier BE, Boos N: Expression and distribution of tumor necrosis factor alpha in human lumbar intervertebral discs: a study in surgical specimen and autopsy controls, *Spine (Phila Pa 1976)* 30:44–53, 2005. discussion 4.

29. Mio F, Chiba K, Hirose Y, et al.: A functional polymorphism in COL11A1, which encodes the alpha 1 chain of type XI collagen, is associated with susceptibility to lumbar disc herniation, *Am J Hum Genet* 81:1271–1277, 2007.

30. Brain WR, Knight GC, Bull JW: Discussion of rupture of the intervertebral disc in the cervical region, *Proc R Soc Med* 41: 509–516, 1948.

31. Hagberg M, Wegman DH: Prevalence rates and odds ratios of shoulder-neck diseases in different occupational groups, *Br I Ind Med* 44:602–610, 1987.

32. Rahim KA, Stambough JL: Radiographic evaluation of the degenerative cervical spine, *Orthop Clin North Am* 23:395–403, 1992.

33. Takamiya Y, Nagata K, Fukuda K, et al.: Cervical spine disorders in farm workers requiring neck extension actions, *J Orthop Sci* 11:235–240, 2006.

34. Kauppila LI: Atherosclerosis and disc degeneration/low-back pain: a systematic review, *Eur J Vasc Endovasc Surg* 37:661–670, 2009.

35. Jacobs B, Ghelman B, Marchisello P: Coexistence of cervical and lumbar disc disease, *Spine (Phila Pa 1976)* 15:1261–1264, 1990.

36. Gore DR, Carrera GF, Glaeser ST: Smoking and degenerative changes of the cervical spine: a roentgenographic study, *Spine J* 6:557–560, 2006.

37. Kelsey JL, Githens PB, Walter SD, et al.: An epidemiological study of acute prolapsed cervical intervertebral disc, *J Bone Surg Am* 66:907–914, 1984.

38. Mundt DJ, Kelsey JL, Golden AL, et al.: An epidemiologic study of sports and weight lifting as possible risk factors for herniated lumbar and cervical discs: the Northeast Collaborative Group on Low Back Pain, *Am J Sports Med* 21:854–860, 1993.

39. Battie MC, Videman T: Lumbar disc degeneration: epidemiology and genetics, *J Bone Surg Am* 88(Suppl 2):3–9, 2006.

40. Pluijm SM, van Essen HW, Bravenboer N, et al.: Collagen type I alpha1 Sp1 polymorphism, osteoporosis, and intervertebral disc degeneration in older men and women, *Ann Rheum Dis* 63: 71–77, 2004.

41. Tilkeridis C, Bei T, Garantziotis S, Stratakis CA: Association of a COL1A1 polymorphism with lumbar disc disease in young military recruits, *J Med Genet* 42e44, 2005.

42. Annunen S, Paassilta P, Lohiniva J, et al.: An allele of COL9A2 associated with intervertebral disc disease, *Science* 285:409–412, 1999.

43. Jim JJ, Noponen-Hietala N, Cheung KM, et al.: The TRP2 allele of COL9A2 is an age-dependent risk factor for the development and severity of intervertebral disc degeneration, *Spine (Phila Pa 1976)* 30:2735–2742, 2005.

44. Kales SN, Linos A, Chatzis C, et al.: The role of collagen IX tryptophan polymorphisms in symptomatic intervertebral disc disease in Southern European patients, *Spine (Phila Pa 1976)* 29:1266–1270, 2004.

45. Karppinen J, Paakko E, Raina S, et al.: Magnetic resonance imaging findings in relation to the COL9A2 tryptophan allele among patients with sciatica, *Spine (Phila Pa 1976)* 27:78–83, 2002.

46. Paassilta P, Lohiniva J, Goring HH, et al.: Identification of a novel common genetic risk factor for lumbar disk disease, *JAMA* 285:1843–1849, 2001.

47. Solovieva S, Lohiniva J, Leino-Arjas P, et al.: Intervertebral disc degeneration in relation to the COL9A3 and the IL-1ss gene polymorphisms, *Eur Spine J* 15:613–619, 2006.

48. Solovieva S, Kouhia S, Leino-Arjas P, et al.: Interleukin 1 polymorphisms and intervertebral disc degeneration, *Epidemiology* 15:626–633, 2004.

49. Virtanen IM, Karppinen J, Taimela S, et al.: Occupational and genetic risk factors associated with intervertebral disc disease, *Spine (Phila Pa 1976)* 32:1129–1134, 2007.

50. Kawaguchi Y, Osada R, Kanamori M, et al.: Association between an aggrecan gene polymorphism and lumbar disc degeneration, *Spine (Phila Pa 1976)* 24:2456–2460, 1999.

51. Roughley P, Martens D, Rantakokko J, et al.: The involvement of aggrecan polymorphism in degeneration of human intervertebral disc and articular cartilage, *Eur Cells Mater* 11:1–7, 2006.

52. Watanabe H, Nakata K, Kimata K, et al.: Dwarfism and age-associated spinal degeneration of heterozygote cmd mice defective in aggrecan, *Proc Natl Acad Sci U S A* 94:6943–6947, 1997.

53. Cheung KM, Chan D, Karppinen J, et al.: Association of the Taq I allele in vitamin D receptor with degenerative disc disease and disc bulge in a Chinese population, *Spine (Phila Pa 1976)* 31:1143–1148, 2006.

54. Jones G, White C, Sambrook P, Eisman J: Allelic variation in the vitamin D receptor, lifestyle factors and lumbar spinal degenerative disease, *Ann Rheum Dis* 57:94–99, 1998.

55. Kawaguchi Y, Kanamori M, Ishihara H, et al.: The association of lumbar disc disease with vitamin-D receptor gene polymorphism, *J Bone Surg Am* 84:2022–2028, 2002.

56. Videman T, Gibbons L E, Battie M C, et al.: The relative roles of intragenic polymorphisms of the vitamin d receptor gene in lumbar spine degeneration and bone density, *Spine (Phila Pa 1976)* 26:E7–E12, 2001.

57. Videman T, Leppavuori J, Kaprio J, et al.: Intragenic polymorphisms of the vitamin D receptor gene associated with intervertebral disc degeneration, *Spine (Phila Pa 1976)* 23:2477–2485, 1998.

58. Takahashi M, Haro H, Wakabayashi Y, et al.: The association of degeneration of the intervertebral disc with 5a/6a polymorphism in the promoter of the human matrix metalloproteinase-3 gene, *J Bone Surg Br* 83:491–495, 2001.

59. Seki S, Kawaguchi Y, Chiba K, et al.: A functional SNP in CILP, encoding cartilage intermediate layer protein, is associated with susceptibility to lumbar disc disease, *Nat Genet* 37:607–612, 2005.

60. Kimura T, Nakata K, Tsumaki N, et al.: Progressive degeneration of articular cartilage and intervertebral discs: an experimental study in transgenic mice bearing a type IX collagen mutation, *Int Orthop* 20:177–181, 1996.

61. Okada E, Matsumoto M, Fujiwara H, Toyama Y: Disc degeneration of cervical spine on MRI in patients with lumbar disc herniation: comparison study with asymptomatic volunteers, *Eur Spine J* 20:585–591, 2011.

62. Kalichman L, Hunter D J: The genetics of intervertebral disc degeneration: associated genes, *Joint Bone Spine* 75:388–396, 2008.

63. Weiler C, Schietzsch M, Kirchner T, et al.: Age-related changes in human cervical, thoracal and lumbar intervertebral disc exhibit a strong intra-individual correlation, *Eur Spine J* 21(Suppl 6):S810–S818, 2012.

64. Sambrook P N, MacGregor A J, Spector T D: Genetic influences on cervical and lumbar disc degeneration: a magnetic resonance imaging study in twins, *Arthritis Rheum* 42:366–372, 1999.

65. Seki S, Kawaguchi Y, Mori M, et al.: Association study of COL9A2 with lumbar disc disease in the Japanese population, *J Hum Genet* 51:1063–1067, 2006.

66. Higashino K, Matsui Y, Yagi S, et al.: The alpha2 type IX collagen tryptophan polymorphism is associated with the severity of disc degeneration in younger patients with herniated nucleus pulposus of the lumbar spine, *Int Orthop* 31:107–111, 2007.

67. Goupille P, Jayson M I, Valat J P, Freemont A J: Matrix metalloproteinases: the clue to intervertebral disc degeneration? *Spine (Phila Pa 1976)* 23:1612–1626, 1998.

68. Morrison N A, Qi J C, Tokita A, et al.: Prediction of bone density from vitamin D receptor alleles, *Nature* 367:284–287, 1994.

69. Uitterlinden A G, Fang Y, Bergink A P, et al.: The role of vitamin D receptor gene polymorphisms in bone biology, *Mol Cell Endocrinol* 197:15–21, 2002.

70. Zmuda J M, Cauley J A, Ferrell R E: Recent progress in understanding the genetic susceptibility to osteoporosis, *Genet Epidemiol* 16:356–367, 1999.

71. Cheung K M, Karppinen J, Chan D, et al.: Prevalence and pattern of lumbar magnetic resonance imaging changes in a population study of one thousand forty-three individuals, *Spine (Phila Pa 1976)* 34:934–940, 2009.

72. de Schepper E I, Damen J, van Meurs J B, et al.: The association between lumbar disc degeneration and low back pain: the influence of age, gender, and individual radiographic features, *Spine (Phila Pa 1976)* 35:531–536, 2010.

73. Samartzis D, Karppinen J, Mok F, et al.: A population-based study of juvenile disc degeneration and its association with overweight and obesity, low back pain, and diminished functional status, *J Bone Surg Am* 93:662–670, 2011.

74. Takatalo J, Karppinen J, Niinimaki J, et al.: Does lumbar disc degeneration on magnetic resonance imaging associate with low back symptom severity in young Finnish adults? *Spine (Phila Pa 1976)* 36:2180–2189, 2011.

75. Samartzis D, Karppinen J, Chan D, et al.: *The association of disc degeneration based on magnetic resonance imaging and the presence of low back pain. Presented at World Forum for Spine Research: Intervertebral Disc, 2010 July 5–8, Montreal, 2010, Canada.*

76. Bogduk N: The innervation of the lumbar spine, *Spine (Phila Pa 1976)* 8:286–293, 1983.

77. Fagan A, Moore R, Vernon Roberts B, et al.: ISSLS prize winner: the innervation of the intervertebral disc: a quantitative analysis, *Spine (Phila Pa 1976)* 28:2570–2576, 2003.

78. Hussain M, Natarajan RN, An HS, Andersson GB: Reduction in segmental flexibility because of disc degeneration is accompanied by higher changes in facet loads than changes in disc pressure: a poroelastic C5-C6 finite element investigation, *Spine J* 10:1069–1077, 2010.

79. Moneta G B, Videman T, Kaivanto K, et al.: Reported pain during lumbar discography as a function of anular ruptures and disc degeneration: a re-analysis of 833 discograms, *Spine (Phila Pa 1976)* 19:1968–1974, 1994.

80. DePalma M J, Ketchum J M, Saullo T: What is the source of chronic low back pain and does age play a role? *Pain Med* 12:224–233, 2011.

81. Carragee E J, Don A S, Hurwitz E L, et al.: 2009 ISSLS Prize Winner. Does discography cause accelerated progression of degeneration changes in the lumbar disc: a ten-year matched cohort study, *Spine (Phila Pa 1976)* 34:2338–2345, 2009.

82. Guzman J, Haldeman S, Carroll L J, et al.: Clinical practice implications of the Bone and Joint Decade 2000-2010 Task Force on Neck Pain and Its Associated Disorders: from concepts and findings to recommendations, *Spine (Phila Pa 1976)* 33(Suppl):S199–S213, 2008.

83. Nilsson N: The prevalence of cervicogenic headache in a random population sample of 20-59 year olds, *Spine (Phila Pa 1976)* 20:1884–1888, 1995.

84. Heller J G: The syndromes of degenerative cervical disease, *Orthop Clin North Am* 23:381–394, 1992.

85. Hogg-Johnson S, van der Velde G, Carroll L J, et al.: The burden and determinants of neck pain in the general population: results of the Bone and Joint Decade 2000-2010 Task Force on Neck Pain and Its Associated Disorders, *Spine (Phila Pa 1976)* 33(Suppl):S39–S51, 2008.

86. Goode A P, Freburger J, Carey T: Prevalence, practice patterns, and evidence for chronic neck pain, *Arthritis Care Res (Hoboken)* 62:1594–1601, 2010.

87. Leino-Arjas P, Viikari-Juntura E, Kaila-Kangas L, Nykyri E, Riihimäki H: Neck pain and chronic neck syndrome, Musculoskeletal Disorders and Diseases in Finland. Results of the Health 2000 Survey. Publications of the National Public Institute B25, 2007.

88. Yin W, Bogduk N: The nature of neck pain in a private pain clinic in the United States, *Pain Med* 9:196–203, 2008.

89. Aprill C, Dwyer A, Bogduk N: Cervical zygapophyseal joint pain patterns. II. A clinical evaluation, *Spine (Phila Pa 1976)* 15:458–461, 1990.

90. Radhakrishnan K, Litchy W J, O'Fallon W M, Kurland L T: Epidemiology of cervical radiculopathy: a population-based study from Rochester, Minnesota, 1976 through 1990, *Brain* 117:325–335, 1994.

91. Holmes A, Wang C, Han Z H, Dang G T: The range and nature of flexion-extension motion in the cervical spine, *Spine (Phila Pa 1976)* 19:2505–2510, 1994.

92. Lind B, Sihlbom H, Nordwall A, Malchau H: Normal range of motion of the cervical spine, *Arch Phys Med Rehabil* 70:692–695, 1989.

93. Montgomery D M, Brower R S: Cervical spondylotic myelopathy: clinical syndrome and natural history, *Orthop Clin North Am* 23:487–493, 1992.

94. Henderson C M, Hennessy R G, Shuey H M Jr, Shackelford E G: Posterior-lateral foraminotomy as an exclusive operative technique for cervical radiculopathy: a review of 846 consecutively operated cases, *Neurosurgery* 13:504–512, 1983.

95. Lunsford L D, Bissonette D J, Zorub D S: Anterior surgery for cervical disc disease. Part 2: Treatment of cervical spondylotic myelopathy in 32 cases, *J Neurosurg* 53:12–19, 1980.

96. Ellenberg M R, Honet J C, Treanor W J: Cervical radiculopathy, *Arch Phys Med Rehabil* 75:342–352, 1994.

97. Gore D R, Sepic S B, Gardner G M, Murray M P: Neck pain: a long-term follow-up of 205 patients, *Spine (Phila Pa 1976)* 12:1–5, 1987.

98. Lees F, Turner J W: Natural history and prognosis of cervical spondylosis, *Br Med J* 2:1607–1610, 1963.

99. Chiles BW 3rd, Leonard MA, Choudhri HF, Cooper PR: Cervical spondylotic myelopathy: patterns of neurological deficit and recovery after anterior cervical decompression, *Neurosurgery* 44:762–769, 1999. discussion 769–770.

100. George B, Gauthier N, Lot G: Multisegmental cervical spondylotic myelopathy and radiculopathy treated by multilevel oblique corpectomies without fusion, *Neurosurgery* 44:81–90, 1999.

101. Kumar VG, Rea GL, Mervis LJ, McGregor JM: Cervical spondylotic myelopathy: functional and radiographic long-term outcome after laminectomy and posterior fusion, *Neurosurgery* 44:771–777, 1999. discussion 777–778.

102. Voskuhl RR, Hinton RC: Sensory impairment in the hands secondary to spondylotic compression of the cervical spinal cord, *Arch Neurol* 47:309–311, 1990.

103. Bucciero A, Vizioli L, Cerillo A: Soft cervical disc herniation: an analysis of 187 cases, *J Neurosurg Sci* 42:125–130, 1998.

104. Citow JS, Macdonald RL: Posterior decompression of the vertebral artery narrowed by cervical osteophyte: case report, *Surg Neurol* 51:495–498, 1999. discussion 498–499.

105. Friedenberg ZB, Miller WT: Degenerative disc disease of the cervical spine, *J Bone Surg Am* 45:1171–1178, 1963.

106. Benneker LM, Heini PF, Anderson SE, et al.: Correlation of radiographic and MRI parameters to morphological and biochemical assessment of intervertebral disc degeneration, *Eur Spine J* 14:27–35, 2005.

107. Daffner SD, Xin J, Taghavi CE, et al.: Cervical segmental motion at levels adjacent to disc herniation as determined with kinetic magnetic resonance imaging, *Spine (Phila Pa 1976)* 34:2389–2394, 2009.

108. Jensen TS, Karppinen J, Sorensen JS, et al.: Vertebral endplate signal changes (Modic change): a systematic literature review of prevalence and association with non-specific low back pain, *Eur Spine J* 17:1407–1422, 2008.

109. Albert HB, Kjaer P, Jensen TS, et al.: Modic changes, possible causes and relation to low back pain, *Med Hypotheses* 70:361–368, 2008.

110. Mann E, Peterson CK, Hodler J: Degenerative marrow (modic) changes on cervical spine magnetic resonance imaging scans: prevalence, inter- and intra-examiner reliability and link to disc herniation, *Spine (Phila Pa 1976)* 36:1081–1085, 2011.

111. Peterson CK, Humphreys BK, Pringle TC: Prevalence of modic degenerative marrow changes in the cervical spine, *J Manipulative Physiol Ther* 30:5–10, 2007.

112. Dillin W, Uppal GS: Analysis of medications used in the treatment of cervical disk degeneration, *Orthop Clin North Am* 23:421–433, 1992.

113. Gross A, Miller J, D'Sylva J, et al.: Manipulation or mobilisation for neck pain, *Cochrane Database Syst Rev* (1):CD004249, 2010.

114. Harris PR: Cervical traction: review of literature and treatment guidelines, *Phys Ther* 57:910–914, 1977.

115. Tan JC, Nordin M: Role of physical therapy in the treatment of cervical disk disease, *Orthop Clin North Am* 23:435–449, 1992.

116. McCray RE, Patton NJ: Pain relief at trigger points: a comparison of moist heat and shortwave diathermy, *J Orthop Sports Phys Ther* 5:175–178, 1984.

117. Fountain FP, Gersten JW, Sengir O: Decrease in muscle spasm produced by ultrasound, hot packs, and infrared radiation, *Arch Phys Med Rehabil* 41:293–298, 1960.

118. Garra G, Singer AJ, Leno R, et al.: Heat or cold packs for neck and back strain: a randomized controlled trial of efficacy, *Acad Emerg Med* 17:484–489, 2010.

119. Pangarkar S, Lee PC: Conservative treatment for neck pain: medications, physical therapy, and exercise, *Phys Med Rehabil Clin N Am* 22:503–520, 2011. ix.

120. Patel KC, Gross A, Graham N, et al.: Massage for mechanical neck disorders, *Cochrane Database Syst Rev* 9:CD004871, 2012.

121. Kay TM, Gross A, Goldsmith CH, et al.: Exercises for mechanical neck disorders, *Cochrane Database Syst Rev* 8:CD004250, 2012.

122. Orr RD, Zdeblick TA: Cervical spondylotic myelopathy: approaches to surgical treatment, *Clin Orthop Relat Res* (359) 58–66, 1999.

123. Wada E, Ohmura M, Yonenobu K: Intramedullary changes of the spinal cord in cervical spondylotic myelopathy, *Spine (Phila Pa 1976)* 20:2226–2232, 1995.

124. Chang KC, Samartzis D, Luk KD, Cheung KM: Cervical spine disease in Asian populations, *Hong Kong Med J* 16:69–70, 2010.

125. Shen FH, Samartzis D: Careful follow-up after "successful" surgery: postoperative spondylolisthesis after anterior cervical corpectomy and fusion with instrumentation, *Surg Neurol* 69:637–640, 2008. discussion 640.

126. Samartzis D, Marco RA, Jenis LG, et al.: Characterization of graft subsidence in anterior cervical discectomy and fusion with rigid anterior plate fixation, *Am J Orthop* 36:421–427, 2007.

127. Perez-Cruet MJ, Samartzis D, Fessler RG: Anterior cervical discectomy and corpectomy. *Neurosurgery* 58:ONS-355-359, discussion ONS-359, 2006.

128. Orndorff DG, Samartzis D, Whitehill R, Shen FH: Traumatic fracture-dislocation of C5 on C6 through a previously solid multilevel anterior cervical discectomy and fusion: a case report and review of the literature, *Spine J* 6:55–60, 2006.

129. Samartzis D, Shen FH, Goldberg EJ, An HS: Is autograft the gold standard in achieving radiographic fusion in one-level anterior cervical discectomy and fusion with rigid anterior plate fixation? *Spine (Phila Pa 1976)* 30:1756–1761, 2005.

130. Samartzis D, Shen FH, Lyon C, et al.: Does rigid instrumentation increase the fusion rate in one-level anterior cervical discectomy and fusion? *Spine J* 4:636–643, 2004.

131. Shen FH, Samartzis D, Khanna N, et al.: Comparison of clinical and radiographic outcome in instrumented anterior cervical discectomy and fusion with or without direct uncovertebral joint decompression, *Spine J* 4:629–635, 2004.

132. Samartzis D, Shen FH, Matthews DK, et al.: Comparison of allograft to autograft in multilevel anterior cervical discectomy and fusion with rigid plate fixation, *Spine J* 3:451–459, 2003.

133. Hodges SD, Castleberg RL, Miller T, et al.: Cervical epidural steroid injection with intrinsic spinal cord damage: two case reports, *Spine (Phila Pa 1976)* 23:2137–2142, 1998. discussion 2141–2142.

134. McLain RF, Fry M, Hecht ST: Transient paralysis associated with epidural steroid injection, *J Spinal Disord* 10:441–444, 1997.

135. McGuire KJ, Harrast J, Herkowitz H, Weinstein JN: Geographic variation in the surgical treatment of degenerative cervical disc disease: American Board of Orthopedic Surgery Quality Improvement Initiative. Part II: candidates, *Spine (Phila Pa 1976)* 37:57–66, 2012.

136. Cloward RB: The anterior approach for removal of ruptured cervical disks, *J Neurosurg* 15:602–617, 1958.

137. Smith GW, Robinson RA: The treatment of certain cervical-spine disorders by anterior removal of the intervertebral disc and interbody fusion, *J Bone Surg Am* 40:607–624, 1958.

138. Rahme R, Boubez G, Bouthillier A, Moumdjian R: Acute swan-neck deformity and spinal cord compression after cervical laminectomy, *Can J Neurol Sci* 36:504–506, 2009.

139. Sim FH, Svien HJ, Bickel WH, Janes JM: Swan-neck deformity following extensive cervical laminectomy: a review of twenty-one cases, *J Bone Surg Am* 56:564–580, 1974.

140. Fountas KN, Kapsalaki EZ, Nikolakakos LG, et al.: Anterior cervical discectomy and fusion associated complications, *Spine (Phila Pa 1976)* 32:2310–2317, 2007.

141. Bernard TN Jr, Whitecloud TS 3rd: Cervical spondylotic myelopathy and myeloradiculopathy: anterior decompression and stabilization with autogenous fibula strut graft, *Clin Orthop Relat Res* (221)149–160, 1987.

142. Emery SE, Bohlman HH, Bolesta MJ, Jones PK: Anterior cervical decompression and arthrodesis for the treatment of cervical spondylotic myelopathy: two to seventeen-year follow-up, *J Bone Surg Am* 80:941–951, 1998.

143. Okada K, Shirasaki N, Hayashi H, et al.: Treatment of cervical spondylotic myelopathy by enlargement of the spinal canal anteriorly, followed by arthrodesis, *J Bone Surg Am* 73:352–364, 1991.

144. Flynn TB: Neurologic complications of anterior cervical interbody fusion, *Spine (Phila Pa 1976)* 7:536–539, 1982.

145. Epstein JA: The surgical management of cervical spinal stenosis, spondylosis, and myeloradiculopathy by means of the posterior approach, *Spine (Phila Pa 1976)* 13:864–869, 1988.

146. Hirabayashi K, Watanabe K, Wakano K, et al.: Expansive open-door laminoplasty for cervical spinal stenotic myelopathy, *Spine (Phila Pa 1976)* 8:693–699, 1983.

147. Robertson JT, Papadopoulos SM, Traynelis VC: Assessment of adjacent-segment disease in patients treated with cervical fusion or arthroplasty: a prospective 2-year study, *J Neurosurg Spine (Phila Pa 1976)* 3:417–423, 2005.

148. Heller JG, Sasso RC, Papadopoulos SM, et al.: Comparison of BRYAN cervical disc arthroplasty with anterior cervical decompression and fusion: clinical and radiographic results of a randomized, controlled, clinical trial, *Spine (Phila Pa 1976)* 34:101–107, 2009.

149. Mummaneni PV, Burkus JK, Haid RW, et al.: Clinical and radiographic analysis of cervical disc arthroplasty compared with allograft fusion: a randomized controlled clinical trial, *J Neurosurg Spine (Phila Pa 1976)* 6:198–209, 2007.

150. Huppert J, Beaurain J, Steib JP, et al.: Comparison between single- and multi-level patients: clinical and radiological outcomes 2 years after cervical disc replacement, *Eur Spine J* 20:1417–1426, 2011.

Cervical Radiculopathy

13

Jonathan Tuttle and Norman Chutkan

CHAPTER PREVIEW

Chapter Synopsis   Cervical radiculopathy is defined as pain with or without a motor, sensory, or reflex deficit that is caused by cervical nerve root compression or irritation. Typically, cervical radiculopathy has a favorable natural history. This chapter reviews the epidemiology, natural history, pathogenesis, and differential diagnosis of the disease.

Important Points   Neural compression resulting in radiculopathy can result from a variety of sources, the most common being cervical spondylosis and herniated nucleus pulposus.

Consensus statements from a review of available evidence indicate that cervical radiculopathy from degenerative processes has a favorable prognosis and tends to be self-limiting.

Symptoms of cervical radiculopathy frequently mimic those of other diseases; therefore, careful history, examination, and imaging are required to confirm the diagnosis.

Careful correlation of history and examination with imaging studies is necessary because asymptomatic degenerative changes in the cervical spine are very common findings in advanced imaging, in particular magnetic resonance imaging.

As a degenerative condition, cervical radiculopathy results most commonly from spondylosis or herniated nucleus pulposus. Cervical radiculopathy can also have other causes, such as tumor, trauma, synovial cysts, meningeal cysts, dural arteriovenous fistulas, or tortuous vertebral arteries. This chapter focuses on spondylosis and herniated nucleus pulposus.

In 1817, Parkinson published the first clinical description of cervical radiculopathy but misunderstood the etiology.[1] In 1926, Elliott published his work describing how neuroforaminal stenosis caused cervical radiculopathy. In 1948 and 1952, Brain published articles on the intervertebral disk and cervical spondylosis.[2,3]

Cervical radiculopathy is defined as pain with or without a motor, sensory, or reflex deficit that is caused by cervical nerve root compression or irritation. The irritation may result in one or more of the following signs and symptoms: loss of strength, neck pain, arm pain, and numbness or paresthesias in a dermatomal or myotomal distribution.

Epidemiology

A population-based study from Rochester, Minnesota, revealed an incidence of cervical radiculopathy of 107.3 per 100,000 men and 63.5 per 100,000 women.[1] In this study population, no cervical radiculopathy was seen is persons who were more than 60 years old. The investigators also found that the C7 nerve root was most often involved, followed by C6.

Natural History

The natural history of cervical radiculopathy was initially studied by Lees and Turner in 1963.[4] These investigators followed two groups of patients: one group with myelopathy and the other with radiculopathy. Fifty-seven patients with cervical radiculopathy were followed for up to 19 years. No patients with radiculopathy became myelopathic, but 25% suffered from persistent or worsening radicular pain.

Gore and associates followed 205 patients with neck pain and no neurologic deficit for a minimum of 10 years.[5] At the final follow-up, one third of these patients had moderate to severe pain that limited their lifestyle. Unfortunately, it is difficult to determine how many of these patients had primarily radicular pain, as opposed to isolated neck pain, despite tabular notation in the article of shoulder, arm, forearm, and hand pain in some of the patients.

A more recent article from the Degenerative Disorders Work Group of the North American Spine Society Evidence-Based Clinical Guideline Development Committee noted methodologic problems with all reviewed studies pertaining to the natural history of cervical radiculopathy.[6] This work group proposed the following consensus statement: "It is likely that for most patients with cervical radiculopathy from degenerative disorders signs and symptoms will be self-limited and will resolve spontaneously over a variable length of time without specific treatment."

Pathophysiology

Most patients with cervical radiculopathy patients present to their physician with symptoms caused by cervical spondylosis and the resultant neuroforaminal stenosis or "hard disk." Cervical spondylosis starts with disk desiccation.[7] The avascular disk loses water because of a decrease in the proteoglycan content in the nucleus pulposus that leads to a reduction of water content from 90% at birth to 74% during the eighth decade of life.[8] This change results in a loss of disk height, microinstability and subsequent osteophyte formation, facet hypertrophy, and ligamentum flavum buckling and hypertrophy. Degeneration of the spine, or spondylosis, may result in neuroforaminal stenosis and potentially, spinal canal stenosis.

The other main cause of cervical radiculopathy is a "soft disk" or herniated nucleus pulposus. This disorder is seen more often than a hard disk in younger patients. Roughly 75% of cervical radiculopathies occur between the ages of 40 and 59 years. Patients in their 40s tend to have more soft disks, and those in their 50s tend to have more hard disks.

Double crush phenomenon occurs less than 1% of the time on the same nerve, according to Morgan and Wilbourn; it is observed when a cervical nerve root is compressed and is accompanied by additional peripheral compression.[9] These investigators found that 3.4% of the time, a patient had either carpal tunnel syndrome or ulnar neuropathy combined with a cervical root lesion. The double crush phenomenon was first reported by Upton and McComas, who hypothesized that it originated from impaired axoplasmic flow that made the distal portion of the nerve more susceptible to compression injury.[10]

Pertinent Examination Findings by Level

Cervical radiculopathies can result from any pathologic condition at the nerve root level.[11] Above the level of C5, diagnosis can be difficult to elucidate based on history and physical examination because examination findings are limited and nonspecific (Fig. 13-1). C2 radiculopathy is characterized by a history of occipital neuralgia in which the patient has suboccipital or auricular pain. The C3 nerve root, which is the smallest cervical root, exits through the largest foramen and is usually not affected by spondylosis. Because C4 radiculopathy may manifest with pain to the posterior neck,

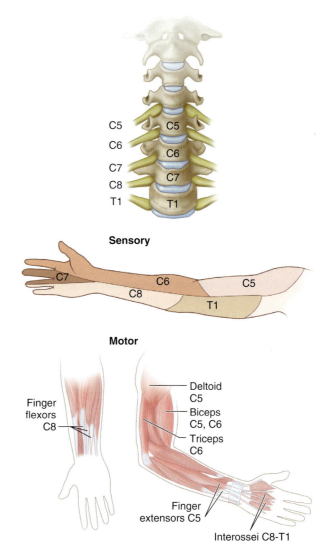

FIGURE 13-1 Cervical root motor and sensory findings by level. (From Benzel EC, editor: *Spine surgery: techniques, complication avoidance, and management,* ed 2, Philadelphia, 2005, Churchill Livingstone, as modified in Shen FH, Shaffrey CI, editors: *Arthritis and arthroplasty: the Spine,* Philadelphia, 2010, Saunders.)

trapezius muscle, and anterior chest, this disorder can sometimes be difficult to differentiate from axial neck pain.

C5 radiculopathy typically causes pain that radiates over the shoulder and into the proximal arm along the lateral aspect of the deltoid muscle (Table 13-1). Examination findings can include deltoid weakness, as well as some biceps muscle weakness. Biceps weakness can also come from C6 radiculopathy because of dual innervation. For C6 radiculopathy, pain, numbness, or tingling may radiate to the thumb and index fingers. Wrist extension, provided by the extensor carpi radialis muscle, is from C6 innervation, and this may be weak. The brachioradialis reflex may be diminished or absent.

C7 radiculopathy may cause pain that radiates to the middle finger or to the interscapular region. The triceps muscle is innervated by C7, and it may be weak. An absent or diminished triceps reflex also indicates C7 radiculopathy.

Table 13-1 Cervical Motor and Sensory Findings by Nerve Root Level

Disk Herniation	Affected Root	Motor Test/Muscle
C4-5	C5	Shoulder abduction/deltoid
C5-6	C6	Elbow flexion/biceps
		Radial wrist extension/extensor carpi radialis longus
C6-7	C7	Elbow extension/triceps
		Finger extension/extensor digitorum communis
C7-T1	C8	Finger flexion/flexor digitorum superficialis and profundus
		Hand intrinsics/interossei (<T1)
T1-2	T1	Hand intrinsics/interossei

Modified from Benzel EC, editor: *Spine surgery: techniques, complication avoidance, and management,* ed 2, Philadelphia, 2005, Churchill Livingstone.

C8 radiculopathy may cause pain radiating to the medial arm and forearm, as well as the ring and little fingers. Hand intrinsic muscles may be weak, and the patient may exhibit the benediction sign in which the ring and little fingers do not fully extend. Rarely, T1 radiculopathy may be present and may cause numbness on the ulnar side of the forearm or atrophy of the dorsal interosseous muscle.

Differential Diagnosis

The differential diagnosis of cervical radiculopathies often includes peripheral neuropathies. Carpal tunnel syndrome, cubital tunnel syndrome, and anterior and posterior interosseous nerve compression can have similar presentations. Table 13-2 may help differentiate one diagnosis from another.

Imaging Studies

Radiography

Radiographs provide information regarding sagittal alignment, fractures, dislocations, and congenital anomalies. Overt or occult instability may be demonstrated by dynamic imaging.[12] Oblique radiographs may be useful for demonstrating neuroforaminal stenosis (Fig. 13-2).

Computed Tomography Myelography or Plain Computed Tomography

This imaging modality provides excellent visualization of previously instrumented levels in which magnetic resonance imaging (MRI) may have too much artifact. It is the test of choice for patients with metal foreign bodies who cannot undergo MRI studies and is excellent at showing ossification of the posterior longitudinal ligament. Computed tomography myelography is invasive and therefore suboptimal for routine imaging in patients who can undergo MRI. A computed tomography scan without myelography is helpful to reveal fractures or dislocations in great detail, as well as uncovertebral hypertrophy and neuroforaminal stenosis (Fig. 13-3).

Table 13-2 Differential Diagnosis

Diagnostic Concern	Diagnostic Clues
C5 versus rotator cuff tear	Intrinsic shoulder problems often are associated with shoulder motion that causes pain and decreased range of motion
C6 or C7 versus carpal tunnel syndrome	Carpal tunnel syndrome is associated with nocturnal dysesthesias in the palmar aspect of the index through ring fingers, and may produce a positive Phalen test result and Tinel sign at the wrist
C7 versus posterior interosseous nerve compression	The posterior interosseous nerve does not have a sensory component; C7 radiculopathy can cause a diminished or absent triceps reflex or weakness
C8 versus anterior interosseous nerve compression	Anterior interosseous nerve entrapment does not cause sensory changes and may produce a positive pinch test in which the terminal phalanges of the thumb and index finger are hyperextended.
C8 versus ulnar entrapment	Ulnar entrapment may produce a positive Phalen test result or Tinel sign at the elbow.

Modified from Abbed KM. Coumans JV: Cervical radiculopathy: pathophysiology, presentation, and clinical evaluation. *Neurosurgery* 60(Suppl 1):S28-S34, 2007.

Magnetic Resonance Imaging

MRI is noninvasive and is the test of choice to evaluate cervical spinal cord compression, tumors, syringomyelia, neuroforaminal stenosis, demyelinating disorders, herniated nucleus pulposus, and myelomalacia. However, careful correlation of the history and examination with imaging studies is necessary because asymptomatic degenerative changes in the cervical spine are very common findings on advanced imaging, in particular MRI.

Adjunct Studies

Electrodiagnostic Studies

Electromyography and nerve conduction velocity studies can supplement imaging data when history and physical examination findings do not seem to correlate with the imaging or when peripheral neuropathy is suspected.

Treatment Options

According to the North American Spine Society clinical guideline, cervical radiculopathy is a disorder that can be treated with conservative management a majority of the time and will resolve. Conservative management options include corticosteroids, nonsteroidal anti-inflammatory drugs, muscle relaxants, cervical traction, cervical isometric exercises, cervical collars, and judicious use of narcotics. The use of cervical injections may be an option in selected patients. However, careful consideration of the associated risks should be considered and discussed with the patient.

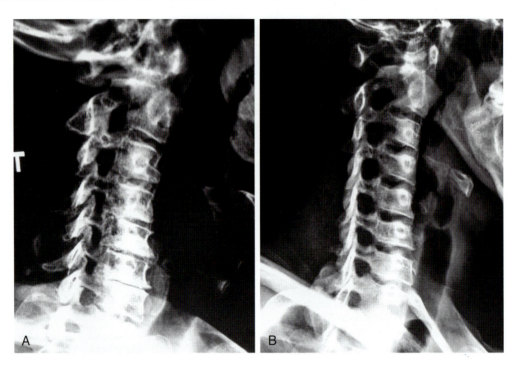

FIGURE 13-2 A and **B,** Oblique radiographs showing neuroforaminal stenosis.

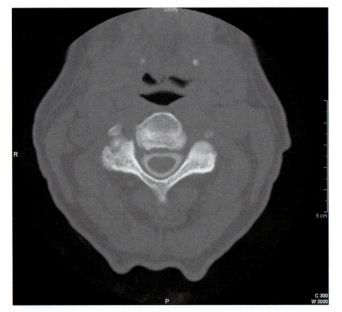

FIGURE 13-3 Computed tomography myelogram depicting neuroforaminal stenosis.

Operative management is covered in depth in other chapters but is usually reserved for patients who have undergone a trial of conservative management that has failed or who have progressively lost motor function or have unbearable pain.[13] The cervical spine can be treated from anterior or posterior approaches, and treatment can involve decompression or decompression and fusion. Another available option is cervical disk arthroplasty.

Conclusion

Cervical radiculopathy is a disorder with a favorable natural history. This chapter reviews the epidemiology, natural history, pathogenesis, and differential diagnosis of the disease. It also discusses specific examination findings and the rationale for selecting imaging modalities related to the diagnosis. Once a diagnosis is achieved, the discussion touches on treatment options; however, examination, imaging, and surgical treatment options are covered in greater depth in other chapters of this text.

REFERENCES

1. Radhakrishnan K, Litchy WJ, O'Fallon WM, Kurland LT: Epidemiology of cervical radiculopathy: a population-based study from Rochester, Minnesota, 1976 through 1990, *Brain* 117:325–335, 1994.
2. Brain WR, Knight GC, Bull JWD: Discussion on rupture of the intervertebral disc in the cervical region, *Proc R Soc Med* 41:509–516, 1948.
3. Brain WR, Northfield D, Wilkinson M: The neurological manifestations of cervical spondylosis, *Brain* 75:187–225, 1952.
4. Lees F, Turner JW: Natural history and prognosis of cervical spondylosis, *Br Med J* 2:1607–1610, 1963.
5. Gore D R, Sepic S B, Gardner G M, Murray M P: Neck pain: a long-term follow-up of 205 patients, *Spine (Phila Pa 1976)* 12:1–5, 1987.
6. Bono C M, Ghiselli G, Gilbert TJ, et al.: An evidence-based clinical guideline for the diagnosis and treatment of cervical radiculopathy from degenerative disorders, *Spine J* 11:64–72, 2011.
7. Ferguson R J, Caplan L R: Cervical spondylitic myelopathy, *Neurol Clin* 3:373–382, 1985.
8. Kraemer I, Kolditz D, Cowin R: Water and electrolyte content of human intervertebral discs under variable load, *Spine (Phila Pa 1976)* 10:69–71, 1985.
9. Morgan G, Wilbourn A: Cervical radiculopathy and coexisting distal entrapment neuropathies: double-crush syndromes? *Neurology* 50:78–83, 1998.
10. Upton A R, McComas A J: The double crush in nerve entrapment syndromes, *Lancet* 2:359–362, 1973.
11. Harrop J S, Hanna A, Silva MT, Sharan A: Neurological manifestations of cervical spondylosis: an overview of signs, symptoms and pathophysiology, *Neurosurgery* 60(Suppl 1):S14–S20, 2007.
12. Abbed K M: Coumans JV: Cervical radiculopathy: pathophysiology, presentation, and clinical evaluation, *Neurosurgery* 60(Suppl 1):S28–S34, 2007.
13. Matz PG, Holly LT, Groff MW, et al.: Indications for anterior cervical decompression for the treatment of cervical degenerative radiculopathy, *J Neurosurg Spine* 11:174–182, 2009.

Cervical Spondylotic Myelopathy

14

Shayan Rahman, Khoi Than, Paul Park, and Frank La Marca

CHAPTER PREVIEW

Chapter Synopsis	Cervical spondylotic myelopathy (CSM) is spinal cord dysfunction accompanying age-related degeneration of the cervical spine. The lack of prospective studies of its natural history and vague clinical symptoms pose difficult challenges for clinicians. This chapter aims to resolve conflicts concerning the pathophysiology, natural history, and various treatment algorithms through evidence based in the current literature.
Important Points	The pathophysiology of CSM relates to spondylotic narrowing of the spinal canal leading to spinal cord compression and dysfunction.
	The natural history is variable and unpredictable.
	The hallmark symptoms of CSM are gait abnormalities and upper motor neuron dysfunction.
	Magnetic resonance imaging is the most useful diagnostic test for differentiating CSM from other disorders; however, care should be taken to correlate findings with the patient's history and examination.
	Surgical decompression is typically reserved for patients with moderate to severe disease or progressive neurologic deterioration.

Cervical spondylotic myelopathy (CSM) is spinal cord dysfunction accompanying age-related degeneration of the cervical spine. CSM is also the most common cause of spinal dysfunction in older adults and is the most common cause of nontraumatic spastic paraparesis and quadriparesis. The underlying pathophysiology of this disease process typically involves compression of the spinal cord leading to upper motor neuron dysfunction, such as hyperreflexia and gait disturbance.[1]

Despite anecdotal reports of the high prevalence of CSM among older adults, accurate data on its epidemiology remain elusive. This insufficiency stems partly from the lack of prospective studies of CSM, but also from the challenges of making accurate and timely diagnoses. CSM often manifests with obscure clinical signs and subtle symptoms. CSM may be overshadowed by other concurrent conditions, such as radiculopathy, or it may masquerade as other diseases, such as amyotrophic lateral sclerosis (ALS) or multiple sclerosis.[2] Furthermore, the natural history appears highly variable and unpredictable.

This chapter aims to describe the current understanding of the pathophysiology and natural history of CSM. A basic understanding of this complex, yet common, degenerative process is necessary before any treatment algorithm is considered.

Pathophysiology

Cervical spondylosis refers to degenerative changes affecting the vertebrae, intervertebral disks, facets, and associated ligaments. Although these changes are most frequently seen with increasing age, other factors associated with an increased risk of spondylotic changes include repeated occupational trauma (e.g., carrying axial loads), genetic predisposition, smoking, and Down syndrome.[3] Despite the widespread presence of cervical spondylosis in the aging spine, most patients do not develop myelopathy because a certain amount of narrowing is tolerated before cervical spinal cord compression becomes a risk. In an anatomic cadaveric study, Arnold noted the strong correlation between sagittal diameter of the spinal canal in cervical spondylosis and the production of myelopathy.[4] The normal sagittal diameter of the spinal canal from C3 to C7 is 17 to 18 mm, whereas the diameter of the cervical spinal cord measures approximately 10 mm. This leaves a compensatory zone of approximately 7 to 8 mm in the anteroposterior dimension that buffers the spinal cord from moderate spondylotic narrowing.[5] A sagittal canal diameter of less than 12 mm has been shown to be a risk factor for myelopathy in patients with cervical spondylosis. Similarly, patients with congenital spinal canal narrowing tolerate far less spondylotic narrowing before spinal cord compression occurs.[6]

The cascade of cervical spine degeneration begins with the loss of integrity of the intervertebral disk. As disks age, the nucleus pulposus fragments, loses water, and collapses. As a result, the central annular lamellae buckle inward, and the external concentric bands of the annulus fibrosis bulge outward. This process leads to disk bulging and loss of disk height, which biomechanically translate to reduced load-bearing capability.[1,5,7] In a large cadaveric study, Christe and colleagues described the histologic changes in aging cervical disks by illustrating variable degrees of cystic degeneration, lamellar disorganization, and radiating tears through the annulus fibrosis.[8] These changes result in increased mechanical stresses at the end plates of the adjacent vertebral body.

Abnormal motions and forces may then lead to subperiosteal bone formation, which creates osteophytic bars that extend along the ventral aspect of the spinal canal. Osteophytic bars may have a biomechanically compensatory effect by stabilizing adjacent vertebrae by increasing the weight-bearing surface of the end plates, which are hypermobile as a result of lost disk material. However, osteophytic bars can also encroach on nervous tissue, thus causing compression of the spinal cord or nerve roots.[9] Severe anterior spinal cord compression can also occur with ossification of the posterior longitudinal ligament (OPLL), observed predominantly in certain Asian populations. In addition, osteophytes may form at the uncovertebral joints and facets and may cause bony hypertrophy that frequently breaches the ventrolateral portion of the intervertebral foramina. Posteriorly in the spinal canal, the ligamentum flavum thickens as it loses tension and folds into the spinal canal as the intervertebral disks lose height.[1,5,7] These static mechanical factors ultimately lead to circumferential narrowing of the spinal canal and potential compromise of the spinal cord, with resulting cervical myelopathy (Fig. 14-1).

In addition to these static mechanical factors, myelopathy results from dynamic mechanical factors. Dynamic factors relate to the fact that normal flexion and extension of the neck can exacerbate existing spinal cord or nerve root irritation, especially in the presence of advanced cervical spondylosis, OPLL, or a congenitally narrow spinal canal. With neck flexion, the spinal cord lengthens and is stretched over ventral osteophytic spurs protruding into the spinal canal. During extension, the ligamentum flavum may buckle into the spinal cord and cause compression of the cord between the ligamentum flavum and the posterior margin of the vertebral body.[10] Using a computerized simulation model based on the mechanical properties of white and gray matter, Ichihara and colleagues measured the stresses on the spinal cord in the presence of dynamic compressive factors. These investigators showed that, in patients with severe canal narrowing, repeated hyperextension of the cervical spine subjects the posterior spinal cord and, to a lesser degree, the anterior spinal cord to high shear stress comparable to that occurring in acute spinal cord injury.[11] These episodic events may partly account for the neuropathologic changes seen in CSM.

Although the primary mechanism of CSM may be compression of nervous tissue by static and dynamic mechanical factors, growing evidence indicates that spinal cord ischemia may also play a role in CSM. Multiple studies have shown that the histopathologic changes seen in CSM are comparable to those observed in isolated spinal cord ischemia.[5] Investigators have established that oligodendroglia are particularly susceptible to the effects of ischemia that contribute to the early demyelination of the corticospinal tracts. In an autopsy series, patients with varying degrees of spinal cord compression also showed damage to the lateral corticospinal tracts similar to that seen in spinal cord ischemia.[12] Hakuda and Wilson published a study on the effects of anterior spinal cord compression and ischemia on the canine cervical spinal cord and found that the effects of vascular insufficiency and compression of the anterior spinal cord are additive, a finding that partially explains the clinical signs in patients with CSM.[13] Most likely, ischemia occurs at the level of the impaired microcirculation and is probably caused by reduced flow in the pial plexuses, as well as by venous congestion and compression of larger vessels, such as the anterior spinal artery.[5,12] Other possible factors in the pathophysiology of CSM include impairment of intracellular energy metabolism, free radical–mediated injury, apoptosis, and cation-mediated cell injury.

Natural History

Despite the high prevalence of CSM, few studies have addressed its natural history. Furthermore, consensus on the natural history of CSM remains elusive even with these published reports. Clark and Robinson published the first natural history study of CSM in 1956. Their review of 120 affected patients demonstrated that CSM caused slow, progressive motor deterioration that occurred with acute exacerbations rather than a steady, unrelenting neurologic decline. In their subset of patients who had no treatment, complete remission never occurred, and spontaneous regression of neurologic deficits was uncommon. Most of those affected were left with permanent but variable degrees of disability.[14] Similarly, Lees and Turner reviewed 44 patients with clinical and radiographic evidence of CSM. More than half the patients were followed for more than 10 years. These investigators concluded that CSM follows a prolonged clinical course, in which an initial phase of deterioration is followed by lengthy periods of stable symptoms.[15]

In the 1970s, Nurick confirmed these earlier reports with his retrospective review of 37 patients treated conservatively. In this study, patients were classified according to 6 grades of disability, based on the degree of difficulty encountered in walking (Table 14-1). Nurick considered CSM a benign disorder in which old age was the only risk factor for progression of symptoms, and he believed that treatment should be reserved for this small subset of patients. Nurick concluded that no significant difference in outcome could be found in the majority of patients treated with surgical decompression as opposed to nonoperative care.[16,17] In contrast, Symon and Lavendar argued that CSM is not a "benign" condition. In their surgical series, 67% of patients demonstrated relentless progression of neurologic deterioration without any static clinical period.[18]

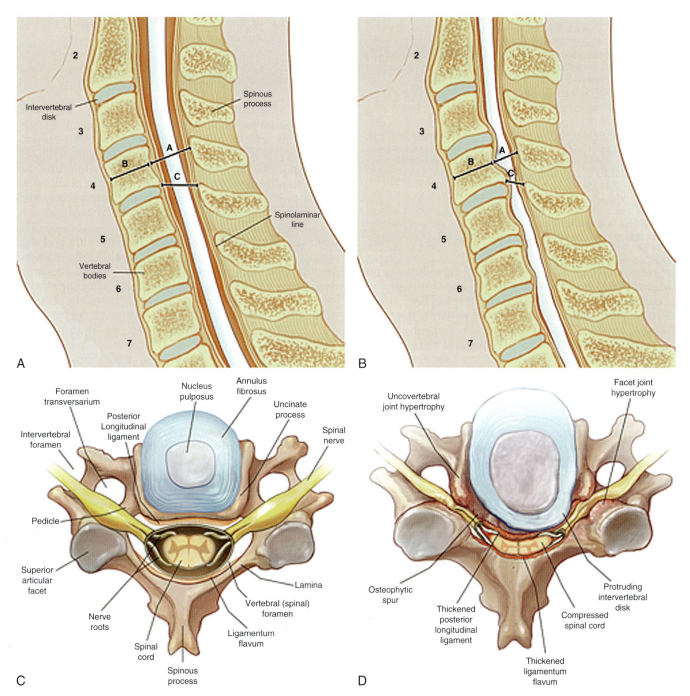

FIGURE 14-1 **A** and **C** show midsagittal and axial views of the normal cervical spine, whereas **B** and **D** show midsagittal and axial views of cervical spinal stenosis result from a combination of a congenitally narrow cervical spinal canal and superimposed cervical spondylosis. In **A** and **B**, *A* represents the antero-posterior spinal canal diameter; *B* is the vertebral body diameter; and *C* is the narrowest spinal canal opening as measured by the distance between the most posterior aspect of a vertebral body, including its osteophytic spur, and the nearest point on the spinolaminar line formed by the junction of the lamina and spinous process. (From Tracy JA, Bartleson JD: Cervical spondylotic myelopathy. *Neurologist* 16:176-187, 2010.)

Like the series by Symon and Lavendar, some more recent studies have maintained that patients treated medically show continual progressive neurologic deterioration. These arguments have been used in support of early intervention for even mildly symptomatic patients. Along these lines, Sadasivian and associates conducted a retrospective evaluation of 22 patients, classified according to the Nurick grades; their findings suggested that the natural history of CSM is one of progressive deterioration with no stabilization of symptoms. These investigators noticed a significant mean delay from the onset of symptoms to diagnosis of 6.3 years, during which patients deteriorated on average by two Nurick grades.[19] Bednarik and colleagues developed a predictive model to determine the risk factors for progression to myelopathy specifically in presymptomatic patients with spinal cord compression. These investigators concluded that electrophysiologic abnormalities of cervical spinal cord dysfunction,

Table 14-1 Nurick Disability Score

Grade	Signs and Symptoms
0	Signs or symptoms of root involvement but no evidence of spinal cord disease
1	Signs of spinal cord disease but no difficulty in walking
2	Slight difficulty in walking that prevented full-time employment
3	Difficulty in walking that prevented full-time employment or the ability to do all housework but that was not so severe as to require someone else's help to walk
4	Ability to walk only with someone else's help or with the aid of a frame
5	Chairbound or bedridden status

Modified from Nurick S: The natural history and the results of surgical treatment of the spinal cord disorder associated with cervical spondylosis. *Brain* 95:101-108, 1972.

together with clinical signs of cervical radiculopathy and magnetic resonance imaging (MRI) hyperintensity, are useful predictors of early progression into CSM. In their retrospective analysis of 45 affected patients, their multivariate model predicted early progression into SCM in 81.4% of cases.[20] Although these studies show merit in elucidating the natural history of CSM, they are nevertheless retrospective studies subject to observation bias and lack standardized outcome measures.

Prospective studies on the effectiveness of surgery in altering the natural history of CSM are few and inconclusive, thus highlighting the difficulty in performing controlled studies in these patients. In their Cochrane review of the role of surgery for CSM, Fouyas and colleagues conducted a meta-analysis to determine whether surgical treatment of cervical radiculopathy or myelopathy is associated with improved outcome as compared with conservative management. Most notably, these investigators reviewed a trial of 49 patients who had mild functional deficits associated with cervical myelopathy and in whom the effects of surgery were compared with those of conservative treatment. Although functional scores were better in the conservatively treated group at 6 months, at 2 years no significant differences were observed between the groups.[21] Similarly, Kadanka and colleagues performed a 3-year prospective randomized study of surgical versus nonsurgical treatment of patients with mild and moderate degrees of CSM. The results showed no discernible difference between the two groups over a 3-year follow-up period. In their discussion, these investigators stated that the degree of success in the treatment of CSM with nonoperative approaches was similar to that observed with surgical intervention.[22]

In contrast, excellent results for surgical management of CSM have been demonstrated in many studies.[22] Sampath and colleagues published the results of a multicenter, prospective trial of 503 nonrandomized patients that found significant improvements in the functional status of patients undergoing surgical intervention in comparison with patients who were conservatively treated. Although the medically treated group was less symptomatic before assignment to treatment, surgically treated patients had better outcomes.[23] Numerous uncontrolled reports have documented substantial improvement after surgical treatment, but well-conducted controlled studies

that document the long-term benefit of surgical decompression are still lacking.

Signs and Symptoms

The clinical symptoms of CSM are often subtle and can be accompanied by signs that are difficult to elicit, thereby making its early diagnosis challenging. Furthermore, isolated myelopathy is relatively rare in patients with cervical spondylosis. Typically, the presentation includes nerve root impingement and radiculopathy (myeloradiculopathy).[1] Besides neurogenic pain, patients may also complain of nonspecific neck stiffness or regional pain secondary to the presence of advanced spondylosis. The hallmark symptoms of CSM are gait abnormalities and weakness or stiffness of the legs. Additionally, patients may present with loss of manual dexterity and abnormal sensations manifesting with problems buttoning clothes or using a zipper or with poor penmanship. Loss of sphincter control and urinary incontinence are rare, but some patients may complain of urgency, frequency, and hesitancy.[5] Confirmation of clinical suspicion is made by a thorough motor, sensory, and reflex examination of every patient, with special attention to signs suggestive of upper motor neuron dysfunction.

The most typical physical examination findings suggest upper motor neuron dysfunction. These include hyperactive deep tendon reflexes, ankle-patellar clonus, spasticity, the Babinski sign, and the Hoffman sign. The Hoffman sign is considered present when sudden extension of the distal interphalangeal joint of the middle finger causes reflexive flexion of the thumb or index finger.[24] An inverted radial reflex occurs when tapping the distal brachioradialis tendon induces reflexive flexion of one or more of the fingers and diminishing of normal wrist extension; this finding is reportedly seen with C5 to C6 level spinal cord compression. The pectoralis muscle reflex can be elicited by tapping the pectoralis tendon in the deltopectoral groove, thus causing adduction and internal rotation of the shoulder if hyperactivity is present. This reflex suggests compression of the upper cervical spine (C2 to C4).[25]

In the lower extremities, the Babinski response, described as the reflexive extension and abduction of the toes after gentle, sharp stimulation of the lateral aspect of the sole of the foot, also suggests upper motor neuron disease. Similarly, more than two beats of clonus after a rapid Achilles stretch is often pathologic as well. These pathologic reflexes, which result from a loss of the inhibitory function of the upper motor neurons, usually describe the spasticity associated with myelopathy. In patients with generalized spasticity, an increased jaw jerk reflex may differentiate an intracranial or metabolic disorder from suspected cervical myelopathy.[5] Therefore, the presence of spasticity is not specific for myelopathy, although it helps corroborate the diagnosis of CSM and warrants further investigation.

Gait disturbance may be extremely subtle and is often the first physical symptom of CSM. Progression often occurs gradually and slowly over time. Early in the disease, the patient may have a subjective sensation of imbalance or subtle incoordination during turns or walking around corners. Other patients may complain of unsteadiness on uneven terrain or an inability to walk distances. Patients with more advanced CSM may demonstrate a stiff or spastic gait. On examination, myelopathic gait is often described as broad based and hesitant. Loss of motor coordination is further demonstrated by difficulty in maintaining balance with toe walking and heel walking.[5] Measuring of walking times and of the number or steps taken over 30 minutes may be an objective, reproducible, and quantitative method of assessing the severity of gait dysfunction. Furthermore, a positive Romberg test is demonstrated by a loss of balance while the patient is standing with the eyes closed and the arms elevated in front of the body. Qualitatively, these findings can suggest the presence and severity of myelopathy.

In terms of motor examination in the upper extremities, patients with CSM most commonly exhibit triceps or hand intrinsic muscle weakness. Severe myelopathy can also result in atrophy of the intrinsic hand musculature. The finger escape sign may suggest weakness in the hand intrinsic muscles. To test for this, patients are asked to hold their fingers extended and adducted. If the ulnar digits drift into abduction and flexion, these patients have a positive finger escape sign. The patients' hand function should also be assessed, in addition to the upper extremity strength assessment. A useful maneuver involves having the patient make and release a fist more than 20 times in 10 seconds. Impairment or clumsiness during this maneuver, the grip release sign, may suggest cervical cord dysfunction.[1,5] In the lower extremities, distal strength is rarely affected without weakness in the more proximal muscle groups. Weakness is most frequently detected in the iliopsoas, followed by the quadriceps femoris. The finding of lower extremity weakness and hyperreflexia without upper extremity symptoms and signs should prompt an investigation of the thoracic spinal cord for other pathologic processes.

Sensory abnormalities in CSM have a variable pattern. Typically, symptoms start in the fingertips, are confined to the hand, and occur in a nonradicular distribution. Loss of vibratory sensation or proprioception in the extremities, particularly the feet, is sometimes the result of damage to the posterior columns and can be one of the early signs of myelopathy. This condition can be detected by tuning fork examination of the great toes or by testing proprioception of the toes or ankles.[24] The Lhermitte sign, which consists of electrical shock–like sensations running down the back and shooting into the limbs during flexion of the neck, may also suggest dysfunction of the posterior columns.[25] This sign is not specific for CSM, however. Spinothalamic sensory loss, when present, usually is asymmetric. The examiner must be aware of other medical comorbidities that can confound the sensory examination, such as diabetes mellitus or other metabolic causes of peripheral neuropathy.

Patients with CSM may also present acutely with a central spinal cord syndrome. This typically occurs when a patient experiences an acute hyperextension injury with preexisting stenosis (congenital or acquired) or

Table 14-2 Modified Japanese Orthopedic Association Score

I. Motor Dysfunction Score of the Upper Extremities	
Inability to move hands	0
Inability to eat with a spoon but ability to move hands	1
Inability to button shirt but ability to eat with a spoon	2
Ability to button shirt with great difficulty	3
Ability to button shirt with slight difficulty	4
No dysfunction	5
II. Motor Dysfunction Score of the Lower Extremities	
Complete loss of motor and sensory function	0
Sensory preservation without ability to move legs	1
Ability to move legs but inability to walk	2
Ability to walk on flat floor with a walking aid (i.e., cane or crutch)	3
Ability to walk up and/or down stairs with hand rail	4
Moderate to significant lack of stability but ability to walk up and/or down stairs without hand rail	5
Mild lack of stability but ability to walk unaided with smooth reciprocation	6
No dysfunction	7
III. Sensation	
Complete loss of hand sensation	0
Severe sensory loss or pain	1
Mild sensory loss	2
No sensory loss	3
IV. Sphincter Dysfunction Score	
Inability to micturate voluntarily	0
Marked difficulty with micturition	1
Mild to moderate difficulty with micturition	2
Normal micturition	3

Modified from Yonenobu K, Abumi K, Nagata K, et al: Interobserver and intraobserver reliability of the Japanese Orthopedic Association scoring system for evaluation of cervical compression myelopathy. *Spine* 26:1890-1894, 2001.

myelopathy, resulting in acute spinal cord compression. The syndrome consists of greater upper extremity weakness than lower extremity weakness, varying degrees of sensory disturbance below the lesion, and myelopathic findings, such as spasticity and urinary retention.[1]

Numerous scales are available for objectively grading the severity of CSM. Nurick developed a widely used grading scale based mainly on the degree of patients' difficulty in ambulating (see Table 14-1). More recently, the Japanese Orthopedic Association (JOA) assessment scale gained popularity because it combines extremity motor function with other CSM symptoms including those related to sensory and bladder function. This scale is most widely used as the modified JOA (mJOA) score, as modified by Benzel and colleagues (Table 14-2). The mJOA score also has been demonstrated to have a high interobserver and intraobserver reliability.[26] Other scales used to measure outcomes in patients with CSM include the Cooper scale, Harsh scale, and Prolo scale. Additionally, general instruments that measure pain (e.g., visual analog scale) and functional status (e.g., the Medical Outcomes Study Short Form-36) are used. Most often, these scales and scores are used in research settings, rather than in everyday clinical practice.

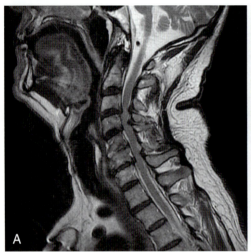 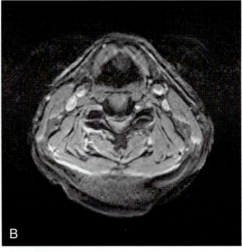

FIGURE 14-2 T2-weighted cervical magnetic resonance imaging demonstrating cervical spondylosis with resultant cervical stenosis and spinal cord compression. (Courtesy Paul Park, MD, University of Michigan, Ann Arbor, Mich.)

Diagnostic Testing

MRI is the most useful diagnostic test and should be ordered for all patients with signs of myelopathy or progressive neurologic deficits. MRI provides multiplanar images and excellent visualization of the spinal cord and surrounding cerebrospinal fluid. It can confirm the diagnosis of CSM, document the extent and severity of the spondylotic changes, and effectively differentiate CSM from other diagnoses. In the setting of myelopathy, the degree of spinal canal stenosis or spinal cord compression can be directly measured. Myelopathic changes within the spinal cord appear as regions of high signal intensity on T2-weighted images. Although the presence of these spinal cord changes does not correlate with treatment outcomes, it may suggest spinal cord compression of longer duration.[27] The examiner must evaluate the integrity of structures surrounding the cervical spinal cord including the disk, facet joints, and ligamentum flavum. The relative contribution of these structures to cervical spinal cord compression helps guide surgical planning (Fig. 14-2).

Computed tomography (CT) myelography is the test of choice in patients who have a contraindication to MRI or in whom MRI data are inconclusive. In addition, CT myelography can be a helpful adjunct to MRI in delineating the osseous anatomy and spinal cord deformation. However, unlike MRI, CT myelography provides poor visualization of pathologic features intrinsic to the spinal cord. Furthermore, CT myelography is more invasive than MRI in that it requires lumbar puncture and administration of radiopaque dye. Neurologic complications include intracranial hypotensive headache, persistent spinal fluid leak, aseptic meningitis, arachnoiditis, contrast allergic reaction, and rare instances of neurologic worsening.[28] Plain CT is not as detailed as MRI or CT myelography, but it can be used as a rough screening tool or to evaluate osseous anatomy for surgical planning.

Plain radiographs, although inexpensive and widely available, have limited utility in diagnosing cervical myelopathy accurately. However, plain films can roughly demonstrate spondylotic changes and suggest spinal canal narrowing. The anteroposterior view may demonstrate uncovertebral joint space narrowing or scoliosis. The lateral view delineates disk space narrowing, the presence of end plate osteophytes, and alterations in sagittal plane alignment. OPLL may be evident as a solid line of bone immediately posterior to the vertebral bodies. Cervical spinal stenosis can be detected on lateral views by using the Torg ratio (the ratio of vertebral body diameter to space available for the spinal cord). A value less than 0.8 or overlap of the spinolaminar line with the posterior edge of the facets suggests significant stenosis.[29] However, studies have found that this ratio correlates poorly with measured cervical spinal canal volume when compared with MRI such that in nearly all cases, advanced imaging is necessary.[30] Flexion and extension radiographs provide dynamic views to assess increased motion of vertebrae at levels with spondylosis or spondylolisthesis. Excessive motion indicates biomechanical instability and may contribute to myelopathic symptoms from dynamic compression of the spinal cord.

Although routinely used during spinal surgery, electrophysiologic studies are not commonly used for diagnosing CSM. However, these studies are sometimes used to exclude specific syndromes that may mimic CSM symptoms, such as peripheral neuropathy, ALS, or multiple sclerosis. Nonspecific abnormalities are often noted on nerve conduction studies (NCSs) and electromyography (EMG) in the setting of CSM. With compression of the anterior spinal cord, damage to anterior horn cells can occur. This can manifest as long-duration, high-amplitude, polyphasic motor units with reduced recruitment on needle EMG examination. Abnormal spontaneous activity such as fibrillations and positive sharp waves can occur if the denervation is subacute or not fully compensated.[5] Compression of either the spinal cord or the motor nerve roots at a particular level produces similar EMG findings. NCSs are important mainly to rule out alternative diagnoses, such as peripheral neuropathy, peripheral nerve entrapment, and brachial plexopathy. In the setting of CSM, results of motor NCSs may be normal because many of the involved cervical levels are not tested on routine NCSs, which usually focus on C8 to T1 innervated muscles in the upper limbs. Although not very sensitive, F-wave latencies may be abnormally prolonged if proximal nerve damage has occurred. Pure sensory radiculopathies and spinal cord syndromes are not well evaluated by standard NCSs. In cases of pure motor dysfunction, comprehensive NCSs and EMG may be needed to diagnose or exclude motor neuron disease, such as ALS. Somatosensory-evoked potentials (SEPs), usually using the median and tibial nerves, may be helpful in assessing the degree of central sensory conduction impairment in CSM.[5] Investigators have suggested that motor-evoked potentials (MEPs) may be more sensitive than SEPs in early myelopathy.

Various laboratory studies may assist in differentiating cervical spondylotic disease as a cause of a patient's symptoms from other causes of radiculopathy and myelopathy. Cyanocobalamin (vitamin B_{12}) levels and a serum rapid plasma reagin assay may help distinguish metabolic and infectious causes of myelopathy from CSM.

Differential Diagnoses

The differential diagnosis of CSM is broad and includes multiple categories that can cause or mimic myelopathy. Furthermore, asymptomatic degenerative spondylosis has a high frequency. Physicians face a difficult clinical challenge that relies on careful assessment of diagnostic testing and physical examination findings. An understanding of the potential causes of myelopathy is crucial in addressing this diagnostic challenge.

Infectious causes of myelopathy include abscess (bacterial, fungal, or tubercular), human immunodeficiency virus–related myelopathy, West Nile virus infection, tropical spastic paraparesis, and tabes dorsalis, among other causes. Risk factors such as immunosuppression, intravenous drug use, hemodialysis, or a history of trauma may suggest an infectious origin.[31] Typically, these patients have evidence of systemic infection, including fever, chills, malaise, and an elevated white blood cell count. Laboratory assays can often identify the inciting infectious agent.

Major vascular lesions that can mimic CSM include spinal cord infarction, spinal cord hematoma, and vascular malformations of the spinal cord. MRI of the cervical spine typically can identify these lesions. Vascular malformations characteristically demonstrate serpiginous flow voids on MRI.[32] Vascular malformations typically occur in the thoracic spinal cord but can cause upper limb symptoms and may be missed if MRI of the thoracic spine is not performed. Often magnetic resonance angiography or conventional spinal angiography may be needed to confirm the diagnosis and plan therapy. Acute spinal cord infarction and hemorrhage typically manifest with an acute onset of symptoms.

Noninfectious inflammatory and demyelinating causes of myelopathy include multiple sclerosis, acute disseminated encephalomyelitis (ADEM), transverse myelitis, and neuromyelitis optica (NMO). These disorders may manifest with acute or subacute myelopathic symptoms. MRI of the cervical spine typically shows an area of patchy T2 hyperintensity in the cervical spinal cord that suggests an inflammatory process. A history of optic neuritis and

the presence of humoral NMO immunoglobulin G antibodies are specific to NMO. Multiple sclerosis typically manifests with multifocal neurologic lesions on neurologic examination and MRI of the brain and spinal cord. ADEM generally has an abrupt or subacute onset of multifocal neurologic manifestations.[5]

Rheumatologic diseases can be associated with inflammatory spinal cord lesions. These disorders include systemic lupus erythematosus, Sjögren syndrome, sarcoidosis, and rheumatoid arthritis. These can usually be differentiated from CSM by radiologic findings and by the presence of nonneurologic manifestations and serologic markers. Patients with rheumatoid arthritis and ankylosing spondylitis are prone to upper cervical spine involvement, including craniocervical and C1 to C2 subluxations with myelopathy.[33] Angiotensin-converting enzyme levels and lung lesions can aid in the diagnosis of sarcoidosis. Syringomyelia can be confused with CSM until diagnostic imaging is performed.

Nutritional and metabolic causes of myelopathy should be suspected when imaging of the spinal cord does not reveal a structural cause. Blood tests and metabolic assays can identify nutritional and metabolic deficiencies. Vitamin B_{12} deficiency can produce subacute combined degeneration primarily affecting dorsal columns and lateral corticospinal tracts.[34] MRI may show increased signal intensity on T2-weighted images in the dorsal columns, but definitive diagnosis requires demonstration of low cobalamin levels and elevated methylmalonic acid and homocysteine levels. Copper deficiency can produce both myelopathy and peripheral neuropathy. Although many patients with copper deficiency myelopathy have normal results of spinal cord imaging, areas of increased signal intensity on T2-weighted images involving the dorsal columns have been reported. Vitamin E deficiency and folic acid deficiency can also result in myelopathy.

Various spinal tumors, including gliomas, meningiomas, neurofibromas, and metastases, can produce myelopathic symptoms either by direct compression or by invasion into nervous tissue. Additionally, tumors involving the vertebral bodies, such as metastatic prostate cancer or multiple myeloma, can cause severe pain, bony destruction, spinal instability, and spinal cord compression. MRI with contrast generally detects the presence of tumors. Meningeal carcinomatosis typically produces a polyradicular pattern of neurologic signs and symptoms. Paraneoplastic disorders can also manifest with myelopathic symptoms and can be associated with various serologic markers. Postradiation myelopathy can occur in patients who have received radiation therapy for malignant disease in which the spinal cord is within the field of treatment. This disorder can occur either early after radiation, when transient sensory symptoms predominate, or months to years after radiation, with mild to severe persistent motor and sensory deficits.[35]

Motor neuron disease, chiefly ALS, can easily be confused with CSM. ALS typically manifests with upper and lower motor neuron signs, as can CSM with concomitant radiculopathy. Fasciculations of the tongue and lack of sensory deficits are particularly useful in differentiating ALS from CSM. EMG can help corroborate the diagnosis.

Nonoperative Treatment

The aggressiveness of treatment should depend on the type and severity of neurologic symptoms and the patient's rate of worsening. Nonoperative treatment is indicated in patients with mild myelopathy (i.e., mild hyperreflexia without functional impairments) or in whom medical comorbidities make the risk of surgery too great.[36] Asymptomatic patients with evidence of cervical spinal cord compression on MRI are also candidates for nonoperative management. For these patients, immobilization and isometric exercises may reduce the neural irritation and provide some relief from myelopathic symptoms.[37] Use of cervical soft collars or rigid bracing is also commonly recommended, though little evidence for its efficacy exists. Furthermore, physical therapy can strengthen the musculature of the neck and reduce biomechanical loads on the cervical spine, thereby slowing spondylotic degeneration. Analgesic medications (i.e., nonsteroidal antiinflammatory drugs) directed at arthritic neck pain may provide symptomatic relief early in the disease course. Neuromodulating medications (i.e., gabapentin or pregabalin) and tricyclic agents (i.e., amitriptyline or nortriptyline) can be tried for persistent neck or upper limb pain. Although epidural steroids and cervical traction are common therapies for radiculopathy, they do not reduce the symptoms of myelopathy. Generally, patients are encouraged to modify their lifestyles and living arrangements to avoid activities that may exacerbate symptoms. More importantly, patients should be counseled about falls and injuries, which may worsen neurologic function because of the relatively higher risk of spinal cord compression following neck hyperextension.[1] Conservatively treated patients should be frequently monitored for progression of symptoms.

Operative Treatment

Surgical indications for CSM vary among spinal surgeons, but most agree that the natural history of CSM seems to be one of persistent deterioration. When considering surgical intervention, the surgeon must consider the severity and rate of neurologic deterioration, the amount of pain, and the magnitude of spinal cord compression seen on imaging studies. Patients should understand that the goal of surgery is to prevent further neurologic deterioration; complete resolution of symptoms rarely occurs, and improvement is highly variable. It is appropriate to offer urgent surgery for patients who show rapid worsening of neurologic function attributable to spondylotic changes. Patients with moderate to severe symptoms, including disruption of gait; changes in bowel, bladder, and sexual function; and significant hand dysfunction should be offered surgery, especially if their symptoms significantly affect their quality of life or employment potential.[1] In a retrospective review of the spinal cord morphometry of myelopathic patients, Fujiwara and colleagues determined that the severity of spinal cord compression has been shown to predict a negative postoperative prognosis.[38] Based on these findings, patients with mild symptoms should be considered surgical candidates only if marked spinal cord compression is evident on imaging studies.

The chief objective of surgery is decompression of the spinal cord and its circulation by expanding the spinal canal. Secondary goals include stabilization of segments where motion can damage the spinal cord and prevention of future spine deformity. The surgical approach is largely guided by the anteroposterior location of the compression, the number of involved levels, the presence of instability, and the sagittal plane alignment.

Anterior Surgery

Anterior cervical approaches include single- or multiple-level anterior diskectomies or corpectomies followed by arthrodesis with autogenous or allogeneic bone grafts. This approach is usually accompanied by the use of anterior instrumentation to prevent graft extrusion and pseudarthrosis. The anterior approach allows for direct decompression of anterior pathologic structures contributing to spinal cord compression. Other advantages of the anterior approach are that it allows for correction of sagittal plane alignment in patients with loss of cervical lordosis. Sagittal plane deformity correction is more difficult to achieve from posterior approaches.[39] Patients with evidence of spinal cord compression solely at the disk levels are candidates for anterior cervical diskectomy and fusion (ACDF). Multilevel ACDFs, requiring multiple bone grafts or cages, increase the number of healing surfaces and thus carry a higher risk of pseudarthrosis. Corpectomy is often considered as a substitute for two-level ACDF to reduce the number of healing surfaces from four to two, with the concomitant theoretical advantage of reducing the risk of pseudarthrosis.[40]

In addition, partial or subtotal corpectomy is indicated when compressive pathologic elements (i.e., osteophyte formation, disk herniation, or OPLL) extend above or below the disk space such that diskectomy alone will not achieve adequate anterior decompression. Partial corpectomy involves removal of a portion of the top or bottom of the vertebral body, whereas subtotal corpectomy involves removal of the entire proximodistal extent of the vertebral body with the exception of the lateral walls, which are left intact to protect the vertebral arteries and to stabilize the graft. The corpectomy defects can then be reconstructed and arthrodesed with a combination of structural bone graft, metal cages, and cancellous bone.[39,40]

Spinal fusion, however, has well-known potential disadvantages. Most notably, fusion leads to loss of natural motion and flexibility, with the potential for accelerated degeneration of adjacent-level disks and the subsequent need for more surgery. As an alternative to spinal fusion surgery, cervical artificial disk replacement is gaining popularity by theoretically avoiding these shortcomings. Although long-term outcomes remain to be defined, artificial disks can potentially reduce damage to nearby disks and joints by reestablishing natural motion and normal distribution of stress along the cervical spine. Arthroplasty has been used for the indication of single-level disk disease from C3 through C7 with intractable radiculopathy or myelopathy.[41]

Posterior Surgery

Posterior approaches are typically indicated in patients with dorsal spinal cord compression, usually from hypertrophy or dynamic buckling of the ligamentum flavum. Other indications include diffuse spinal canal stenosis, multilevel spondylosis, or OPLL. A relative contraindication to posterior decompression is the presence of preoperative kyphosis, especially with anterior compression unless the kyphosis can be corrected. To treat anterior disorders with posterior decompression, the spinal cord must shift dorsally in the thecal sac, which is less likely in the setting of a kyphotic spine. Compared with long anterior exposures, posterior decompressions tend to be technically less demanding and do not place key anterior structures, such as the esophagus, trachea, and recurrent laryngeal nerve, at risk.[5] However, posterior approaches have a higher rate of wound complications, are more painful for the patient, and typically have a longer recovery period. The posterior surgical options include laminectomy with or without fusion and laminoplasty.

Historically, single- or multiple-level laminectomy had been regarded as the standard posterior procedure for the treatment of CSM. Laminectomy, however, fell into relative disfavor because of well-known postoperative sequelae, such as the development of kyphosis, segmental instability, perineural adhesions, increased progression of OPLL, and late neurologic deterioration.[42] Currently, laminectomy alone has a very narrow indication, and it should probably be offered only to patients with single-level posterior compressive lesions and normal sagittal plane alignment.

Adding fusion to the laminectomy theoretically reduces some of the disadvantages associated with laminectomy alone. In a retrospective review of patients treated with laminectomy and fusion, Kumar and colleagues concluded that rigid stabilization minimized the postoperative complications commonly seen with laminectomy alone. Among their 25 patients who were followed up for more than 2 years, 76% had improved myelopathy scores, and none had late neurologic deterioration or evidence of postoperative kyphosis.[42] Furthermore, stabilization of the cervical spine decreases flexion motion, which could cause intermittent trauma to the spinal cord over any residual anterior compression that may be present.

Although laminectomy with fusion may deter the progression of spondylosis, it does so at the expense of reduced spinal motion. Laminoplasty was developed in the 1980s to address the shortcomings of fusion. The technique was originally developed to reduce postoperative instability while maintaining normal cervical motion. Both techniques have the common goal of expanding the area of the spinal canal, but laminoplasty procedures do so by preserving the posterior elements, which serve as anchors for muscle reattachment. The "open door" laminoplasty and its variations involve opening the posterior arch on one side with a contralateral hinge. The "French door" laminoplasty involves opening the lamina in the midline with bilateral hinges.[43-45]

One theoretical advantage of muscular reattachment is the maintenance of cervical stability and alignment. This occurs by preventing cervical muscle atrophy by allowing natural neck motion. Some investigators have theorized that this procedure additionally helps reduce postoperative neck pain in comparison with patients who undergo fusion. However, few comparative reports are available on these two techniques, nor have many long-term follow-up reviews on laminoplastic surgery been published. In a matched cohort analysis of laminoplasty and laminectomy with fusion, Heller and colleagues suggested that laminoplasty could be preferable to laminectomy with fusion for CSM. These investigators found greater objective clinical improvement (Nurick score) in patients' function, as well as radiographic evidence of improved cervical alignment, in the laminoplasty-treated patients when compared with those treated with laminectomy and fusion.[46,47] The study, however, was limited in its relatively small number of patients and lack of long-term follow-up. Yonenobu and colleagues retrospectively looked at various outcome measures in patients treated with laminoplasty for CSM. Their results show that laminoplasty techniques on average resulted in a loss of approximately 30% to 50% of cervical mobility.[48] However, this finding compares favorably with techniques involving multiple-level arthrodesis in which the goal of surgery is the elimination of all motion. Despite the theoretical advantages of laminoplasty, significant results that document its long-term benefit when compared with laminectomy with fusion are still lacking.

Anterior and Posterior Surgery

Combined anterior and posterior approaches may be indicated in patients with severe sagittal plane kyphosis and multilevel stenosis. Posterior arthrodesis and instrumentation have also been used to augment an anterior construction in patients with significant unstable factors, such as two- or three-level corpectomies that were associated with laminectomy or poor bone quality.[49-51] The anterior procedure is aimed at restoring sagittal plane alignment and spinal cord decompression, whereas the goal of the posterior procedure is to provide enhanced stability to minimize anterior graft complications and enhance the chances of arthrodesis. Typically, this entails a multiple-level corpectomy with a long strut graft staged with lateral mass screws with plate or rod fixation. The strong dorsal and ventral fixation is helpful in resisting translation and torsion of the spine, reducing graft-related complications, and increasing fusion rates.[52-54]

Conclusions

CSM typically results from age-related spondylosis and can cause severe, irreversible symptoms from spinal cord compression. It continues to be a very common source of disability in older adults. The diagnosis and treatment of CSM remain elusive despite numerous studies on the pathophysiology and natural history of this disorder. A broad differential diagnosis combined with a high frequency of asymptomatic degenerative spondylosis creates a diagnostic challenge. The astute physician must detect sometimes subtle physical examination findings, such as such as walking difficulty, loss of fine motor control of the hands, and hyperreflexia, and must subsequently confirm the diagnosis with appropriate radiologic evaluation.

Treatment for CSM has relied largely on surgical decompression of the spinal cord for patients with moderate to severe disease. The surgical approach is guided by the anteroposterior location of the compression, the number of involved levels, the presence of instability, and the overall sagittal plane alignment. The anterior surgical approach has the advantages of direct decompression of the spinal cord with the ability to correct a sagittal plane deformity. Posterior surgical decompression alone tends to be technically less demanding but requires sagittal plane lordosis. Laminectomy and fusion comprise an alternative option for selected patients who have lost the normal cervical lordosis. Anterior and posterior surgery is reserved for patients with complex kyphotic sagittal plane deformities and for those with poor bone quality. Predictive factors for good surgical outcomes remain elusive, and further research must be performed.

REFERENCES

1. Baron EM, Young W: Cervical spondylotic myelopathy: a brief review of its pathophysiology, clinical course, and diagnosis, *Neurosurgery* 60(Suppl 1):35–42, 2007.
2. Burgerman R, Rigamonti D, Randle JM, et al.: The association of cervical spondylosis and multiple sclerosis, *Surg Neurol* 38:265–270, 1992.
3. Crandall PH, Batzdorf U: Cervical spondylotic myelopathy, *J Neurosurg* 25:57–66, 1966.
4. Arnold JG: The clinical manifestations of spondylochondrosis (spondylosis) of the cervical spine, *Ann Surg* 141:872–889, 1955.
5. Bohlman HH, Emery SE: The pathophysiology of cervical spondylosis and myelopathy, *Spine (Phila Pa 1976)* 13:843–846, 1988.
6. Murone I: The importance of the sagittal diameters of the cervical spinal canal in relation to spondylosis and myelopathy, *J Bone Joint Surg Br* 56:30–36, 1974.
7. Tracy JA, Bartleson JD: Cervical spondylotic myelopathy, *Neurologist* 16:176–187, 2010.
8. Christe A, Laubli R, Guzman R, et al.: Degeneration of the cervical disc: histology compared with radiography and magnetic resonance imaging, *Neuroradiology* 47:721–729, 2005.
9. Hoff JT, Wilson CB: The pathophysiology of cervical spondylotic radiculopathy and myelopathy, *Clin Neurosurg* 24:474–487, 1977.
10. Young WF: Cervical spondylotic myelopathy: a common cause of spinal cord dysfunction in older persons, *Am Fam Physicians* 62:1064–1073, 2000.
11. Ichihara K, Taguchi T, Sakuramoto I, et al.: Mechanism of the spinal cord injury and cervical spondylotic myelopathy: new approach based on the mechanical features of the spinal cord white and gray matter, *J Neurosurg Spine* 99:278–285, 2003.
12. Gledhill RF, Harrison BM, McDonald WI: Demyelination and remyelination after acute spinal cord compression, *Exp Neurol* 38:472–487, 1973.
13. Hakuda AS, Wilson C: Experimental cervical myelopathy: effects of compression and ischemia on the canine cervical cord, *J Neurosurg* 37:631–652, 1972.
14. Clark E, Robinson PK: Cervical myelopathy: a complication of cervical spondylosis, *Brain* 79:483–510, 1956.
15. Lees F, Turner JW: Natural history and prognosis of cervical spondylosis, *Br Med J* 2:1607–1610, 1963.
16. Nurick S: The natural history and the results of surgical treatment of the spinal cord disorder associated with cervical spondylosis, *Brain* 95:101–108, 1972.
17. Nurick S: The pathogenesis of the spinal cord disorder associated with cervical spondylosis, *Brain* 95:87–100, 1972.
18. Symon L, Lavendar P: The surgical treatment of cervical spondylotic myelopathy, *Neurology* 17:117–127, 1967.
19. Sadasivian KK, Reddy RP, Albright JA: The natural history of cervical spondylotic myelopathy, *Yale J Biol Med* 66:235–242, 1993.
20. Bednarik J, Kadanka Z, Dusek L, et al.: Presymptomatic spondylotic cervical myelopathy: an updated predictive model, *Eur Spine J* 17:421–431, 2008.
21. Fouyas IP, Statham PF, Sandercock PA: Cochrane review on the role of surgery in cervical spondylotic radiculomyelopathy, *Spine (Phila Pa 1976)* 27:736–747, 2002.
22. Kadanka Z, Mares M, Bednarik J, et al.: Approaches to spondylotic cervical myelopathy: conservative versus surgical results in a 3-year follow-up study, *Spine (Phila Pa 1976)* 27:2205–2210, 2002.
23. Sampath P, Bendebba M, Davis JD, Ducker TB: Outcome of patients treated for cervical myelopathy, *Spine (Phila Pa 1976)* 25:670–676, 2000.
24. Denno JJ, Meadows GR: Early diagnoses of cervical spondylotic myelopathy: a useful clinical sign, *Spine (Phila Pa 1976)* 16:1353–1355, 1991.
25. Ono K, Ebara S, Fuji T, et al.: Myelopathy hand: new clinical signs of cervical cord damage, *J Bone Joint Surg Br* 69:215–219, 1987.
26. Yonenobu K, Abumi K, Nagata K, et al.: Interobserver and intraobserver reliability of the Japanese Orthopedic Association scoring system for evaluation of cervical compression myelopathy, *Spine (Phila Pa 1976)* 26:1890–1894, 2001.
27. Morio Y, Yamamoto K, Kuranobu K, et al.: Does increased signal intensity of the spinal cord on MR images due to cervical myelopathy predict prognosis? *Arch Orthop Trauma Surg* 113:254–259, 1994.
28. Arvin B, Kalsi-Ryan S, Karpova A, et al.: Post-operative magnetic resonance imaging can predict neurological recovery following surgery for cervical spondylotic myelopathy: a prospective study with blinded assessments, *Neurosurgery* 69:362–368, 2011.
29. Furlan JC, Kalsi-Ryan S, Kailaya-Vasan A, et al.: Functional and clinical outcomes following surgical treatment in patients with cervical spondylotic myelopathy: a prospective study of 81 cases, *J Neurosurg Spine* 14:348–355, 2011.
30. Shafaie FF, Wippold FJ II, Gado M, et al.: Comparison of computed tomography myelography and magnetic resonance imaging in the evaluation of spondylotic myelography and radiculopathy, *Spine (Phila Pa 1976)* 24:1781–1785, 1999.
31. Torg JS, Pavlov H, Genuario SE, et al.: Neurapraxia of the cervical spinal cord with transient quadriplegia, *J Bone Joint Surg Am* 68:1354–1370, 1986.
32. Prasad SS, O'Malley M, Caplan M, et al.: MRI Measurements of the cervical spine and their correlation to Pavlov's ratio, *Spine (Phila Pa 1976)* 28:1263–1268, 2003.
33. Berger JR, Sabet A: Infectious myelopathies, *Semin Neurol* 22:133–142, 2002.
34. Atkinson JL, Miller GM, Krauss WE, et al.: Clinical and radiographic features of dural arteriovenous fistula, a treatable cause of myelopathy, *Mayo Clin Proc* 76:1120–1130, 2001.
35. Shen FH, Samartzis D, Jenis LG, et al.: Rheumatoid arthritis: evaluation and surgical management of the cervical spine, *Spine J* 4:689–700, 2004.
36. Maamar M, Mezalek ZT, Harmouche H, et al.: Contribution of spinal MRI for unsuspected cobalamin deficiency in isolated subacute combined degeneration, *Eur J Intern Med* 19:143–145, 2008.
37. Rampling R, Symonds P: Radiation myelopathy, *Curr Opin Neurol* 11:627–632, 1998.
38. Matsumoto M, Chiba K, Ishikawa M, et al.: Relationships between outcomes of conservative treatment and magnetic resonance imaging findings in patients with mild cervical myelopathy caused by soft disc herniation, *Spine (Phila Pa 1976)* 26:1592–1598, 2001.
39. Murphy MJ, Lieponis JV: Nonoperative treatment of cervical spine pain. In Sherk HH, Cervical Spine Research Society, editors: *The cervical spine*, Philadelphia, 1989, Lippincott, pp 670–677.
40. Fujiwara K, Yonenobu K, Ebara S, et al.: The prognosis of surgery for cervical compression myelopathy: an analysis of the factors involved, *J Bone Joint Surg Br* 71:393–398, 1989.
41. Smith GW, Robinson RA: The treatment of certain cervical-spine disorders by anterior removal of the intervertebral disc and interbody fusion, *J Bone Joint Surg Am* 40:607–624, 1958.
42. Connolly ES, Seymour RJ, Adams JE: Clinical evaluation of anterior cervical fusion for degenerative cervical disc disease, *J Neurosurg* 23:431–437, 1965.
43. Heller JG, Sasso RC, Papadopoulos SM, et al.: Comparison of BRYAN cervical disc arthroplasty with anterior cervical decompression and fusion: clinical and radiographic results of randomized, controlled, clinical trial, *Spine (Phila Pa 1976)* 39:101–107, 2009.

44. Anderson PA, Matz PG, Groff MW, et al.: Laminectomy and fusion for the treatment of cervical degenerative myelopathy: Joint Section on Disorders of the Spine and Peripheral Nerves of the American Association of Neurological Surgeons and Congress of Neurological Surgeons, *J Neurosurg Spine* 11:150–156, 2009.

45. Ryken TC, Heary RF, Matz PG, et al.: Cervical laminectomy for the treatment of cervical degenerative myelopathy: Joint Section on Disorders of the Spine and Peripheral Nerves of the American Association of Neurological Surgeons and Congress of Neurological Surgeons, *J Neurosurg Spine* 11:142–149, 2009.

46. Kumar VG, Rea GL, Mervis LJ, et al.: Cervical spondylotic myelopathy: functional and radiographic long-term outcome after laminectomy and posterior fusion, *Neurosurgery* 44:771–777, 1999.

47. Matz PG, Anderson PA, Groff MW, et al.: Cervical laminoplasty for the treatment of cervical degenerative myelopathy: Joint Section on Disorders of the Spine and Peripheral Nerves of the American Association of Neurological Surgeons and Congress of Neurological Surgeons, *J Neurosurg Spine* 11:157–169, 2009.

48. Inoue H, Ohmori K, Ishida Y, et al.: Long-term follow-up review of suspension laminotomy for cervical compression myelopathy, *J Neurosurg* 85:817–823, 1996.

49. Heller JG, Edwards CC, Murakami H, Rodts GE: Laminoplasty versus laminectomy and fusion for multilevel cervical myelopathy: an independent matched cohort analysis, *Spine (Phila Pa 1976)* 26:1330–1336, 2001.

50. Mummaneni PV, Kaiser MG, Matz PG, et al.: Cervical surgical techniques for the treatment of cervical spondylotic myelopathy: Joint Section on Disorders of the Spine and Peripheral Nerves of the American Association of Neurological Surgeons and Congress of Neurological Surgeons, *J Neurosurg Spine* 11:130–156, 2009.

51. Yonenobu K, Hosono N, Iwasaki M, et al.: Laminoplasty versus subtotal corpectomy: a comparative study of results in multisegmental cervical spondylotic myelopathy, *Spine (Phila Pa 1976)* 17:1281–1284, 1992.

52. Highsmith JM, Dhall SS, Haid RW, et al.: Treatment of cervical stenotic myelopathy: a cost and outcome comparison of laminoplasty versus laminectomy and lateral mass fusion, *J Neurosurg Spine* 14:619–625, 2011.

53. Han K, Lu C, Li J, et al.: Surgical treatment of cervical kyphosis, *Eur Spine J* 20:523–536, 2010.

54. Song KJ, Johnson JS, Choi BR, et al.: Anterior fusion alone compared with combined anterior and posterior fusion for the treatment of degenerative cervical kyphosis, *J Bone Joint Surg Br* 92:1548–1552, 2010.

15

Cervical Deformity and Treatment Algorithms

Justin K. Scheer, Yoon Ha, Vedat Deviren, Sang-Hun Lee, William R. Sears, and Christopher P. Ames

CHAPTER PREVIEW

Chapter Synopsis	Cervical deformity is disruption of normal cervical alignment. This chapter focuses on the different causes of cervical deformity, normative data, and deformity evaluation and examination and presents various treatment options for the proper management of these debilitating conditions.
Important Points	Disruption of normal cervical lordosis can result in loss of horizontal gaze and resulting mechanical neck pain.
	Main etiologic factors in cervical spine deformity can be divided into primary, inflammatory, degenerative, and iatrogenic causes.
	Careful history and examination and thorough imaging are important for the assessment, diagnosis, and surgical planning in patients with cervical spine deformities.
	Surgical treatment may be indicated in patients with severe mechanical neck pain, neurologic compromise, and progressive deformity causing significant disability such as dysphagia or loss of horizontal gaze.
	Considerations for anterior, posterior, and/or combined circumferential procedures are based on the patient's pathologic process and the surgeon's familiarity with and preference for the surgical techniques.

Normal Cervical Lordosis

To understand cervical spine alignment and deformity treatment properly, several basic concepts must be understood:

1. The significant mass of the head is supported by the cervical spine, and significant deviation from normal alignment increases cantilever loads and muscular activity.
2. The flexible, mobile cervical segment is connected to the relatively fixed thoracic spine.
3. The T1 inclination determines the amount of subaxial lordosis required to maintain the center of gravity of the head in a balanced position.
4. The T1 inclination varies depending on global spinal alignment as measured by the sagittal vertical axis (SVA) and by inherent upper thoracic kyphosis.
5. The radiographic parameters that affect health-related quality of life scores are not well defined compared with global and pelvic parameters in thoracolumbar deformity.[1-4] Chin-brow to vertical angle (CBVA), cervical SVA (C2 SVA), and regional cervical lordosis should all be considered in preoperative planning

strategies involving standing 36-inch radiographs in which the external auditory canal (approximation of head center of mass) to the femoral head is visible.

In asymptomatic normal volunteers, cervical standing lordosis is greatest at C1 to C2, and little lordosis exists in the lower cervical levels (Table 15-1).[5] Approximately 75% of total cervical lordosis is taken at C1 to C2. Mean total cervical lordosis is approximately −40 degrees, with, on average, the occiput-C1 segment being kyphotic (Fig. 15-1).[5] Only 6 degrees (15%) occurs at the lowest three cervical levels (C4 to C7) (see Table 15-1).[5] Furthermore, no difference is noted between asymptomatic men and women in total cervical lordosis, and a positive correlation exists with cervical lordosis and increasing age.[5,6] The average odontoid-C7 plumb line distance ranges from 15 to 17 ± 11.2 mm (see Table 15-1).[5]

Anatomically and biomechanically, the cranium and cervical spine are placed over the thoracic inlet, a fixed bony circle that is composed of the T1 vertebral body, the first ribs on both sides, and the upper part of the sternum. The sagittal balance of the cranium and cervical spine may possibly be influenced by the shape and orientation of the thoracic inlet to obtain a balanced, upright posture

Table 15-1 Normal Cervical Spinal Values in Asymptomatic Adults from the Literature*

Segmental Cervical Angles[5]		C2-C7 Lordosis[6]		
Level	Angle (Degree)	Age Group (yr)	Men (Degree)	Women (Degree)
C0-C1	2.1 ± 5.0	20-25	16 ± 16	15 ± 10
C1-C2	−32.2 ± 7.0	30-35	21 ± 14	16 ± 16
C2-C3	−1.9 ± 5.2	40-45	27 ± 14	23 ± 17
C3-C4	−1.5 ± 5.0	50-55	22 ± 15	25 ± 11
C4-C5	−0.6 ± 4.4	60-65	22 ± 13	25 ± 16
C5-C6	−1.1 ± 5.1			
C6-C7	−4.5 ± 4.3			
C2-C7	−9.6			
Total (C1-C7)	−41.8			
Cervical Sagittal Vertical Axis[5]				
Odontoid marker at C7	15.6 ± 11.2 mm			
Odontoid marker at sacrum	13.2 ± 29.5 mm			

*Values presented as the means ± SD and the negative sign indicates lordosis in the segmental values.

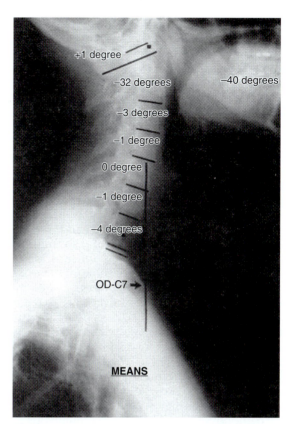

FIGURE 15-1 Cervical standing lateral radiograph displaying the cervical lordosis angles in asymptomatic normal adults. *OD,* Odontoid. (From Hardacker JW, Shuford RF, Capicotto PN, Pryor PW: Radiographic standing cervical segmental alignment in adult volunteers without neck symptoms. *Spine (Phila Pa 1976)* 22:1472-1480, 1997. discussion 1480.)

and horizontal gaze, similar to the pelvic incidence in the pelvis.[7] The authors have found linkage of significant correlation from the thoracic inlet angle to the cranial offset and craniocervical alignment.[7] The ratio of the C0-C2 to C2-C7 angles to total cervical lordosis was 77%:23%, and the ratio of cervical to cranial tilting to T1 slope was 70%:30% in asymptomatic individuals.[7]

Neck tilting was maintained at approximately 45 degrees to minimize energy expenditure of the neck muscles. These results indicate that a small thoracic inlet angle makes the small T1 slope to maintain physiologic neck tilting and makes the small cervical spine lordotic angle, and vice versa. According to the study, the thoracic inlet angle and the T1 slope may be used as parameters to evaluate sagittal balance, predict physiologic alignment, and guide deformity correction of the cervical spine.[7]

Pathophysiology (Epidemiology, Pathophysiology, Natural History, and Differential Diagnoses)

Cervical spine lordosis is required for sagittal plane alignment because it counteracts thoracic kyphosis, aids in maintaining a neutral global SVA, and keeps the center of gravity of the head over the spine.[8,9] Any disruption of cervical lordosis leads to a loss of horizontal gaze and severe mechanical neck pain, which can be very debilitating both physically and mentally to the patient.

Deformities of the cervical spine present many challenges to the surgeon, one of which is determining the ideal treatment option. The most common type of cervical

spine deformity occurs in the sagittal plane as a kyphotic deformity, whereas malalignment in the coronal plane is much less common.[10-12] Furthermore, the most common type of cervical kyphotic deformity is iatrogenic, specifically after multiple-level laminectomy, with an incidence of 20%.[12-14] The primary goals of the various treatment options are to restore cervical sagittal alignment and thus improve horizontal gaze, reduce neck pain, and, if the deformity is severe enough, improve swallowing and respiration.[2,10] This chapter focuses on the different causes of cervical deformity and presents various treatment options for the proper management of these debilitating conditions.

Etiologic Factors

The causes of common cervical spine deformities may be characterized in terms of four broad categories: primary, inflammatory, degenerative, and iatrogenic.[10] Primary deformities of the cervical spine include congenital scoliosis, skeletal dysplasias, and neurofibromatosis. The exact origin of congenital scoliosis remains unclear; however, many factors have been implicated, such as genetics, drugs, chemicals, vitamin deficiency, and environmental factors.[10,15] These factors cause physiologic injury during the early embryonic period before the development of cartilage and bone. This injury leads either to failure of the vertebrae to form completely or to failure of segmentation (nonfusions of phenotypically normal-appearing vertebrae). These malformations in the vertebrae result in curvature of the spine and may continue to be progressive during the growth of the child.

Cervical spinal deformities caused by systemic inflammatory arthritic conditions tend to be a result of rheumatoid arthritis (RA) or ankylosing spondylitis. RA is a common autoimmune disorder; approximately 2 million people in the United States are affected, and it is the most common inflammatory disorder of the cervical spine.[16,17] The current theory of the etiology of RA is an immune response against synovial cells. The immune response causes destruction of cartilage, ligaments, tendons, and bone, and it leads to ligamentous laxity and bone erosion. The upper cervical spine is the most commonly affected because the occipital-C1 and C1-C2 joints are primarily synovial. Three types of deformities result: atlantoaxial instability or subluxation; superior migration of the odontoid; and subaxial subluxation, usually at multiple levels. Atlantoaxial instability is caused by erosion of the C1-C2 joint and may be classified as reducible, partially reducible, or fixed; all classes of instability affect treatment. The superior migration of the odontoid is also the result of erosion of the C1-C2 joint and the occipital-C1 joint that causes vertical height reduction between the brainstem and C2. The multiple-level subaxial subluxations all combine to produce significant cervical kyphosis, which may need surgical correction.

The pathophysiology of ankylosing spondylitis (AS) is similar to that of RA in that AS is a chronic inflammatory disease; however, AS is characterized by ossification of the joints and ligaments and typically affects the axial spine.[17,18] The initial onset is localized to the sacroiliac joint, from which it progresses superiorly to the lumbar spine and then to the cervical spine. Inflammation of the annulus fibrosus causes squaring of the vertebral bodies and formation of bridging osteophytes. Furthermore, inflammation of the apophysial joints with ossification of the adjacent ligaments leads to complete fusion of the spinal column. During this process, lumbar and cervical lordosis is lost, and significant cervical kyphosis may develop as the disease progresses. Eventually, the patient may develop a chin-on-chest deformity with a severe loss of horizontal gaze. Despite the increased bony fusion and appearance on radiographs, the spine may be osteoporotic as a result of stress shielding, and this possibility must be considered during surgical planning.

Cervical spondylosis is a form of degenerative etiology resulting in cervical deformity.[10,19] Three main symptomatic complexes associated with cervical spondylosis are neck pain, radiculopathy, and myelopathy. The primary pathogenesis of cervical spondylosis leading to cervical deformity lies within intervertebral disk desiccation. This process leads to biochemical changes within the disk that cause the nucleus pulposus to lose elasticity and to become smaller and more fibrous. This change shifts the primary weight-bearing mechanism to the annulus fibrosus, causes it to bulge posteriorly into the spinal canal, and thus reduces intervertebral disk height. The initial loss of height occurs anteriorly, which ultimately produces a positive feedback loop of increased anterior weight bearing leading to cervical kyphotic deformity.[10,19] Changes in cervical spine biomechanics cause the peripheral fibers of the annulus fibrosus and Sharpey fibers to be dissected away from the vertebral body edges and the posterior longitudinal ligament to buckle and peel off the vertebral bodies. The annular disk herniation, ligamentous laxity, and degenerative changes all lead to progressive cervical kyphosis, abnormal cervical spine movement, and neck pain.

The most common cause of cervical spine deformity is iatrogenic, of which the most common type is postlaminectomy kyphosis.[13,20] The natural biomechanics of the spine relies on a lordotic curvature in which the posterior columns withstand approximately 65% of the load and the anterior columns 35%. Thus, the posterior neural arch is responsible for most of the load transmission down the cervical spine, and removal of this structure causes a significant loss of stability. Initially, performing extensive multiple-level laminectomies does not immediately destabilize an intact spine. However, the added instability with losing the posterior arch–facet complex causes a shift in load bearing from the posterior column to the anterior column. Over time, this shift places added stress on the cervical musculature that requires constant contraction to maintain an upright head posture. This results in fatigue and pain. Cervical kyphosis occurs as the load is shifted anteriorly, and as the disks and vertebral bodies become wedged, it progresses to greater imbalance (Fig. 15-2, A).

Progressive cervical kyphosis has also been associated with myelopathy. The deformity leads to draping of the spinal cord against the vertebral bodies, thus increasing longitudinal cord tension because the spinal cord is tethered by the dentate ligaments and the cervical nerve roots.[13,20] As the curve becomes greater over time, the spinal cord becomes compressed and flattened.[21] The anterior and posterior margins of the cord compress, whereas the lateral margins expand. During tethering of the spinal cord, the intramedullary pressure increases.[22-24] This compression leads to neuronal loss and demyelination of the spinal cord.[21] Furthermore, mechanical compression has significant adverse angiogenic effects. The small feeder blood vessels on the spinal cord become flattened, thus leading to a loss of blood supply. The number of vessels and the network size are greatly reduced, with interruption and abnormal arrangement of the blood vessels.[21] As the kyphotic angle increases, these changes become more pronounced, especially on the anterior side, which is exposed directly to the mechanical compression.[21] Greater spinal cord tension increases intramedullary cord pressure,[22-25] and it has been shown to lead to apoptosis in animal models.[21] Decompression alone, even ventral decompression, that does not decrease spinal cord tension induced by kyphosis may therefore not result in optimal outcomes.[21]

Decision-Making Process and Algorithms

Assessment

The primary goals during the preoperative assessment of a patient with a cervical kyphotic deformity are to

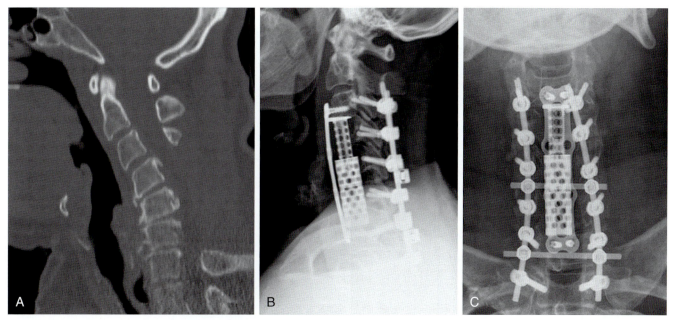

FIGURE 15-2 Case example of flexible postlaminectomy kyphosis. Preoperative computed tomography scan (**A**) showing cervical kyphosis following multiple-level laminectomy and postoperative lateral (**B**) and anteroposterior (**C**) radiographs showing the correction.

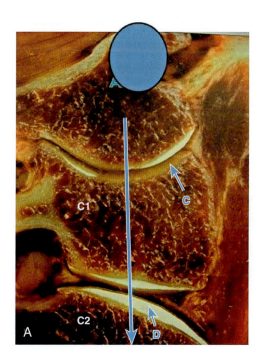

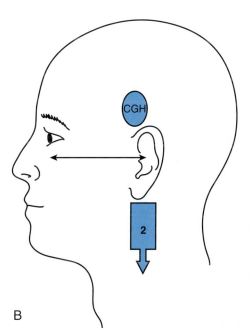

FIGURE 15-3 **A,** Sagittal cut through a cadaver cervical spine illustrating the center of gravity of the head (CGH; *blue oval*) being transmitted through C1 and C2 (*blue plumb line*). C, Superior endplate of C1. D, Superior endplate of C2. **B,** A schematic highlighting the location of the CGH in relation to the ear and the C2 plumb line.

determine the ideal amount of correction and to ascertain where along the spine the correction should be applied. Currently, no clear indications exist for the correct amount of cervical lordosis to be obtained postoperatively; however, a general rule of completely correcting the cervical kyphosis to neutral has been accepted.[12] Current research is likely to define cervical sagittal parameters similar to C7 SVA but instead measured on standing 3-foot films from C2 or the head center of mass (Fig. 15-3).

The initial evaluation of the patient includes a complete medical history and physical examination. Many of these patients are high-risk surgical patients, and pertinent history (i.e., smoking, use of nonsteroidal antiinflammatory drugs) can be used to tailor treatment. The physical examination component should include assessing the patient while he or she is standing upright with hips and knees fully extended and in the sitting and supine positions. The sitting position removes the effect of lumbar and pelvic or hip deformity, and the supine position can be used to assess the rigidity of semirigid curves under the direct effect of gravity.

The CBVA is measured preoperatively and postoperatively using the CBVA method (Figs. 15-4 and 15-5). This angle is measured between the chin-brow line and

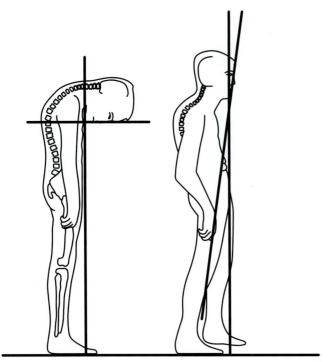

FIGURE 15-4 Artist's rendering of the chin-brow vertical angle (CBVA) measurement method.

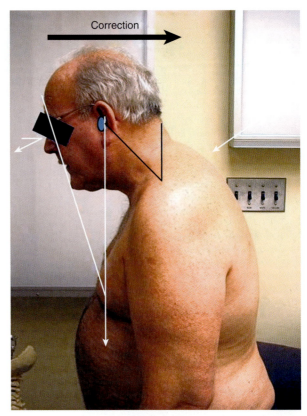

FIGURE 15-5 The chin-brow vertical angle (CBVA) measurement method portrayed on a clinical photograph.

the vertical line with the patient standing with the hips and knees extended and the neck in its neutral or fixed position. Based on this angle, the size of the wedge to be removed posteriorly can be determined. Despite lying flat, patients with fixed primary cervical deformity have persistent cervical flexion (Fig. 15-6), whereas patients with thoracic, lumbar, or hip deformities correct in the sitting or supine positions.

Following the physical examination, initial radiographic evaluation includes 36-inch standing plain x-ray films and dynamic flexion and extension cervical plain x-ray films (Fig. 15-7). The 36-inch standing film allows for global spinal assessment, whereas the dynamic films aid in determining the presence of any atlantoaxial instability and the relative flexibility of the spine.

Further radiographic studies, such as computed tomography (CT) and magnetic resonance imaging, are usually performed to assess osseous landmarks for instrumentation and spinal cord tethering or impingement. CT scans are used to determine extent of facet fusion and osteophytic bridging at the disk to determine the need for osteotomy anteriorly and posteriorly in a fixed deformity.

Nonoperative Treatment

The indications for surgery are not well defined and remain controversial. The patient may attempt several conservative treatment options before considering surgical intervention. Conservative treatment of cervical deformity is primarily aimed at reducing symptoms, usually targeting pain. Some options include physical therapy, chiropractic care, cervical traction, brace therapy, steroid injections, and nonsteroidal antiinflammatory agents. Surgical treatment may be indicated in patients with severe mechanical neck pain, neurologic compromise,

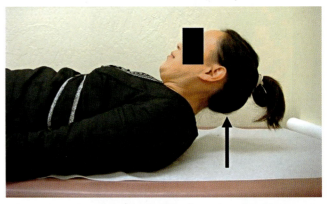

FIGURE 15-6 Clinical photograph of the supine physical examination component demonstrating a patient with fixed cervical kyphosis.

and progressive deformity causing significant disability such as dysphagia or loss of horizontal gaze.

Patients who present with cervical camptocormia (head ptosis or neck drop) have a flexible deformity of the spine in the sagittal plane that is corrected on lying supine.[26] The various causes of camptocormia include amyotrophic lateral sclerosis (ALS), different myopathies, parkinsonian disorders, and idiopathic conditions.[26] Thus, the initial workup of a patient with camptocormia (or other flexible deformity) should include appropriate electromyography and nerve conduction studies to rule out primary myopathy or ALS. Furthermore, patients should be referred to physical therapy before treatment with surgical correction and fusion is considered.

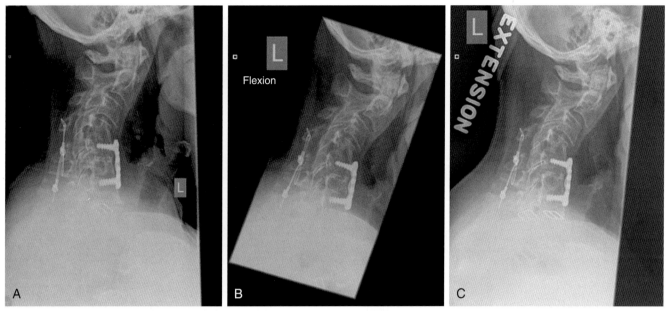

FIGURE 15-7 A, Preoperative lateral radiograph of a patient with fixed cervical kyphosis. Dynamic radiographs assessing the extent of rigidity by flexion (**B**) and extension (**C**).

Cervical traction may be used to attempt deformity correction before surgical intervention. Generally, 3 to 5 days of traction may be sufficient to reduce the deformity.[12] If the deformity is not reduced following 5 days of traction, further traction is unlikely to benefit the patient. In addition to the traction, muscle relaxants may also be used to aid in the reduction. If successful reduction of the cervical kyphosis does occur, posterior fixation and fusion may be used to prevent the deformity from progressing.

Operative Treatment

Evaluation of the flexibility of the cervical spine may determine the surgical intervention needed. If the spine is flexible, an anterior-alone or posterior-alone correction strategy may be used. If the spine is rigid without ankylosed facets, an anterior-alone strategy may be used. If the spine is rigid with ankylosed facets, a combination of anterior and posterior strategies may be used to correct the deformity.

The anterior-alone strategy allows for correction of the deformity as well as instrumentation to maintain the correction. It uses both posture and biomechanics to obtain the cervical lordosis needed. The patient is placed in the supine position with the head slightly extended. After exposure, anterior release, including disk and osteophytes, is performed, and distraction pins are placed in the vertebral bodies to allow for segmental extension of the vertebral bodies and thus cervical lordosis. Anterior release is usually by means of diskectomy because multiple lordosing diskectomies are generally more effective than a single long corpectomy at creating lordosis. Following release and distraction, struts and/or lordotic cages or grafts may be placed to facilitate bone fusion. Finally, a plate is contoured to the desired lordosis and is fixed anteriorly to the cervical spine. Lordotic plates can be used to generate additional lordosis by using a three-point bending technique to "pull" the spine up to the

plate once the plate is fixed at the ends. This technique relies on flexibility of the spine after diskectomy and anterior osteotomy.

When the cervical deformity is rigid with ankylosed facets, a combined anterior and posterior strategy may be employed.[27] The side of correction is chosen first, and the contralateral side is then released. Generally, the posterior strategy is performed first, with placement of screws and facetectomy and Smith-Peterson osteotomy. The patient is turned to the supine position, for disk release, anterior osteotomy, and lordotic plating. The patient is then turned prone, and instrumentation and posterior compression are applied. In certain patients with significant fixed subaxial kyphosis, it may be advantageous to perform an anterior osteotomy first, including release of the vertebral arteries from the foramen transversarium, followed by posterior osteotomy and correction with head manipulation after circumferential release. For this technique, we prefer the halo ring over the Mayfield clamp to allow a better grip on the head during manual reduction. Usually, more lordosis is possible using an anterior release followed by posterior correction compared with a posterior release followed by an anterior fixation because generally it is possible to generate more lordosis from the posterior position.

If the cervical deformity is very kyphotic and rigid with ankylosed facets, an osteotomy or combination of osteotomies may be used to correct the deformity. Traditionally, the Smith-Petersen osteotomy has been used to correct cervical spinal deformities in the sagittal plane. This type of osteotomy may be used when less than 30 degrees of correction is needed.[28] The Smith-Petersen osteotomy does have a few significant limitations. First, the patient may need multiple osteotomies at different levels to obtain the desired correction. Having multiple osteotomies increases the risk of pseudarthrosis. Second, a flexible anterior column (or the creation of an anterior

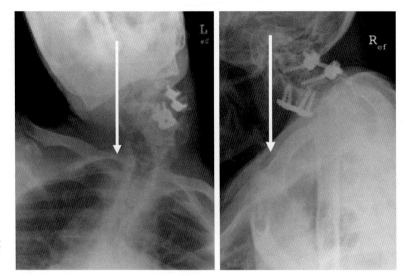

FIGURE 15-8 Left, Anteroposterior radiograph showing coronal malalignment. **Right,** Lateral radiograph showing sagittal malalignment.

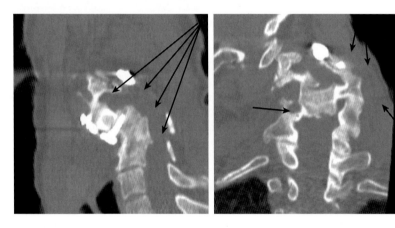

FIGURE 15-9 Left, Sagittal computed tomography (CT) image showing severe cervical sagittal malalignment (*arrows*). **Right,** Anteroposterior CT showing severe coronal malalignment (*arrows*).

osteotomy) is necessary to obtain complete closure. This generally requires an anterior and posterior approach unless osteoclasis is possible, as in cases of AS. Simmons popularized the Smith-Petersen osteotomy (opening wedge), thus allowing for a posterior-only approach in patients with AS.[29,30] In patients with anterior bridging osteophytes and a calcified anterior longitudinal ligament, such as in AS, controlled anterior osteoclasis to create an opening wedge in addition to the modified Smith-Petersen osteotomy may be performed.[29,30] This technique is frequently used for chin-on-chest deformities in AS.[29,30]

If the patient has a rigid deformity and requires greater than 15-degree correction and correction of cervical sagittal imbalance, cervical or cervicothoracic pedicle subtraction osteotomy (PSO) may be used.[31,32] The PSO is increasingly used and can correct large kyphotic deformities. It is a posterior-only approach that allows for all three spinal columns to contact on closure of the osteotomy. This feature increases the likelihood of successful fusion and biomechanical stability.[31,33] PSO also can be used in nonankylosed patients in whom anterior osteoclasis is not likely to occur. Furthermore, PSO allows for controlled closure. If neurologic injury is a concern, PSO may be an appropriate option. However, it is a technically demanding procedure.

Coronal cervical deformities may be isolated or occur in combination with sagittal deformities. Patients with fixed multiplanar deformities may require large three-column osteotomies to correct the spine in both planes and to decompress the spinal cord and nerves (Figs. 15-8 and 15-9). A 540-degree circumferential osteotomy or possibly a cervical vertebral column resection may be used (Fig. 15-10 shows a case example of cervical scoliosis).[34]

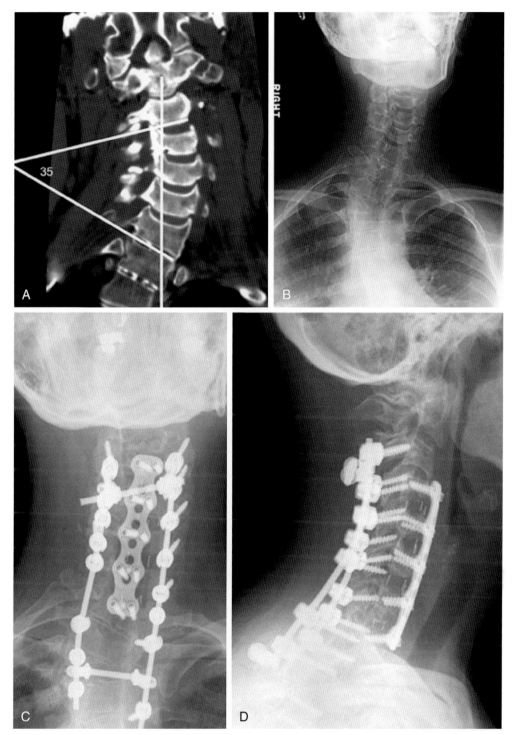

FIGURE 15-10   Case example of cervical scoliosis. This 41-year-old woman with severe neck pain and right arm radicular pain had a previous thoracic fusion for scoliosis at age 14 years and then instrumentation removal at age 25 years for pain. Preoperative computed tomography (CT) scan (**A**) showing measurement of a 35-degree coronal curve and anteroposterior radiograph (**B**). Postoperative anteroposterior (**C**) and lateral (**D**) radiographs showing correction of the coronal malalignment.

REFERENCES

1. Bridwell KH, Baldus C, Berven S, et al.: Changes in radiographic and clinical outcomes with primary treatment adult spinal deformity surgeries from two years to three- to five-years follow-up, *Spine (Phila Pa 1976)* 35:1849–1854, 2010.
2. Glassman SD, Bridwell K, Dimar JR, et al.: The impact of positive sagittal balance in adult spinal deformity, *Spine (Phila Pa 1976)* 30:2024–2029, 2005.
3. Schwab F, Farcy JP, Bridwell K, et al.: A clinical impact classification of scoliosis in the adult, *Spine (Phila Pa 1976)* 31:2109–2114, 2006.
4. Schwab FJ, Smith VA, Biserni M, et al.: Adult scoliosis: a quantitative radiographic and clinical analysis, *Spine (Phila Pa 1976)* 27:387–392, 2002.
5. Hardacker JW, Shuford RF, Capicotto PN, Pryor PW: Radiographic standing cervical segmental alignment in adult volunteers without neck symptoms, *Spine (Phila Pa 1976)* 22:1472–1480, 1997. discussion 1480.
6. Gore DR, Sepic SB, Gardner GM: Roentgenographic findings of the cervical spine in asymptomatic people, *Spine (Phila Pa 1976)* 11:521–524, 1986.
7. Lee SH, Seo EM, Suk KS, et al: The influence of thoracic inlet alignment on the craniocervical sagittal balance in asymptomatic adults. Presented at the 38th Annual Meeting of the Cervical Spine Research Society, Charlotte, North Carolina, 2010.
8. Beier G, Schuck M, Schuller E, Spann W: *Determination of physical data of the head. I. Center of gravity and moments of inertia of human heads, report no. A333080, Munich, West Germany.* Office of Naval Research, 1979.
9. Roussouly P, Nnadi C: Sagittal plane deformity: an overview of interpretation and management, *Eur Spine J* 19:1824–1836, 2010.
10. Chi JH, Tay B, Stahl D, Lee R: Complex deformities of the cervical spine, *Neurosurg Clin N Am* 18:295–304, 2007.
11. Mummaneni PV, Deutsch H, Mummaneni VP: Cervicothoracic kyphosis, *Neurosurg Clin N Am* 17:277–287, 2006. vi.
12. Steinmetz MP, Stewart TJ, Kager CD, et al.: Cervical deformity correction, *Neurosurgery* 60:S90–S97, 2007.
13. Albert TJ, Vacarro A: Postlaminectomy kyphosis, *Spine (Phila Pa 1976)* 23:2738–2745, 1998.
14. Kaptain GJ, Simmons NE, Replogle RE, Pobereskin L: Incidence and outcome of kyphotic deformity following laminectomy for cervical spondylotic myelopathy, *J Neurosurg* 93:199–204, 2000.
15. Hensinger RN: Congenital scoliosis: etiology and associations, *Spine (Phila Pa 1976)* 34:1745–1750, 2009.
16. Nguyen HV, Ludwig SC, Silber J, et al.: Rheumatoid arthritis of the cervical spine, *Spine J* 4:329–334, 2004.
17. Reiter MF, Boden SD: Inflammatory disorders of the cervical spine, *Spine (Phila Pa 1976)* 23:2755–2766, 1998.
18. Etame AB, Than KD, Wang AC, et al.: Surgical management of symptomatic cervical or cervicothoracic kyphosis due to ankylosing spondylitis, *Spine (Phila Pa 1976)* 33:E559–E564, 2008.
19. Shedid D, Benzel EC: Cervical spondylosis anatomy: pathophysiology and biomechanics, *Neurosurgery* 60:S7–S13, 2007.
20. Deutsch H, Haid RW, Rodts GE, Mummaneni PV: Postlaminectomy cervical deformity, *Neurosurg Focus* 15:E5, 2003.
21. Shimizu K, Nakamura M, Nishikawa Y, et al.: Spinal kyphosis causes demyelination and neuronal loss in the spinal cord: a new model of kyphotic deformity using juvenile Japanese small game fowls, *Spine (Phila Pa 1976)* 30:2388–2392, 2005.
22. Iida H, Tachibana S: Spinal cord intramedullary pressure: direct cord traction test, *Neurol Med Chir (Tokyo)* 35:75–77, 1995.
23. Jarzem PF, Quance DR, Doyle DJ, et al.: Spinal cord tissue pressure during spinal cord distraction in dogs, *Spine (Phila Pa 1976)* 17:S227–S234, 1992.
24. Tachibana S, Kitahara Y, Iida H, Yada K: Spinal cord intramedullary pressure: a possible factor in syrinx growth, *Spine (Phila Pa 1976)* 19:2174–2178, 1994. discussion 2178–2179.
25. Kitahara Y, Iida H, Tachibana S: Effect of spinal cord stretching due to head flexion on intramedullary pressure, *Neurol Med Chir (Tokyo)* 35:285–288, 1995.
26. Umapathi T, Chaudhry V, Cornblath D, et al.: Head drop and camptocormia, *J Neurol Neurosurg Psychiatry* 73:1–7, 2002.
27. Wang VY, Aryan H, Ames CP: A novel anterior technique for simultaneous single-stage anterior and posterior cervical release for fixed kyphosis, *J Neurosurg Spine* 8:594–599, 2008.
28. Gill JB, Levin A, Burd T, Longley M: Corrective osteotomies in spine surgery, *J Bone Joint Surg Am* 90:2509–2520, 2008.
29. Simmons ED, DiStefano RJ, Zheng Y, Simmons EH: Thirty-six years experience of cervical extension osteotomy in ankylosing spondylitis: techniques and outcomes, *Spine (Phila Pa 1976)* 31:3006–3012, 2006.
30. Simmons EH: The surgical correction of flexion deformity of the cervical spine in ankylosing spondylitis, *Clin Orthop Relat Res*(86)132–143, 1972.
31. Deviren V, Scheer JK, Ames CP: Technique of cervicothoracic junction pedicle subtraction osteotomy for cervical sagittal imbalance: report of 11 cases, *J Neurosurg Spine* 15:174–181, 2011.
32. Samudrala S, Vaynman S, Thiayananthan T, et al.: Cervicothoracic junction kyphosis: surgical reconstruction with pedicle subtraction osteotomy and Smith-Petersen osteotomy. Presented at the 2009 Joint Spine Section meeting: clinical article, *J Neurosurg Spine* 13:695–706, 2010.
33. Scheer JK, Tang JA, Buckley JM, et al.: Biomechanical analysis of osteotomy type and rod diameter for treatment of cervicothoracic kyphosis, *Spine (Phila Pa 1976)* 36:E519–E523, 2011.
34. Ames CP, Weber MH, Tay BK, et al.: Circumferential osteotomy for fixed cervical sagittal imbalance: a novel surgical technique, *Operative Neurosurg*, 2011.

Ossification of the Posterior Longitudinal Ligament

16

Katsushi Takeshita

CHAPTER PREVIEW

Chapter Synopsis   Ossification of the posterior longitudinal ligament (OPLL) has unique characteristics in multiple lesions from the cervical spine to the lumbar spine and in its gradual extension of ossification. The clinical course resembles that of spondylosis. However, in some patients, extremely severe compression of the spinal cord can occur. The purpose of this chapter is to describe the epidemiology, pathophysiology, diagnosis, and treatment of patients with OPLL.

Important Points   OPLL can involve the entire spine and result in multiple-level, severe neural compression.

The ossification can extend into the dura.

OPLL probably has both genetic and environmental components.

Radiographic classification of OPLL can be difficult, and advanced imaging is typically required.

Computed tomography (CT) and CT myelography provide better assessment of the degree of ossification and associated neural compression.

Magnetic resonance imaging can provide additional information on involvement of the neurovascular structures.

Surgical management is typically indicated in the symptomatic patient with OPLL.

Laminoplasty remains the main surgical option for the treatment of OPLL; however, it may be contraindicated in patients with significant kyphosis.

The anterior approach may provide better results in patients with severe compression.

The chosen surgical approach should be individualized to the patient's pathologic process and the surgeon's preference and experience.

Tsukimoto's first report of ossification of the posterior longitudinal ligament (OPLL) described compression of the spinal cord in the cervical spine secondary to progressive OPLL.[1] Because most studies of OPLL were initially from Japan, OPLL was once termed "the Japanese disease." However, as more reports from both Eastern and Western countries became available and analyses of case series from other Asian countries increased, it became clear that all contemporary spinal surgeons must be aware of OPLL.

OPLL imposes a unique burden on patients as well as on physicians as compared with cervical spondylotic myelopathy. In patients with a strong tendency to ossification, OPLL can extend all the way from the upper cervical spine down to the lower lumbar spine, with resulting multiple-level severe neural compression (Fig. 16-1). Furthermore, ossification of the dura with resulting spinal cord dysfunction can be common in OPLL and can pose challenges for both the medical treatment and surgical management of this disorder. The purpose of this chapter is to describe the epidemiology, pathophysiology, diagnosis, and treatment of patients with OPLL.

Epidemiology

Prevalence

Morbidity of OPLL in Japan has been reported at 1.9% to 3.2%. Similar or smaller percentages of morbidity in other Asian countries have been reported: 2.1% to 3%

in Taiwan, 0.8% to 1.8% in China, 1.5% in the Philippines, 0.95% in Korea, and 0.8% in Singapore. Studies in Europe and the United States have found far less morbidity: 0.1% to 1.3% in the United States, 1.7% in Italy, and 0.1% in Germany.[2] Symptomatic OPLL is speculated to affect 20% to 50% of persons with OPLL, and myelopathic OPLL is found in 29% to 40% of patients with symptomatic OPLL. Cervical OPLL accounts for 70% of all OPLL cases and sometimes accompanies thoracic or lumbar OPLL.

Natural History

Progression of Ossification

Ossification is often found in people who are more than 40 years old. This ossification develops in an axial direction and/or a longitudinal axis. Progression of ossification is more active in younger persons than in older adults. Progression of ossification continues after surgical treatment (Fig. 16-2).

Progression of Neurologic Symptoms

In a large cohort study,[2] 304 patients with no neurologic findings on their first visit were treated conservatively. Myelopathy developed in 55 (17%) of patients with a follow-up of 10 to 30 years, and these patients had a higher range of motion or severe stenosis (>60%) in the cervical spine. Another study observed 21 patients with a small space available for the spinal cord (<12 mm).[3] With a follow-up of 4.2 years on average, only one patient exhibited deteriorated neurologic symptoms, and no patient changed to surgical treatment.

These studies indicate that preventive surgery is not always necessary in patients with slight to mild myelopathy even when compression to the spinal cord is substantial. However, the potential risk of spinal cord injury (SCI), if significant, supports the use of preventive surgery. In a retrospective survey of 453 patients with cervical SCI, Chikuda and colleagues reported that OPLL was found in 106 (23%) patients.[4] OPLL is a significant risk factor for SCI, at least in Japan, after considering the 1.9% to 3.2% prevalence of OPLL. Most (75%) patients with SCI

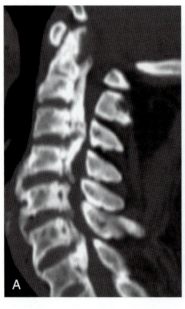
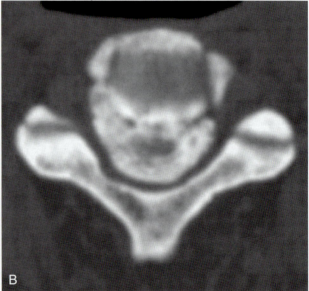

FIGURE 16-1 Massive OPLL with a mixed type. As for surgery, meticulous decompression under neuromonitoring is mandatory not only from the anterior approach but also from the posterior approach. **A,** Reconstructed sagittal computed tomography (CT) image. **B,** Axial CT image.

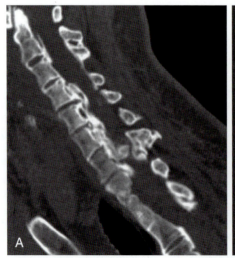
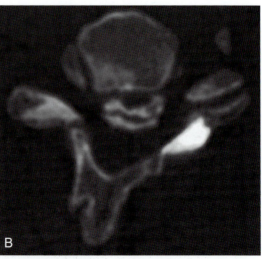

FIGURE 16-2 This man experienced nine surgical procedures: two in the cervical spine, five in the thoracic spine, and two in the lumbar spine. Imaging was obtained just before the last surgical procedure. **A,** Reconstructed sagittal imaging. **B,** Progression of OPLL after the first laminoplasty.

are unaware of their OPLL before injury. As a result, in some countries where asymptomatic OPLL may be highly prevalent in the general population, advocates have proposed instituting a screening program to identify unrecognized OPLL, although it is unclear whether awareness of the disease can actually decrease the incidence of SCI. Regardless, surgeons should educate their patients on the potential risks of SCI associated with incidental falls and other accidental injuries.

Pathophysiology

OPLL is an ectopic ossification. From histologic findings, endochondral ossification forms the majority of ossification, although intramembranous ossification is sometimes observed.[5] Hypertrophy of the posterior longitudinal ligament often precedes ossification. The posterior longitudinal ligament has deep and superficial layers, and ossification usually starts at the attachment of the deep layer to the posterior vertebral body. In some cases, ossification may first develop at the posterior aspect of the vertebral body.

Ossification of the dura, a unique pathologic feature of OPLL, is sometime observed and may result from extension of the bone-forming process with ossification into the neighboring dura. As for the spinal cord, tissue necrosis and cavity formations expand from the central parts of the gray matter to the ventral parts of the posterior column. A triangular deformity of the spinal cord with a less than 60% of normal in more than one segment appeared to be associated with severe and irreversible pathologic changes.

Genetics

Genetic inheritance of OPLL has been validated from various studies. In a nationwide pedigree survey in Japan, 23% of families and 29% of siblings had OPLL among 347 patients. Koga and Sakou and their associates studied the genetics of OPLL. These investigators reported an association between OPLL and some haplotypes in chromosome 6. Following these studies, these investigators performed linkage analysis of 91 sib pairs and found two candidate genes: collagen α2 (XI) (*COL11A2*) and retinoic X receptor β (*RXRβ*).[6] The former gene, *COL11A2*, which encodes collagen α2 (XI), a fibril-forming minor collagen of chondrocytes, seems clinically more important. Another team performed a genome-wide linkage study of 142 sib pairs and found an association of *COL6A1* and OPLL.[7] Other proposed candidate genes are nucleotide pyrophosphatase (NPPS), bone morphogenetic protein-2 (BMP-2), transforming growth factor-β, B crystalline, cadherin, BMP-4, proteoglycan 1, osteopontin, parathyroid hormone receptor 1, insulin-like growth factor-I, estrogen receptor, and interleukin-1β.

Environmental Factors and Comorbidities

Mechanical stress is regarded as one main cause of progression of ossification. Mechanical stress increases production of various proteins and cytokines such as alkaline phosphatase, BMPs, and osteopontin at the site of ossification.

Diabetes is associated with OPLL. Insulin-like growth factor-I and insulin receptors are suspected to play a key role in the formation of OPLL. Akune and colleagues showed that the insulin secretory response was associated with the extent of OPLL ligament.[8] Hypoparathyroidism and hypophosphatemic rickets are also factors in OPLL.

Diagnosis

Imaging

Cervical OPLL is categorized into four groups from lateral radiographs: the continuous type, the mixed type, the segmental type, and the localized type (Fig. 16-3). One type of OPLL can develop into another after elongation or fusion of ossification. The continuous type and the mixed type have common properties, and they are often regarded as a single group. Genetic study also validated this affinity between a continuous type and a mixed type.

The accuracy of the radiographic classification is not high because ossification is often fuzzy. Computed tomography (CT) is the best imaging modality to evaluate the ossification. The presence of a double layer of ossification called the "double-layer sign" usually indicates ossification of the dura (Fig. 16-4). Identification

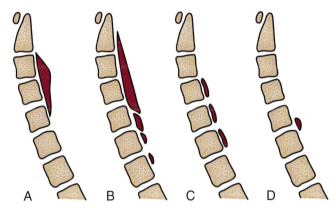

FIGURE 16-3 Classification of ossification of the posterior longitudinal ligament. **A,** Continuous type. **B,** Mixed type. **C,** Segmental type. **D,** Localized type.

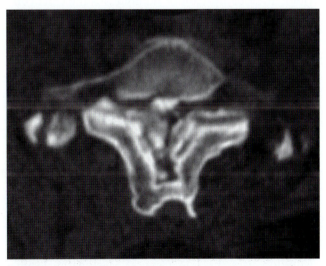

FIGURE 16-4 This man had recurrence of myelopathy 10 years after laminoplasty at another institution. The double-layer sign indicated ossification of the dura, which was confirmed during an anterior surgical procedure.

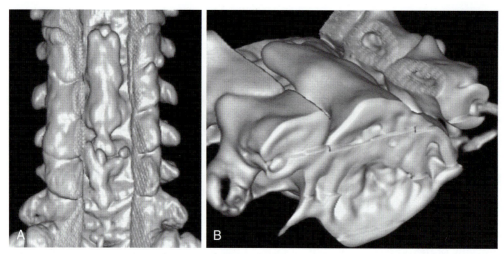

FIGURE 16-5   Reconstructed imaging helps surgeons to grasp the complicated picture of ossification. **A,** Dorsal view. Virtual laminectomy visualizes the mixed type of ossification. **B,** Dorsal oblique view. Occupation of the ossification into the spinal canal and foraminal stenosis are intuitively recognized.

of ossification of the dura is important because resection of the ossification can result in cerebrospinal fluid leaks during anterior decompressions. Although not necessary, reconstructed three-dimensional CT images may demonstrate the ossification more intuitively (Fig. 16-5).

Magnetic resonance imaging (MRI) can depict the neural structures more clearly than can other imaging modalities. In addition, MRI can provide information on the spinal cord caliber, location of compression, and evidence of intrinsic cord signal abnormalities. Although ossification can be evaluated on MRI, frequently it appears to be imaged "larger." Therefore, compression of the neural structure from ossification as seen on MRI may be prone to be overexpressed and appear greater than it is. In these particular cases, CT and/or CT myelogram can provide better assessment of the associated ossification and neural involvement.

Symptoms and Outcomes

Symptoms of OPLL are similar to those of cervical spondylotic myelopathy. Pain or numbness is the chief complaint, followed by motor palsy. In a national multicenter study,[9] Fujiwara and associates evaluated 80 patients with OPLL who received conservative treatment. Pain intensity was 44 ± 30/100, and the Neck Disability Index (NDI) was 26.8% ± 16.8%, outcomes similar to those observed in spondylotic myelopathy. Neurologic symptoms consist of loss of proficient movement of the arms and hands; instability with walking, with a spastic or ataxic gait; and problems with urination.

As for neurologic assessment, Japanese Orthopaedic Association (JOA), or modified JOA score, is most popular and commonly used, followed by the Nurick grade. Patient-reported outcomes have become mandatory in the assessment of any medical treatment, and the Medical Outcomes Study Short Form-36 and NDI have been the major tools in cervical spine evaluation. Because neither scale is specific for myelopathy, the author's institution uses the JOA Cervical Myelopathy Evaluation Questionnaire (JOACMEQ) for the evaluation of myelopathy.[10]

Differential Diagnoses

The differential diagnosis of OPLL includes any other disorder that can result in cervical myelopathy, and it can include primary and secondary diseases of the brain and intrinsic spinal cord disorders. The differential diagnosis of other more common extradural sources of spinal cord compression includes other heterotopic ossification processes.

Hyperostosis is relative disease, and a patient who has hyperostosis in other skeletal sites is diagnosed with diffuse idiopathic skeletal hyperostosis (DISH). Calcification of the yellow ligament is a different entity (Fig. 16-6), and surgical treatment is performed exclusively from the posterior approach.

Treatment

Nonoperative Treatment

The principles of treatment of cervical myelopathy can be directly applied to OPLL. The symptomatic patient with OPLL has few contraindications to surgery. Although many different modalities are available, little long-term evidence supports the benefits of nonoperative treatment. Therefore, conservative management is essentially reserved for patients who are medically or otherwise unable to tolerate a surgical intervention.

The use of a cervical collar is most popular (Fig. 16-7), and other options include bed rest and traction. However, it can take several days for patients to obtain relief of symptoms; furthermore, Nakamura and associates demonstrated that conservative treatment cannot result in good neurologic recovery in myelopathic patients with severe symptoms.[11] Medications are a frequent choice for the management of pain. Nonsteroidal antiinflammatory drugs (NSAIDs) are typically effective only for slight or mild pain. Moderate or severe pain usually has an inflammatory or neuropathic component, for which high-dose steroids or anticonvulsant drugs such as pregabalin and carbamazepine may be more effective. Although

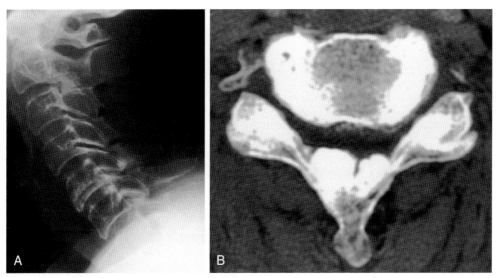

FIGURE 16-6   This woman had ossification of the posterior longitudinal ligament, as well as calcification of the yellow ligament in the lower cervical spine. **A,** An oval shadow is seen at the ventral interlaminar space of C5-C6. **B,** Bilateral calcification inside the yellow ligament.

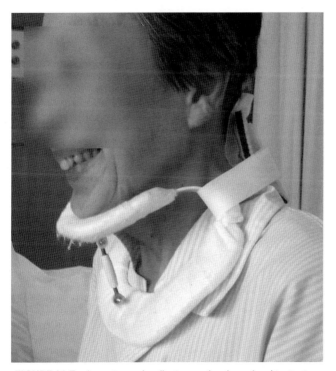

FIGURE 16-7   A concise neck collar invented at the authors' institution.

somewhat controversial, injection therapy may be the best modality for severe pain from radiculopathy. However, the role of injections in the management of myelopathy has not been supported.

Operative Treatment

Patients with OPLL who have severe or progressive myelopathy are candidates for surgical treatment. Preventive or prophylactic surgery for OPLL remains controversial and may be a relative indication in patients with severe spinal cord compression irrespective of their symptoms. This view is based on concern for the increased risk of SCI after relatively minor trauma.

An anterior approach with extirpation of the ossification is expected to achieve maximum recovery of neurologic function (Fig. 16-8). Several studies showed that anterior surgery, compared with posterior surgery, resulted in better clinical results in myelopathic patients with severe compression of the spinal cord.

However, in the treatment of extremely large and long ossifications, anterior decompression can be technically demanding, and even in the most skilled hands, patients remain at risk for cerebrospinal fluid leakage, dysphagia, recurrent laryngeal nerve palsy, and other complications associated with cervical surgery. If a cerebrospinal fluid leak is a high concern because of ossified dura, the "floating method," which leaves a bony shell just anterior to the involved arachnoid membrane and the spinal cord, can be a better strategy than complete extirpation of the OPLL. To remove the ossification safely, neuromonitoring is mandatory, and the author's institution often adopts a computer navigation system for extirpation (Fig. 16-9).[12]

Posterior surgery is an alternative: laminectomy or laminoplasty with or without posterior instrumentation. Laminectomy alone has been abandoned because of the high risk of kyphosis progression. Laminoplasty is the mainstay for most patients with OPLL (Fig. 16-10). The reported JOA recovery rate by laminoplasty is 47.3% to 60.0%. Long-term follow-up studies demonstrated that neurologic recovery was maintained for more than 10 years.

Neck pain, a main drawback of laminoplasty, was observed in 60% of patients.[13] In the retrospective survey of cervical surgery in the author's institution of 103 patients with OPLL who underwent laminoplasties, 47% had neck pain that was greater than 2/10 grade, and 26% had neck pain that was greater than 4/10 grade. In the author's cohort study, neck pain decreased in 26.3%, was unchanged in 47.4%, and increased in 21.1% of 19 patients with OPLL (unpublished data).

Postoperative motor paresis of an upper extremity, often called C5 nerve root palsy, is another concern after

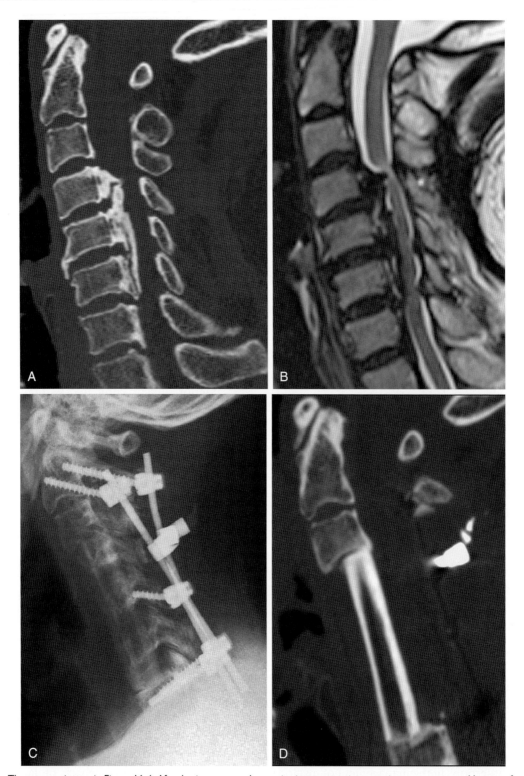

FIGURE 16-8   The same patient as in Figure 16-4. After laminectomy and posterior instrumentation, anterior corpectomy and bone graft were performed. **A,** Preoperative reconstructed sagittal imaging. **B,** Preoperative T2-weighted magnetic resonance imaging. **C,** Postoperative lateral radiograph. **D,** Postoperative reconstructed sagittal imaging.

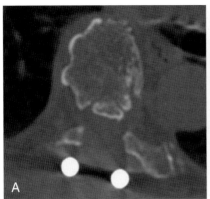
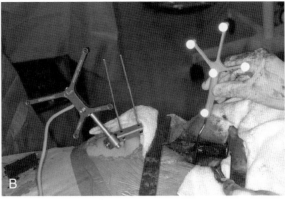
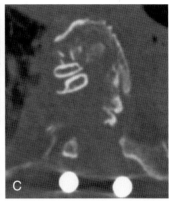

FIGURE 16-9   Thoracic ossification of the posterior longitudinal ligament (OPLL). A computer navigation system is used to facilitate decompression and placement of pedicle screws in difficult cases from the cervical spine to the lumbar spine. **A,** Preoperative axial computed tomography (CT) image before an anterior surgical procedure. This strategy for thoracic OPLL is posterior decompression and fusion at first, followed by anterior surgery, which is performed only when the index surgery is not effective. **B,** Under registration by a navigation probe on the *right.* A reference arc on the left was connected to Steinmann pins, which were temporally fixed to the vertebral bodies. **C,** Postoperative axial CT image.

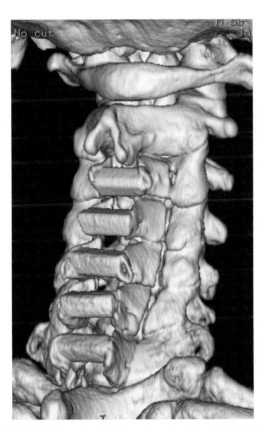

FIGURE 16-10   Reconstructed three-dimensional imaging of laminoplasty.

laminoplasty. From a review article of surgical procedures for OPLL, the incidence of motor palsy after laminoplasty ranged from 0% to 30% (average, 4.7%).[14] In a national multicenter study, Seichi and colleagues analyzed neurologic complications in 581 patients with OPLL after laminoplasty procedures at 27 hospitals in Japan.[15] Motor paresis of an upper extremity was detected in 23 patients (4.0%): proximal paresis in 16 and distal paresis in 7. Seven patients among 23 with upper motor paresis did not regain full recovery.

However, an equivalent ratio of C5 nerve root palsy was reported from an analysis of anterior surgery. Mochizuki and Hashimoto and their colleagues analyzed 91 patients who underwent anterior surgical procedures for OPLL and found that 9 (9.7%) patients developed C5 nerve root palsy.[3] A review article also found a similar degree of C5 nerve root palsy after anterior surgery (1.6% to 12.1%; average, 4.3%).

Additional posterior instrumentation prevents kyphosis progression (Fig. 16-11). However, a higher percentage of C5 nerve root palsy has been reported, and the author's impression is that patients have greater axial pain than with laminoplasty alone.

Choice of Surgical Approaches

Although laminoplasty remains the mainstay for the surgical management of OPLL, it has limitations. Traditionally, OPLL with kyphosis has been considered a contraindication to laminoplasty. A kyphotic spine may not allow for the necessary posterior spinal cord drift to escape the anterior compression from the OPLL. Severe preoperative neck pain is another relative contraindication because postoperative neck pain can be worse after laminoplasty. Several surgeons have investigated imaging parameters by which surgeons can estimate the surgical effect of posterior decompression (Table 16-1).

Regardless, the choice of the surgical treatment should be tailored to the individual patient. In addition to the foregoing parameters, the patient's profile and symptoms must be considered: age, severity of symptoms, history of surgery, physical and mental status, and comorbidities. The surgeon's preference also must be considered. A treatment algorithm is shown in Figure 16-12.

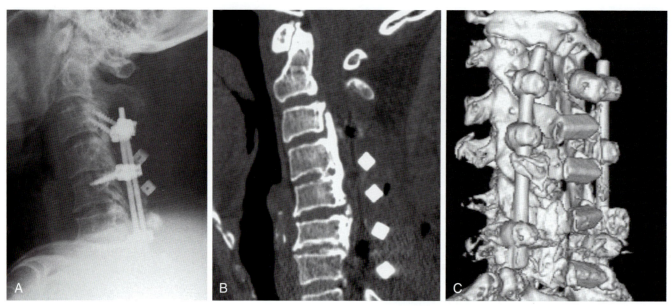

FIGURE 16-11 Laminoplasty and posterior instrumentation. **A,** Postoperative lateral radiograph. **B,** Sagittal view reconstructed from computed tomography. Hydroxyapatite spacers for split interspinous processes are seen. **C,** Reconstructed three-dimensional view.

Table 16-1 Imaging Parameters to Indicate Limitation of Posterior Surgery

Investigators	Modality	Criteria	Comment
Fujiyoshi[16]	X-p	Ossification protrudes dorsally over the K-line (a line that connects the midpoints of the spinal canal at C2 and C7)	Confirmed from retrospective study
Gwinn[17]	X-p	Ossification protrudes dorsally over the simple straight line drawn from the dorsal caudal aspect of the C2 vertebral body to the dorsal caudal aspect of the C7 vertebral body.	
Suda[18]	X-p	Local kyphosis >13 degrees	Analysis in spondylotic myelopathy
Seichi[19]	CT	OPLL thickness >7.2 mm	No correlation with motor JOA score
Iwasaki[20]	CT	Occupying ratio >60% and/or hill-shaped ossification	Confirmed from comparative study

CT, Computed tomography; *JOA,* Japanese Orthopaedic Association; *OPLL,* ossification of the posterior longitudinal ligament.

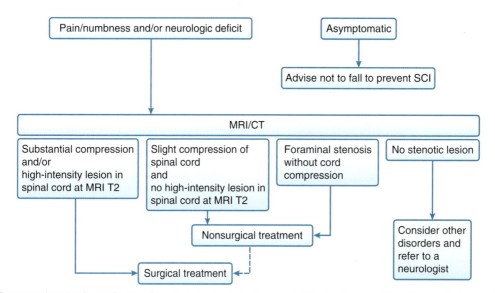

FIGURE 16-12 Treatment algorithm for ossification of the posterior longitudinal ligament. This algorithm considers only neurologic symptoms. *CT,* Computed tomography; *MRI,* magnetic resonance imaging; *SCI,* spinal cord injury.

REFERENCES

1. Tsukmoto H: A case report - autopsy of syndrome of compression of spinal cord owing to ossification within spinal canal of cervical spine, *Arch Jpn Chir* 29:1003–1007, 1960.
2. Matsunaga S, Sakou T, Taketomi E, Komiya S: Clinical course of patients with ossification of the posterior longitudinal ligament: a minimum 10-year cohort study, *J Neurosurg* 100(Suppl): 245–248, 2004.
3. Mochizuki M, Aiba A, Hashimoto M, et al.: Cervical myelopathy in patients with ossification of the posterior longitudinal ligament, *J Neurosurg Spine* 10:122–128, 2009.
4. Chikuda H, Seichi A, Takeshita K, et al.: Acute cervical spinal cord injury complicated by pre-existing ossification of the posterior longitudinal ligament: a multi-center study, *Spine (Phila Pa 1976)* 36:1453–1458, 2011.
5. Tsuzuki N: Review of histopathological studies on OPLL of the cervical spine, with insights into the mechanism. In Yonenobu K, Nakamura K, Toyama Y, editors: *OPLL: ossification of the posterior longitudinal ligament*, ed 2, Tokyo, 2006, Springer, pp 41–47.
6. Koga H, Sakou T, Taketomi E, et al.: Genetic mapping of ossification of the posterior longitudinal ligament of the spine, *Am J Hum Genet* 62:1460–1467, 1998.
7. Tanaka T, Ikari K, Furushima K, et al.: Genomewide linkage and linkage disequilibrium analyses identify *COL6A1*, on chromosome 21, as the locus for ossification of the posterior longitudinal ligament of the spine, *Am J Hum Genet* 73:812–822, 2003.
8. Akune T, Ogata N, Seichi A, et al.: Insulin secretory response is positively associated with the extent of ossification of the posterior longitudinal ligament of the spine, *J Bone Joint Surg Am* 83:1537–1544, 2001.
9. Fujiwara N, Takeshita K, Kawaguchi H, et al.: *Pain and numbness in OPLL and their associated factors: 2008 report on the ossification of the spinal ligaments of the Japanese Ministry of Public Health and Welfare*, Tokyo, pp 17–38, 2009. [in Japanese].
10. Fukui M, Chiba K, Kawakami M, et al.: JOA back pain evaluation questionnaire (JOABPEQ)/JOA cervical myelopathy evaluation questionnaire (JOACMEQ): the report on the development of revised versions April 16, 2007. The Subcommittee of the Clinical Outcome Committee of the Japanese Orthopaedic Association on Low Back Pain and Cervical Myelopathy Evaluation, *J Orthop Sci* 14:348–365, 2009.
11. Nakamura K, Kurokawa T, Saita K, et al.: Multiple-level compression myelopathy: concomitant asymptomatic cervical compression adversely affects surgical outcome for thoracic compression myelopathy, *J Spinal Disord* 9:500–504, 1996.
12. Seichi A, Takeshita K, Kawaguchi H, et al.: Image-guided surgery for thoracic ossification of the posterior longitudinal ligament: technical note, *J Neurosurg Spine* 3:165–168, 2005.
13. Hosono N, Yonenobu K, Ono K: Neck and shoulder pain after laminoplasty: a noticeable complication, *Spine (Phila Pa 1976)* 21:1969–1973, 1996.
14. Cardoso MJ, Koski TR, Ganju A, Liu JC: Approach-related complications after decompression for cervical ossification of the posterior longitudinal ligament, *Neurosurg Focus* 30:E12, 2011.
15. Seichi A, Hoshino Y, Kimura A, et al.: Neurological complications of cervical laminoplasty for patients with ossification of the posterior longitudinal ligament: a multi-institutional retrospective study, *Spine (Phila Pa 1976)* 36:E998–E1003, 2011.
16. Fujiyoshi T, Yamazaki M, Kawabe J, et al.: A new concept for making decisions regarding the surgical approach for cervical ossification of the posterior longitudinal ligament: the K-line, *Spine* 33(26):E990–E993, 2008.
17. Gwinn DE, Iannotti CA, Benzel EC, et al.: Effective lordosis: analysis of sagittal spinal canal alignment in cervical spondylotic myelopathy, *J Neurosurg Spine* 11(6):667–672, 2009.
18. Suda K, Abumi K, Ito M, et al.: Local kyphosis reduces surgical outcomes of expansive open-door laminoplasty for cervical spondylotic myelopathy, *Spine* 28(12):1258–1262, 2003.
19. Seichi A, Chikuda H, Kimura A, et al.: Intraoperative ultrasonographic evaluation of posterior decompression via laminoplasty in patients with cervical ossification of the posterior longitudinal ligament: correlation with 2-year follow-up results, *J Neurosurg Spine* 13(1):47–51, 2010.
20. Iwasaki M, Okuda S, Miyauchi A, et al.: Surgical strategy for cervical myelopathy due to ossification of the posterior longitudinal ligament: Part 2: Advantages of anterior decompression and fusion over laminoplasty, *Spine* 32(6):654–660, 2007.

SECTION 3

Trauma

Occipitocervical and Upper Cervical Spine Fractures

17

Carlo Bellabarba, Richard J. Bransford, and Jens R. Chapman

CHAPTER PREVIEW

Chapter Synopsis

The occipitocervical junction consists of structurally important osseous and ligamentous complexes that stabilize the skull base to the spine. Compromise of either the complex bony or ligamentous complex places the integrity of the occipitocervical junction at risk. Because of the proximity of neurovascular structures, acute loss of occipitocervical structural integrity carries a high mortality. This chapter reviews the classification system, imaging, surgical indications, and treatment options available for management of various occipitocervical injury patterns.

Important Points

Because of the complex anatomy and high degree of mobility of the occipitocervical junction, stability of this region depends on the ligamentous integrity as much as on the bony anatomy.

Bony and ligamentous injuries can result in a wide range of instability patterns in the occipitocervical junction.

Given the proximity of the neurovascular structures in this area, loss of structural integrity can result in significant morbidity and mortality.

Clinical and Surgical Pearls

Most occipital condyle factures can be managed nonoperatively; however care should be taken to ensure that they are not part of a wider instability pattern, such as occipitocervical dissociation.

Assessing the integrity of the transverse alar ligament is vital to determining C1-C2 stability.

Type II odontoid fractures are at highest risk of pseudarthrosis; however, surgical stabilization remains controversial.

Clinical and Surgical Pitfalls

A high index of suspicion is necessary for the diagnosis and treatment of occipitocervical injuries.

Occipitocervical dissociations may manifest with minimal bony radiographic and computed tomography findings. Careful assessment of the associated soft tissue shadows and use of magnetic resonance imaging as indicated can help identify these injuries.

Most traumatic isthmic spondylolistheses of C2 can be treated nonoperatively; however care should be taken to identify the IIA subtype that is at higher risk of progression of deformity and neurologic compromise.

If surgical stabilization is undertaken, identification of the location of the neurovascular structures, in particular the vertebral artery, can help dictate the surgical technique and approach.

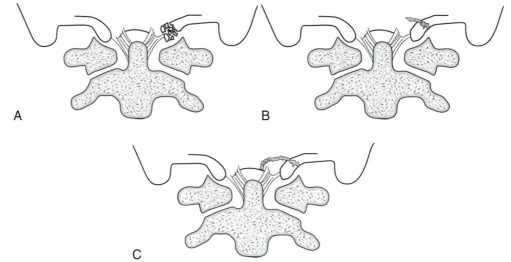

FIGURE 17-1 Anderson and Montesano classification of occipital condyle fractures.[1] **A,** Type I injuries are comminuted, stable impaction fractures caused by axial loading. **B,** Type II injuries are impaction or shear fractures extending into the base of the skull and are usually stable. **C,** Type III injuries are alar ligament avulsion fractures and represent unstable distraction injuries of the craniocervical junction. (From Smorgick Y, Fischgrund JS: Occipitocervical injuries. *Semin Spine Surg* 25:14-22, 2013.)

The occipitocervical junction consists of structurally important osseous and ligamentous complexes that stabilize the skull base to the spine and encase vital neurovascular structures.

The high susceptibility of the occipitocervical junction to traumatic injury is largely related to the lever arm forces of the spine on the immobile skull base combined with a reliance on ligamentous rather than bony structures for stability.

This complex anatomic arrangement is maintained by specialized C1 and C2 bony segments interconnected by an incompletely understood ligamentous system that, if compromised, places the structural integrity of the occipitocervical junction at risk.

Because of the proximity of neurovascular structures, sudden loss of occipitocervical structural integrity carries a high mortality. However, improved trauma care has dramatically increased the likelihood of survival and has shifted the burden of responsibility to the spine surgeon for appropriate diagnosis and treatment of such life-threatening injuries.

This chapter focuses primarily on six upper cervical fracture types, which may coexist: (1) occipital condyle fractures, (2) occipitocervical dissociation, (3) fractures of the atlas (C1), (4) C1-C2 instability patterns, (5) odontoid (C2) fractures, and (6) traumatic spondylolisthesis (hangman fracture) of C2.

Occipital Condyle Fractures

Injury Classification

Although often stable, occipital condyle fractures may be highly unstable if they are associated with bony avulsion of major craniocervical stabilizers. Anderson and Montesano described the following classification system distinguishing mainly bony involvement, as opposed to more ligamentous involvement (Fig. 17-1)[1]:

- Type I: Stable, comminuted axial loading injuries
- Type II: Potentially unstable injuries caused by a shear mechanism that result in an oblique fracture extending from the condyle into the skull base

- Type III: Unstable alar ligament avulsion fractures that result in a transverse fracture of the occipital condyle and may represent a component of occipitocervical dissociation

Lower amount of fracture displacement, greater degree of apposition, and larger fragment size have been proposed as criteria for healing of occipital condylar fractures.[2] Overall, occipital condyle fractures are usually benign. Nonetheless, any occipital condyle fracture should be considered a possible component of occipitocervical dissociation.

Radiographic Evaluation

Occipital condyle fractures are difficult to visualize on plain radiographs. They are most easily characterized with computed tomography (CT) imaging. Magnetic resonance imaging (MRI) plays a role primarily in establishing whether type III odontoid fractures are associated with extensive ligamentous injury and occipitocervical instability.

Indications for Surgery

Operative treatment of occipital condyle fractures is generally reserved for type III injuries that represent alar ligament avulsions and result in occipitocervical instability (Fig. 17-2). Surgical indications are therefore equivalent to those described later for occipitocervical dissociation (Table 17-1).

Treatment and Outcomes

Type I and most type II occipital condyle fractures are treated nonoperatively, with a rigid cervical collar. Because type I injuries can result in considerable articular incongruity, the outcome often depends on the presence or absence of symptomatic posttraumatic arthritis, which may result in neck pain, occipital headaches, restricted occipitocervical motion, and torticollis. Palsy of closely associated cranial nerves (IX, X, XI, XII) has also been described. Type II and isolated type III injuries generally pose less risk of posttraumatic arthritis because of the lower likelihood of articular incongruity. However, if these injuries are components of craniocervical

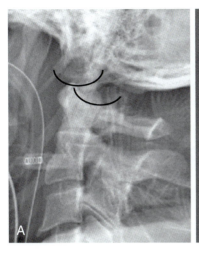
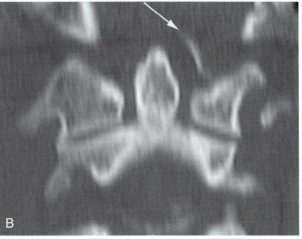

FIGURE 17-2 Type III occipital condyle fracture as a component of craniocervical dissociation. The lateral cervical spine radiograph (**A**) shows dislocation of the atlanto-occipital joints in a 48-year-old man involved in a high-speed motor vehicle collision. The coronal computed tomography image (**B**) illustrates an associated avulsion fracture of the left occipital condyle (*arrow*), resulting in functional incompetence of the attached alar ligament.

Table 17-1 Occipital Condyle Fractures

Injury Type	Distinguishing Characteristics	Significance and Treatment
I	Comminuted fracture	Usually stable injury treated with cervical collar or possibly halo vest for severe collapse
II	Extension of basilar skull fracture	Cervical collar unless associated with occipitocervical dissociation
III	Avulsion fracture of alar ligament insertion	Cervical collar unless associated with occipitocervical dissociation

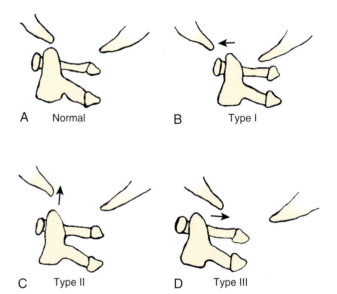

FIGURE 17-3 The Traynelis classification of craniocervical dislocation. **A,** Normal atlanto-occipital alignment. **B,** Type I: anterior displacement. **C,** Type II: distraction injury. **D,** Type III: posterior displacement. (Redrawn from Traynelis VC, Marano GD, Dunker RO, Kaufman HH: Traumatic atlanto-occipital dislocation: case report. *J Neurosurg* 65:863-870, 1986. In Herkowitz HN, Garfin SR, Eismont FJ, Bell GR, editors: *Rothman-Simeone the spine,* ed 6, Philadelphia, 2011, Saunders.)

or occipitocervical dissociation, the prognosis is worse (see later).

Occipitocervical Dissociation

Classification

Traynelis and associates identified three occipitocervical dissociation patterns based on the direction of displacement of the occiput relative to the cervical spine (Fig. 17-3).[3] However, the extreme instability of these injuries renders the position of the head relative to the neck completely arbitrary and more dependent on external forces than on any intrinsic injury characteristic. A directionally based classification therefore seems to have little inherent value.

A classification that reflects injury severity and quantifies the stability of the occipitocervical junction would provide greater clinical significance with regard to treatment and prognosis. Signs of instability are translation or distraction of more than 2 mm in any plane,[4] neurologic injury, and concomitant cerebrovascular trauma.[5] However, patients with minimally displaced occipitocervical injuries may have less easily recognized unstable occipitocervical dissociative injuries and therefore must

be segregated into the following two groups: (1) patients with relatively stable injuries who can be treated nonoperatively and (2) patients with highly unstable but partially reduced injuries who require operative stabilization in spite of a misleadingly low degree of displacement. Distinguishing between these two possible clinical situations by the use of manual traction testing (see later) can be useful in patients with minimally displaced injuries with evidence of extensive occipitocervical injury (ligamentous injury, soft tissue swelling, neurologic or cerebrovascular abnormalities). Surgical stabilization can be reserved for patients with type II and III injuries of the occipitocervical junction, which are defined as dissociations according to the Harborview classification system (Table 17-2).[6]

Table 17-2 Harborview Classification of Craniocervical Injuries

Stage	Description of Injury
I	MRI evidence of injury to craniocervical osseoligamentous stabilizers Craniocervical alignment within 2 mm of normal Distraction of ≤2 mm on provocative traction radiograph
2*	MRI evidence of injury to craniocervical osseoligamentous stabilizers Craniocervical alignment within 2 mm of normal Distraction of >2 mm on provocative traction radiograph
3*	Craniocervical malalignment of >2 mm on static radiographic studies

MRI, Magnetic resonance imaging.
*These injuries are defined as craniocervical dissociation.

Radiographic Evaluation

Lateral Cervical Spine Radiography

Injuries to the upper cervical spine are notoriously difficult to detect with plain radiographs, for several reasons. Because the x-ray beam is directed toward the midcervical spine, the parallax effect at the occipitocervical junction precludes proper visualization of the upper cervical articulations. Other structures, such as the mastoid air cells, may also obscure the relevant upper cervical anatomy. Because of the rarity of occipitocervical injuries relative to other types of cervical spine injuries, decreased vigilance is also likely to be a factor.

Various radiographic lines have been established in an attempt to measure occipitocervical alignment indirectly. Of these, the Harris lines have been the most useful in helping to identify occipitocervical dissociation injuries (Fig. 17-4).[7] Either a basion-dens interval (BDI) or a basion-axial interval (BAI) greater than 12 mm is highly likely to represent an occipitocervical distraction injury. These lines are not as specific as they are sensitive, and a study demonstrated that one third of patients in a series of 48 consecutive survivors of occipitocervical dissociation had normal BAI and BDI values.[8] An additional clue may be provided by examining the soft tissue shadows because patients with occipitocervical dissociation invariably have a large amount of soft tissue injury and extensive prevertebral swelling extending up to the occipitocervical junction.

Computed Tomography

CT, now commonly used as a routine screening test for cervical spine injury, also allows for more accurate Harris line measurements and has the advantage of enabling the examiner to visualize the occipitocervical and atlantoaxial joints directly to assess for subluxation. Even the slightest asymmetry or distraction of the atlanto-occipital joints should be viewed with suspicion because these joints usually have a displacement tolerance of 2 mm or less.

An additional clue to the presence of an unstable occipitocervical injury can be provided by detecting avulsion fractures of the alar ligament, which along with the tectorial membrane, serves as one of the two primary stabilizers of the occipitocervical junction. These avulsion

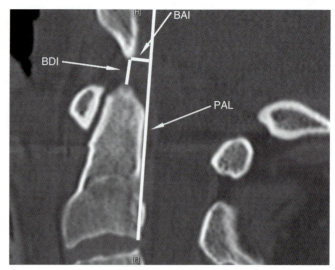

FIGURE 17-4 Harris radiographic lines for assessing occipitocervical alignment: If either the basion-dens interval (BDI) or the basion-axial interval (BAI) is greater than 12 mm long on sagittal computed tomography or lateral radiographic measurement, occipitocervical dissociation should be suspected. Because these measurements are more sensitive than they are specific, normal parameters do not exclude the presence of occipitocervical dissociation. *PAL,* Posterior axial line.

fractures generally consist of bony avulsions from the origin of the alar ligament on the inferomedial aspect of the occipital condyle and are classified as type III occipital condyle fractures according the classification of Anderson and Montesano (see Fig. 17-1). Avulsion fractures may also occur at the alar ligament insertion on the odontoid process and are classified as type I odontoid fractures according to Anderson and D'Alonzo.[9]

Distraction is often seen at both the occiput-C1 and C1-C2 joints because the primary stabilizers of the occipitocervical junction extend from the occiput to C2. Highly unstable occipitocervical injuries can have an unsettlingly benign appearance on CT imaging. Once again, extensive soft tissue swelling can generally be seen on CT evaluation and should provide an important clue. Any finding suggestive of a significant occipitocervical injury should be further evaluated with MRI.

Magnetic Resonance Imaging

MRI generally demonstrates increased T2-weighted signal intensity within the occiput-C1 and C1-C2 articulations. Definitive evidence of disruption of the alar and tectorial ligaments can sometimes be seen, although making this determination may be difficult. Evaluation of the spinal cord and brainstem parenchyma may reveal injuries ranging from mild edema and increased T2-weighted signal intensity to the presence of intraspinal hematoma or even transection. Epidural fluid collections representing hematoma or cerebrospinal fluid are commonly seen, as is the presence of subdural hematoma. Extensive soft tissue swelling extending to the occipitocervical finding is a universal finding and is easily identified on MRI.

Computed Tomography Angiography and Magnetic Resonance Angiography

Evaluation of a large series of survivors of occipitocervical dissociation demonstrated a high likelihood of vertebral

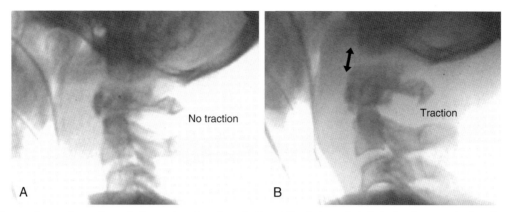

FIGURE 17-5 Provocative traction radiographs for staging of craniocervical instability. **A,** Lateral cervical spine fluoroscopic view shows minimal (1-mm) subluxation with increased signal intensity at the atlantoaxial joints on computed tomography and magnetic resonance imaging, respectively (not shown). Note extensive soft tissue swelling anterior to the occipitocervical junction. **B,** Manual traction using cranial tongs under live fluoroscopy demonstrates greater than 2 mm of widening of the atlantoaxial joints (*double arrow*) with no obvious sensation of a solid end point. This positive traction test result confirms an unstable occipitocervical ligamentous injury that requires operative stabilization, defined as Harborview type II occipitocervical dissociation. (From Bucholz RW, Heckman JD, Court-Brown C, et al, editors: *Rockwood and Green's fractures in adults*, ed 6, Philadelphia, 2006, Lippincott Williams & Wilkins, p 1445.)

artery or internal carotid injury with occipitocervical distractive injury; this combination affected approximately two thirds of patients.[9] Although most of these injuries among survivors were thought to be asymptomatic, prior knowledge of an existing vascular injury may help dictate perioperative management of the patient or the fixation strategy used for definitive stabilization. For example, the surgeon may consider the use of lower-risk C2 fixation, such as the use of translaminar screws, if preoperative vascular evaluation suggests the presence of contralateral vertebral artery compromise. The treatment of asymptomatic vascular injuries in this region remains controversial, with proponents for observation alone, for aspirin therapy, and for anticoagulation with warfarin.

Dynamic (Traction) Views

Traction views under specific, controlled conditions have been advocated by some investigators for a selected group of patients in whom the diagnosis of occipitocervical dissociation is uncertain.[6] Although these patients have generally been identified as having upper cervical spine injuries, they are generally noted to have minimal displacement of the occiput-C1-C2 articulations with only equivocal evidence of true occipitocervical dissociation.

The authors' preference is to perform traction testing in the operating room by using live fluoroscopic evaluation with electrodiagnostic monitoring. This test is treated as a precursor to definitive fixation. Therefore, the patient is given general anesthesia, with preparations made to proceed with posterior occipitocervical fixation in the event of a positive test result. Mayfield or Gardner-Wells tongs are applied after baseline electrodiagnostic signals have been obtained. The C-arm is oriented to obtain a true lateral view of the upper cervical spine. Guided by live fluoroscopy, the surgeon applies gradually increasing manual traction to the cranial tongs. Some surgeons prefer applying progressive 5-pound weights to the tongs, but manual traction provides important proprioceptive feedback.

Whether a traction test result is negative or positive is not usually in question. With a negative test result, a firm

end point is felt almost immediately by the surgeon performing the distraction. Progressively greater amounts of traction cause only minimal distraction of no greater than 2 mm. The occipitocervical junction is therefore deemed stable, and surgical intervention is aborted in favor of treatment with external immobilization.

In the event of a positive test result, distraction greater than 2 mm occurs quickly and with minimal traction. No semblance of an end point can be detected by the surgeon applying traction. Obviously, continuing the distraction beyond the minimum necessary required to demonstrate occipitocervical instability has little value. Once occipitocervical dissociation is confirmed, the surgeon proceeds with posterior occipitocervical instrumented arthrodesis.

Indications for Surgery

Displacement of greater than 2 mm at the atlanto-occipital joint, either on static imaging studies or with provocative traction testing (Fig. 17-5; see Table 17-2), and the presence of neurologic injury are indications for occipitocervical stabilization. Particularly in the presence of neurologic deficits, stabilization is performed as early as reasonably possible.

Treatment and Outcomes

Because occipitocervical dissociation is fatal in most cases, few meaningful descriptions of treatment results are available. More recent series suggest that one of the primary challenges is to make an accurate and timely diagnosis; reports note delayed diagnosis in 30% to 50% of patients and a higher likelihood of preoperative neurologic worsening in patients with diagnostic delay.[6] Once the diagnosis has been confirmed, the focus is shifted toward provisional stabilization until definitive surgical intervention can be performed.

The most appropriate form of provisional stabilization is controversial and depends on many factors, including the timing of surgery, the degree of initial displacement, and the patient's neurologic status, body habitus, and associated injuries. Possible options include one or more of the following: rigid cervical collar immobilization;

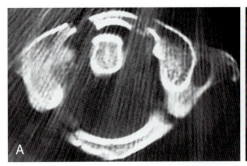 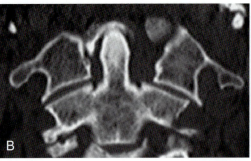 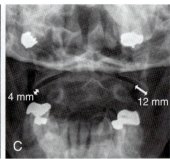

FIGURE 17-6 C1 Jefferson fracture with transverse alar ligament (TAL) injury in a 71-year-old woman. Axial (**A**) and coronal (**B**) computed tomography images demonstrate a four-part C1 ring fracture with initially 4 mm of combined overhang of the C1 lateral masses. The subsequent upright open-mouth anteroposterior radiograph (**C**) demonstrates an increase in combined lateral mass overhang to 16 mm, thus indicating rupture of the TAL. The recommended treatment is C1-C2 posterior arthrodesis.

halo immobilization; taping of the head to sandbags on both sides; and the use of Trendelenburg positioning, if tolerated, to minimize distraction. Finally, definitive surgical intervention generally consists of posterior occipitocervical instrumented fusion, which is done as early as reasonably possible, taking into account the patient's physiologic condition.

Posterior occipitocervical fixation, extending from the occiput to at least C2, is the definitive treatment for occipitocervical dissociation. The authors recommend the use of electrodiagnostic monitoring with prepositioning baselines and the use of Mayfield tongs for turning patients with this highly unstable injury into the prone position. Rigid craniocervical fusion techniques using screw and plate constructs with suboccipital- and sublaminar-cabled structural graft have resulted in fusion rates approaching 100%; the largest reported series of patients treated in this manner showed no incidence of hardware failure or need for revision surgical procedures for reasons of instability.[6,8] Potential technical problems include the following: malreduction, which may result in neurologic worsening; possible penetration of the inner cortex of the skull, which can lead to injury to neural or vascular structures; and vertebral artery injury.

Treatment outcomes in survivors of occipitocervical dissociation depend on the type and severity of associated injuries (particularly intracranial injuries and cerebrovascular injury), the severity of neurologic deficits, and the timeliness with which the diagnosis of craniocervical dissociation is recognized and treated.

Fractures of the Atlas (C1)

Classification

Atlas fractures (C1) can occur in isolation or in conjunction with other injuries, typically of the axis, in 40% to 44% of cases.[10] Instability invariably equates with the presence of transverse alar ligament (TAL) insufficiency, which can be diagnosed either by direct means, such as by identifying bony avulsion on CT scan or ligament rupture on MRI, or indirectly by identifying widening of the lateral masses with a 7-mm or greater lateral overhang relative to the lateral masses of C2 on the open-mouth anteroposterior (AP) view on plain radiographs (Fig. 17-6).[11]

Levine and Edwards described a useful four-part classification system: (1) posterior arch fractures, (2) lateral mass fractures, (3) isolated anterior arch fractures, and (4) bursting-type fractures.[12] As mentioned earlier, the extent of lateral mass separation, which reflects the integrity of the TAL, is more relevant than the number of fracture fragments.

Particular fracture orientations within the fracture subdivisions described by Levine and Edwards can manifest in an atypical fashion. Although the horizontal anterior arch fractures of C1 are typically stable, Vilela and coworkers reported a series of five atypical cases in which this fracture was a subtle sign of more severe occipitocervical instability.[13] Bransford and associates also reported that patients with sagittally oriented unilateral lateral mass fractures are at risk of delayed deformity and severe pain.[14] The authors show good results with the technique of direct fixation of the C1 ring for stabilization of these fractures (Fig. 17-7).[15]

Radiographic Evaluation

Plain Radiography

The open-mouth AP view is the most helpful in evaluating fractures of the atlas because it allows for the assessment of lateral overhang of the lateral masses. The rule of Spence suggests that a combined overhang of both sides of 7 mm or greater is indirect evidence of TAL injury (see Fig. 17-6).[11] Lateral radiographs are useful for detecting posterior arch fractures, unusual variants such as horizontal anterior arch fractures, and any widening of the atlantodens interval (ADI). Particular attention should be paid to both the anterior and posterior ADIs.

Computed Tomography

CT is the most effective imaging technique for evaluating atlas fractures. It provides details of specific fracture patterns, the extent of lateral mass separation and overhang, and the presence of TAL avulsion fractures that may have implications on stability. It also allows for evaluation of surrounding structures and identification of odontoid fractures, which are commonly associated with C1 fractures but may be difficult to detect on plain radiographs.

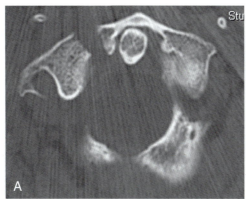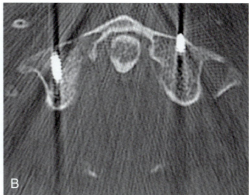

FIGURE 17-7 Direct repair of C1 lateral mass fracture. **A,** Axial computed tomography (CT) image of a right lateral mass fracture with an associated posterior arch fracture (not seen on this image) in a young male patient who had survived an airplane crash. **B,** Postoperative axial CT image shows direct repair of the C1 fracture with C1 lateral mass screws connected by a transverse bar. The indications for this procedure have not been well established, but the primary benefit appears to be in sagittal plane fractures of the lateral mass adjacent to the insertion of the transverse alar ligament in association with posterior arch fractures.

Magnetic Resonance Imaging

Other than for evaluation of associated injuries, including spinal cord injury, the primary benefit of MRI in atlas fractures is the opportunity it provides for identifying intrasubstance tears of the TAL.

Indications for Surgery

Most C1 fractures can be treated nonoperatively. Indications for operative management are related mainly to the loss of TAL integrity, as suggested by combined lateral mass displacement of 7 mm or more, which introduces the potential for progressive lateral mass separation, C1-C2 instability, and pseudarthrosis.[11] Halo or rigid cervical collar immobilization alone may be insufficient to maintain acceptable alignment in these patients. If upright radiographs show further lateral mass displacement or an anterior ADI greater than 3 mm, patients must be treated either with prolonged recumbency in cranial tong traction or with operative stabilization, generally with posterior C1-C2 fixation (Table 17-3).

Treatment and Outcomes

Nonoperative treatment, generally in patients without evidence of TAL compromise, consists of either rigid collar or halo vest immobilization, depending on the surgeon's preference. Severe complications are rare. However, with nonoperatively treated fractures, patients have a 17% fracture nonunion rate and an 80% incidence of residual neck pain, possibly because of posttraumatic arthritis. Severe malunion of unstable atlas fractures may result in painful torticollis, requiring realignment and posterior occipitocervical fusion.

Surgical stabilization options consist of C1-C2 transarticular screw fixation or segmental C1-C2 screw and rod fixation. The latter method provides the opportunity to correct the C1 lateral mass widening by approximating the two rods with a cross connector, a procedure that must be performed with a reduction clamp before instrumentation if using the transarticular technique.

Internal fixation of the C1 ring, by simply reapproximating the lateral masses to each other through lateral mass screws connected to a transversely oriented rod (see Fig. 17-7), is a useful option that theoretically

Table 17-3	C1 Fractures	
Injury Type	**Distinguishing Characteristics**	**Treatment**
Stable	Posterior arch fracture	Rigid collar
	Anterior arch fracture	Rigid collar
	C1 ring fracture with <7 mm combined lateral mass displacement	Rigid collar or halo vest
Unstable	C1 ring fracture with ≥7 mm of overall C1 lateral mass displacement	Traction followed by halo vest versus C1-C2 posterior arthrodesis
	Anterior arch fracture with posterior displacement relative to the odontoid	Halo vest versus C1-C2 posterior arthrodesis

preserves C1-C2 motion. A potential problem with direct repair of an unstable C1 fracture is that the associated TAL deficiency may result in persistent C1-C2 instability. However, unlike in shear or distractive injuries, the axial loading mechanism that causes TAL rupture in displaced C1 ring fractures allows secondary restraints to remain intact, thus minimizing any remaining atlantoaxial translational instability once the atlas has been stabilized.[16]

Atlantoaxial Instability

Classification

Instability of the atlantoaxial joint may result from an injury to the dens, rupture of the alar ligaments or the TAL, or secondary to fracture of the C1 ring, which commonly involves the lateral masses. This discussion focuses primarily on TAL rupture with translational instability of the atlantoaxial complex, with some discussion of rotational injuries.

The TAL can rupture secondary to bony avulsion from C1, or it can sustain a midsubstance tear, with implications on classification and treatment. Although traumatic causes of injury to the TAL are discussed, one should be aware that chronic ligamentous attenuation or rupture may be manifest in congenital, infectious, or inflammatory conditions. An extremely rare mechanism is a rostrally directed force leading to rupture of the alar and apical ligaments with posterior dislocation in which the anterior arch is dislocated posterior to the dens.[17]

Rotatory injuries of the atlantoaxial joint are uncommon entities that also deserve mention. These are rare in adults and usually result from high-energy vehicular trauma. These injuries are quite different from the more commonly seen subluxations in children that can result from trauma or pharyngeal infection and often are self-limiting. Adults with this injury have commonly sustained bilateral C2 lateral mass fractures secondary to the flexion and rotation mechanism.[18]

Three atlantoaxial instability patterns may manifest either as isolated or combined injuries:

- Type A injuries are rotationally displaced in the transverse plane. These deformities are usually nontraumatic.
- Type B injuries are translationally unstable in the sagittal plane as a result of TAL insufficiency.
- Type C injuries are distractive injuries that represent a variant of craniocervical dissociation.

Type A Injuries

Rotational displacement of the atlantoaxial motion segment is most commonly nontraumatic and will therefore not be described in much detail. However, traumatic causes have been described and range in severity from mild rotational subluxation to complete dislocation of the atlantoaxial lateral masses (Fig. 17-8).[19]

Type B Injuries

Translational atlantoaxial instability is the result of TAL insufficiency. The index of suspicion must be heightened if plain radiographs or CT scans show the ADI to be wider than 3 mm. Treatment of these highly unstable injuries depends on differentiating a ligamentous tear (type I) from a bony avulsion injury (type II) (Fig. 17-9).[10]

Type C Injuries

Distractive atlantoaxial injuries, or atlantoaxial dissociations, constitute a variant of occipitocervical dissociation because the disrupted primary ligamentous stabilizers—the alar ligaments and tectorial membrane—extend from C2 to the occiput (Fig. 17-10). These injuries frequently coexist with overt atlanto-occipital distraction injuries. The index of suspicion must be raised if distraction is noted on imaging studies or if the Harris lines are longer than 12 mm.

Radiographic Evaluation

Plain Radiography

Lateral radiographs demonstrate an abnormal relationship of C2 and the odontoid process with C1. In type B (translational) injuries, this relationship manifests as an

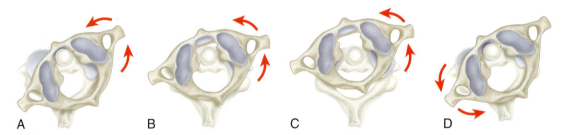

FIGURE 17-8 Fielding and Hawkins classification of rotational (type A) atlantoaxial instability. **A,** Type I. **B,** Type II. **C,** Type III. **D,** Type IV. (From Warner WC: Pediatric cervical spine. In Canale ST, Beaty JH, editors: *Campbell's operative orthopaedics,* ed 12, Philadelphia, 2013, Saunders.)

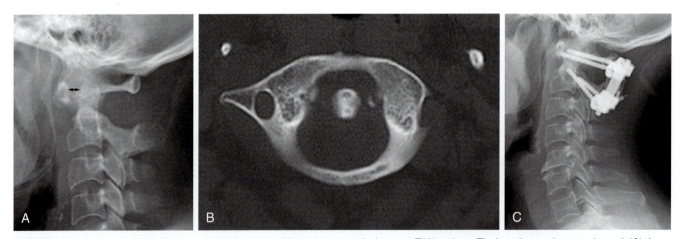

FIGURE 17-9 Translational (type B) atlantoaxial subluxation with bony transverse alar ligament (TAL) avulsion. The lateral cervical spine radiograph (**A**) shows widening of the atlantodens interval (*double arrow*) and of the distance between the posterior elements of C1 and C2. The axial computed tomography image (**B**) shows an avulsion fracture at the left TAL insertion. Open reduction and posterior instrumented C1-C2 arthrodesis were performed (**C**). (From Bucholz RW, Heckman JD, Court-Brown C, et al, editors: *Rockwood and Green's fractures in adults,* ed 6, Philadelphia, 2006, Lippincott Williams & Wilkins, p 1446.)

increase in the anterior ADI, which in a normal radiograph is usually 3 mm wide or less. Type C (distractive) injuries demonstrate widening of the C1-C2 articulations and an abnormal relationship of the odontoid process with the foramen magnum (see the previous discussion of Harris lines). Type A (rotational) injuries show a more global abnormality in the architecture of the C1-C2 complex.

The open-mouth AP odontoid view is not particularly helpful for translational injuries, but it can reveal the distractive findings associated with C1-C2 injuries and is particularly useful for identifying the asymmetry between the odontoid and the C1 lateral masses in rotational injuries. Any significant asymmetry between the lateral ADI on either side suggests a rotational deformity.

Computed Tomography

The CT scan further clarifies the relationship between the atlas and the axis. It is particularly useful in identifying avulsion fractures of the TAL insertions onto the C1 lateral masses and thereby helps distinguish type IB from type IIB injuries and may determine whether operative or nonoperative treatment is recommended.

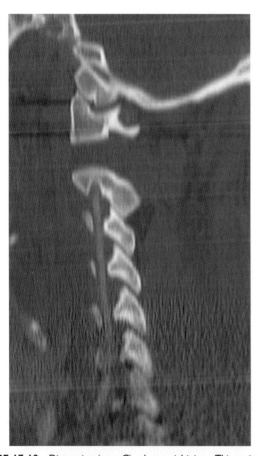

FIGURE 17-10   Distractive (type C) atlantoaxial injury. This sagittal computed tomography image through the C0-C1 and C1-C2 articulations shows an upper cervical distractive injury, with wide displacement across the C1-C2 articulation. Also visible is subtle associated C0-C1 anterior subluxation. Because the major stabilizing ligaments of the occipitocervical junction extend from the foramen magnum to C2, distractive injuries at either of these two joints frequently result in instability at the adjacent articulation. (From Bucholz RW, Heckman JD, Court-Brown C, et al, editors: *Rockwood and Green's fractures in adults*, ed 6, Philadelphia, 2006, Lippincott Williams & Wilkins, p 1447.)

CT imaging is also useful in characterizing more complex rotational injuries, which are often associated with lateral mass fractures of C1 and C2, as well as other injuries.

Magnetic Resonance Imaging

Although intrasubstance tears of the TAL are often difficult to detect, MRI can provide direct visualization of these injuries.

Vascular Study

Either CT or MR angiography is recommended for evaluation of distractive injuries of the upper cervical spine, such as type C atlantoaxial injuries.

Indications for Surgery

Translational Instability

Type B fractures are highly unstable injuries that generally require posterior atlantoaxial arthrodesis. However, in the presence of bony avulsion, successful healing may occur in 74% of patients with a period of recumbent traction followed by immobilization in a halo or sternal occipital mandibular immobilizer (SOMI).[10] An ADI greater than 3 mm on flexion radiographs after 3 months of immobilization constitutes a failure of closed treatment and indicates the need for atlantoaxial arthrodesis.

Distraction Injuries

Type C distraction injuries of C1-C2 with 2 mm or more of displacement require surgical stabilization. This injury is analogous to occipitocervical dissociation at the atlanto-occipital joint and should be treated using similar guidelines.

Rotational Injuries

Adults with rotational injuries that result from high-energy trauma often have associated C1 and C2 lateral mass fractures or ligamentous injuries that require surgical stabilization. An attempt at closed reduction with traction, followed by mobilization in a collar or halo, is warranted when the integrity of the major osseoligamentous stabilizers is preserved, with careful follow-up and a low threshold for surgical intervention in the event of subsequent loss of alignment (Table 17-4).

Treatment and Outcomes

An attempt at nonoperative care with a halo vest orthosis may be warranted in patients with type IIB injuries, which are translational injuries with associated TAL avulsion. Most patients with traumatic TAL insufficiency require operative stabilization, most commonly with posterior C1-C2 arthrodesis.

The authors' preferred methods for atlantoaxial fusion involve either posterior transarticular screw fixation and direct decortication and bone grafting of the C1-C2 joints, augmented with a modified Gallie-cabled structural bone graft, or the use of interconnected C1 lateral mass and C2 pedicle screw fixation. In cases of anomalous vertebral artery anatomy, in which these forms of C2 instrumentation are deemed either unsafe or technically implausible, C2 translaminar screws can be used as an alternative,

Table 17-4 Atlantoaxial Injuries

Injury Type	Distinguishing Characteristics	Treatment
A	Rotation centered on the dens; TAL usually intact	Closed reduction and immobilization; beware of associated fractures
B	Translation between C1 and C2 with TAL disruption	Type 1 (midsubstance TAL tear): C1-C2 arthrodesis. Type 2 (TAL avulsion fracture): halo vest versus C1-C2 arthrodesis
C	Distraction injury	Open reduction and posterior instrumented arthrodesis

TAL, Transverse alar ligament.

although they render placement of structural bone grafting more difficult, if not impossible.

The prognosis is largely contingent on neurologic status at the time of injury. Because a severe neurologic injury at this level is incompatible with life as a result of cardiorespiratory compromise, patients who survive the injury generally have a favorable neurologic profile and prognosis. The results of posterior atlantoaxial arthrodesis are favorable, with pseudarthrosis rates of less than 5%.[20] Potentially serious intraoperative complications include the risk of vertebral artery injury, the incidence of which has been reported as 2% or lower per C2 transarticular or pedicle screw.[21] Although the risk is very low, because of their proximity to the anterior aspect of the lateral mass, bicortical C1 lateral mass screws may injure the internal carotid artery and hypoglossal nerve.[22]

Odontoid Fractures

Classification

The most widely used classification system is the three-part classification of Anderson and D'Alonzo (Fig. 17-11).[9]

- Type I injuries are bony avulsions of the alar ligament and represent a component of craniocervical dissociation.
- Type II injuries occur at the odontoid waist and have the highest propensity for pseudarthrosis.
  - A Type IIA subtype consists of a highly unstable, segmentally comminuted fracture.[23]
- Type III fractures extend into the cancellous vertebral body and have wider, well-vascularized cancellous fracture surfaces.

Radiographic Evaluation

Plain Radiography

Displaced fractures of the odontoid process are generally identifiable on plain lateral radiographs. However, particularly in older patients with poor bone quality, advanced degenerative changes, and more subtle degrees of displacement, odontoid fractures can be difficult to identify with plain radiographs alone.

Computed Tomography

CT clearly demonstrates the fracture pattern and degree of displacement and offers the detail required to classify these injuries properly. Other subtle findings such as the presence and extent of comminution and of associated fractures, such as C1 ring fractures, can help dictate the most appropriate treatment plan.

Magnetic Resonance Imaging

In the absence of neurologic injury, MRI of odontoid fractures is of limited value. If odontoid fracture is suspected, simultaneous rupture of the TAL, which is an obvious contraindication to odontoid screw fixation, can potentially be confirmed with MRI. With the uncommon subset of odontoid fractures associated with worrisome distractive injury (usually a type III fracture pattern), MRI demonstrates extensive ligamentous disruption with increased T2-weighted signal intensity and widening of the C1-C2 articulation and disruption of the posterior atlantoaxial membrane.

Indications for Surgery

Treatment of type I odontoid fractures relates to their impact on occipitocervical stability, which is previously discussed.

Surgical indications for type II odontoid fractures remain controversial. Fractures for which surgical stabilization can clearly be advocated include fractures with distractive patterns of displacement and those associated with spinal cord injury. Relative indications include multiple injuries, associated closed head injury, initial displacement greater than 4 mm, angulation of more than 10 degrees,[24] delayed presentation (>2 weeks), multiple risk factors for nonunion, the inability to treat with a halo because of advanced age or body habitus,[25] associated cranial or thoracoabdominal injury, other medical comorbidities, and the presence of associated upper cervical fractures.

Operative stabilization of type III injuries is not commonly required, but it is warranted in patients with spinal cord injury or distractive instability patterns (Fig. 17-12). Relative indications include highly displaced irreducible fractures, displaced injuries in patients who cannot be treated with a halo, and fractures with initial displacement of 5 mm or more, which have a high potential for nonunion (Table 17-5).

Treatment and Outcomes

In patients with favorable bone quality and an appropriate body habitus, noncomminuted fractures with a fracture pattern that is either transverse or has anterosuperior to posteroinferior obliquity are ideal for anterior odontoid screw fixation.[26] In patients with extensive fracture comminution, compromised bone quality, fracture obliquity from anteroinferior to posterosuperior, or technical constraints to anterior odontoid screw trajectory, the authors favor posterior atlantoaxial fusion using either transarticular screw fixation or segmental C1-C2 screw and rod fixation (see Fig. 17-12). In general, odontoid screw fixation is not recommended in the older population. Proper patient selection helps avoid the complications that have been reported in up to 28% of patients who undergo anterior odontoid screw fixation.[27]

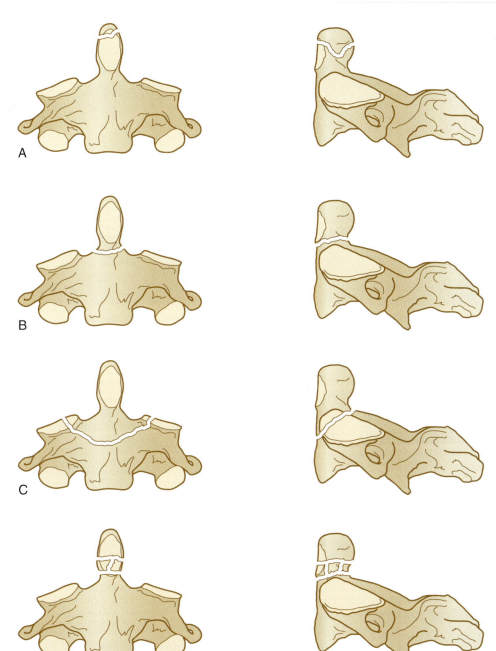

FIGURE 17-11 Anderson and D'Alonzo's odontoid fracture classification.[9,23] **A,** Type I fractures of the odontoid tip represent alar ligament avulsions. **B,** Type II fractures occur at the odontoid waist, above the C2 lateral masses. **C,** Type III fractures extend below the odontoid waist to involve the body and lateral masses of C2. **D,** Hadley added the type IIA fracture with segmental comminution at the base of the odontoid.

Delayed unions or pseudarthroses occur in approximately 10% of nonoperatively treated patients.[28] In acute or ununited type III fractures, posterior C1-C2 arthrodesis is the surgical treatment method of choice because anterior odontoid screw fixation has a high failure rate in type III odontoid fractures.[26]

The treatment of odontoid fractures, both operative and nonoperative, is associated with significant morbidity and mortality. In-hospital mortality rates for older patients with type II odontoid fractures range from approximately 10% to 42%.

Primary neurologic injury or secondary deterioration rarely occurs with odontoid fractures. Fracture nonunion and missed injuries are the most common complications. Subtly displaced injuries in older patients can be particularly difficult to detect on plain radiographs. With type II odontoid fractures, displacement greater than 4 mm or angulation of more than 9 degrees has been associated with nonunion rates of 22% to 54%. Other risk factors include age greater than 60 years and delay in treatment.[24] Nonoperative treatment of type III odontoid fractures with the use of a halo is associated with pseudarthrosis rates from 9% to 13%.[28]

An overall perioperative complication rate of up to 28% and a nonunion rate of 10% have been described with odontoid screw fixation (Fig. 17-13).[27] If surgical stabilization of type III odontoid fractures is undertaken, it should consist of atlantoaxial fixation because excessively high failure rates (55%) have been reported for odontoid screw fixation.[26] C1-C2 posterior fusions

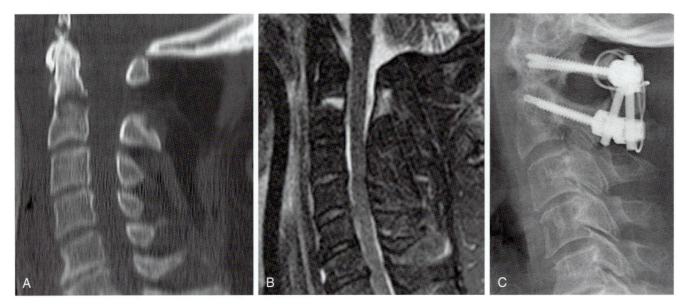

FIGURE 17-12   Type III odontoid fracture with distraction. Sagittal computed tomography (**A**) and magnetic resonance imaging (**B**) show a distracted type III odontoid fracture. This atlantoaxial distractive injury is associated with extensive ligamentous disruption, as illustrated by the increased signal intensity between C1 and C2 posteriorly on MRI. A lateral radiograph 3 months after posterior instrumented C1-C2 arthrodesis (**C**) shows restoration of odontoid and atlantoaxial alignment. (From Stannard JP, Schmidt AH, Kregor PJ, editors: *Surgical treatment of orthopaedic trauma*, New York, 2007, Thieme, p 113.)

Table 17-5   Odontoid Fractures

Injury Type	Distinguishing Characteristics	Treatment
I	Avulsion at alar ligament insertion	Treated surgically if associated with occipitocervical dissociation
II	Fracture at waist of odontoid process	High risk of nonunion; options include halo vest versus anterior odontoid screw versus posterior C1-C2 arthrodesis, depending on displacement, fracture pattern, and bone quality
III	Fracture extending into cancellous bone within C2 vertebral body	Halo versus cervical collar; distraction injuries require posterior C1-C2 arthrodesis

have reported nonunion rates of 4% or less using transarticular screw and wired structural bone graft constructs.[20] Vertebral artery injury is generally reported as occurring at a rate of less than 2% per transarticular or pedicle screw placement and appears to be decreasing in concert with expansion of options for posterior C2 instrumentation and an increasing ability to tailor fixation specifically to each patient's individual anatomy.[21]

Traumatic Spondylolisthesis of the Axis (Hangman Fractures)

Classification

Traumatic spondylolisthesis of the axis, or the hangman fracture, is classified by the modification by Levine and Edwards[29] and by Starr and Eismont[30] of the original classification by Effendi and associates[31] into three primary injury types and two atypical subtypes (Fig. 17-14):

- Type I: Minimally displaced (≤3 mm), relatively stable fractures of the pars interarticularis that result from hyperextension and axial loading
  - Type IA: Atypical unstable lateral bending fractures that are obliquely displaced, with a fracture through one pars and more anteriorly into the body on the contralateral side (Fig. 17-15)
- Type II: Displaced injuries (>3 mm) that occur when a flexion force follows the initial hyperextension and axial loading insult; these may visible only on upright radiographs if they are spontaneously reduced on supine imaging
  - Type IIA: Unstable injury with associated C2-C3 disk and interspinous ligament disruption caused by a flexion-distraction mechanism, in which kyphosis is the prevailing deformity rather than translation (Fig. 17-16)
- Type III: Highly unstable injuries in which the pars interarticularis fractures are associated with dislocation of the C2-C3 facet joints

Radiographic Evaluation

Plain Radiography

Traumatic spondylolisthesis is generally appreciated as anterolisthesis of the C2 vertebral body relative to C3 on lateral radiographs. Upright lateral radiographs are necessary to confirm the presence of a type I injury, as opposed to a type II injury that has reduced into a more anatomic alignment on prior supine imaging. The type IIA subtype is suspected in injuries having relatively little anterolisthesis relative to the degree of

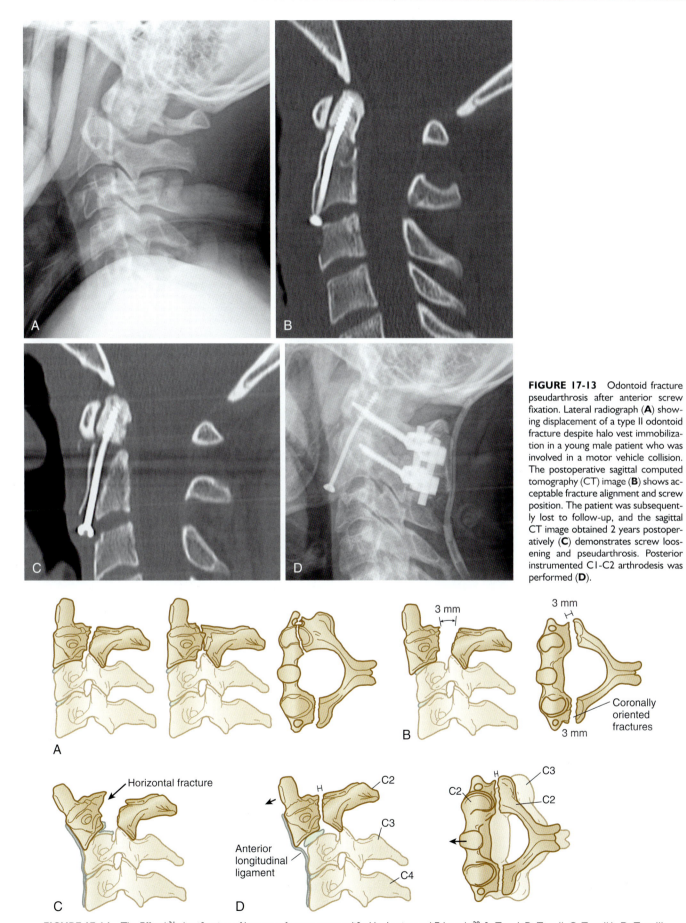

FIGURE 17-13 Odontoid fracture pseudarthrosis after anterior screw fixation. Lateral radiograph (**A**) showing displacement of a type II odontoid fracture despite halo vest immobilization in a young male patient who was involved in a motor vehicle collision. The postoperative sagittal computed tomography (CT) image (**B**) shows acceptable fracture alignment and screw position. The patient was subsequently lost to follow-up, and the sagittal CT image obtained 2 years postoperatively (**C**) demonstrates screw loosening and pseudarthrosis. Posterior instrumented C1-C2 arthrodesis was performed (**D**).

FIGURE 17-14   The Effendi[31] classification of hangman fractures as modified by Levine and Edwards.[29] **A,** Type I. **B,** Type II. **C,** Type IIA. **D,** Type III.

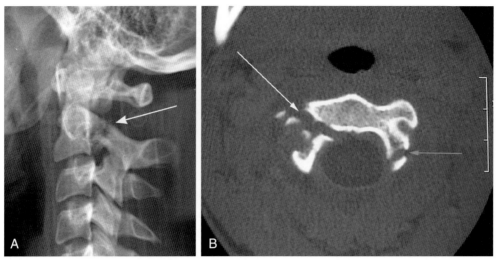

FIGURE 17-15 Type IA "atypical" traumatic spondylolistheses of C2. The fracture lines are not collinear on the lateral view, thus giving the impression of an elongated pars (*arrow*) on the lateral radiograph (**A**). Axial computed tomography scan (**B**) shows the usual position of a pars interarticularis fracture (*gray arrow*) on one side and an atypical contralateral fracture extending into the vertebral body and foramen transversarium (*white arrow*). Displacement of the vertebral body fracture at the spinal canal results in a higher likelihood of spinal cord injury with type IA injuries than with other type I or II injuries. (From Stannard JP, Schmidt AH, Kregor PJ, editors: *Surgical treatment of orthopaedic trauma*, New York, 2007, Thieme, p 115.)

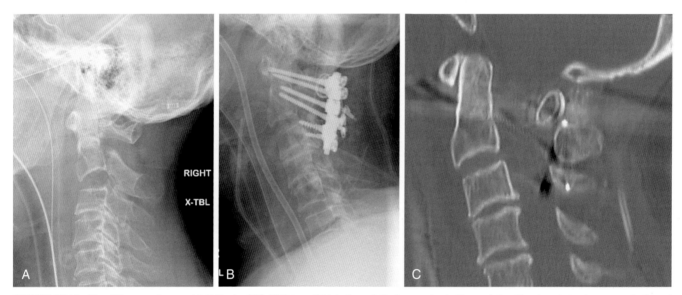

FIGURE 17-16 Type IIA traumatic spondylolisthesis of C2. With type IIA injuries, relatively more kyphotic angulation than translation is seen on the lateral cervical spine radiograph (**A**). The C2-C3 segment must be stabilized because of the extensive disk disruption. Although interfragmentary screws were placed across the C2 pars interarticularis fractures bilaterally, the instrumentation was extended to C1 in this particular patient because of his advanced age and osteoporosis, as seen on the postoperative lateral radiograph of the cervical spine (**B**) and the sagittal computed tomography image (**C**). *X-TBL*, Cross-table. (From Bucholz RW, Heckman JD, Court-Brown C, et al, editors: *Rockwood and Green's fractures in adults*, ed 6, Philadelphia, 2006, Lippincott Williams & Wilkins, p 1454.)

kyphotic angulation, although exact numeric parameters have not been definitively established. C2-C3 facet dislocation is readily recognizable in type III injuries. Most injuries can be classified based on plain radiographs alone.

Computed Tomography

CT can be useful in delineating the exact fracture pattern in more atypical injuries and in evaluating the vertebral artery foramen anatomy when planning for surgical intervention. For atypical injuries with neurologic deficits, CT imaging can provide information on the source of spinal cord compression.[30]

Magnetic Resonance Imaging

In the absence of neurologic deficits, MRI seemingly has little role in the evaluation of traumatic spondylolisthesis. Although the extent of C2-C3 disk injury can usually be inferred from the appearance of plain films and CT images, in some situations, particularly in patients with atypical injury pattern, evaluation of the integrity of the C2-C3 disk may be warranted to evaluate the need for operative intervention.

Vascular Study

Either CT or MR angiography is recommended for evaluation of injuries with involvement of the vertebral

Table 17-6 Traumatic Spondylolisthesis of the Atlas (Hangman Fractures)

Injury Type	Distinguishing Characteristics	Treatment
I	Displacement <3 mm Fracture through arch of C2	Rigid cervical collar
IA	Atypical fracture involving C2 arch on one side and vertebral body on other side; often involves vertebral artery foramen	Often associated with spinal cord injury; usually treated with halo; may require surgery if severely displaced or associated with spinal cord injury; fixation options include C2-C3 ACDF, C2-C3 PSIF, C1-C3 PSIF, or, rarely, combined anterior and posterior approach
II	Displaced fracture of C2 arch	Halo
IIA	Fracture of C2 arch associated with flexion-distraction mechanism and C2-C3 disk disruption greater kyphosis than translation	C2-C3 PSIF versus C1-C3 PSIF versus C2-C3 ACDF
III	Fracture of C2 arch associated with C2-C3 facet joint dislocation	Often associated with spinal cord injury; treated with posterior open reduction and C2-C3 versus C1-C3 PSIF

ACDF, Anterior cervical diskectomy and fusion; *PSIF,* posterior instrumented fusion.

foramen, which is a common occurrence with traumatic C2 spondylolisthesis.

Indications for Surgery

Operative stabilization is rarely indicated for traumatic spondylolisthesis of the axis.[32] Most injuries can be treated with 12 weeks of external immobilization using a rigid collar for type I (and most IA) injuries and a halo vest for most type II fractures.[31] Surgical intervention is recommended for type IIA injuries because the kyphotic alignment generally cannot be effectively controlled with external immobilization. Traction is contraindicated, given that it accentuates the kyphotic deformity and can result in neurologic compromise from the progression of deformity. Type III injuries are generally irreducible by traction and require operative reduction and stabilization (Table 17-6).

Treatment and Outcomes

Most injuries can be treated effectively with a rigid collar or halo immobilization; the pseudarthrosis rate is low, on the order of 5%.[29] Acute postadmission mortality after hangman fractures is as low as 2% to 3%.[33] Associated upper cervical injuries (15%), subaxial injuries (23%), and head injuries usually have a greater effect on prognosis than does the C2 fracture itself. Neurologic injury occurs in only 3% to 10% of patients, but certain subtypes are at much higher risk.[29,32] Because of the presence of facet dislocation, type III injuries pose the highest risk of neurologic injury, with a reported incidence of up to 60%.[34] Type IA fractures have a 33% incidence of associated spinal cord injury, probably secondary to the spinal canal compromise that occurs with fracture displacement in this atypical oblique fracture pattern (see Fig. 17-15). Type IA injuries also have a greater potential for vertebral

artery injury because of common foramen transversarium involvement.[30]

Surgical treatment is generally reserved for atypical (type IA), type IIA, and type III fractures, which constitute a greater treatment challenge as a result of their atypical fracture orientation, the amount of displacement, or the associated ligamentous injury. The usefulness of direct osteosynthesis for type II hangman fractures has been questioned because nonoperative treatment is so effective and because this technique does not address the associated injury to the C2-C3 intervertebral disk.

For the treatment of type IA and IIA fractures, options for minimizing the number of fused levels include C2-C3 anterior cervical diskectomy and fusion (ACDF)[35] with plating (Fig. 17-17), as opposed to posterior C2-C3 instrumented fusion, which also requires direct osteosynthesis of the pars interarticularis fracture with C2 pars or pedicle screws (Fig. 17-18). The disadvantage of anterior C2-C3 ACDF is that it compromises the anterior longitudinal ligament and anterior annulus, the only remaining intact major ligamentous structures at C2-C3. Dysphagia, dysphonia, and swallowing difficulties are also relatively common with anterior upper cervical exposures, and access to the C2-C3 level anteriorly can be challenging.

Posterior stabilization is more versatile and stable, but unless adequate purchase can be achieved across the fractured C2 pars interarticularis, loss of atlantoaxial motion results from the need to extend fixation to C1 (see Fig. 17-16).

Stabilization options for type III injuries include posterior C1-C3 fusion, posterior C2-C3 fusion using lag screws across the fracture at C2 (see Fig. 17-18), and anterior C2-C3 ACDF only in the unusual event that reduction occurs by closed methods.

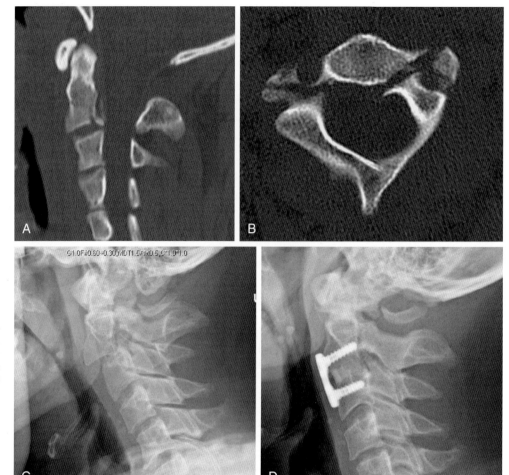

FIGURE 17-17 Anterior cervical diskectomy and fusion (ACDF) for treatment of atypical hangman fracture. Sagittal (**A**) and axial (**B**) computed tomography images demonstrate an atypical hangman fracture variant (type IA) extending into the vertebral body, with comminution associated with posterior C1 arch fracture. Increased angulation and translation on the upright lateral radiograph (**C**) despite halo vest immobilization resulted in treatment with C2-C3 ACDF, as noted on the lateral radiograph obtained 6 months postoperatively (**D**).

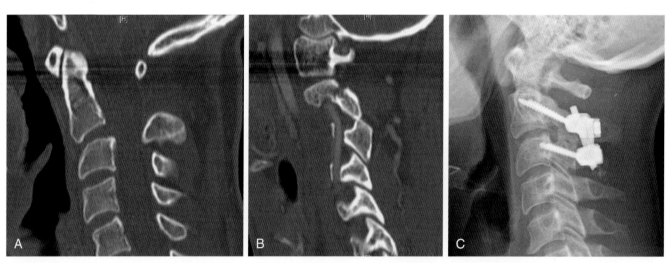

FIGURE 17-18 Unusual variant of type III traumatic spondylolisthesis of C2 with a unilateral perched facet, as seen on sagittal computed tomography images (**A** and **B**). As with most type III injuries, the facet dislocation could not be reduced by closed means. It was treated with urgent open reduction and C2-C3 posterior instrumented arthrodesis, relying on simultaneous direct osteosynthesis of the C2 pars interarticularis fracture as demonstrated on the postoperative lateral radiograph (**C**).

REFERENCES

1. Anderson PA, Montesano PX: Morphology and treatment of occipital condyle fractures, *Spine (Phila Pa 1976)* 13:731–736, 1988.
2. Hanson JA, Deliganis AV, Baxter AB, et al.: Radiologic and clinical spectrum of occipital condyle fractures: retrospective review of 107 consecutive fractures in 95 patients, *AJR Am J Roentgenol* 178:1261–1268, 2002.
3. Traynelis VC, Marano GD, Dunker RO, Kaufman HH: Traumatic atlanto-occipital dislocation: case report, *J Neurosurg* 65:863–870, 1986.
4. Dvorak J, Schneider E, Saldinger P, Rahn B: Biomechanics of the craniocervical region: the alar and transverse ligaments, *J Orthop Res* 6:452–461, 1988.
5. Song WS, Chiang YH, Chen CY, et al.: A simple method for diagnosing traumatic occlusion of the vertebral artery at the craniovertebral junction, *Spine (Phila Pa 1976)* 19:837–839, 1994.
6. Bellabarba C, Mirza SK, West GA, et al.: Diagnosis and treatment of craniocervical dislocation in a series of 17 consecutive survivors during an 8-year period, *J Neurosurg Spine* 4:429–440, 2006.
7. Harris JH Jr, Carson GC, Wagner LK, Kerr N: Radiologic diagnosis of traumatic occipitovertebral dissociation: 2. Comparison of three methods of detecting occipitovertebral relationships on lateral radiographs of supine subjects, *AJR Am J Roentgenol* 162:887–892, 1994.
8. Bellabarba C, Bransford RJ, Chapman JR: Timing to diagnosis and neurological outcomes in 48 consecutive craniocervical dissociation patients: proceedings of the 26th Annual Meeting of the North American Spine Society, *Spine J* 11(Suppl):57S, 2011.
9. Anderson LD, D'Alonzo RT: Fractures of the odontoid process of the axis, *J Bone Joint Surg Am* 56:1663–1674, 1974.
10. Dickman CA, Greene KA, Sonntag VK: Injuries involving the transverse atlantal ligament: classification and treatment guidelines based upon experience with 39 injuries, *Neurosurgery* 38:44–50, 1996.
11. Spence KF Jr, Decker S, Sell KW: Bursting atlantal fracture associated with rupture of the transverse ligament, *J Bone Joint Surg Am* 52:543–549, 1970.
12. Levine AM, Edwards CC: Fractures of the atlas, *J Bone Joint Surg Am* 73:680–691, 1991.
13. Vilela MD, Bransford RJ, Bellabarba C, Ellenbogen RG: Horizontal C-1 fractures in association with unstable distraction injuries of the craniocervical junction, *J Neurosurg Spine* 15:182–186, 2011.
14. Bransford R, Falicov A, Nguyen Q, Chapman J: Unilateral C-1 lateral mass sagittal split fracture: an unstable Jefferson fracture variant, *J Neurosurg Spine* 10:466–473, 2009.
15. Bransford R, Chapman JR, Bellabarba C: Primary internal fixation of unilateral C1 lateral mass sagittal split fractures: a series of 3 cases, *J Spinal Disord Tech* 24:157–163, 2011.
16. Fielding JW, Cochran GB, Lawsing JF, Hohl M: Tears of the transverse ligament of the atlas: a clinical and biomechanical study, *J Bone Joint Surg Am* 56:1683–1691, 1974.
17. Neumann U, Urbanski H, Riedel K: Posterior atlantoaxial dislocation without fracture of the odontoid: a case report, *J Bone Joint Surg Am* 85:1343–1346, 2003.
18. Weisskopf M, Naeve D, Ruf M, et al.: Therapeutic options and results following fixed atlantoaxial rotatory dislocations, *Eur Spine J* 14:61–68, 2005.
19. Fielding JW, Hawkins RJ: Atlanto-axial rotatory fixation (fixed rotatory subluxation of the atlanto-axial joint), *J Bone Joint Surg Am* 59:37–44, 1977.
20. Haid RW, Subach BR, McLaughlin MR, et al.: C1-C2 transarticular screw fixation for atlantoaxial instability: a 6-year experience, *Neurosurgery* 49:65–68, 2001.
21. Bransford RJ, Russo AJ, Freeborn M, et al.: Posterior C2 instrumentation: accuracy and complications associated with four techniques, *Spine (Phila Pa 1976)* 36:E936–E943, 2011.
22. Currier BL, Maus TP, Eck JC, et al.: Relationship of the internal carotid artery to the anterior aspect of the C1 vertebra: implications for C1-C2 transarticular and C1 lateral mass fixation, *Spine (Phila Pa 1976)* 33:635–639, 2008.
23. Hadley MN, Browner CM, Liu SS, Sonntag VK: New subtype of acute odontoid fractures (type IIA), *Neurosurgery* 22:67–71, 1988.
24. Clark CR, White AA 3rd: Fractures of the dens: a multicenter study, *J Bone Joint Surg Am* 67:1340–1348, 1985.
25. Bednar DA, Parikh J, Hummel J: Management of type II odontoid process fractures in geriatric patients: a prospective study of sequential cohorts with attention to survivorship, *J Spinal Disord* 8:166–169, 1995.
26. Apfelbaum RI, Lonser RR, Veres R, Casey A: Direct anterior screw fixation for recent and remote odontoid fractures, *J Neurosurg* 93(Suppl):227–236, 2000.
27. Etter C, Coscia M, Jaberg H, Aebi M: Direct anterior fixation of dens fractures with a cannulated screw system, *Spine (Phila Pa 1976)* 16(Suppl):S25–S32, 1991.
28. Apuzzo ML, Heiden JS, Weiss MH, et al.: Acute fractures of the odontoid process: an analysis of 45 cases, *J Neurosurg* 48:85–91, 1978.
29. Levine AM, Edwards CC: Traumatic lesions of the occipitoatlantoaxial complex, *Clin Orthop Relat Res (239)*:53–68, 1989.
30. Starr JK, Eismont FJ: Atypical hangman's fractures, *Spine (Phila Pa 1976)* 18:1954–1957, 1993.
31. Effendi B, Roy D, Cornish B, et al.: Fractures of the ring of the axis: a classification based on the analysis of 131 cases, *J Bone Joint Surg Br* 63:319–327, 1981.
32. Francis WR, Fielding JW, Hawkins RJ, et al.: Traumatic spondylolisthesis of the axis, *J Bone Joint Surg Br* 63:313–318, 1981.
33. Greene KA, Dickman CA, Marciano FF, et al.: Acute axis fractures: analysis of management and outcome in 340 consecutive cases, *Spine (Phila Pa 1976)* 22:1843–1852, 1997.
34. Levine AM, Edwards CC: The management of traumatic spondylolisthesis of the axis, *J Bone Joint Surg Am* 67:217–226, 1985.
35. Tuite GF, Papadopoulos SM, Sonntag VK: Caspar plate fixation for the treatment of complex hangman's fractures, *Neurosurgery* 30:761–764, 1992.

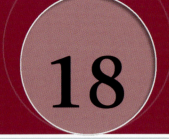

18 Subaxial Cervical Spine Injuries

Kelley Banagan and Frank M. Phillips

CHAPTER PREVIEW

Chapter Synopsis	Injuries to the subaxial cervical spine comprise the majority of cervical spine injuries annually. Since 2000, novel classification systems have been developed to provide a uniform method of characterizing subaxial cervical spine injuries and to help guide treatment. Surgical intervention is aimed at restoring mechanical stability and improving neurologic outcome. The surgical approach largely depends on the mechanism of injury, the location of the pathologic features, and the nature of the fracture. This chapter reviews the classification system, radiographic evaluation, and surgical management of traumatic injuries to the subaxial cervical spine.
Important Points	Subaxial cervical spine injuries represent the majority of cervical spine trauma.
	The Subaxial Injury Classification (SLIC) system was developed in an effort to streamline information about injury pattern, treatment, and prognosis.
	The SLIC system is based on injury morphology, the status of the diskoligamentous complex, and the neurologic status of the patient.
	Magnetic resonance imaging should be used in the obtunded patient to evaluate for potential subaxial cervical spine injuries.
	The goals of surgical treatment of traumatic subaxial cervical spine injuries are mechanical stability and neural decompression.
	The location of the pathologic features and the morphology of the fracture dictate the operative approach.

Of the more than 1 million acute spine injuries that occur annually in the United States, 50,000 are fractures of the bony spinal column and 11,000 include injury to the spinal cord. Trauma to the cervical spine accounts for nearly 50% of all spine injuries and results in almost half of the estimated spinal cord injuries.[1] The subaxial spine accounts for the majority of the injuries: 65% of fractures and 75% of all dislocations. However, despite the prevalence of these injuries, their classification, management, and treatment can vary widely among surgeons.

From a functional standpoint, the cervical spine can be divided into two distinct regions: the craniocervical junction (occiput to C2) and the subaxial cervical spine (C3 to C7). The craniocervical junction consists of unique anatomic structures. It obtains stability primarily through ligamentous attachments, and the joints have a lower degree of intrinsic stability to provide a more substantial range of motion. The subaxial spine has a higher degree of intersegmental stability. Secondary to variations in anatomy of the cervical spine are injury patterns characteristic to each region. Recognition of the specific injury patterns facilitates diagnosis and treatment.[2]

Injury Classification and Pathophysiology

In 1970, Sir Frank Holdsworth created the first comprehensive classification system for spinal column injuries based on his experience with more than 2000 patients; he recognized the importance of the posterior ligamentous complex in determining stability.[1] In 1982, Allen and colleagues proposed a classification system of subaxial cervical spine injuries based on plain radiographs in which mechanism of injury was inferred from the recoil position of the spine. Six categories were originally described: compressive flexion, vertical compression, distractive flexion, compressive extension, distractive extension, and lateral flexion. Harris then modified the system to incorporate rotational vectors in flexion and extension. The six mechanisms described were flexion, flexion and rotation, hyperextension and rotation, vertical compression, extension, and lateral flexion. Each mechanism was further subdivided to determine the severity of the injury with respect to the primary vector; the goal was to indicate the degree of tissue damage and instability. Both systems are comprehensive, but they are rarely used because of their complexity and the difficulty in correlating the subtypes and injury severity.[2]

A novel classification system, the Subaxial Injury Classification (SLIC), was developed in an effort to convey information about injury pattern, treatment considerations, and prognosis. The system consists of three components: (1) injury morphology, (2) integrity of the diskoligamentous complex (DLC), and (3) neurologic status of the patient. Injury morphology is determined by the pattern of spinal column disruption on imaging studies.

Injury Morphology

Within the SLIC system, injury morphology is divided into three categories: compression, distraction, and translation or rotation. *Compression* is a visible loss of height through part of or the entire vertebral body or by disruption through the end plate. This morphology includes traditional compression fractures and burst fractures, sagittal and coronal plane fractures, and teardrop or flexion compression fractures. Undisplaced or minimally displaced lateral mass and facet fractures are categorized as compression-type injuries, and they are likely the result of a lateral compression mechanism.[3]

Distraction is defined as an anatomic dissociation in the vertical axis, and it signifies a greater degree of destruction and potential instability. This injury pattern commonly involves ligamentous disruption that propagates through the disk space or the facet joints. A hyperextension injury disrupting the anterior longitudinal ligament and widening the anterior disk space also represents a distractive pattern of injury.[3]

Translation or rotation injuries have radiographic evidence of horizontal displacement of one part of the subaxial spine relative to another. By definition, both anterior and posterior structures are disrupted, and a high degree of instability is present. A relative angulation of greater than 11 degrees has been the suggested threshold for rotation. Unilateral and bilateral facet fracture-dislocations, fracture separation of the lateral mass or a "floating" lateral mass, and bilateral pedicle fractures are also examples of translational injuries.[3]

Diskoligamentous Complex

The DLC is represented by the anterior and posterior longitudinal ligaments and by the posterior ligaments (ligamentum flavum, interspinous ligament, supraspinous ligament, and facet capsule). The integrity of the DLC is postulated to be directly proportional to spinal stability.

The facet joint capsules are the strongest anatomic structure posteriorly, whereas anteriorly the anterior longitudinal ligament is strongest. Therefore, abnormal facet alignment, characterized by articular apposition of less than 50% or diastasis of more than 2 mm through the facet joint, can be considered an absolute indication of DLC disruption. Another absolute indication of DLC

disruption is abnormal widening of the anterior disk space on neutral or extension radiographs.

The interspinous ligament is the weakest ligament in the subaxial cervical spine. Consequently, radiographic evidence of interspinous process widening indicates incompetence of the DLC only if lateral flexion radiographs demonstrate abnormal facet alignment or angulation of greater than 11 degrees at the involved interspace.[3]

Neurologic Status

The neurologic status of the patient can be an indicator of the degree of spinal column injury and can influence the decision whether the patient should undergo surgical intervention, in particular if new neurologic deficits are present. In the SLIC system, neurologic status is defined as intact, root injury, complete cord injury, or incomplete cord injury. Continued cord compression exists as a modifier in those patients with either complete or incomplete spinal cord injuries. In patients with translational or rotational injuries, assessment of spinal cord compression is made after attempted reduction of the injury.[3]

Application of the Subaxial Injury Classification System

Within the SLIC system are three injury axes: morphology, DLC, and neurologic status.[3] A numeric value is generated from each axis, and the tally of the three numbers is the SLIC score; the larger the number, the more severe the injury. The score can be used to guide treatment, but it should not be used in isolation. Both the descriptive information on which the scoring is based and the final score itself are necessary to understand the injury fully and to make treatment decisions (Table 18-1).

Radiographic Evaluation

Determining mechanical stability of the cervical spine is of paramount importance to prevent further

Table 18-1 Subaxial Injury Classification and Scoring System

	Points
Morphology	
No abnormality	0
Compression	1
Burst	2
Distraction	3
Rotation or translation	4
Diskoligamentous Complex	
Intact	0
Indeterminate	1
Disrupted	2
Neurologic Status	
Intact	0
Root injury	1
Complete cord injury	2
Incomplete cord injury	3
Presence of continued cord compression in the setting of spinal cord injury	+1

Modified from Vaccaro AR, Fehlings MG, Dvorak MF, editors: *Spine and spinal cord trauma: evidence-based management*, New York, 2011, Thieme.

displacement and late deformity, either of which can cause pain or neurologic dysfunction. In most cases, mechanical instability manifests as abnormal alignment or static deformity on routine radiographic studies. Based on cadaveric studies, White and Punjabi and their colleagues defined cervical spine instability as follows: (1) destruction of either all the anterior or all the posterior elements, thereby rendering them unable to function; (2) more than 3.5 mm of displacement of one vertebra in relation to another anteriorly or posteriorly; and (3) greater than 11 degrees of rotational difference between adjacent vertebra.[4]

Anteroposterior, lateral, and open-mouth odontoid views are the traditional radiographic views for symptomatic patients after traumatic cervical spine injury. The reported sensitivity of the three-view series for detecting injury to the subaxial spine has been reported to range from 53% to 83%.[5,6] In selected patients, upright radiographs may help identify more subtle instability patterns. The role of dynamic flexion-extension radiographs to determine instability is limited in the acute setting because of pain, muscle spasm, and limited cervical excursion. Thin-cut computed tomography with sagittal and coronal reconstructions has been more widely used in the acute trauma setting to identify fractures and dislocations, and this may be a more sensitive tool for detecting acute injuries.[5]

MRI may be more beneficial for evaluating for more subtle forms of instability, in particular for assessing ligamentous integrity. However, although MRI is sensitive in identifying ligamentous injury, the clinical significance of these findings is controversial, and decisions should therefore be based on the patient's entire clinical picture. Because MRI has a moderate positive predictive value of detecting ligamentous injury, it can lead to a high number of false-positive results. Thus, direct evidence of a posterior ligamentous complex injury shown by MRI should not be used in isolation to assess mechanical stability or determine a treatment plan.[7] MRI may be most useful in the evaluation of an obtunded patient or uncooperative patient in whom physical examination is not possible. Finally, when surgery is contemplated, MRI can provide valuable information on the location and degree of stenosis, the presence of associated epidural hematoma, and evidence of spinal cord signal change and intraspinal edema or hemorrhaging.

Surgical Treatment

The treatment of subaxial cervical trauma is based on the fracture pattern, the suspected mechanism of injury, spinal alignment, the neurologic injury, and expected long-term stability.[3] Determining the need for surgical intervention in the cervical spine can be difficult. Algorithms that correlate treatment with classification systems have been developed, but the vast spectrum of injury makes strict surgical indications difficult.

The fundamental principles of operative intervention are to maximize ultimate neurologic function through neural decompression and to restore spinal alignment and stability while preserving motion segments when possible. In general, the choice of surgical approach,

whether anterior or posterior, is based on the location of the pathologic features and the extent of instability. Combined anterior and posterior approaches may be necessary if the extent of the injury warrants them.[2]

Ultimately, no single surgical management has been determined for all subaxial spine injuries, and considerations should be individualized to the injury, the associated comorbidities of the patient, and the surgeon's experience and preference.

Compression and Burst Injuries

Compression and burst injuries to the subaxial spine typically are caused by axial loading. These injuries can result in end plate and vertebral body injury with or without disruption of the DLC. Neurologic status and the presence of residual spinal cord compression typically dictate treatment.

In burst-type fractures in which bone is retropulsed into the spinal canal and causes neurologic injury, anterior corpectomy and stabilization comprise the preferred treatment (Figs. 18-1 to 18-3). This treatment allows for direct removal of the impinging bone and realignment and stabilization of the cervical spine. In the presence of intact posterior elements, anterior decompression (corpectomy), fixation, and strut graft provide adequate stability.[8]

Aebi and colleagues reported on 22 patients with burst or teardrop injuries who were treated with anterior bisegmental bone grafting and plating, with a mean follow-up

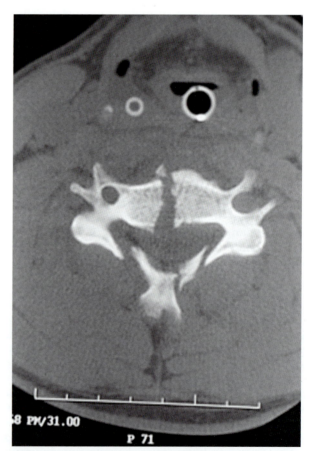

FIGURE 18-1 Axial view computed tomographic scan of a C5 burst fracture in a 23-year-old man who was involved in a motorcycle collision in which he was ejected from the motorcycle at 65 mph.

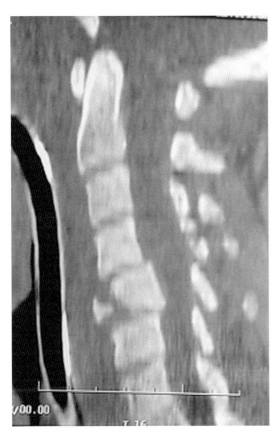

FIGURE 18-2 Sagittal view computed tomographic scan of a C5 burst fracture.

of 40 months. These investigators concluded that anterior bone grafting and plating comprise a safe and reliable treatment option for these injuries.[9]

Distraction Injuries

Hyperextension distraction injuries typically occur in the stiff spondylotic or ankylosed spine and can be highly unstable. These injuries occur through distraction in the anterior column with sequential propagation through the middle and posterior columns. Radiographically, this injury is typically seen with distraction through the anterior column, usually with a gaped open disk space. The presence of posterior element fractures is typically the result of posterior compression of the lamina or facet joints. Because these injuries are generally highly unstable, they are frequently associated with an incomplete central spinal cord injury.[8] A widened disk space may be the only apparent radiographic abnormality, and computed tomography may reveal bilateral pedicle fractures. Patients with ankylosing spondylitis are the paradigm for this injury pattern, although this injury is also observed in patients with near ankylosis secondary to advanced degenerative spondylosis[2] (Figs. 18-4 to 18-6).

Surgical management of these lesions should be customized to the patient, the specific injury, and the surgeon's preference. When injuries occur through a spondylotic and ankylosed spine, posterior segmental stabilization may be necessary to achieve adequate fixation points above and below the injury and thus provide adequate spinal stability. Because these injuries act

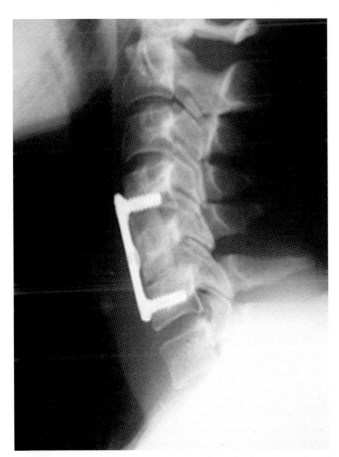

FIGURE 18-3 Lateral view postoperative radiograph of a patient with a C5 burst fracture treated with anterior decompression and stabilization.

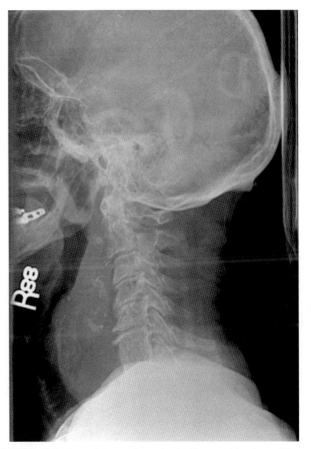

FIGURE 18-4 Lateral view radiograph of a 75-year-old patient with pre-existing spondylosis who was involved in a head-on motor vehicle collision.

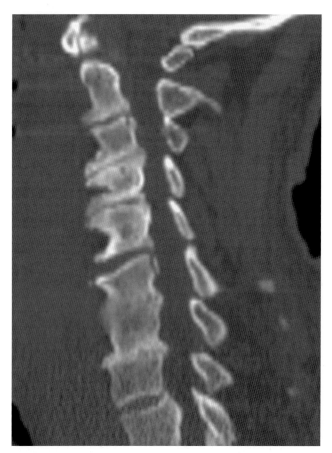

FIGURE 18-5 Sagittal view computed tomographic scan revealing disk space widening in a patient with spondylosis who was involved in a motor vehicle collision and sustained a hyperextension injury.

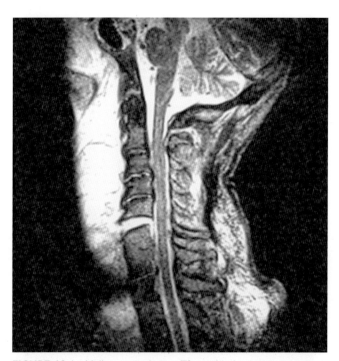

FIGURE 18-6 Midline sagittal view T2-weighted magnetic resonance image revealing disk space widening and edema in the posterior ligamentous structures of a patient with ankylosis who sustained a hyperextension injury.

as "long bone fractures," single-level fixation above and below the fracture may not be sufficient. In addition, the presence of osteoporosis in these patients can make anterior fixation difficult (Fig. 18-7).

Depending on the degree of anterior distraction, a staged or same-day anterior stabilization and fusion procedure to provide anterior column support can be considered. However, if adequate fixation is achieved posteriorly and solid fusion is achieved, an anterior procedure is not always required, even in patients with significant anterior distraction.

In patients with a distractive extension injury and a normal, mobile, nonankylosed spine, consideration of isolated anterior diskectomy and fusion with plate fixation alone may be sufficient. Conversely, in the case of focal or fixed kyphosis, or anterior compression from disk protrusion or a spondylotic bar, anterior surgical decompression and fusion are indicated.[8]

Flexion Injuries

In contradistinction to distraction injuries, hyperflexion injuries begin with distraction of the posterior elements that sequentially propagates anteriorly. In these cases, disruption of the supraspinous and interspinous ligaments with injury to the facet and facet joint can result in injuries ranging from nondisplaced unilateral facet fractures and lateral mass separations to complete bilateral facet fracture-dislocations.

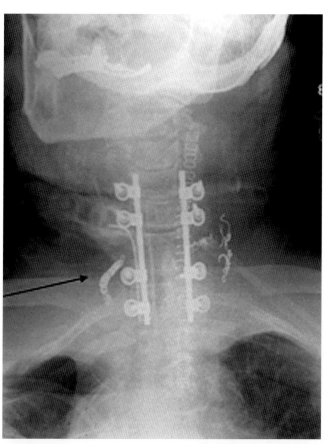

FIGURE 18-7 Postoperative lateral view radiograph of a patient with spondylosis who sustained a hyperextension injury and was treated with posterior stabilization (*arrow*).

The role of closed reduction and traction before operative intervention for facet subluxations or dislocations is controversial and warrants discussion. It can dictate the decision whether to perform an anterior or a posterior procedure initially. One of the main controversies focuses on whether MRI is necessary before reducing facet dislocations to assess for the presence of an occult herniated disk.

In 1991, Eismont and associates reported on 6 of 86 patients seen between 1980 and 1987 who sustained a fracture or dislocation of a cervical facet with associated disk herniation and spinal cord compression. These investigators recommended MRI to rule out a herniated nucleus pulposus in patients with worsening neurologic symptoms or neurologic deficit after the injury, in patients for whom closed reduction would be difficult, and in patients undergoing operative intervention.[10] In contrast, Vadera and colleagues from Thomas Jefferson University in Philadelphia maintained that baseline MRI in an awake, alert, cooperative patient is unnecessary before closed reduction, provided the patient is closely monitored neurologically during the reduction. These investigators asserted that postreduction MRI is necessary to determine the presence of a herniated nucleus pulposus and to help define the appropriate operative approach.[11]

Regardless of whether prereduction MRI is performed, reduction of dislocated facets is the most effective way to decompress the spinal cord, and it should be done as expeditiously as possible in patients presenting with neurologic deficits. The decision whether to use open or closed reduction depends on the patient's presentation, the institutional resources, and the physician's experience and preference. Closed reduction is contingent on an awake, alert, and cooperative patient. For closed reduction to be successful, the circumstances must be such that the area of interest can be radiographed and serial neurologic examinations can be performed on the patient. In these instances, closed reduction is warranted, and MRI likely is unnecessary. Closed reduction is accomplished by adding sequential weight to skull tongs or a halo ring. Serial radiographs and neurologic examinations are performed as increasing weight is applied.[12,13] In most cases, reduction can be obtained with a weight of 80 pounds or less, although the use of up to 140 pounds of traction has been reported.

When MRI reveals a disk fragment dorsal to the posterior cortex of the caudal vertebral body with a facet dislocation or subluxation, an anterior diskectomy-decompression procedure is preferred before reduction of the dislocation. This procedure may be followed by anterior reduction of the facet dislocation and placement of an interbody graft and an anterior cervical plate. Because this injury is primarily a posterior ligamentous lesion, complete apposition of the facets, placement of a trapezoidal interbody graft, and contouring of the plate into lordosis optimize the stability of the construct.

Razack and associates conducted a 6-year retrospective study of patients who were treated at a single institution and who had traumatic cervical bilateral facet fracture-dislocations. All fracture-dislocations that could be aligned with traction were later stabilized with anterior cervical diskectomy and fusion. Twenty-two patients were

followed up for an average of 32 months. At final follow-up, all patients had evidence of radiographic fusion.[14] If anterior reduction of the dislocation cannot be safely accomplished, a graft is placed in the disk space after diskectomy, and posterior reduction and stabilization are performed. If the graft displaces during the reduction maneuver, repeat placement of the graft anteriorly may be required. The use of an antikick plate can be considered and may reduce the risk of graft displacement during the posterior reduction maneuver.

When facet dislocation without a herniated disk is treated surgically, anterior or posterior stabilization is possible (Figs. 18-8 to 18-10). The choice of procedure may be influenced by available equipment and the surgeon's preference. However, consideration of anterior issues, such as the risk of dysphagia and potential injury to visceral structures, should be weighed against the additional muscle dissection and wound infection risk of posterior procedures.[8] In addition, performing the surgical procedure anteriorly avoids the need for positioning the patient prone with an unstable cervical spine. One clinical situation in which anterior fixation may be beneficial is fracture of the facet and ipsilateral pedicle, or lateral mass separation. In this injury, only a single-level fusion would be possible anteriorly, whereas posteriorly a multiple-level fusion would be required.[2]

Other specific considerations for anterior fixation for the management of unilateral or bilateral facet injuries

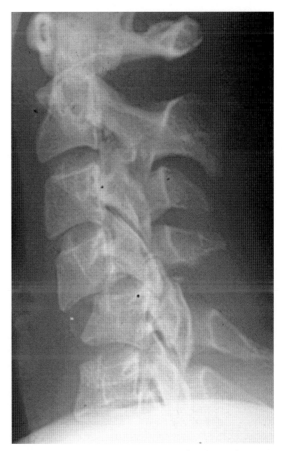

FIGURE 18-8 Lateral view radiograph of C4-C5 bilateral facet dislocation in a patient injured during a diving accident. At presentation, the injury was classified as C4 American Spinal Injury Association grade A.

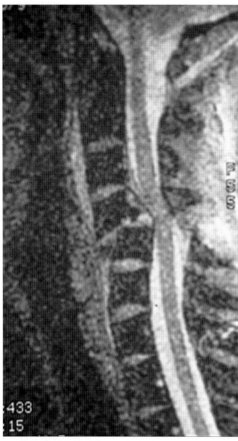

FIGURE 18-9   Sagittal view T2-weighted magnetic resonance image of C4-C5 bilateral facet dislocation.

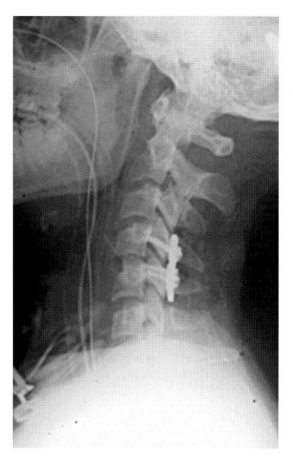

FIGURE 18-10   Postoperative lateral view radiograph of a patient with C4-C5 bilateral facet dislocation treated with posterior stabilization with lateral mass screws.

include careful preoperative imaging to evaluate for subtle vertebral end plate fractures or displaced fractures of the facet joints, for which consideration of circumferential fixation may be necessary, and consideration given to multiple-level anterior fixation to achieve adequate initial spinal stability. Another potential pitfall of anterior fixation is placement of too large an anterior graft. This situation can cause neurologic injury through a stretch-type mechanism and can distract the facet joints at the level of injury.

Spinal Cord Injury Secondary to Hyperextension Injuries without Mechanical Instability

Spinal cord injuries after hyperextension-type injuries without mechanical instability comprise another subset of subaxial spinal injuries and are considered briefly here. These patients are different from those with distraction injuries described earlier. Most notably, the hallmark presentation of these patients is acute neurologic deficit without mechanical instability. Typically, these are older patients with baseline spinal stenosis from degenerative spondylosis who sustain hyperextension injury typically from a low-energy injury such as a ground-level fall or a fall down a flight of stairs.

Although any spinal cord injury pattern can occur, the most common is the central cord syndrome, with greater neurologic involvement of the upper than the lower extremity. This syndrome typically occurs secondary to compression of the spinal cord between the disko-osteophytic complex anteriorly and the hypertrophied ligamentum flavum and facet capsule posteriorly. As a result, these patients can have neurologic instability or deficit without mechanical instability.

Optimal timing for the surgical management of these lesions is controversial. Some investigators previously suggested a benefit to early decompression, whereas others suggested that as long as the spine is stable and the patient is neurologically intact or improving, initial observation is an acceptable treatment option. In general, if a patient presents with profound and static neurologic deficits, surgical intervention is warranted. Similarly, patients with neurologic deficits and the presence of mechanical instability do not fall into this group, and early surgical intervention should be considered as well.

Chen and associates conducted a prospective study of 37 patients with cervical spondylosis and incomplete spinal cord injury after minor neck trauma. These investigators evaluated surgical and nonsurgical treatment in these 37 patients. More than 60% of the patients had neurologic recovery of a muscle grade or higher, but recovery was found to be faster in those treated operatively.[15] Guest and colleagues compared clinical outcomes in 50 patients who presented with traumatic central cord syndrome and underwent early (<24 hours) and late (>24 hours) surgical intervention. These investigators found that in patients with central cord syndrome secondary to acute disk herniation or fracture-dislocation, early surgical intervention resulted in greater overall motor improvement.[16] However, the study population evaluated by Guest and associates included patients with both mechanically stable and unstable conditions.

REFERENCES

1. Patel AA, Hurlbert RJ, Bono CM, et al.: Classification and surgical decision making in acute subaxial cervical spine trauma, *Spine (Phila Pa 1976)* 35(Suppl 21):S228–S234, 2010.
2. Banagan K, Gelb D: Surgical management of cervical spine fractures. In Bridwell KH, editor: *The textbook of spinal surgery*, Philadelphia, 2011, Lippincott Williams & Wilkins.
3. Vaccaro AR, Hulbert RJ, Patel AA, et al.: The subaxial cervical spine injury classification system: a novel approach to recognize the importance of morphology, neurology, and integrity of the disco-ligamentous complex, *Spine (Phila Pa 1976)* 32:2365–2374, 2007.
4. White AA 3rd, Johnson RM, Panjabi MM, Southwick WO: Biomechanical analysis of clinical stability in the cervical spine, *Clin Orthop Relat Res (109)*85–96, 1975.
5. Mathen R, Inaba K, Munera F, et al.: Prospective evaluation of multislice computed tomography versus plain radiographic cervical spine clearance in trauma patients, *J Trauma* 62:1427–1431, 2007.
6. West OC, Anbari MM, Pilgram TK, Wilson AJ: Acute cervical spine trauma: diagnostic performance of single-view versus three-view radiographic screening, *Radiology* 204:819–823, 1997.
7. Rihn JA, Fisher C, Harrop J, et al.: Assessment of the posterior ligamentous complex following acute cervical spine trauma, *J Bone Joint Surg Am* 92:583–589, 2010.
8. Dvorak MF, Fisher CG, Fehlings MG, et al.: The surgical approach to subaxial cervical spine injuries: an evidence-based algorithm based on the SLIC classification system, *Spine (Phila Pa 1976)* 32:2620–2629, 2007.
9. Aebi M, Zuber K, Marchesi D: Treatment of cervical spine injuries with anterior plating. Indications, techniques, and results, *Spine (Phila Pa 1976)* 16(Suppl 3):S38–S45, 1991.
10. Eismont FJ, Arena MJ, Green BA: Extrusion of an intervertebral disc associated with traumatic subluxation or dislocation of cervical facets: case report, *J Bone Joint Surg Am* 73:1555–1560, 1991.
11. Vadera S, Ratliff J, Brown Z, et al.: Management of cervical facet dislocations, *Semin Spine Surg* 19:250–255, 2007.
12. Grant GA, Mirza SK, Chapman JR, et al.: Risk of early closed reduction in cervical spine subluxation injuries, *J Neurosurg* 90(Suppl 1):13–18, 1999.
13. Wiseman DB, Bellabarba C, Mirza SK, Chapman J: Anterior versus posterior surgical treatment for traumatic cervical spine dislocation, *Curr Opin Orthop* 14:174–181, 2003.
14. Razack N, Green BA, Levi AD: The management of traumatic cervical bilateral facet fracture-dislocations with unicortical anterior plates, *J Spinal Disord* 13:374–381, 2000.
15. Chen T, Dickman CA, Eleraky M, Sonntag V: The role of decompression for acute incomplete cervical spinal cord injury in cervical spondylosis, *Spine (Phila Pa 1976)* 23:2398–2403, 1998.
16. Guest J, Eleraky MA, Apostolides PJ, et al.: Traumatic central cord syndrome: results of surgical management, *J Neurosurg* 97(Suppl 1):25–32, 2002.

19 Spinal Cord Injuries and Syndromes

Dave J. Seecharan and Paul M. Arnold

CHAPTER PREVIEW

Chapter Synopsis   Spinal cord injury (SCI) is a serious worldwide health problem, often resulting in significant morbidity and permanent neurologic deficits. The American Spinal Injury Association (ASIA) impairment scale can be used to classify the extent of the injury and can also serve as a predictor of neurologic outcome. Several common discrete clinical syndromes are associated with incomplete SCI and cover a broad range of neurologic dysfunction. This chapter reviews the classification, the common incomplete spinal cord syndromes, and the conus medullaris and cauda equina syndromes.

Important Points   ASIA uses a standardized protocol to assess patients with traumatic SCIs to define a neurologic level.

Spinal shock identifies the period of spinal cord dysfunction after a traumatic injury that results in complete loss of motor, sensory, and reflex function below the level of injury.

The significance of spinal shock lies in that determination of the presence of complete versus incomplete SCI, and therefore ultimate prognosis, is impossible during this period.

Neurogenic shock should not be confused with spinal shock; its occurrence is secondary to disruption of the sympathetic pathway, and it manifests as hypotension with bradycardia.

Central cord syndrome is the most common SCI and manifests with quadriparesis with upper greater than lower extremity involvement.

Brown-Séquard syndrome manifests with ipsilateral hemiplegia, ipsilateral loss of proprioception, and contralateral loss of pain and temperature secondary to spinal cord hemisection.

Anterior spinal cord syndrome manifests with complete motor paralysis and loss of pain and temperature sensation with sparing of proprioception and vibration sense secondary to injury to the anterior spinal cord from direct trauma or vascular injury typically to the anterior spinal artery.

Posterior spinal cord syndromes manifest with preservation of motor and pain and temperature with loss of proprioception and vibration sense below the level of injury.

Conus medullaris and cauda equina syndromes are two complex clinical neurologic disorders that are seen with injury to the terminal elements of the spinal cord.

Classification of Spinal Cord Injury

Spinal cord injury (SCI) can be assessed using the International Standards for Neurological Classification of Spinal Cord Injury (ISCSCI), developed by the American Spinal Injury Association (ASIA). This standardized protocol can be used to assess patients with traumatic SCI and to define a neurologic level of injury.[1] This standardized system can be used not only as a framework for classification of injuries but also as a predictor of neurologic and functional outcomes, as well as long-term prognosis.[2] The ASIA standard is applicable only to traumatic SCI and should not be used for the assessment of nontraumatic SCI.

The ASIA assessment consists of a neurologic evaluation of a sensory point within 28 dermatomes on both the right and left sides of the body and an evaluation of muscle strength within 10 myotomes on both sides of the body. The sensory level refers to the most caudal segment of the spinal cord with intact sensory function on both sides of the body. In a similar fashion, the motor level refers to the most caudal myotome that has motor strength of 3 out of 5 or better, with normal strength 5 out of 5 in the level above. The neurologic level of injury is the most caudal level at which both motor and sensory levels are intact. Patients with no neurologic injury have a score of 100 (grade 5 muscle strength, 10 myotomes, left and right sides).

Using the ASIA impairment scale, SCI is classified into levels A to E, in descending order of severity. Complete SCI (ASIA A) is defined as the absence of sensory and motor function in the most caudal sacral segment of the spinal cord. In comparison, incomplete injury (ASIA B to E) is defined as partial preservation of sensory or motor function below the neurologic level, including the most caudal sacral segment. ASIA B is defined as intact sensory function below the neurologic level extending through the sacral segments without intact motor function. ASIA C is defined as intact motor function below the neurologic level, with strength in most key muscles below the level at less than 3 out of 5. ASIA D is defined as intact motor function below the neurologic level, with strength in most key muscles below the injured level greater than 3 out of 5. A patient with completely intact sensory and motor function would be considered ASIA E.

The testing of the most caudal sacral function at S4 to S5 is critical to assessing the extent of the injury within this assessment protocol. Sacral sensation may be assessed by pinprick or light touch sensation at the anal mucocutaneous junction, as well as deep anal sensation with digital rectal examination. The presence of sacral sensation in the absence of distal motor function (sacral sparing) may indicate an incomplete SCI and therefore prognosticate a better potential for neurologic recovery. Motor function at this level is tested by the presence of voluntary contraction of the external anal sphincter on digital examination. The integrity of the connections between neurons within the spinal cord at this level can be monitored by testing for the polysynaptic bulbocavernosus reflex. In normal individuals, involuntary contraction of the rectal sphincter occurs with pinching of the glans penis or by tugging on an indwelling Foley catheter (normal or present bulbocavernosus reflex). The absence of this reflex indicates disruption of supraspinal inputs to the outflow tracts of the lower spinal cord and suggests spinal shock.

The assessment of complete versus incomplete SCI is confounded by the presence of spinal shock, which is a transient period immediately following an injury. Spinal shock manifests as flaccid paralysis, complete loss of sensation, and complete areflexia below the level of the injury. These initial symptoms are followed by a period of hypertonia and spasticity, as well as a variable return of motor and sensory function. The initial phase of spinal shock usually lasts between 24 and 72 hours and can be monitored by assessing the bulbocavernosus reflex.

The dysfunction seen in the initial phase of spinal shock results from a loss of excitatory input to alpha and gamma motor neurons, interneurons, and preganglionic sympathetic neurons from supraspinal centers, as well as increased spinal inhibition secondary to reduced descending inhibition of spinal inhibitory pathways. The spinal neurons, which are isolated from supraspinal input, retain their synaptic contacts from reflex afferents and interneurons and over time acquire new contacts from sprouting of neurons. This feature accounts for the spasticity and hyperreflexia that develop in the later stages of spinal shock.[3]

The return of the bulbocavernosus reflex usually marks the end of the initial phase of spinal shock. Therefore, the determination of complete versus incomplete SCI cannot be made during spinal shock, and the prognosis for recovery should be delayed until return of bulbocavernosus reflex and the end of spinal shock. In the uncommon event that the bulbocavernosus reflex does not return (conus medullaris injury or direct injury to the S3 and lower reflex arc), then the end of spinal shock can be assumed to be after 72 hours from the time of the initial injury.

Spinal shock should be differentiated from neurogenic shock. Neurogenic shock is caused by disruption of the sympathetic pathways within the brain or spinal cord that results in unopposed vagal tone and increased vascular dilatation, with a consequent decrease in systemic vascular resistance. In this situation, hypotension, bradycardia, and hypothermia result. This autonomic dysfunction is most often observed in spinal injuries above the T6 level.

Central Cord Syndrome

Central cord syndrome (CCS) is the most common type of incomplete SCI. It manifests as symmetric incomplete quadriparesis, which disproportionately affects the upper extremities relative to the lower extremities. Sensory impairment is variable, and urinary retention is common.

CCS commonly occurs as a result of hyperextension injury in the presence of previous underlying cervical spondylosis. Injury occurs from posterior compression of the spinal cord by buckling of the ligamentum flavum or by anterior compression by osteophytes. It may also be associated with fracture and disruption of the structural spinal elements in which anteroposterior compressive forces direct the greatest damage to the central portions of the spinal cord parenchyma (Fig. 19-1).

The pathophysiology of this syndrome is thought to be related to the somatotopic organization of the corticospinal tract within the spinal cord. The lamination of the corticospinal tract is organized such that the sacral components are the most lateral, with the lumbar, thoracic, and cervical components advancing medially toward the central spinal canal. Damage to axons traveling within the spinal cord may stem from concussive forces causing contusion of the spinal cord and stasis of axoplasmic flow resulting in edema. Autopsy studies in patients with CCS found hemorrhage in the central portion of the spinal cord, a finding that favors a worse neurologic outcome; however, more recent histopathologic studies

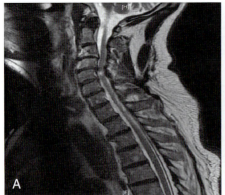 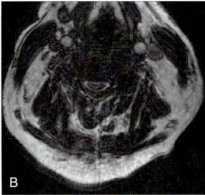 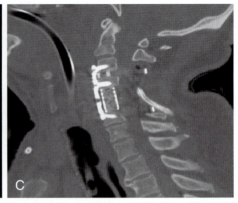

FIGURE 19-1 A 57-year-old man suffered a fall from a tree. He presented with bilateral upper and lower extremity weakness, with very weak hand grip strength. Sagittal (**A**) and axial (**B**) magnetic resonance images show severe cervical spinal cord stenosis, with signal change in the spinal cord. The patient suffered central cord syndrome. He underwent an anterior and posterior procedure within 24 hours of injury (**C**), and he recovered nearly all motor function.

demonstrated that the damage seen in CCS is predominantly white matter injury.[4]

Early surgical treatment of CCS is still somewhat controversial. Several studies showed benefits of early surgical intervention to decompress the spinal cord in patients with radiographic compression on magnetic resonance imaging or abnormal signal intensity within the spinal cord. In patients without a definite structural lesion or signal abnormality on magnetic resonance imaging, a favorable neurologic prognosis can be predicted following nonsurgical treatment, with significant recovery occurring by 6 weeks. Patients with severe initial neurologic damage and older patients tend to show poorer recovery.[5-8]

Brown-Séquard Syndrome

Brown-Séquard syndrome (BSS) manifests with ipsilateral hemiplegia, ipsilateral loss of proprioception, and contralateral loss of pain and temperature. BSS usually occurs from penetrating trauma resulting in physiologic hemisection of the spinal cord; however, this syndrome may also be caused by blunt trauma or other spinal disease processes, including hematoma, syringomyelia, neoplasms, myelitis, demyelinating disease, and disk herniation.

The distinct neurologic findings in BSS are secondary to disruption of three separate neural pathways within the spinal cord. Damage to fibers within the descending lateral corticospinal tracts and the ascending dorsal columns, both of which decussate in the medulla, results in ipsilateral hemiplegia and ipsilateral loss of proprioception, respectively. Disruption of the fibers running in the ascending lateral spinothalamic tract, which decussate within three levels of the dorsal root entrance, results in the contralateral loss of pain and temperature sensation.

Management of BSS is usually nonsurgical and focuses primarily on rehabilitation, with surgical indications reserved for patients with spinal instability or spinal cord compression.[9] For patients participating in a comprehensive rehabilitation program, BSS carries a relatively good prognosis, and many patients show almost full recovery of motor function within 3 to 6 months.[10,11]

Anterior Spinal Cord Syndrome

Anterior spinal cord syndrome (ASCS) manifests with complete motor paralysis and loss of pain and temperature sensation, with sparing of proprioception and vibration sense. Motor loss in ASCS tends to affect the lower extremities to a greater extent than the upper extremities. ASCS is usually the result of injury causing hyperflexion and axial loading. It can also be seen in the setting of central disk herniations, fracture-dislocation injuries, vascular lesions or injuries to the anterior spinal artery, compression fractures, and other lesions that compress the ventral aspect of the spinal canal.

The pathophysiology of ASCS results from damage that occurs primarily within the anterior two thirds of the spinal cord and that affects the corticospinal tract and spinothalamic tracts, thus causing motor paralysis and loss of pain and temperature sensation, respectively. The posterior third of the spinal cord containing the dorsal columns is usually uninvolved and accounts for the sparing of proprioceptive and vibration sense. Damage to the anterior portion of the spinal cord can occur by direct insult to the anterior cord itself or by vascular insufficiency related to insult to the anterior spinal artery and its vascular territory within the spinal cord.

ASCS carries the least favorable prognosis of the spinal cord syndromes; only 10% to 15% of patients will show functional recovery. Good prognostic signs include incomplete loss of pain and temperature sensation and progressive recovery of neurologic function within the first 24 hours.[12] Surgical intervention for ASCS is usually reserved for injuries with radiographic demonstration of persistent cord compressive or spinal instability. Several studies showed that early intervention for decompression (surgery within 24 hours of injury) does not provide improved outcome over delayed intervention (surgery after >24 hours).[13,14]

Posterior Spinal Cord Syndrome

Posterior spinal cord syndrome (PSCS) manifests with preservation of motor function, pain, and temperature,

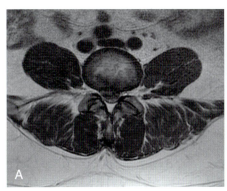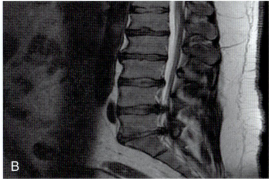

FIGURE 19-2   A 38-year-old man was at work and had a sudden onset of low back pain, bilateral lower extremity pain and weakness, and urinary incontinence. Axial (**A**) and sagittal (**B**) magnetic resonance imaging revealed a large herniated disk at L4-L5. The patient underwent emergency diskectomy within 24 hours of symptoms. He regained all lost neurologic function except some right lower extremity numbness.

but loss of proprioception and vibration sense below the level of the injury. PSCS is the most uncommon spinal cord syndrome. Damage to the posterior portion of the spinal cord can occur by direct insult or can be secondary to injury to the posterior spinal arteries. Although these patients typically are able to ambulate, because they lack proprioception and vibratory sense, they often require direct visualization of their feet to walk. As a result, these patients are usually unable to ambulate in the dark. One uncommon cause of PSCS, tabes dorsalis, typically results from injury to the posterior spinal cord secondary to infections such as syphilis.

Conus Medullaris and Cauda Equina Syndrome

Conus medullaris syndrome (CMS) and cauda equina syndrome (CES) are two complex clinical neurologic disorders that are seen with injury to the terminal elements of the spinal cord. The spinal cord terminates in the conus medullaris, the tapered caudal segment of the cord. The nerve roots of the lower lumbar and sacral spine descend from the conus to form the cauda equina before they exit the spinal canal through their respective neuroforamina. The conus medullaris usually terminates between the levels of the T11 and L1 vertebral bodies, and, as such, damage often occurs in association with thoracolumbar injuries at these levels. The spinal cord and nerve roots in this area are vulnerable to injury because of their location at the thoracolumbar junction, a transitional area between the rigid kyphotic thoracic spine and the more mobile lordotic lumbar spine. CMS and CES are caused by lesions that compress the conus medullaris and nerve roots, such as herniated disk, bone fragment, hematoma, infection, or tumor; the most common cause is disk herniation.

The nerve fibers traveling in this region of the spine are responsible for function of the bladder, bowels, genitals, and lower extremities. Patients typically present with a combination of lower back and leg pain, lower extremity paralysis and paresthesias, saddle anesthesia, and bowel and bladder dysfunction.

Several features distinguish CMS from CES. In CMS, deficits are usually symmetric and tend to affect the lower

extremities bilaterally. Patients often present with symptoms of spinal cord compression and upper motor neuron dysfunction such as hyperreflexia and spasticity and even fasciculations. The spinal levels affected in CMS are usually T11 to L1. In contrast, in CES, deficits are usually asymmetric and unilateral, and they affect a single extremity. Moreover, patients present with radiculopathy and lower motor neuron signs such as areflexia and atrophy secondary to compression of the nerve roots. CES usually affects the levels below L1 (Fig. 19-2).

Bowel and bladder dysfunction is a typical finding in both CMS and CES, and it initially manifests with constipation, as well as difficulty in initiating micturition. These symptoms then progress to fecal incontinence and painless urinary retention with overflow incontinence. Physical examination usually reveals an enlarged, palpable bladder and decreased rectal tone and sensation. Patients may also have loss of the bulbocavernosus reflex.

CMS and CES have comparable outcomes. Most patients show improvement in motor function and ambulatory status with a varying degree of residual bowel and bladder dysfunction. The most meaningful indicator of recovery is the initial severity of the neurologic deficit; patients with incomplete injuries are the most likely to show improvement. Surgical intervention provides the benefits of shorter hospital stays and earlier rehabilitation over conservative management. Surgical decompression and stabilization from a posterior approach have the same outcome as an anterior approach, with the benefits of reduced morbidity and familiarity of the surgeon with the procedure.[15] Anterior decompression may offer a potential benefit over the posterior approach in regard to the return of bladder function, specifically with delayed interventions.[15]

Timing of surgical decompression in CMS and CES remains a controversial topic. A review of the literature suggests that CES is a diagnostic and surgical emergency, and surgical treatment within a 24-hour window is desirable for preservation of function. Worse outcomes have been demonstrated when decompression is delayed for more than 48 hours. Few data have evaluated the outcome of decompressive surgery within the 24- to 48-hour time frame.[16]

REFERENCES

1. Maynard FM Jr., Bracken MB, Creasey G, et al.: International standards for neurological and functional classification of spinal cord injury: American Spinal Injury Association, *Spinal Cord* 35:266–274, 1997.
2. Burns AS, Ditunno JF: Establishing prognosis and maximizing functional outcomes after spinal cord injury: a review of current and future directions in rehabilitation management, *Spine (Phila Pa 1976)* 26(Suppl):S137–S145, 2001.
3. Ditunno JF, Little JW, Tessler A, Burns AS: Spinal shock revisited: a four-phase model, *Spinal Cord* 42:383–395, 2004.
4. Li X-F, Dai L-Y: Acute central cord syndrome: injury mechanisms and stress features, *Spine (Phila Pa 1976)* 35:E955–964, 2010.
5. Nowak DD, Lee JK, Gelb DE, et al.: Central cord syndrome, *J Am Acad Orthop Surg* 17:756–765, 2009.
6. Ishida Y, Tominaga T: Predictors of neurologic recovery in acute central cervical cord injury with only upper extremity impairment, *Spine (Phila Pa 1976)* 27:1652–1658, 2007.
7. Song J, Mizuno J, Inoue T, Nakagawa H: Clinical evaluation of traumatic central cord syndrome: emphasis on clinical significance of prevertebral hyperintensity, cord compression, and intramedullary high-signal intensity on magnetic resonance imaging, *Surg Neurol* 65:117–123, 2006.
8. McKinley W, Santos K, Meade M, Brooke K: Incidence and outcomes of spinal cord injury clinical syndromes, *J Spinal Cord Med* 30:215–224, 2007.
9. Kohno M, Takahashi H, Yamakawa K, et al.: Postoperative prognosis of Brown-Séquard-type myelopathy in patients with cervical lesions, *Surg Neurol* 51:241–246, 1999.
10. Miranda P, Gomez P, Alday R, et al.: Brown-Séquard syndrome after blunt cervical spine trauma: clinical and radiological correlations, *Eur Spine J* 16:1165–1170, 2007.
11. Roth EJ, Park T, Pang T, et al.: Traumatic cervical Brown-Séquard and Brown-Séquard–plus syndromes: the spectrum of presentations and outcomes, *Paraplegia* 29:582–589, 1991.
12. Foo D, Subrahmanyan TS, Rossier AB: Post-traumatic acute anterior spinal cord syndrome, *Paraplegia* 19:201–205, 1981.
13. Vaccaro AR, Daugherty RJ, Sheehan TP, et al.: Neurologic outcome of early versus late surgery for cervical spinal cord injury, *Spine (Phila Pa 1976)* 22:2609–2613, 1997.
14. Levi L, Wolf A, Rigamonti D, et al.: Anterior decompression in cervical spine trauma: does the timing of surgery affect the outcome? *Neurosurgery* 29:216–222, 1991.
15. Kingwell SP, Curt A, Dvorak MF: Factors affecting neurological outcome in traumatic conus medullaris and cauda equina injuries, *Neurosurg Focus* 25:E7, 2008.
16. Shapiro S: Medical realities of cauda equina syndrome secondary to lumbar disk herniation, *Spine (Phila Pa 1976)* 25:348–351, 2000.

Traumatic Arterial Injuries: Diagnosis and Management

20

Chris A. Cornett, Gregory Grabowski, and James D. Kang

CHAPTER PREVIEW

Chapter Synopsis   Vertebral artery injuries (VAIs) are becoming increasingly recognized as more screening protocols are being used. Angiography is the gold standard, but many centers are using computed tomography angiography (CTA) or magnetic resonance angiography (MRA) as the initial screening study. Treatment is recommended for all patients with symptomatic injuries. Treatment of asymptomatic injuries remains controversial, and treatments should be individualized to each particular situation.

Important Points   Traumatic VAIs have an incidence of 0.5% in all patients who have sustained blunt trauma.

Among patients with traumatic VAIs, 70% will have an associated cervical spine fracture.

Most VAIs occur after motor vehicle accidents or falls, and they occur in the second segment of the vertebral artery (V2).

Angiography is the gold standard study for diagnosis of VAI.

Many centers are now using CTA or MRA as a screening study.

Treatments include observation, antiplatelet agents, anticoagulation, and endovascular interventions.

Symptomatic injuries should be treated.

Treatment of asymptomatic injuries is controversial and should be individualized for each case.

Background

Vertebral artery injury (VAI) secondary to blunt trauma has become an increasingly discussed topic. Initially, these injuries were thought to be extremely rare events with minimal significance. However, studies using rigorous screening protocols demonstrated that VAIs occur with some regularity (the overall incidence in blunt trauma is approximately 0.5%) and can be associated with significant morbidity.[1,2] Some of these investigators argued that routine anticoagulation is effective and should be considered for patients with these injuries. However, other studies concluded that no compelling evidence exists to recommend treatment of asymptomatic traumatic blunt VAIs (BVIs).[3,4]

Incidence and Risk Factors

Although the overall incidence of VAI in patients who have sustained blunt trauma is approximately 0.5%, the incidence is certainly higher in certain subsets of patients. Seventy percent of patients with traumatic VAIs have an associated cervical spine fracture.[5] Cervical spine injuries associated with increased VAI include subluxations and dislocations, fractures involving the transverse foramen, and fractures of the upper cervical spine (C1-C3) (Fig. 20-1).[6] Other patients considered at higher risk and potentially requiring screening include those with basilar skull fractures, significant facial fractures, cervical hematomas, neurologic examination findings inconsistent with head computed tomography (CT) scans, or lateralizing neurologic examination findings.

In general, most traumatic BVIs occur after high-energy mechanisms, often with rapid deceleration. Most of these injuries occur after motor vehicle accidents, after falls, or when pedestrians are struck by vehicles. Another rarely cited reason for BVI is chiropractic manipulation. In a large review of published case reports from 1934 to 2003, Ernst found 26 published fatalities associated with chiropractic manipulation.[7] At least 6 of these deaths were

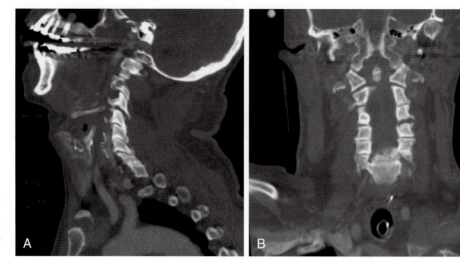

FIGURE 20-1 Sagittal (**A**) and coronal (**B**) computed tomography (CT) images showing facet diastasis at C3-C4 on the *left*, in a patient who was later diagnosed with a vertebral artery injury on CT angiography.

believed to have resulted from vertebral artery dissection. The true incidence of such events is difficult to estimate, however. Aside from traumatic BVI, the other major category of traumatic VAI includes penetrating injuries, such as gunshot wounds and lacerations. Traumatic VAIs from lacerations have a high mortality rate related to bleeding.

Relevant Arterial Anatomy

Arteries such as the vertebral artery each have three main layers that comprise the vessel wall. The intima is composed of endothelial cells. The next layer out is the media, which contains the smooth muscle cells that allow contraction of the vessel lumen. The outer layer is the adventitia, which is composed of collagen bundles. The adventitia also contains the vasa vasorum, or vessels to the vessels.

The vertebral artery usually starts from the subclavian artery and then enters the transverse foramen, usually at C6. This first segment, before the artery enters the transverse foramen, is known as V1. V2 is the second segment, as the artery travels superiorly through the transverse foramen at each level, usually from C6 to C1. The third segment is located from the transverse foramen of C1 to where the artery enters the dura. The fourth segment is from the dural entry site to where it joins the basilar artery. Most traumatic injuries to the vertebral arteries occur at the second (V2) or third (V3) segment, often related to cervical injury at these regions. Investigators have demonstrated that the vertebral artery and nerve root are encased in a fibroligamentous band at the level of the intertransverse space, and this band attaches to the lateral side of the uncinate.[8] Perhaps this tethering of the vertebral artery to the bone helps explain why trauma in this region can easily cause arterial injury.

Types and Classification of Vertebral Artery Injuries

Intimal flaps occur when the intima of the vessel has a tear, which can cause a flap to protrude into the vessel lumen. When the intima is injured and bleeding occurs

BOX 20-1 Types of Injuries

1. Intimal flap
2. Dissection
3. Pseudoaneurysm
4. Occlusion
5. Transection

Table 20-1 Classification of Injuries

Grade I	<25% stenosis of vessel from intramural clot or dissection, or wall irregularity
Grade II	>25% stenosis of vessel from intramural clot or dissection, or raised flap or intraluminal clot
Grade III	Pseudoaneurysms
Grade IV	Occlusions
Grade V	Transections

into the vessel wall, *dissection* can occur. The blood that collects within the vessel wall can cause narrowing of the vessel lumen. When blood is forced through the vessel wall and causes a hematoma, which can cavitate, a *pseudoaneurysm* may form. Pseudoaneurysms can also effectively narrow the vessel lumen. *Occlusions* are complete blockages of the artery. *Transections* are complete arterial divisions (Box 20-1).

Biffl and colleagues developed a grading scale for injuries that has been used for classification of traumatic VAIs.[9] Grade I includes an irregularity of the vessel wall or an intramural dissection or clot that causes less than 25% stenosis of the vessel. Grade II signifies 25% or more stenosis of the vessel as a result of an intramural clot or dissection, or an intraluminal thrombus or raised intimal flap is seen. Grade III is a pseudoaneurysm. Grade IV includes occlusions of the vessel, and grade V represents a vessel transection (Table 20-1).

Sequelae of Vertebral Artery Injury

The range of outcomes for traumatic BVIs is wide. Many patients are asymptomatic and have no adverse effects of their injury. Other patients can have visual changes, significant stroke, or death. Neurologic deficit can result from decreased posterior brain circulation (vertebrobasilar insufficiency), clot formation with embolization downstream, obstruction of posterior inferior cerebellar blood flow, and anterior spinal artery compromise that causes subsequent spinal cord ischemia.[5]

Symptoms of dizziness, ataxia, decreased level of consciousness, or visual disturbances can all be evidence of vertebrobasilar insufficiency. More significant ischemia can occur with posterior stroke if collateral flow is not adequate. Collateral flow is extremely important because some patients with bilateral vertebral artery occlusion have no permanent neurologic deficit because they have sufficient collateral flow.

Diagnosis

Whether aggressive screening for traumatic VAIs is beneficial is debated. Nonetheless, common injuries for which patients who have sustained trauma are screened include significant soft tissue injury of the neck, cervical spine fractures or subluxations, facial trauma, unexplained neurologic findings, and skull base fractures; patients with Horner syndrome also undergo screening (Box 20-2).[10]

Catheter angiography has long been considered the gold standard to evaluate a VAI fully (Fig. 20-2). However, as with all invasive studies, it does carry some inherent risks. In a study by Miller and associates, a 3% complication rate was seen for arteriography (4 of 146).[2] These investigators reported one femoral artery dissection, one groin hematoma, one episode of contrast nephropathy, and one thalamic infarct.

Many centers are now trying to use faster, less invasive studies to screen for these injuries. Although CT angiography (CTA) and magnetic resonance angiography (MRA) were considered inadequate for screening in the past, newer technology has improved the effectiveness of these modalities (Fig. 20-3).[11-13] Additionally, the time to diagnosis of injury is significantly less using these modalities, and the potential for complications is also less. Eastman and associates showed a reduced time to diagnosis of blunt cerebrovascular injury from 31.2 hours after admission with angiography to just 2.65 hours with CTA. This study also showed that a CTA-based screening protocol and interdisciplinary treatment guidelines reduced the time to diagnosis of blunt cerebrovascular injuries by 12-fold while actually reducing their institution's stroke rate 4-fold.[11] Therefore, many institutions have gone to less invasive initial screening methods for these injuries and use angiography as needed when further information or clarification is required.

Treatment

Treatment of these injuries is controversial at best, as described later in the discussion of outcomes among treated and untreated patients. However, if treatment is determined to be necessary, several options exist. Some authors have recommended the use of systemic heparin in all patients who have no contraindications.[1] When a heparin drip is contraindicated, antiplatelet agents, low-dose

BOX **20-2**   **When to Consider Screening**

1. Cervical spine fractures (upper cervical fractures, transverse foramen injury, subluxations or dislocations)
2. Unexplained neurologic examination findings
3. Significant facial fractures or injury
4. Fractures of the skull base
5. Significant soft tissue injury of the neck
6. Penetrating trauma
7. Horner syndrome

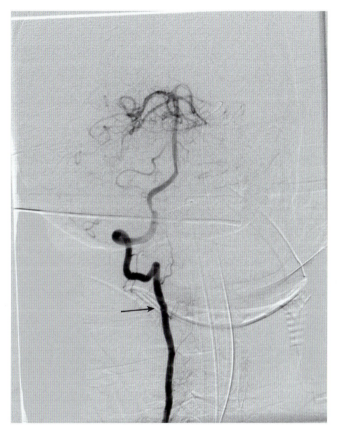

FIGURE 20-2 Angiography image from a patient with a grade I vertebral artery injury. Note the subtle change (*arrow*), which is difficult to appreciate on this still image.

subcutaneous heparin, or low-molecular-weight heparin may be used.[1] If absolutely no anticoagulation can be given, observation is an option as well.

Other investigators have stratified treatment based on the grade of arterial injury along with the relative risk of anticoagulation. Eastman and co-workers described general treatment guidelines based on those factors.[11] Their different treatment recommendations, in increasing order, were observation, antiplatelet therapy, delayed antiplatelet therapy, anticoagulation, embolization, and surgical intervention (Table 20-2).

As endovascular treatments continue to evolve and improve, they are becoming reasonable options for treatment in selected patients. In a study of six patients treated for traumatic VAIs, five of six dissections and pseudoaneurysms were successfully treated with endovascular therapy by using stents and coils.[14] The other patient in this study had a vertebral artery transaction treated with coil

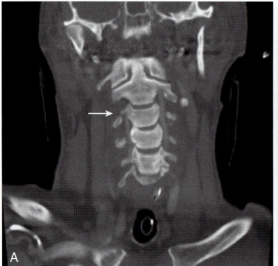
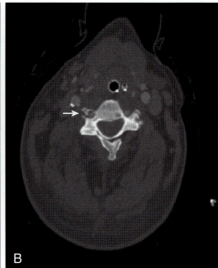

FIGURE 20-3 A, Coronal computed tomography angiography (CTA) of a patient with a fracture through the foramen transversum and decreased proximal flow of the right vertebral artery (*arrow*). **B,** Axial CTA showing the vertebral artery within a fractured transverse foramen (*arrow*).

Table 20-2 Example of Treatment Guidelines

Grade	Anticoagulation Risk	Treatment Recommendation
I	High	None
I	Low	Antiplatelet
II	High	None versus delayed antiplatelet
II	Low	Antiplatelet versus anticoagulation
III	High	Antiplatelet
III	Low	Anticoagulation
IV	High	Angiographic embolization
IV	Low	Antiplatelet with or without anticoagulation
V	High	Surgical versus angiographic
V	Low	Surgical versus angiographic

embolization. In this small series, no delayed neurologic or vascular complications were noted, and no recurrent lesions were seen during follow-up.[14]

Additional studies have stressed the importance of follow-up imaging in these patients. A study by Biffl and colleagues found that 61% of patients with blunt cerebrovascular injuries required a change in management based on follow-up angiography.[15] These investigators found that although higher-grade injuries remained unchanged for the most part, grade I and II injuries changed frequently with follow-up imaging.

Outcomes

Whether traumatic VAIs should be specifically treated remains controversial. A commonly cited study by Biffl and associates found a stroke incidence of 24% and a death rate incidence of 8% attributable to VAI.[1] These investigators found that anticoagulation with systemic heparin was associated with improved stroke and neurologic outcomes. However, only seven patients were treated with observation, and that treatment was chosen because those patients had absolute contraindications

to receiving heparin. Other investigators also found that screening and treatment reduced stroke rate in these patients.[10,11]

In a contrasting viewpoint, a study by Berne and Norwood of more than 8000 patients who had sustained blunt trauma found a BVI-related mortality rate of 7%.[4] Of the 44 patients with a VAI, 3 died. The investigators determined that 2 of these deaths were not preventable. The other patient could not be anticoagulated secondary to intracranial hemorrhage, and this was deemed the only potentially preventable BVI-related death in this study. These investigators stated that despite using an aggressive screening protocol on more than 8000 patients with individualized treatments for BVI, only 1 preventable death occurred, in a patient with intracranial hemorrhage. These investigators were unable to conclude that screening or treatment improved outcomes for these patients.

A literature review in 2008 on this topic found that few would argue with treatment of symptomatic injuries, but that the type of treatment is debatable.[5] Moreover, the investigators believed that it was unclear whether a need existed to screen for or treat asymptomatic injuries based on the available literature because no good level 1 evidence was available on this topic.

A study by Taneichi and co-workers using MRA at initial presentation and follow-up found that vertebral artery occlusion is rarely symptomatic because the collateral blood supply through the contralateral vertebral artery, as well as the circle of Willis, is sufficient.[12] These investigators also related the mechanism of cervical spine injury to the potential for restoration of blood flow. They found that the potential for restoration of blood flow was higher in compressive types of injuries than in distractive injuries. None of the 11 patients in this study underwent anticoagulation, including a patient who had bilateral occlusion. This patient had some transient blurry vision, but none of the patients in this study had any permanent neurologic deficits.

Therefore, based on the available literature and the paucity of level 1 studies on this topic, the optimal treatment recommendations for traumatic BVIs remains somewhat unclear. Most surgeons would agree that symptomatic injuries should receive some type of treatment, and that treatment must be individualized to the particular patient's situation. Treatment of asymptomatic injuries remains a more controversial topic. Studies have been published that argue for and against treatment, with both improved outcomes and no difference in outcomes reported. The best available literature indicates that it is prudent to screen high-risk individuals, and that treatment decisions should be made on an individual basis, depending on the particular patient's situation and risk factors.

Another issue that remains controversial is treatment of an unstable cervical spine injury in the setting of a coexistent traumatic VAI. Historically, the cervical spine injury has been treated before any specific treatment for the VAI. If the artery is injured unilaterally, this may lead to an alteration in the fixation scheme of a cervical injury that requires surgery. The surgeon may elect to not place the uninjured artery at risk of intraoperative injury. Alternatively, the unstable cervical spine injury may be treated with a halo vest initially or indefinitely while the VAI is being treated with anticoagulation. The senior author of this chapter encountered a case in which the cervical spine injury was treated surgically even though the patient had a traumatic VAI. This particular patient did have a stroke perioperatively from the VAI and ultimately died. Because management of these clinical situations remains unclear and controversial, management considerations should ultimately be individualized to the patient and based on the surgeon's experience and preference.

Conclusions

Traumatic VAIs are being recognized more commonly now that screening of high-risk patients is performed in many centers. Roughly 0.5% of all patients who have sustained blunt trauma will have a traumatic VAI. Certain patients are at higher risk, including patients with cervical spine injuries. Approximately 70% of all patients with traumatic VAIs will have an associated cervical spine fracture. Although angiography remains the gold standard imaging study, many centers are now using less invasive initial screening studies such as CTA

and MRA. Treatment options for these injuries include observation, antiplatelet agents, anticoagulation, and endovascular interventions. At this time, few would argue with treatment of symptomatic injuries, but the treatment of asymptomatic injuries remains controversial. Treatments for these patients must be made on a case-by-case basis.

REFERENCES

1. Biffl WL, Moore EE, Elliot JP, et al.: The devastating potential of blunt vertebral arterial injuries, *Ann Surg* 231:672–681, 2000.
2. Miller PR, Fabian TC, Bee TK, et al.: Blunt cerebrovascular injuries: diagnosis and treatment, *J Trauma* 51:279–286, 2001.
3. Spaniolas K, Velmahos GC, Alam HB, et al.: Does improved detection of blunt vertebral artery injuries lead to improved outcomes? Analysis of the National Trauma Data Bank, *World J Surg* 32:2190–2194, 2008.
4. Berne JD, Norwood SH: Blunt vertebral artery injuries in the era of computed tomographic angiographic screening: incidence and outcomes from 8292 patients, *J Trauma* 67:1333–1338, 2009.
5. Fassett DR, Dailey AT, Vaccara AR: Vertebral artery injuries associated with cervical spine injuries: a review of the literature, *J Spinal Disord Tech* 21:252–258, 2008.
6. Cothren CC, Moore EE, Biffl WL, et al.: Cervical spine fracture patterns predictive of blunt vertebral artery injury, *J Trauma* 55:811–813, 2003.
7. Ernst E: Deaths after chiropractic: a review of published cases, *Int J Clin Pract* 64:1162–1165, 2010.
8. Lu J, Ebraheim NA: The vertebral artery: surgical anatomy, *Orthopedics* 22:1081–1085, 1999.
9. Biffl WL, Moore EE, Offner PJ, et al.: Blunt carotid arterial injuries: implications of a new grading scale, *J Trauma* 47:845–853, 1999.
10. Miller PR, Fabian TC, Croce MA, et al.: Prospective screening for blunt cerebrovascular injuries. Analysis of diagnostic modalities and outcomes, *Ann Surg* 236:386–395, 2002.
11. Eastman AL, Muraliraj V, Sperry JL, Minei JP: CTA-based screening reduces time to diagnosis and stroke rate in blunt cervical vascular injury, *J Trauma* 67:551–556, 2009.
12. Taneichi H, Suda K, Kajino T, Kaneda K: Traumatically induced vertebral artery occlusion associated with cervical spine injuries: prospective study using magnetic resonance angiography, *Spine (Phila Pa 1976)* 30:1955–1962, 2005.
13. Stein DM, Boswell S, Sliker CW, et al.: Blunt cerebrovascular injuries: does treatment always matter? *J Trauma* 66:132–144, 2009.
14. Lee YJ, Ahn JY, Han IB, et al.: Therapeutic endovascular treatments for traumatic vertebral artery injuries, *J Trauma* 62:886–891, 2007.
15. Biffl WL, Ray CE, Moore EE, et al.: Treatment-related outcomes from blunt cerebrovascular injuries: importance of routine follow-up arteriography, *Ann Surg* 235:699–707, 2002.

Sanjitpal S. Gill

CHAPTER PREVIEW

Chapter Synopsis	Cervical cord neurapraxia and stingers can create significant angst in players, coaches, families, and spectators. Avoidance of permanent injury is tantamount. Effective postinjury management of the injured athlete by medical personnel either on the field or in the hospital setting can reduce the risk of secondary neurologic injury. This chapter covers the mechanisms, examination, imaging, and management of stingers and transient paresis.
Important Points	Sporting events are the fourth most common cause of spinal cord injury and the second most common cause of spinal cord injury in the first 3 decades of life.
	Football is associated with the highest number of direct catastrophic injuries for any sport reported and with a significant number of stingers or brachial plexus injuries.
	Burners and stingers are injuries to the brachial plexus that typically result in unilateral arm symptoms.
	Transient quadripareses are injuries to the spinal cord that usually cause bilateral extremity symptoms.
	Return to play is controversial and should be individualized to the patient; however, neurologic deficits, length of symptoms, and static and dynamic imaging should be included in the decision-making process.
	Prevention though coaching of proper techniques, in particular tackling and blocking in football, along with athlete education remains paramount.

Sporting events comprise the fourth most common cause of spinal cord injury, after motor vehicle accidents, violence, and falls. Additionally, sports injuries comprise the second most common cause of spinal cord injury in the first 3 decades of life, and 7% of all new cases of spinal cord injury are related to athletic activities. In the United States, football is one of the most popular sports, with more than 1.2 million high school participants during the 2001 to 2002 academic year. Approximately 200,000 individuals engage in college and professional play each year.[1] Unfortunately, football is associated with the highest number of direct catastrophic injuries for any sport reported to the National Center for Catastrophic Sports Injury Research (NCCSIR), and it is also associated with a significant number of stingers or brachial plexus injuries.[2] Other sports that have been implicated in spinal cord injuries include ice hockey, wrestling, diving, skiing, snowboarding, rugby, cheerleading, and baseball.

The NCCSIR characterizes catastrophic sports injury as "any severe spinal, spinal cord, or cerebral injury incurred during participation in a school/college sponsored sport," and these injuries are further subdivided into direct or indirect.[3] Direct injuries result from participation in the sport, such as trauma from a collision or impact, whereas indirect injuries arise from failure from exertion, such as heat stroke or arrhythmia. Indirect injuries are characterized by medical issues, which include cardiopulmonary diseases such as arrhythmias and hypertrophic cardiomyopathy. Concussions are currently not classified as catastrophic injuries by the NCCSIR, but they can cause lifelong disability.

Burners and Stingers (Brachial Plexopathy)

Burners and stingers are injuries to the brachial plexus that arise from traction, compression, and direct trauma. The brachial plexus consists of the cervical nerve roots from C5 to T1, and the most commonly affected roots are the upper plexus roots of C5 and C6[4] (Fig. 21-1). Stingers are the most common cervical spine injury in athletes and are notoriously prevalent in contact and collision sports. As many as 65% of college football players have reported sustaining a stinger in their 4-year career.

Symptoms include reversible, unilateral upper extremity pain, numbness, and weakness, but neurologic symptoms rarely follow a strict dermatomal distribution. The symptoms typically resolve within minutes of the injury.

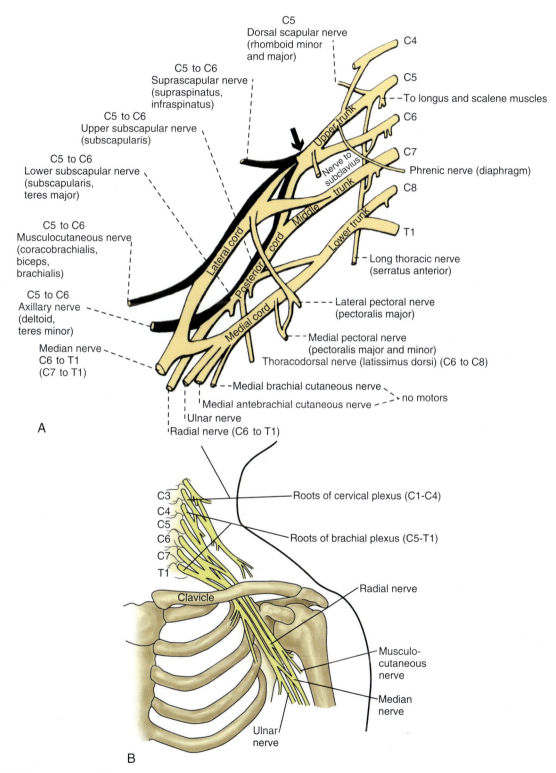

FIGURE 21-1 The upper trunk of the brachial plexus is often involved with stingers and burners with resultant weakness of the deltoid, biceps, and rotator cuff muscles. The clavicle and chest wall are juxtaposed structures to the brachial plexus. (**A,** Modified DeLee JC, Drez D Jr, Miller MD, editors: *DeLee and Drez's orthopaedic sports medicine,* vol 1, ed 2, Philadelphia, 2003, Saunders, p 797; **B,** Copyright William B. Westwood, 1997. In Miller MD, Hart JA, MacKnight JM, editors: *Essential orthopaedics,* Philadelphia, 2010, Saunders, p 488.)

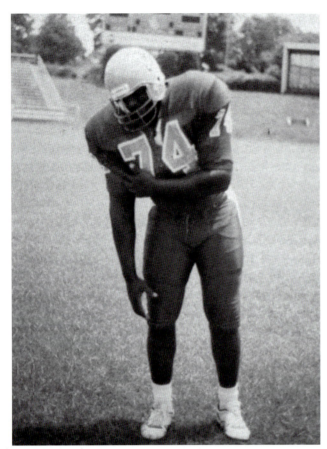

FIGURE 21-2 Common presentation of dead arm syndrome in which the contralateral arm supports the weight of the affected arm as a result of pain or muscle weakness. (From Pritchard JC: Football and other contact sports injuries: diagnosis and treatment. In Buschbacher RM, Braddom RL, editors: *Sports medicine and rehabilitation: a sport specific approach*, Philadelphia, 1994, Hanley & Belfus, p 172.)

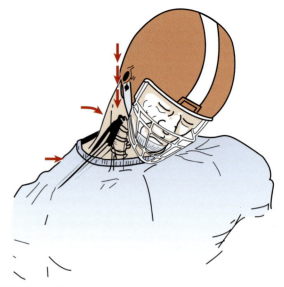

FIGURE 21-3 Classic ipsilateral extension and lateral deviation mechanism of brachial plexopathy. (From Warren WL, Bailes JE: On the field evaluation of athletic neck injury. *Clin Sports Med* 17:99-110, 1998. In Miller MD, editor: *SMART! Sports medicine assessment and review textbook*, Philadelphia, 2010, Saunders.)

Table 21-1 Calculation of Mean Subaxial Space Available for the Cord Index

| Level | Diameter (mm) | | |
	Canal	Cord	Difference (Δ)
C3	11.2	7.8	3.4
C4	10.3	7.8	2.5
C5	10.3	7.8	2.5
C6	11.4	7.0	4.4
Average			3.2

From Olson DE, McBroom SA, Nelson BD, et al: Unilateral cervical nerve injuries: brachial plexopathies. *Curr Sports Med Rep* 6:43-49, 2007.

Transient inability to use the arm actively, termed *dead arm syndrome,* can exist in addition to paresthesias of the entire arm (Fig. 21-2). If the symptoms are bilateral, concern for transient quadriparesis should be raised.

The injury characteristically has three main etiologic patterns: (1) traction, (2) compression, and (3) direct trauma to the brachial plexus. Traction of the plexus from sudden shoulder depression with lateral head deviation is more common in younger athletes without fully developed neck musculature.[5] The compression mechanism from extension, ipsilateral deviation, and rotation to the affected side is more typical in mature athletes as a result of developmental foraminal stenosis and foraminal osteophytes (Fig. 21-3). Finally, direct trauma from a direct blow or compression from the shoulder pad and the superomedial border of the scapula (Erb point) can injure the brachial plexus.

During examination of patients who have sustained stingers, recreation of the direction of the injury can trigger arm symptoms. The Spurling test with cervical extension, lateral flexion to the injured side, and gentle axial compression can reproduce arm symptoms. Similarly, ipsilateral shoulder depression and contralateral head deviation can produce symptoms if the original mechanism was a traction injury to the brachial plexus. Additionally, a Tinel sign may be present on palpation of the Erb point. The athlete may attempt to splint the affected

arm with the contralateral extremity because of the nondermatomal motor deficit that occurs with stingers. The clavicle and spinous processes of the cervical spine should also be palpated to help evaluate for coexisting trauma.[6]

Imaging of patients with stingers includes an anteroposterior view to assess coronal alignment and a lateral view to assess for decreased cervical lordosis from cervical perimuscular spasm that often accompanies brachial plexopathy. Additionally, oblique views may be helpful to evaluate the caliber of the cervical foramina. However, flexion and extension views of the cervical spine have limited utility in the acute posttraumatic setting.

Magnetic resonance imaging (MRI) is helpful in evaluating for suspected spinal cord or nerve root injury. Herniated cervical disks, foraminal or canal stenosis, and spinal cord edema are also clearly visualized on MRI. Greenberg and colleagues demonstrated the mean subaxial space available for the cord index as a predictor of chronic stinger syndrome.[7] At every level of the subaxial spine from C3 to C6, the difference between the space available for the spinal cord and the cord anteroposterior diameter is averaged over the four levels. An index value of less than 4.3 mm has been demonstrated to correlate with a 13-fold increase in the risk of developing multiple stingers, or chronic stinger syndrome (Table 21-1).

The use of computed tomography (CT) and CT myelogram is typically not necessary and may be reserved mainly for patients who cannot tolerate or undergo MRI. CT may have some benefit in patients with congenital stenosis or substantial cervical spondylosis who sustain a spinal cord injury. In these patients, CT scan with or without myelography can help identify whether the cervical neuroforaminal stenosis is secondary to bony or soft tissue compression. As would be expected, in the patient with suspect brachial plexus disorders, CT has a limited role and typically provides insufficient imaging information, whereas CT myelography does not identify the injury because the pathologic process is beyond the neuroforamen and within the brachial plexus.

The utility of electromyography and nerve conduction studies has been called into question. As many as 80% of patients show electromyographic abnormalities more than 5 years after the onset of a stinger. However, persistent symptoms 2 to 4 weeks after the injury may warrant electromyographic studies to help with evaluation and long-term assessment of the injury. Red flags that warrant further testing include bilateral symptoms, lower extremity involvement, painful range of motion, axial tenderness, persistent burning, neurologic deficit, and altered consciousness. These findings may suggest other injuries such as the following: cervical spine injury; cervical cord neurapraxia (CCN), especially if the symptoms are bilateral; clavicle fracture; and cervical disk herniations. In addition, rotator cuff injury, first rib stress fracture, thoracic outlet syndrome, and Parsonage-Turner syndrome should be included in the differential diagnosis.[8]

Initial treatment of stingers and burners should include removing the athlete from play until symptoms resolve completely and cervical spine injury can be excluded. Treatment is largely supportive, including physical therapy and possibly a sling to relieve traction on the brachial plexus. A focused rehabilitation program should include restoration of strength in the upper extremity and cervical spine. Emphasis should also be placed on proper posture, including chin-tuck exercises and cervical retraction.

The prognosis is based on the severity of the injury, which can be graded from least severe (*neurapraxia*) to more severe (*neurotmesis*). With neurapraxia, the most common variant of stingers, all nerve structures remain intact, and symptoms typically resolve in minutes, although they may take as long as 6 weeks. Intermediate injury, termed *axonotmesis*, occurs with axonal disruption in which wallerian degeneration takes place distal to the injury site. Recovery is usually complete, but it may take months because an intact epineurium allows axonal regrowth at a rate of approximately 1 mm per day. Severe injuries (neurotmesis) arise with complete disruption of axons, endoneurium, perineurium, and epineurium. The prognosis is often variable, and complete loss of function is common.

Athletes should not be allowed to return to competition without a full, pain-free cervical arc of motion because this is paramount in preventing more serious spinal cord injury. On return to contact sports, the use of neck rolls, such as a neck-shoulder-cervical orthosis (cowboy collar) or pads at the base of the neck in football players, can help minimize recurrences of stingers.[9] Unfortunately, the long-term implications of recurrent stingers are unknown at present.

Cervical Spinal Cord Neurapraxia (Transient Quadriparesis)

Transient quadriplegia, spinal cord concussion, and CCN are terms often used interchangeably to signify a transient neurologic episode associated with sensory changes with or without motor deficits or complete paralysis in at least two extremities. Hyperflexion, hyperextension, and axial loading are frequently the purported mechanisms of injury.

Symptoms can include loss of strength and sensation in the arms and legs. Bilateral burning pain (dysesthesias) or bilateral tingling (paresthesias) that can occur with CCN should not be confused with similar unilateral symptoms found in patients with burners or stingers.[10] Based on criteria for the definition of the disease, the symptoms are transient, usually lasting between 15 minutes and 36 hours. Because of significant underreporting and the transient nature of this disease, the true prevalence of CCN is difficult to determine. Torg and Pavlov diligently tried to determine the incidence of CCN.[11] In a population of 39,377 athletes exposed during the 1984 National Collegiate Athletic Association season, the reported incidence of transient paresthesias in all four extremities was 6.0 per 10,000, whereas the incidence of paresthesias associated with transient quadriplegia was 1.3 per 10,000 in a single football season. Thus, the cumulative incidence of CCN was 7.3 per 10,000 in a single collegiate football season.

The natural concern with CCN is permanent quadriplegia. Most of the data for permanent quadriplegic events have been compiled from injuries sustained while playing football. The incidence of spinal cord injury peaked from 1971 to 1975, when the National Football Head and Neck Injury Registry compiled 259 (4.14 of 100,000) cervical fracture-dislocations and 99 cases (1.58 of 100,000) of quadriplegia.[12] Defense players accounted for 71% of the injuries, and making the tackle accounted for 69% of the injuries. The defensive back (35.4%), the linebacker (10.3%), and the kickoff special team (8.1%) sustained the majority of the injuries.[13]

The increase in catastrophic cervical spinal trauma coincided with the development of improved helmet technology as a result of the false sense of security from increased head protection. Indeed, a decrease in fatalities from intracranial hemorrhage occurred, but players started altering their blocking and tackling techniques and increasingly lowered their head as a battering ram. Studies demonstrated that anywhere from 25% to 88% of quadriplegia cases occurred from improper tackling techniques as a result of an axial load to the head and cervical spine.

The top of the helmet often became the first point of impact during on-field collisions, and, in 1976, the National Collegiate Athletic Association banned head-first contact (also known as spear tackling) (Fig. 21-4). Over the ensuing decade, the rate of permanent spinal cord injuries progressively decreased. When the rule

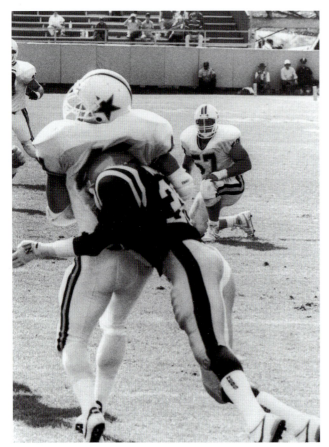

FIGURE 21-4 Football player using spear-tackling techniques against an opponent. (From Torg JS, Guille JT, Jaffe S: Current concepts review: injuries to the cervical spine in American football players. *J Bone Joint Surg Am* 84:112-122, 2002.)

banning spear tackling was instituted in 1976, the annual rate of permanent quadriplegia was 2.24 per 100,000 high school football participants and 10.66 per 100,000 collegiate football players. By 1984, the rate decreased to 0.38 per 100,000 and 0 per 100,000 in high school and college respectively. More recent data show a rate of 0.33 per 100,000 and 1.33 per 100,000 in 2002 for high school and collegiate football, respectively[13] (Figs. 21-5 and 21-6).

CCN continues to be controversial with respect to classification (duration of symptoms), management (steroids, bracing), and return-to-play criteria. Additionally, a causal link between CCN and permanent quadriplegia is difficult to determine and equally difficult to prove. The association between stenosis and quadriplegia was documented by Eismont and colleagues.[14] These investigators demonstrated a higher likelihood of quadriplegia with cervical fracture or fracture-dislocation in patients with preexisting cervical stenosis. Other investigators also described relatively minor trauma, such as falls or minor motor vehicle collisions, that could lead to permanent quadriplegia in people with marked developmental stenosis of the cervical spine.[15,16]

Cervical stenosis has often been denoted by a Torg-Pavlov ratio (space available for the spinal canal divided by the sagittal diameter of the vertebral body) of less than 0.8 on static lateral radiographs of the cervical spine (Fig. 21-7). Unfortunately, static radiographs do not take into account the dynamic stenotic effects of disk bulging and ligamentum flavum infolding with flexion and extension of the neck. However, Torg and colleagues previously reported that the occurrence of CCN and a subsequent injury resulting in quadriplegia are not related.[17] In that study, Torg and associates showed that the overall

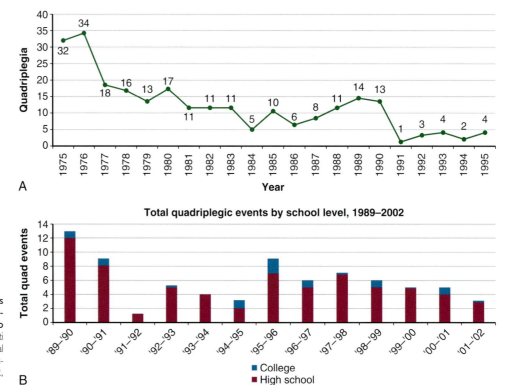

FIGURE 21-5 Total quadriplegic events from 1975 to 1995 (**A**) and total quadriplegic events by school level from 1989 to 2002 (**B**). (Data from Boden BP, Tacchetti RL, Cantu RC, et al: Catastrophic cervical spine injuries in high school and college football players. *Am J Sports Med* 34:1223-1232, 2006.)

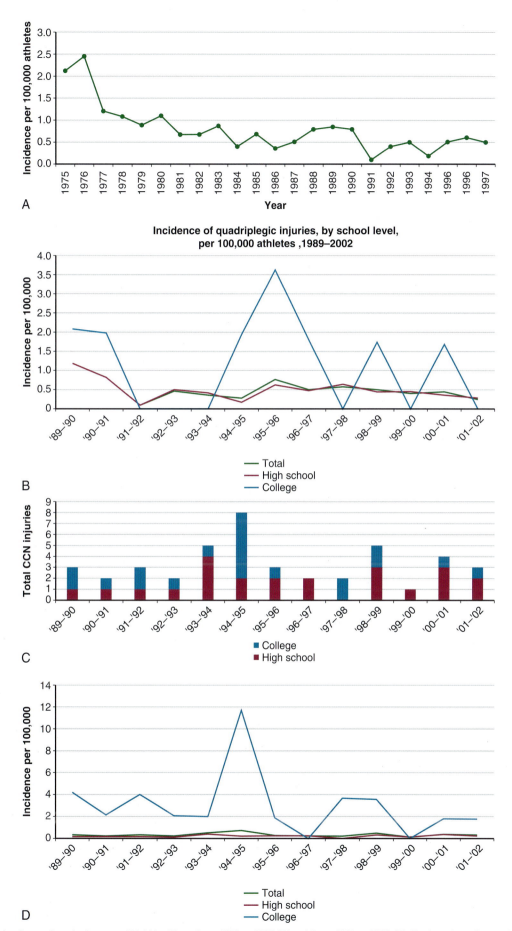

FIGURE 21-6 Incidence of quadriplegia per 100,000 athletes from 1975 to 1997 (**A**) and from 1989 to 2002 (**B**). Total number of cervical cord neurapraxia (CCN) football injuries at the high school and college levels reported to the National Center for Catastrophic Sports Injury Research per school year from 1989 to 1990 to 2001 to 2002 (**C**), and the annual incidence of high school, college, and total football CCN injuries per 100,000 participants from 1989 to 2002 (**D**). (**A** and **B,** Data from Gill SS, Boden BP: The epidemiology of catastrophic spine injuries in high school and college football. *Sports Med Arthrosc Rev* 16:2-6, 2008; **C** and **D,** Data from Boden BP, Tacchetti RL, Cantu RC, et al: Catastrophic cervical spine injuries in high school and college football players. *Am J Sports Med* 34:1223-1232, 2006.)

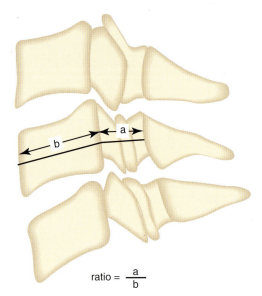

$$\text{ratio} = \frac{a}{b}$$

FIGURE 21-7 Torg-Pavlov ratio. *a* is the distance from the midpoint of the posterior aspect of the vertebral body to the nearest point on the corresponding spinolaminar line. *b* is the anteroposterior width of the vertebral body. (From Torg JS, Pavlov H, Gennuario SE, et al: Neurapraxia of the cervical spinal cord with transient quadriplegia. *J Bone Joint Surg Am* 68:1354-1370, 1986. As redrawn in DeLee JC, Drez D Jr, Miller MD, editors: *DeLee and Drez's orthopaedic sports medicine*, ed 3, Philadelphia, 2009, Saunders.)

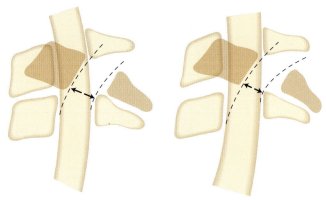

FIGURE 21-8 Extremes of flexion and extension can create spinal cord compression between the posteroinferior portion of the vertebral body above and the anterosuperior lamina of the vertebra below due to the pincer mechanism. (From Thomas BE, McCullen GM, and Yuan HA: Cervical spine injuries in football players. *J Am Acad Orthop Surg* 7:338-347, 1999. As redrawn in DeLee JC, Drez D Jr, Miller MD, editors: *DeLee and Drez's orthopaedic sports medicine*, ed 3, Philadelphia, 2009, Saunders.)

recurrence of CCN with athletes who returned to play was 56%, but only 63 of 109 athletes (58%) returned to contact sports in this study after a single episode of CCN. Furthermore, the risk of recurrence was shown to be highly predictable, with increasing recurrent episodes of CCN associated with decreased sagittal canal diameter. The occurrence of more than one episode of CCN was deemed to be a contraindication to return to play.

Because of the low overall incidence of quadriplegia (≈1 in 192,000 participants), whether athletes with a CCN episode have a higher rate of quadriplegia when they returned to play is still unknown. To make a definitive statement, a study with a high rate of athletes with a history of CCN who returned to play would be required. Additionally, possible randomization to return to play and no return may be necessary after a CCN event to express the likelihood of quadriplegia after the transient paresis episode definitively.

Brigham and Adamson described permanent, partial spinal cord injury in a professional football player with a prior CCN event and preexisting congenital spinal stenosis.[18] The athlete continued to have mild, bilateral upper extremity dysesthesias 2 years after the injury and was taking gabapentin for symptomatic relief. Historically, Torg and colleagues stated that CCN is not an antecedent symptom for permanent spinal cord injury even in patients with preexisting cervical stenosis.[17] Reconciling these data with Brigham and Adamson's work, including data from Boden, Tacchetti, and Cantu that demonstrate permanent spinal cord injury after CCN, is important.[13] In the example described by Boden and associates, the athlete had a variant of a permanent Brown-Séquard spinal cord injury with ipsilateral motor loss and contralateral pain and temperature disruption after he had a previous CCN episode. The athlete's spinal canal width was 12 mm. Based on Torg's definition of stenosis, only

plain radiographs were used to calculate the Torg-Pavlov ratio, in which an overly large vertebral body, possibly in a larger athlete, could lead to a spurious finding of stenosis. Thus, cervical stenosis may not have even been present in some athletes in the database of Torg and colleagues.

Currently, more emphasis is being placed on "dynamic" or "functional" stenosis whereby the space available for the spinal canal is measured on MRI examinations so disk bulging and ligamentum flavum hypertrophy can be taken into account during surveys for cervical canal narrowing. Additionally, the role of dynamic stenosis, or the pincer function, is also more clearly evaluated with cervical MRI examinations obtained in flexion and extension to reproduce the status of the neck during the true mechanism of the injury. With the pincer mechanism, the spinal cord can be impinged by the vertebral body cranially and the posterior elements caudally, or vice versa[19] (Fig. 21-8). Further reconciliation can also be attributed to the extremely low incidence of quadriplegia (1 in 192,000 participants), as well as to the relative attrition rate of athletes' returning to contact sports after a CCN episode. Thus, these two glaring dilemmas in CCN make counseling of athletes on returning to sport extremely difficult.

Return-to-play guidelines have been plagued by significant disagreement in the literature and also by the variable nature of the disease, including duration, severity, and neurologic sequelae of the injury. At the minimum, each case of CCN should be evaluated individually. The initial on-field evaluation should focus on the presence or absence of neck pain or extremity symptoms, grading of the neurologic findings, and evaluation for unilateral or bilateral symptoms. Banerjee, Palumbo, and Fadale created an excellent algorithm for the primary neurologic survey of the injured athlete (Fig. 21-9).[19] Treatment of CCN focuses on regaining strength and correction of tackling (football) or checking (hockey, lacrosse) methods, with an emphasis on "see what you hit" or "heads-up" technique.

Relative and absolute contraindications to return to play include ligamentous instability, significant degenerative disease, intervertebral disk disease with spinal cord compression, MRI evidence of cord edema or defects,

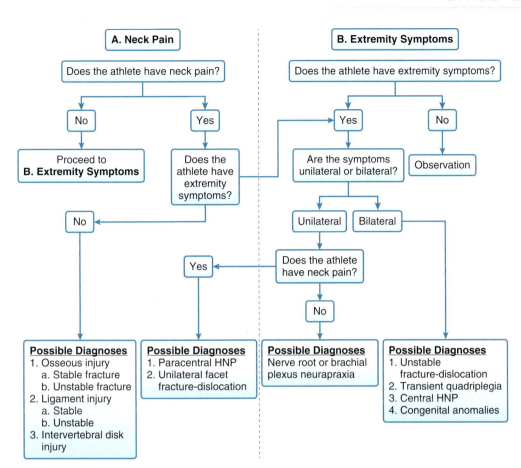

FIGURE 21-9 Algorithm for on-field evaluation of cervical spine injury. *HNP,* Herniated nucleus pulposus. (Redrawn from Banerjee R, Palumbo MA, Fadale PD: Catastrophic cervical spine injuries in the collision sport athlete. Part 1. Epidemiology, functional anatomy, and diagnosis. *Am J Sports Med* 32:1077-1087, 2004.)

neurologic symptoms lasting longer than 36 hours, and more than one recurrence of CCN. Watkins and associates developed a cervical spine injury rating scale that attempts to classify the severity of the injury based on three criteria[20]: (1) neurologic deficit, (2) duration of neurologic deficit, and (3) central diameter of the neural canal (Table 21-2). Based on the total score from these three categories, the athlete's risk of further injury can be stratified into minimal, moderate, or severe. However, once again, the authors stress the need for individual evaluation of each case. In addition, Torg and co-workers defined a clear inverse relationship with the potential recurrence of CCN based on both the Torg-Pavlov ratio and the MRI disk level canal diameter (Fig. 21-10); these data can also assist in athlete counseling.[21]

Conclusions

CCN and stingers can create significant angst in players, coaches, families, and spectators. Proper athlete education on the avoidance of head-down tackling, blocking, or checking techniques must be provided, and strict adherence to the playing rules designed to prevent craniocervical injuries must be enforced during practice and competition. At-risk individuals such as defensive backs, linebackers, special teams personnel, and pole vaulters or athletes who engage in high-risk activities such as individuals who perform tackles, check from behind, use spear-tackling methods, or build pyramids in

Table 21-2 Return-to-Play Risk Stratification for Cervical Cord Neurapraxia

Criterion	Point Value*
Neurologic Deficit	
Unilateral arm numbness or dysesthesia, loss of strength	1
Bilateral upper extremity loss of motor and sensory function	2
Loss of motor and sensory function in arm, leg, and trunk on one side of body	3
Transient quadriparesis	4
Transient quadriplegia	5
Duration of Neurologic Deficit	
<5 min	1
<1 hr	2
<24 hr	3
<1 wk	4
>1 wk	5
Central Diameter of Neural Canal	
>12 mm	1
10-12 mm	2
10 mm	3
8-10 mm	4
8 mm	5

*A total score for all three criteria of less than 6 points represents minimal risk; 6 to 10 points, moderate risk; 10 to 15 points, severe risk.

From Watkins RG, Dillin WH, Maxwell J: Cervical spine injuries in football players. *Spine State Art Rev* 4:391-408, 1990.

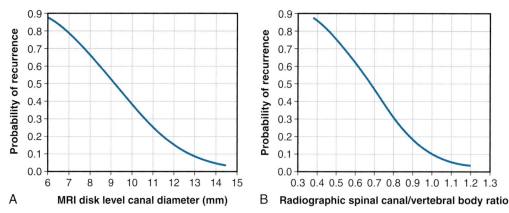

FIGURE 21-10 Inverse probability of recurrence of cervical cord neurapraxia based on magnetic resonance imaging (MRI) sagittal diameter (**A**) and the Torg-Pavlov ratio (**B**). (Redrawn from Torg JS, Corcoran TA, Thibault LE, et al: Cervical cord neurapraxia: classification, pathomechanics, morbidity, and management guidelines. *J Neurosurg* 87:843-850, 1997.)

cheerleading formations may require additional education and monitoring.[3]

Avoidance of permanent injury is tantamount. The annual aggregate cost of treating an athlete with spinal cord injury was estimated at $700 million in 1995,[22] without factoring the emotional component of the injury on the player and family. In 2011, the average per person yearly expediture ranged from $334,170 in the first year and $40,589 in each subsequent year for patients with an incomplete spinal cord injury when compared to $1,023,924 in the first year and $177,808 for each subsequent year for patients with C1-C4 quadriplegia. Additionally, the total annual cost attributed to spinal cord injury in the United States is approximately $14.5 billion.[23] Effective postinjury management of the injured athlete by medical personnel either on the field or in the hospital setting can reduce the risk of secondary neurologic injury. Further research and evaluation of functional and dynamic stenosis and the relationship with subsequent paresthesias and spinal cord syndromes may provide answers to questions on treatment and return-to-play criteria.

REFERENCES

1. Gill S S, Boden B P: The epidemiology of catastrophic spine injuries in high school and college football, *Sports Med Arthrosc Rev* 16:2–6, 2008.
2. National Center for Sports Injury Research: *NCCSIR twelfth annual report: fall 1982-spring 2000*, Chapel Hill, NC, 2005, National Center for Sports Injury Research.
3. Boden B P: Direct catastrophic injury in sports, *J Am Acad Orthop Surg* 13:445–454, 2006.
4. Olson D E, McBroom S A, Nelson B D, et al.: Unilateral cervical nerve injuries: brachial plexopathies, *Curr Sports Med Rep* 6:43–49, 2007.
5. Kasow D B, Curl WW: "Stingers" in adolescent athletes, *Instr Course Lect* 55:711–716, 2006.
6. Feinberg J H: Burners and stingers, *Phys Med Rehabil Clin N Am* 11:771–784, 2000.
7. Greenberg J, Leung D, Kendall J: Predicting chronic stinger syndrome using the mean subaxial space available for the cord index, *Sports Health J* 3:264–267, 2011.
8. Safran M R: Nerve injury about the shoulder. Part 2. Long thoracic nerve, spinal accessory nerve, burners/stingers, thoracic outlet syndrome, *Am J Sports Med* 32:1063–1076, 2004.
9. Weinberg J, Rokito S, Silber J S: Etiology, treatment, and prevention of athletic "stingers", *Clin Sports Med* 22:493–500, 2003.
10. Torg J S, Pavlov H, Gennuario S E, et al.: Neurapraxia of the cervical spinal cord with transient quadriplegia, *J Bone Joint Surg Am* 68:1354–1370, 1986.
11. Torg J S, Pavlov H: Cervical spinal stenosis with cord neurapraxia and transient quadriplegia, *Clin Sports Med* 6:115–133, 1987.
12. Torg J S, Quendenfeld TC, Burstein A, et al.: National Football Head and Neck Injury Registry: report on cervical quadriplegia, 1971 to 1975, *Am J Sports Med* 7:127–132, 1979.
13. Boden B P, Tacchetti R L, Cantu RC, et al.: Catastrophic cervical spine injuries in high school and college football players, *Am J Sports Med* 34:1223–1232, 2006.
14. Eismont F J, Clifford S, Goldberg M, et al.: Cervical sagittal spinal canal size in spinal injury, *Spine (Phila Pa 1976)* 9:663–666, 1984.
15. Matsumoto K, Wakahara K, Sumi H, et al.: Central cord syndrome in patients with Klippel-Feil syndrome resulting from winter sports: report of 3 cases, *Am J Sports Med* 34:1685–1689, 2006.
16. Firoozna H, Ahn J H, Rafii M, et al.: Sudden quadriplegia after a minor trauma: the role of preexisting stenosis, *Surg Neurol* 23:165–168, 1985.
17. Torg J S, Corcoran TA, Thibault L E, et al.: Cervical cord neurapraxia: classification, pathomechanics, morbidity, and management guidelines, *J Neurosurg* 87:843–850, 1997.
18. Brigham C D, Adamson TE: Permanent partial cervical spinal cord injury in a professional football player who had only congenital stenosis, *J Bone Joint Surg Am* 85:1553–1556, 2003.
19. Banerjee R, Palumbo M A, Fadale PD: Catastrophic cervical spine injuries in the collision sport athlete. Part 1. Epidemiology, functional anatomy, and diagnosis, *Am J Sports Med* 32:1077–1087, 2004.
20. Watkins R G, Dillin WH, Maxwell J: Cervical spine injuries in football players, *Spine State Art Rev* 4:391–408, 1990.
21. Torg J S, Guille J T, Jaffe S: Current concepts review: injuries to the cervical spine in American football players, *J Bone Joint Surg Am* 84:112–122, 2002.
22. Devivo M J: Causes and costs of spinal cord injury in the United States, *Spinal Cord* 35:809–813, 1997.
23. Ma VY, Chan L, Carruthers K J: Incidence, prevalence, costs, and impact on disability of common conditions requiring rehabilitation in the United States: stroke, spinal cord injury, traumatic brain injury, multiple sclerosis, osteoarthritis, rheumatoid arthritis, limb loss, and back pain, *Arch Phys Med Rehabil* 95(5): 986–995.e1, 2014 May doi: 10.1016/j.apmr.2013.10.032. Epub 2014 Jan 21. Review. PMID:24462839.

Spinal Tumors, Infections, and Inflammatory Conditions

Primary Tumors of the Spinal Cord

Camilo A. Molina, Byung M. (Jason) Yoon, Ziya L. Gokaslan, and Daniel M. Sciubba

CHAPTER PREVIEW

Chapter Synopsis

Primary tumors of the spinal cord comprise 5% to 15% of all central nervous system (CNS) tumors. They can be divided into two main categories based on anatomic origin: intradural extramedullary or intramedullary spinal cord tumors. Different tumors can result in different findings on clinical examination and imaging. Definitive diagnosis, however, typically involves examination of histologic features of the tumor. Careful assessment of symptoms, tumor location, and tumor type is critical because it dictates management, which can involve chemotherapy, radiation, or surgical intervention. This chapter discusses the anatomic distribution, presentation, diagnosis, and management of the most common types of primary intradural extramedullary and intramedullary spinal cord tumors.

Important Points

Primary tumors of the spinal cord can be categorized as intradural extramedullary and intramedullary spinal cord tumors.

Common intradural extramedullary tumors include meningioma, schwannoma, and neurofibroma.

Common intramedullary spinal cord tumors include ependymoma and astrocytoma.

Different tumors have characteristic findings on magnetic resonance imaging that can help determine the type of tumor.

Definitive diagnosis typically involves examination of the histologic features of the tumor.

Management of primary tumors involves medical, radiation, or surgical therapy, alone or in combination.

Spinal cord tumors account for an estimated 5% to 15% of all central nervous system (CNS) tumors, with an incidence of 0.5 to 2.5 cases per 100,000.[1-3] Among these, nearly 50% are primary intradural spinal cord tumors. Intradural spine tumors are divided into two main categories based on the anatomic origin of the lesion: intradural extramedullary spinal cord tumors (IESCTs), arising from within the spinal cord; and intramedullary spinal cord tumors (ISCTs), originating from the dura but located within the subarachnoid space.[1,4]

IESCTs account for 80% of intraspinal tumors in adults and 65% to 70% of intraspinal tumors in children. The two most common types of IESCTs are nerve sheath tumors (NSTs) (30%) and meningiomas (25%). Because NSTs arise from perineural cells and Schwann cells, the two most common NSTs are schwannomas and neurofibromas; schwannomas account for approximately 65% of NSTs.[5] Most NSTs are sporadic, but they are also common in the setting of inherited disorders such as neurofibromatosis type I (NF-1) and type 2 (NF-2). Sporadic NSTs usually arise in the fifth to seventh decade, whereas those in the setting of neurofibromatosis arise during childhood or early adulthood.[6] Meningiomas originate from arachnoidal cells along the neuraxis and are also commonly associated with neurofibromatosis. However, only 10% of meningiomas arise external to the cranial fossa.[7]

ISCTs account for 20% of intraspinal tumors in adults and 30% to 35% of intraspinal tumors in children.[3] The two most common ISCTs are ependymomas (60%) and astrocytomas (30%). Ependymomas mainly arise in adults in approximately the third or fourth decade, and astrocytomas usually appear in children during the first decade. Given the predominant prevalence of ependymomas and astrocytomas, investigators believe that most ISCTs are of glial origin[1,3] This chapter discusses the anatomic distribution, presentation, diagnosis, and management of the most common types of spinal cord tumors, including both IESCTs and ISCTs.

Intradural Extramedullary Spinal Cord Tumors

Presentation

IESCTs have a nonspecific clinical presentation that includes axial back or neck pain, as well as radicular or myelopathic signs and symptoms. Associated pain is usually most intense in the evening and morning. The specific symptoms of IESCTs mainly depend on the level involved and have no specific anatomic distribution. A study performed by Slin'ko and Al-Qashqish,[4] however, examined 360 patients with IESCTs over an 11-year period and classified tumor location on both the axial and the longitudinal axis. The investigators found that on the longitudinal axis, most IESCTs occurred within the thoracic spine, followed by the cervical and lumbar spine, respectively. On the axial axis, the investigators determined that most lesions occurred on the dorsolateral division, followed, respectively, by the ventrolateral, dorsal, and ventral divisions.[4]

In the case of NSTs, radicular sensory signs are the first to follow pain. Patients have pain because NSTs characteristically arise in the dorsal sensory roots. Radiculopathy with motor deficits is not common, even during involvement of functional roots of the cervical or lumbar spine. However, myelopathic motor signs manifest once the tumor achieves a critical mass, thus resulting in spinal cord compression. The myelopathy has no distinctive symptoms and may include signs such as Brown-Séquard syndrome (ipsilateral hemiplegia with ipsilateral fine touch sensory deficit and contralateral pain and temperature sensory deficit, and upper motor neuron involvement such as upward plantar reflex, hyperreflexia, and clonus). Chronicling the time progression of symptoms is important because rapidly worsening signs and symptoms indicate the presence of a fast-growing, aggressive tumor such as a malignant NST (MNST).[1] Similarly, the presentation of spinal meningiomas is nonspecific and includes signs and symptoms such as progressive lower extremity numbness and weakness. Furthermore, many spinal meningiomas are often asymptomatic as a result of their slow growth and are discovered only incidentally during an imaging study or at autopsy.[8]

Diagnosis

The two most common types of IESCTs are NSTs and meningiomas. The diagnosis of IESCTs is best made using magnetic resonance imaging (MRI) because plain radiography, computed tomography (CT), and CT with myelography do not provide sufficient delineation of an intradural neoplasm. However, when MRI is contraindicated, CT with myelography is the imaging modality of choice.

Of primary importance is determining whether the neoplasm is intramedullary or extramedullary. Extramedullary neoplasms have the following characteristics on MRI: displacement and compression of the spinal cord, expansion of the thecal sac, and a menisci-like interface with the cerebrospinal fluid. Intramedullary neoplasms are characterized by expansion of the spinal cord.

Most IESCTs are isointense to the spinal cord on T1-weighted imaging and hyperintense on T2-weighted images. Furthermore, IESCTs typically enhance with contrast on T1-weighted imaging (Fig. 22-1). NSTs produce unique "target lesions" on MRI that correspond to the pathologic anatomy of the lesion. Despite the optimal ability of MRI to delineate the anatomic interface between the spinal cord and the neoplasm, this modality cannot provide a definitive diagnosis; the differential diagnosis also includes meningiomas, extramedullary ependymomas, mixed cell gliomas, hemangiomas, and cavernous hemangiomas. Definitive diagnosis is usually not made until pathologic examination of the surgical specimen. Patients with a positively identified IESCT should undergo further MRI of the remaining neuraxis to search for additional lesions, particularly in the setting of neurofibromatosis.[2,9]

Nerve Sheath Tumors

The three most common types of NSTs are schwannomas, neurofibromas, and MNSTs. Schwannomas are the most common type of NST. Although most often classified as IESCTs, schwannomas can also be present extradurally. On imaging, schwannomas are most commonly seen encompassing the dorsal sensory root of the lumbar and cervical spine. One common but nonspecific finding on imaging is invasion of the prevertebral space and neural foramina in a "dumbbell"-shaped fashion (see Fig. 22-1, A). This finding is commonly accompanied by erosion of the posterior aspect of the vertebral body and widening of the spinal canal, particularly when the tumor has been present for a long time. Patients with NF-2 should be evaluated for additional lesions because these patients often have multiple schwannomas along the neuraxis.[1,2,9]

Neurofibromas can be distinguished from schwannomas by their ability to encase nerve roots; schwannomas typically exhibit asymmetric growth resulting in nerve root displacement. When visualized on MRI, neurofibromas are often fusiform or rounded. Consistent with other IESCTs, they are isointense and hyperintense on T1- and T2-weighted MR imaging, respectively (see Fig. 22-1, B). Additionally, homogeneous intense enhancement can be observed with gadolinium injection (see Fig. 22-1, B). Patients with NF-1 may harbor numerous plexiform neurofibromas and should be evaluated for such. Furthermore, patients with NF-1 have an increased risk of malignant transformation of their neurofibromas to MNSTs. MNSTs originate most often from dedifferentiated neurofibromas in the setting of NF-1 or from sporadic neurofibromas. MNSTs are characterized by their rapid growth and should be suspected when imaging demonstrates large increases in tumor size over short periods of time.

Meningiomas

Meningiomas originate from the arachnoidal cells of the dura and thus can occur anywhere along the neuraxis. Only 10% of meningiomas occur below the cranial fossa, and they are most often located on the dorsolateral aspect of the thoracic region. Meningiomas usually manifest as

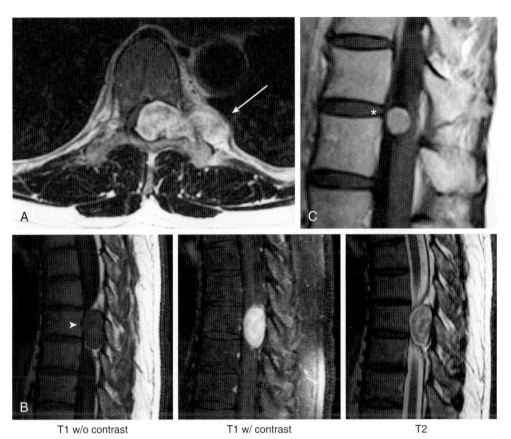

FIGURE 22-1 Examples of intradural extramedullary spinal cord tumors. **A,** Axial view on T2-weighted magnetic resonance imaging showing a "dumbbell"-shaped schwannoma (*arrow*). **B,** Schwannoma (*arrowhead*) typically enhances with contrast on T1-weighted imaging and is hyperintense on T2-weighted imaging. *w/,* with; *w/o,* without. **C,** Meningioma (*asterisk*) similarly enhances with contrast on T1-weighted imaging.

T1 w/o contrast   T1 w/ contrast   T2

solitary lesions, except in patients who also have NF-2. As with other IESCTs, meningiomas are isointense on T1-weighted imaging and hyperintense on T2-weighted imaging (see Fig. 22-1, *C*). However, the hyperintensity on T2-weighted imaging is usually milder than that seen with other IESCTs such as NSTs. Similar to other IESCTs, meningiomas enhance positively with contrast enhancement on T1-weighted imaging (see Fig. 22-1, *C*). Although uncommon, signal changes caused by spinal cord compression may also be visualized.[2] CT imaging may demonstrate bone erosion and remodeling in addition to calcifications within the neoplasm.[10]

Management and Prognosis

IESCTs are ideally managed by complete microsurgical excision. Selection of surgical access to IESCTs should be made after considering all the following: the region of tumor location, the axial plane location of the tumor, and the extent of spread. For example, IESCTs with predominantly ventral locations can be difficult to access and thus may not be amenable to complete tumor resection. In such a case, residual neoplasm can be managed by fractionated radiation therapy or radiosurgery.

NSTs of small size, dumbbell shape, and limited spread (i.e., occupying only the neural foramen) can be surgically managed through dorsolateral access. However, NSTs that demonstrate significant ventral growth through the neural foramen require ventrolateral access irrespective of the spinal level involved.[4] Schwannomas are distinguished from neurofibromas in that they do not encase

nerve roots but rather displace nerve roots, thus making nerve root preservation easier. Generally, if a tumor is large or extends into the extradural space, motor stimulation is employed to assess motor root involvement. In the absence of motor root involvement (i.e., dorsal root involvement or a thoracic root excluding T1 that forms part of the brachial plexus), the entire root can be sacrificed. However, if root involvement is present, the root should be preserved, and the surgeon should attempt to dissect it free from the tumor.[11] Meningiomas commonly adhere to dura, and thus dural resection is often required to achieve complete resection.[10] Cerebrospinal fluid leak, albeit rare, is the most common surgical complication in the management of IESCTs.[4]

Fractionated radiation therapy or radiosurgery can also be considered acceptable as the primary intervention in the setting of recurrent tumors following previous surgical extraction, tumor presence in multiple locations, the absence of significant spinal instability, and any other surgical contraindication.[4]

General positive prognostic factors in the setting of an IESCT include early diagnosis before the appearance of severe neurologic symptoms, complete tumor excision, young age, minor spinal cord compression, the absence of intraoperative spinal cord retraction, and optimal microsurgical technique. In addition, certain prognostic factors are specific to tumor type. Patients with sporadic NSTs who undergo complete tumor resection can remain disease free and, at the least, maintain their preoperative level of neurologic function. However, patients with

NSTs in the setting of neurofibromatosis have a high incidence of both recurrent tumors and new tumors. Furthermore, neurofibromas in patients with NF-1 can undergo malignant transformation to MNSTs, which have a poor prognosis. MNSTs are often not amenable to complete resection and involve leptomeningeal spread, with an average life expectancy of less than 1 year.[12] Analogous to patients with sporadic NSTs, patients with sporadic, slow-growing meningiomas can experience a recurrence-free life span with a neurologically stable prognosis. Younger patients more commonly have aggressive meningiomas with higher rates of recurrence.[2]

Intramedullary Spinal Cord Tumors

Presentation

The presentation of ISCTs cannot be characterized by a particular corollary of signs and symptoms. The average onset of signs and symptoms is 2 years, but the presentation has a wide range, from a rapid 14 days to an insidious onset reported to last as long as several years. Patients who present with a recent onset of symptoms may report that the symptoms began following a trivial injury. Presenting symptoms include localized pain, radicular pain, paresthesia, dysesthesia, spasticity, incontinence, Brown-Séquard syndrome, and extremity weakness. The most common symptom is nocturnal pain that is often described as gnawing and unremitting. A common symptom in children with ISCTs is failure to achieve developmental milestones.[9] Signs include local tenderness, sensory deficits, hyperreflexia, clonus, and gait stiffening. In addition, children may present with kyphoscoliosis and torticollis.[3]

Diagnosis

Similar to IESCTs, ISCTs are best diagnosed by MRI because conventional radiographic imaging (including CT) is not optimal for visualizing these tumors. However, conventional radiography may help increase the suspicion of an ISCT, particularly when a long-standing ISCT in a child results in mild flattening and erosion of the pedicles, as well as a widened spinal canal.

The MRI study should include both T1- and T2-weighted imaging series with gadolinium enhancement. CT with myelography should be employed in patients who are not candidates for MRI.[3] ISCTs are characterized by expansion of the spinal cord and associated polar cysts; however, definitive diagnosis requires pathologic confirmation.

Anatomic distribution is nonspecific. Both ependymomas and astrocytomas can occur anywhere throughout the spinal cord. However, studies have shown that ependymomas have a predilection for the caudal spinal cord, with 50% of ependymomas arising in the lumbosacral cord or filum terminale and the remaining 50% occurring nonpreferentially along the cervical or thoracic spinal cord.[13] ISCTs can be focal, encompassing only a few centimeters of spinal cord, or diffusely spread along the longitudinal axis of the spinal cord (Fig. 22-2).[3]

Ependymomas

Ependymomas are the most common ISCTs in adults. The three main subsets of ependymomas are cellular, myxopapillary, and anaplastic. Cellular ependymomas are most often located in the cervical spine. On T1-weighted MRI, they are isointense to hypointense, whereas on T2-weighted MRI, they are hyperintense. They originate from the ependymal lining of the central canal, thus giving them a concentric appearance on imaging. In addition, cellular ependymomas often display a polar syrinx (see Fig. 22-2).[3]

Myxopapillary ependymomas are most commonly benign and localize most often to the filum terminale and conus medullaris. They differ from other ependymomas morphologically and biologically and often resemble chordomas or chondrosarcomas; immunohistochemical analysis is frequently required for differentiation. Myxopapillary ependymomas manifest in younger individuals, in comparison with cellular ependymomas, and are also more common in male patients.[14] They display large variations in size and are associated with scalloping of the vertebral body and enlargement of the neural foramina. On T1-weighted imaging, myxopapillary ependymomas are most often isointense or hypointense; however, in some instances, they have displayed hyperintensity on T1-weighted imaging because of hemorrhage or their mucin content. On T2-weighted imaging, these tumors are most often hyperintense. Polar cysts are also common findings in myxopapillary ependymomas.[1]

On imaging, anaplastic ependymomas may be distinguished by their larger size, numerous cysts, and heterogeneous postcontrast enhancement.[2] Anaplastic ependymomas are uncommon, comprising only 5% of all ependymomas, but they are characterized by anaplastic features (i.e., vascular proliferation, mitotic figures, cellular pleomorphism, and necrosis) on histologic analysis. Patients experience higher rates of tumor recurrence and decreased rates of survival.[9]

Astrocytomas

The second most common type of ISCT is the astrocytoma, which most commonly localizes to the cervical spine. The two main types of astrocytomas are pilocytic and diffuse fibrillary. Pilocytic astrocytomas are low-grade, well-circumscribed, benign lesions that are clinically not aggressive. Diffuse fibrillary astrocytomas are nonencapsulated lesions that may exhibit an aggressive clinical course in up to one third of cases; these tumors can be distinguished by their enhancement patterns on MRI. Pilocytic astrocytomas enhance intensely with gadolinium, whereas diffuse fibrillary astrocytomas enhance minimally on gadolinium (see Fig. 22-2).[15]

Management and Prognosis

Optimal management of an ISCT involves maximal tumor resection without causing further neurologic deficit. The most significant prognostic factor for a patient with an ISCT is tumor histology because the histologic features of the tumor are most closely correlated with the feasibility of achieving complete tumor resection. Patients with low-grade ISCTs such as cellular ependymomas and pilocytic astrocytomas can undergo complete tumor resection, given the delineated and circumscribed lesion anatomic features characteristic of such tumors. In contrast, patients with aggressive ISCTs such as anaplastic

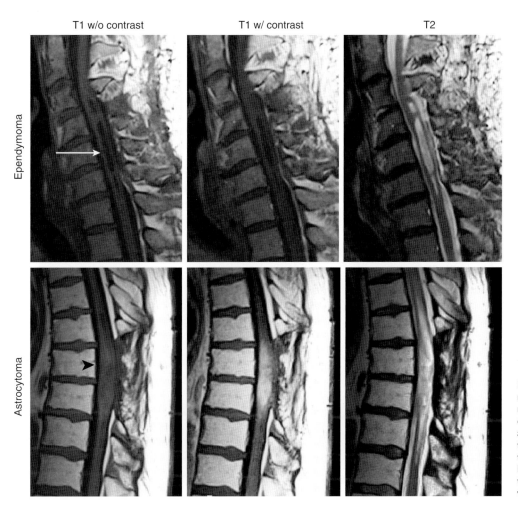

T1 w/o contrast   T1 w/ contrast   T2

Ependymoma

Astrocytoma

FIGURE 22-2 Examples of intramedullary spinal cord tumors. Magnetic resonance imaging of a cervical ependymoma (*arrow*) and thoracic astrocytoma (*arrowhead*) shows contrast enhancement with the astrocytoma but not with the ependymoma. Ependymomas are typically hyperintense on T2-weighted imaging. *w/*, with; *w/o*, without.

ependymomas or diffuse fibrillary astrocytomas have poorer prognosis because of the infiltrative nature of these tumors.

A retrospective trial conducted at the Mayo Clinic in Rochester, Minnesota, over 43 years examined 136 patients with astrocytomas and found that although pilocytic astrocytomas were associated with higher rates of survival than their diffuse fibrillary counterparts, no survival association was noted with the extent of resection. The study investigators determined that the most important positive prognostic factor was low tumor grade (World Health Organization grade I). In addition, they also determined the following to be positive prognostic factors: prolonged (>180 days) onset of symptoms, tumor location other than the cervical spinal cord, and decreased tumor involvement along the longitudinal axis of the spinal cord.[3,15]

Adjuvant therapy often accompanies surgical management. However, evidence demonstrating the efficacy of adjuvant radiation therapy in the setting of ISCTs is inconclusive. Currently, adjuvant radiation therapy is recommended for patients in whom complete resection of the ISCT is unattainable. In the setting of high-grade lesions such as diffuse fibrillary astrocytomas, adjuvant radiation therapy is almost always administered, given the evidence demonstrating improved outcome in such patients.[15]

The main contraindication to adjuvant radiation therapy is prior radiation to the same location. Furthermore, administering radiation therapy should be carefully considered because it is not without potential complications or side effects, such as spinal kyphosis, subluxation, secondary neoplasm, radionecrosis, spinal cord edema, and impaired wound healing.[3,9] Stereotactic radiosurgery is also a potential treatment avenue that is currently undergoing rapid advances. Although this modality is currently most often employed for the treatment of extramedullary tumors, it has been increasingly employed to treat ISCTs, given its ability to deliver a high radiation dose while minimizing radiation of collateral tissues. However, no conclusive evidence is available to establish radiosurgery as a prime management modality.[3]

Chemotherapy use is typically reserved for the management of recurrent or metastatic ISCTs. However, no conclusive evidence exists to establish the use of chemotherapy in these circumstances. Nonetheless, certain treatment regimens have been reported to have activity against these ISCTs. Examples of these treatment regimens include, but are not limited to, carboplatin with vincristine and lomustine, vincristine, and procarbazine. The use of chemotherapeutic regimens should be weighed against their potential complications and side effects, such as life-threatening sepsis, myelosuppression, ototoxicity, nephrotoxicity, vomiting, and nausea.

REFERENCES

1. Abul-Kasim K, Thurnher MM, McKeever P, Sundgren PC: Intradural spinal tumors: current classification and MRI features, *Neuroradiology* 50:301–314, 2008.
2. Beall DP, Googe DJ, Emery RL, et al.: Extramedullary intradural spinal tumors: a pictorial review, *Curr Probl Diagn Radiol* 36:185–198, 2007.
3. Bowers DC, Weprin BE: Intramedullary spinal cord tumors, *Curr Treat Options Neurol* 5:207–212, 2003.
4. Slin'ko EI, Al-Qashqish II: Intradural ventral and ventrolateral tumors of the spinal cord: surgical treatment and results, *Neurosurg Focus* 17:ECP2, 2004.
5. el-Mahdy W, Kane PJ, Powell MP, Crockard HA: Spinal intradural tumours. Part I: extramedullary, *Br J Neurosurg* 13:550–557, 1999.
6. Klekamp J, Samii M: Surgery of spinal nerve sheath tumors with special reference to neurofibromatosis, *Neurosurgery* 42:279–289, 1998; discussion 289–290.
7. Antinheimo J, Sankila R, Carpen O, et al.: Population-based analysis of sporadic and type 2 neurofibromatosis–associated meningiomas and schwannomas, *Neurology* 54:71–76, 2000.
8. Whittle IR, Smith C, Navoo P, Collie D: Meningiomas, *Lancet* 363:1535–1543, 2004.
9. Molina CA, Gokaslan ZL, Sciubba DM: Spinal tumors. In Norden AD, Reardon DA, Wen PCY, editors: *Primary central nervous system tumors*, New York, 2011, Humana Press, p 529.
10. Lee JW, Lee IS, Choi KU, et al.: CT and MRI findings of calcified spinal meningiomas: correlation with pathological findings, *Skeletal Radiol* 39:345–352, 2010.
11. Lot G, George B: Cervical neuromas with extradural components: surgical management in a series of 57 patients, *Neurosurgery* 41:813–820, 1997; discussion 820–822.
12. Seppala MT, Haltia MJ: Spinal malignant nerve-sheath tumor or cellular schwannoma? A striking difference in prognosis, *J Neurosurg* 79:528–532, 1993.
13. Waldron JN, Laperriere NJ, Jaakkimainen L, et al.: Spinal cord ependymomas: a retrospective analysis of 59 cases, *Int J Radiat Oncol Biol Phys* 27:223–229, 1993.
14. Sonneland PR, Scheithauer BW, Onofrio BM: Myxopapillary ependymoma: a clinicopathologic and immunocytochemical study of 77 cases, *Cancer* 56:883–893, 1985.
15. Minehan KJ, Brown PD, Scheithauer BW, et al.: Prognosis and treatment of spinal cord astrocytoma, *Int J Radiat Oncol Biol Phys* 73:727–733, 2009.

Primary Bony Tumors of the Cervical Spine

23

Jason C. Eck, Ahmad Nassr, and Bradford L. Currier

CHAPTER PREVIEW

Chapter Synopsis Most lesions in the cervical spine are metastatic; primary bone tumors are rare. The goals of treatment vary from palliation to cure. It is vital to recognize primary tumors *before* an operation, to achieve the best possible outcome. Surgical treatment of these lesions is complex because of the unique anatomy of the neck and cervical spine. Benign and malignant tumors often require markedly different approaches. A pretreatment biopsy is essential; the location of the biopsy should be planned in conjunction with all surgeons who may be involved in the patient's care. Management with a multidisciplinary team can yield good results in patients with surgically resectable lesions. This chapter reviews the diagnosis and treatment of primary benign and malignant tumors of the cervical spine.

Important Points Primary bone tumors of the cervical spine are rare.

Recognition of these unique tumors is essential because management often depends on the pathologic features, the tumor's location, and involvement of local anatomy.

Biopsy is frequently necessary to confirm the suspected diagnosis.

Biopsy should allow for adequate tissue for diagnosis while avoiding contamination of the surrounding tissue.

Management with a multidisciplinary team can yield good results.

Primary bone tumors of the cervical spine remain relatively rare but potentially devastating conditions. Most cervical spine tumors are the result of metastatic spread from remote sites. Fortunately, most primary cervical spine bone tumors are benign. However, given the possibility of cortical disruption and local tumor growth into surrounding vital structures, even benign tumors can be problematic. Primary malignant tumors of the cervical spine are very rare but have a poor prognosis because most of these tumors cannot be excised with wide margins.

For most patients with primary cervical spine tumors, the presenting symptom is localized pain. The pain is typically of insidious onset and is located in the posterior neck or occipital area. Neurologic findings are less common on initial presentation because of the slow progression of many of these tumors. Pain can be the result of cortical expansion, microfracture of the trabeculae, gross pathologic fracture, or compression of the spinal cord or exiting nerve roots. Motor weakness in a specific nerve root distribution can occur with nerve root compression, whereas generalized weakness can occur with epidural compression of the spinal cord. Bowel and bladder dysfunction and signs of myelopathy are rare findings, but they can manifest in later stages with more severe spinal cord compression.

Following the appropriate patient evaluation including medical history, physical examination, imaging, and laboratory studies, the surgeon must often obtain a tissue biopsy to confirm the suspected diagnosis. The biopsy technique should allow for collection of adequate tissue for diagnosis while avoiding contamination of the surrounding tissues. Unfortunately, this crucial portion of the process is frequently not given sufficient consideration or is performed inappropriately. The location of the biopsy specimen should be determined on the basis of imaging studies. The specimen should be taken from the most accessible location, with the fewest risks to adjacent structures, and the entire biopsy tract should be maintained in line with the planned surgical excision so it can be removed en bloc with the tumor if necessary. The biopsy should be performed at the medical center responsible for the definitive treatment to reduce the risks of the following: contamination of the surrounding tissues; inadequate sample size; inexperience of the pathology staff in bone tumors,[1] which can lead to a delay in diagnosis; tumor recurrence; and the need for more extensive surgical procedures.

These tumors present a significant challenge to the treating clinician. Consultation with appropriate specialists including internal medicine and medical and radiation oncology is necessary to provide the patient with the best treatment plan. An understanding of the natural history of the condition, along with the risks and benefits of complementary treatment options including chemotherapy and radiation therapy, is essential. This chapter introduces the diagnosis and treatment of primary cervical spine tumors. Specific benign and malignant tumors are discussed individually.

Benign Cervical Spine Tumors

Aneurysmal Bone Cyst

An aneurysmal bone cyst is a nonneoplastic lesion that can be aggressive and expansile. Its origin remains uncertain, and it can occur as a solitary lesion or in combination with other tumors, including giant cell tumor, chondroblastoma, chondromyxoid fibroma, and fibrous dysplasia. It is most commonly found in children, with a peak incidence in the second decade of life. A slight female predominance is seen. The most common locations are the spinal column and the long bones.

Of those cysts that affect the spine, 70% are located in the thoracolumbar spine, with only 25% in the cervical spine.[2] They are often found in the posterior elements including the lamina, spinous process, and pedicles. Patients often present with vague complaints of pain, stiffness, and swelling. The slow growth of the lesion and the vague initial symptoms often lead to a delayed diagnosis.

Radiographic features include an expansile lesion with a thin rim of calcification. The cysts have a characteristic "soap bubble appearance" resulting from bony trabeculae and septa. Involvement of multiple vertebral levels is possible, as are pathologic fractures. Computed tomography (CT) scans can reveal multiple fluid-filled cavities. Magnetic resonance imaging (MRI) scans can reveal heterogeneous signals with fluid-fluid levels best seen on T2-weighted images (Fig. 23-1). Despite characteristic imaging, biopsy is necessary to confirm the diagnosis and to differentiate this cyst from other lesions with similar imaging findings, including giant cell tumor and telangiectatic osteosarcoma.

Historically, treatment of aneurysmal bone cysts was intralesional excision with curettage and bone grafting. Because of high rates of local recurrence with this technique, complete surgical resection is recommended with short segment posterior spinal fusion.[3] Preoperative angiography is useful to identify the vascular supply, and preoperative embolization can reduce the risk of bleeding. Although surgical excision is typically considered the treatment of choice for accessible lesions, other treatment options include percutaneous intralesional injection and repeated embolization. Intralesional injection of calcitonin and methylprednisolone is reported to stimulate ossification of the cyst, increase the formation of cancellous bone, and reduce angiogenesis.[4] Repeated, selective arterial embolization procedures have been reported as the potential definitive treatment for aneurysmal bone cysts of the cervical spine that are not amenable to surgical excision.[5] Although it is possible in some cases to avoid the need for surgical intervention, this technique requires multiple embolization procedures over a prolonged time and carries the risk of embolic complications.

Giant Cell Tumor

Giant cell tumors are common primary bone tumors, but they occur infrequently in the spine above the sacrum. Although these tumors are benign, they can become locally aggressive and metastasize to the lung in up to 14% of cases.[6] A slight female predominance is noted, and the tumors are most commonly found in the third and fourth decades of life. Local, progressive pain in the posterior neck and shoulder is the most common presenting symptom. The diagnosis is often delayed because of the insidious onset of symptoms. Patients can present with radicular symptoms resulting from nerve root compression, and paraparesis or paralysis can occur rarely. Neurologic findings are much more common in patients with giant cell tumors of the cervical spine than with other benign cervical spine lesions.

Characteristic imaging findings include osteolysis and cortical expansion without a marked sclerotic border. A large soft tissue component with a thin sclerotic rim may be visible. Pathologic fractures are relatively common at presentation. The lesions can involve a single vertebra or multiple vertebrae, but the intervertebral space is spared. MRI reveals a hypointense signal on T1-weighted images and a hyperintense signal on T2-weighted images. Biopsy is necessary to confirm the diagnosis.

Although results in the long bone are very successful, results for giant cell tumors of the spine are less promising.[7] Various treatment options have been recommended for cervical spine giant cell tumors depending on the location, involvement of surrounding vital structures, and the patient's neurologic symptoms. These options include arterial embolization, curettage, surgical excision, radiation therapy, and cryotherapy. Because of the high risk of recurrence, en bloc surgical excision remains the preferred treatment when possible. Local tumor recurrence following intralesional excision is up to 70%; even in cases of attempted en bloc excision, the risk of recurrence is high, up to 31%.[6]

Osteoid Osteoma

Osteoid osteomas are primary bone-producing tumors that are most commonly found in the long bones, but up to 25% can be found in the spine. These tumors are most commonly found in the first 3 decades of life, and they have a male predominance. The lumbar spine is the most common location in the spine, followed by the thoracic and cervical spine. As a result, cervical spine osteoid osteomas are relatively rare. The most common presenting symptom is pain that is worse at night and is frequently relieved with aspirin or other antiinflammatory medications. Less commonly, neurologic symptoms or a progressive deformity can occur.

Radiographically, osteoid osteomas are commonly found in the posterior elements including the lamina, pedicle, and spinous process. Involvement of the vertebral body is less common. These lesions may be difficult to identify on plain radiographs initially because of their small size. CT scans can be useful for identification of the lesions and show a characteristic osteoid-producing nidus of cells surrounded by a sclerotic halo less than 2 cm in

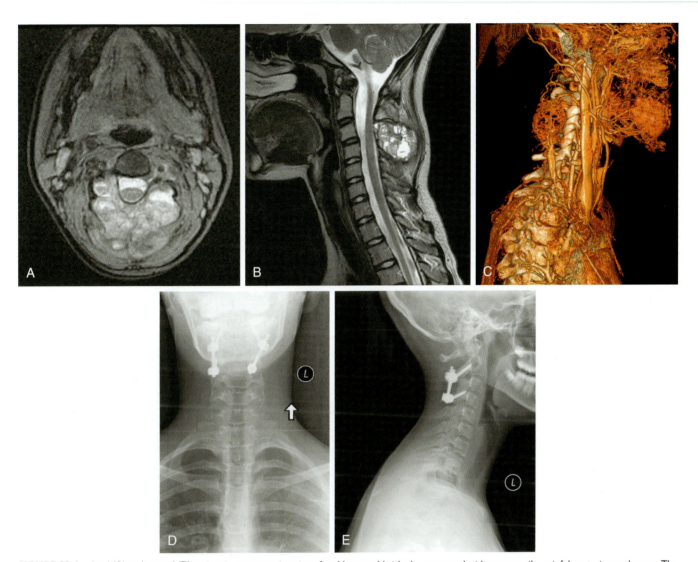

FIGURE 23-1   Axial (**A**) and sagittal (**B**) magnetic resonance imaging of an 11-year-old girl who presented with an expansile, painful posterior neck mass. The images revealed a large mass originating from the posterior elements of C3 with soft tissue expansion and fluid-fluid levels consistent with an aneurysmal bone cyst. **C**, Computed tomography angiography revealed the extremely vascular nature of the tumor with large feeding vessels. Her symptoms failed to improve following two embolization procedures, and surgical excision and stabilization from C2 to C4 were performed. Postoperative anteroposterior (**D**) and lateral (**E**) radiographs are shown.

diameter. MRI can identify the surrounding reactive tissue and is useful in patients with neurologic compression. Technetium bone scans can help localize the lesion by revealing a focal, intense region of increased uptake.

Most osteoid osteomas can be effectively managed conservatively. In patients with intractable pain or progressive deformity, surgical excision is recommended. Lesions that are distant from the neural elements and vascular structures may be amenable to radiofrequency or cryoablation procedures. The need for surgical stabilization following excision is based on the location and amount of bone excised and the subsequent degree of stability. The recurrence rate is approximately 4.5%, but no risk of malignant transformation exists.[8]

Osteoblastoma

Osteoblastomas are similar to osteoid osteomas in many ways. Osteoblastomas are larger than osteoid osteomas and are generally more than 2 cm in diameter. They are also more common in male patients and occur during adolescence and early adulthood. The most common presenting symptom is pain, but it is less responsive to aspirin and other antiinflammatory medications than in patients with osteoid osteomas. Progressive deformity is less frequent with osteoblastomas compared with osteoid osteomas.

Osteoblastoma has radiographic appearance similar to that of osteoid osteoma, except for the larger size of the osteoblastoma. Because of the larger size, osteoblastoma is often easier to detect on plain radiographs. Osteoblastomas are also more likely to continue to expand with potential involvement of the paraspinous tissues and neurologic compromise (Fig. 23-2).

Osteoblastomas often do not respond well to conservatively treatment alone, and the treatment of choice is surgical excision. The risk of local tumor recurrence is higher (15% to 50%) than that of osteoid osteoma, and risk for malignant transformation also exists.[8] Because of the larger size and need for complete excision, surgical stabilization is typically required following excision. A biopsy of

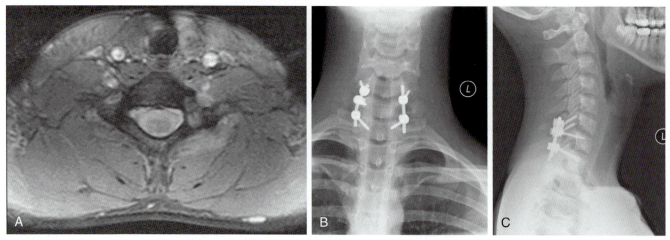

FIGURE 23-2 A, Axial magnetic resonance imaging of a 15-year-old male patient who presented with neck and left arm pain and subjective weakness. The image reveals a lytic lesion in the left C7 pedicle with extension into the lateral mass and vertebral body. Biopsy and imaging were consistent with osteoblastoma. After conservative treatment failed, the patient underwent surgical excision and stabilization from C6 to T1. Postoperative anteroposterior (**B**) and lateral (**C**) radiographs are shown.

FIGURE 23-3 Axial computed tomography (**A**) and magnetic resonance imaging (**B**) of a 41-year-old man with a 1-year history of left periscapular and shoulder pain. The images revealed a lytic, expansile mass involving the posterior elements of T1 on the left, with a large amount of mineralized matrix. The lesion was thought to be most consistent with an osteoblastoma. Unfortunately, the final biopsy results revealed an osteoblastic osteosarcoma.

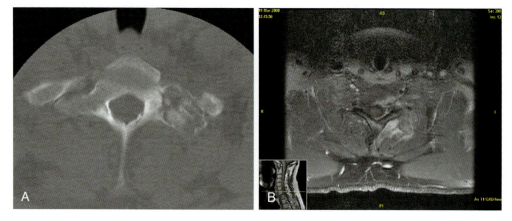

the lesion should precede surgical excision because a primary sarcoma may mimic an osteoblastoma (Fig. 23-3).

Malignant Primary Bone Tumors

Chordoma

Chordomas are rare primary malignant tumors of the spine that account for approximately 4% of primary bone tumors. They typically affect either the sacrococcygeal or the upper cervical regions. They arise from notochordal remnants and are slow-growing tumors. The most common presenting symptom is pain. Because of the vague initial complaints and slow growth, these tumors often have a delayed diagnosis. Local extension of cervical spine chordomas can manifest as a pharyngeal or lateral soft tissue mass. Other potential presenting symptoms include dysphasia or dysphonia resulting from pharyngeal compression, visual disturbances, headaches, endocrinopathies, nasal disturbances, and neurologic deficits secondary to spinal cord or nerve root compression.[9]

Plain radiographs can identify a large, destructive lesion, often with a large, associated soft tissue mass. MRI scans reveal a destructive lesion of the vertebral body associated with a large, well-defined soft tissue mass that is hyperintense on T2-weighted images and heterogeneous with contrast enhancement. CT scans reveal an encapsulated lesion with fine septations and may demonstrate cortical destruction. CT scans are indispensable in surgical planning for resection and stabilization (Fig. 23-4).

The treatment of choice for chordomas is complete en bloc surgical resection.[10] However, because of the involvement of crucial adjacent structures, this procedure is often extremely difficult or impossible in the cervical spine. Another factor limiting the feasibility of en bloc resection is the consistency of the tumor mass. Chordomas are typically gelatinous and can spread along adjacent muscles including the longus colli muscle. This makes en bloc resection with wide margins without tumor breakage and spilling more difficult (Fig. 23-5).

Histologically, chordomas have a characteristic physaliphorous cell that has a central nucleus surrounded by a large vacuolated cytoplasm. Chordomas appear as a combination of physaliphorous cells with a myxoid matrix with positive staining for keratin, epithelial membrane antigen, and S-100 protein (Fig. 23-6).

As with all surgical treatment of tumors, extensive preoperative planning is crucial for management of chordomas. If the vertebral arteries are involved, angiographic studies can identify the presence of collateral blood flow

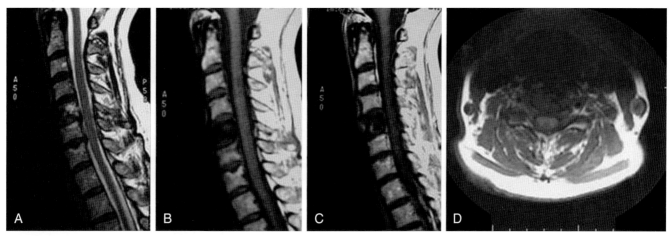

FIGURE 23-4 A 51-year-old woman with biopsy-proved chordoma involving C5. **A,** T2-weighted magnetic resonance imaging showed diffuse increased signal within the C5 vertebral body. **B,** Decreased signal was noted in T1-weighted images. **C,** The lesion did not enhance with gadolinium contrast. **D,** Axial T1-weighted image shows no spinal cord compression or foraminal involvement. (From Currier BL, Papagelopoulos PJ, Krauss WE, et al: Total en bloc spondylectomy of C5 vertebra for chordoma. *Spine [Phila Pa 1976]* 32:E294-E299, 2007.)

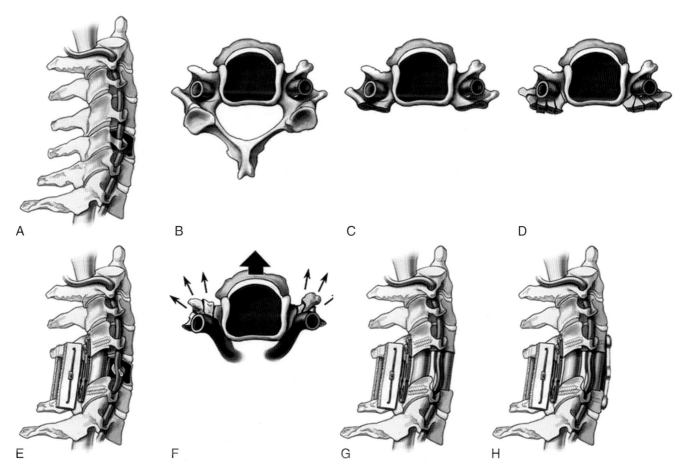

FIGURE 23-5 **A** to **H,** Drawings of the operative technique for treatment of chordoma. **A** and **B,** The tumor (*black*) was contained in the vertebral body of C5. **C,** A total C5 laminectomy was performed removing the C5 lamina in one piece. The lateral masses at C5 were removed by cutting across the pedicle with a medium-sized T saw. **D,** The remaining rim of bone posterior to the vertebral foramen was excised. **E,** Two strut grafts were placed posteriorly fixed with titanium cables to the spinous processes of C4 and C6. Two 13-mm three-hole titanium plates were fixed with 4-0 cancellous screws at the lateral masses of C4 and C6. **F,** Diskectomies at C4-C5 and C5-C6 were performed. Dissection continued between the vertebral arteries and vertebral body and the joints of Luschka. The vertebral arteries were completely freed from the C5 vertebral body and anterior tubercles. The C5 vertebral body was removed anteriorly. An iliac crest tricortical strut graft was placed anteriorly (**G**), and a plate was fixed with four screws to the anterior aspect of the vertebral bodies at C4 and C6 (**H**). (From Currier BL, Papagelopoulos PJ, Krauss WE, et al: Total en bloc spondylectomy of C5 vertebra for chordoma. *Spine [Phila Pa 1976]* 32:E294-E299, 2007.)

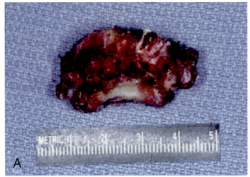
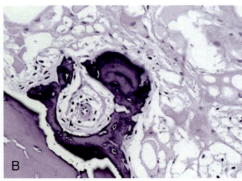

FIGURE 23-6 A, Macroscopic appearance of the removed chordoma specimen. **B,** High-power (×80) histologic appearance of the chordoma showing "physaliphorous" cells with slight cytologic atypia. (From Currier BL, Papagelopoulos PJ, Krauss WE, et al: Total en bloc spondylectomy of C5 vertebra for chordoma. *Spine [Phila Pa 1976]* 32:E294-E299, 2007.)

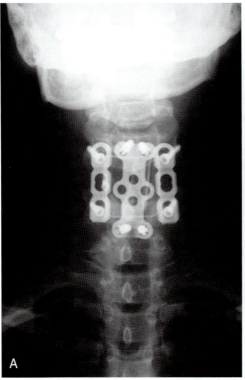
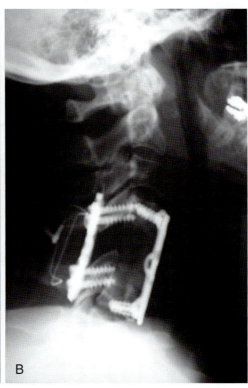

FIGURE 23-7 Anteroposterior (**A**) and lateral (**B**) views 9 years after surgical treatment of chordoma show solid spine fusion and no instability. Mild degenerative changes were noted at C6 to C7. (From Currier BL, Papagelopoulos PJ, Krauss WE, et al: Total en bloc spondylectomy of C5 vertebra for chordoma. *Spine [Phila Pa 1976]* 32:E294-E299, 2007.)

and determine whether sacrifice of one side is possible. Determining the optimal surgical approach is based on the specific location of the tumor and involvement of adjacent structures. Possibilities include retropharyngeal, submandibular, and transmandibular approaches. Consultation with specialists in otorhinolaryngology, facial plastic surgery, or maxillofacial surgery may be beneficial. Despite careful planning and meticulous surgical technique, major complications are common.

Adjuvant radiation therapy has been beneficial in reducing the risk of recurrence and metastatic spread of the tumor. A major limitation in the use of traditional radiation therapy for cervical spine chordomas is the risk to adjacent structures, including the spinal cord. Advanced radiation therapy methods such as proton beam therapy and radiosurgery have shown increased efficacy with decreased associated risk by allowing for increased doses of radiation to be delivered to a specific, focal location, with less exposure to the surrounding tissues. The 5-year overall survival rates range from 60% to 70%, and the 10-year survival rates decrease to 35% to 40%[11] (Figs. 23-7 and 23-8).

Osteosarcoma

Osteosarcoma of the spine is most common in the lumbosacral vertebral bodies, but it can occur less frequently in the cervical spine. The peak age of presentation is during the second and third decades of life, although secondary osteosarcoma caused by transformation of another tumor occurs more commonly in patients more than 50 years old.

Radiographic features of osteosarcoma depend on the histologic cell types and the amount of osteoid production. Lesions can be lytic, sclerotic, or mixed and often are associated with a periosteal reaction, cortical disruption, and soft tissue expansion. The vertebral body is typically affected, with or without involvement of the posterior elements. Distinguishing osteosarcoma from other more common benign tumors, including osteoblastoma or chondroblastoma, is crucial (Fig. 23-9).

Treatment of osteosarcoma consists of neoadjuvant chemotherapy, excision, and stabilization, followed by adjuvant chemotherapy. Despite aggressive treatment, the median survival is less than 2 years because of the frequent inability to obtain resection with wide surgical margins and subsequent tumor recurrence.

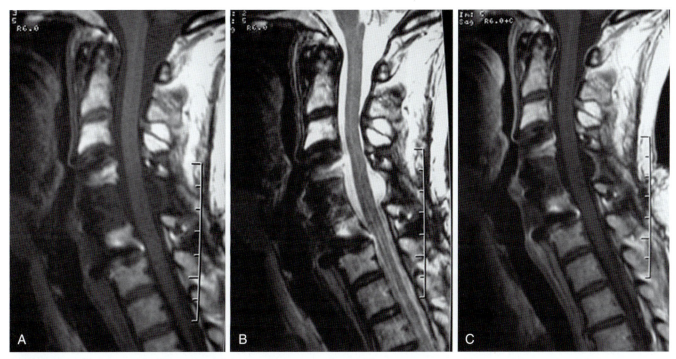

FIGURE 23-8 T1-weighted (**A**), T2-weighted (**B**), gadolinium contrast–enhanced (**C**) magnetic resonance imaging reveals no evidence of recurrent tumor in this patient who underwent surgical treatment of chordoma. (From Currier BL, Papagelopoulos PJ, Krauss WE, et al: Total en bloc spondylectomy of C5 vertebra for chordoma. *Spine [Phila Pa 1976]* 32:E294-E299, 2007.)

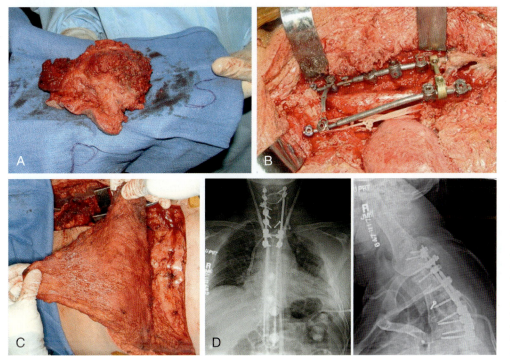

FIGURE 23-9 Final pathologic examination from the patient in Figure 23-3 revealed an osteoblastic osteosarcoma. The patient received adjuvant chemotherapy with a subsequent revised tumor resection and stabilization procedure. **A,** The gross tumor specimen is shown. **B,** A posterior instrumented reconstruction was performed with iliac crest graft from C5 to T4. **C,** A latissimus dorsi muscle flap was elevated for soft tissue coverage. **D,** Final radiographs.

Chondrosarcoma

Chondrosarcomas are most commonly found in the pelvis, femur, humerus, and ribs, but they can less frequently occur in the spine. The thoracic spine is the most common location in the spine, but rare occurrences have been reported in the cervical spine. These tumors typically are derived from either cartilaginous structures or bony tissues derived from cartilage precursors. The peak age at presentation is 45 years. These slow-growing and low-grade tumors often have a delayed diagnosis. Localized pain is the most common presenting symptom. In patients with higher-grade lesions or with a delayed diagnosis, neurologic symptoms are possible. Palpable soft tissue masses can also be present.

Typical radiographic features include a large, centrally based, destructive lesion with areas of flocculent calcification. In lower-grade lesions, scalloping of the cortex is noted, whereas in higher-grade lesions, cortical erosion

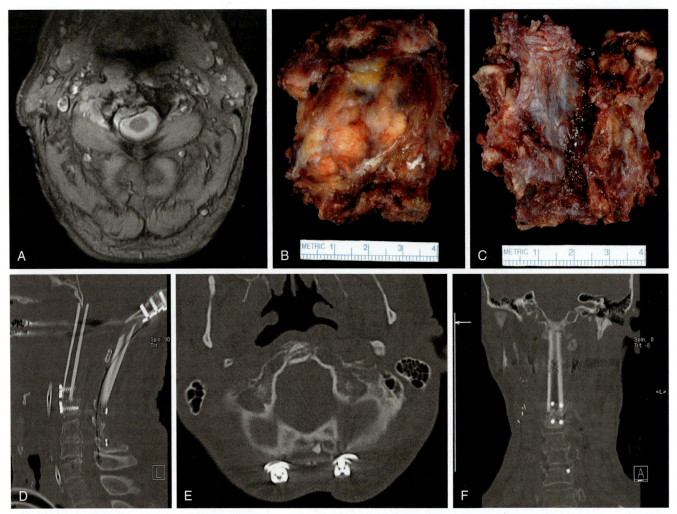

FIGURE 23-10   A 67-year-old man with a C2 chordoma treated with en bloc excision of C1 to C3 including the right vertebral artery and the C2 and C3 nerve roots and reconstruction. **A,** T2-weighted axial magnetic resonance imaging at C2 revealing involvement of the right vertebral artery. **B** and **C,** Resected specimen. **D,** Postoperative midsagittal computed tomography (CT) scan demonstrating resection and reconstruction with vascularized fibular graft anteriorly from the clivus to C4 and posterior iliac grafting with instrumentation from the occiput to C7. **E** and **F,** Follow-up axial and coronal CT scan images showing incorporation of the vascularized fibula graft at the clivus and C4.

with soft tissue expansion may be present. Although CT scans can provide more detailed information on the cortical outlines of the lesion, spinal canal involvement and soft tissue expansion are best seen on MRI.

As opposed to other sarcomas, chondrosarcomas are not responsive to either chemotherapy or traditional radiation therapy, although proton beam therapy has been shown to be more effective. Treatment consists of en bloc surgical excision and stabilization when possible. Adjuvant proton beam therapy can reduce the risk of tumor recurrence or distant metastasis.

Ewing Sarcoma

Ewing sarcoma is most commonly found in the pelvis and femur; involvement of the spine is less common. Most cases with involvement of the spine are from metastases, but primary Ewing sarcoma of the spine can occur. Most cases in the spine involve the sacrum, followed by the lumbar spine and the thoracic spine. The cervical spine is the least common location. The most common presenting symptom is pain, but up to 40% of patients can present with neurologic signs and symptoms.[4] Ewing sarcoma has a slight male predominance.

Initially, radiographs may reveal only very subtle changes and can lead to a delayed diagnosis. Most patients have a lytic lesion with involvement of the posterior elements and extension into the vertebral body. More than 90% of the tumors have expansion into the vertebral canal that accounts for the common neurologic findings.

Treatment of Ewing sarcoma of the spine includes a combination of chemotherapy, surgical excision, and radiation therapy. Despite aggressive treatment, the 5-year survival rate is approximately 50%.[12]

Conclusions

Although primary bony tumors of the cervical spine are rare, their recognition is essential for the practicing spinal surgeon. Imaging characteristics of a lesion can lead to a narrow differential diagnosis, but biopsy is almost always needed to confirm this diagnosis. Management of these lesions often involves complex approaches and a multidisciplinary team approach to yield good results (Fig. 23-10). The expertise of an institution that manages many of these lesions is invaluable because patients with tumors that are treated by an oncologically sound approach have a better outcome and a higher rate of long-term survival.

REFERENCES

1. Mankin HJ, Mankin CJ, Simon MA: The hazards of the biopsy, revisited, *J Bone Joint Surg Am* 78:656–663, 1996.
2. Weinstein JN, McLain RJ: Primary tumors of the spine, *Spine (Phila Pa 1976)* 12:843–851, 1987.
3. Papagelopoulos PJ, Currier BL, Shaughnessy WJ, et al.: Aneurysmal bone cyst of the spine: management and outcome, *Spine (Phila Pa 1976)* 23:621–628, 1988.
4. Gladden ML Jr, Gillingham BL, Hennrikus W, Vaughan LM: Aneurysmal bone cyst of the first vertebrae in a child treated with percutaneous intralesional injection of calcitonin and methyl-prednisolone: a case report, *Spine (Phila Pa 1976)* 25:527–530, 2000.
5. Mohit AA, Eskridge J, Ellenbogen R, Shaffrey CI: Aneurysmal bone cyst of the atlas: successful treatment through selective arterial embolization. Case report, *Neurosurgery* 55:E1001–E1005, 2004.
6. Martin C, McCarthy EF: Giant cell tumor of the sacrum and spine: series of 23 cases and a review of the literature, *Iowa Orthop J* 30:69–75, 2010.
7. Hart RA, Boriani S, Biagini R, et al.: A system for surgical staging and management of spine tumors: a clinical outcome study of giant cell tumors of the spine, *Spine (Phila Pa 1976)* 22:1773–1783, 1997.
8. Zileli M, Cagli S, Basdemir G, Ersahin Y: Osteoid osteomas and osteoblastomas of the spine, *Neurosurg Focus* 15:5, 2003.
9. Nicoucar K, Rausch T, Becker M, Dulguerov P: Cervical chordoma with retropharyngeal extension presenting with impaired voice, *Tumori* 94:873–876, 2008.
10. Currier BL, Papagelopoulos PJ, Krauss WE, et al.: Total en bloc spondylectomy of C5 vertebra for chordoma, *Spine (Phila Pa 1976)* 32:E294–E299, 2007.
11. McMaster ML, Goldstein AM, Bromley CM, et al.: Chordoma: incidence and survival patterns in the United States, 1973-1995, *Cancer Causes Control* 12:1–11, 2001.
12. Ilaslan H, Sundaram M, Unni KK, Dekutoski MB: Primary Ewing's sarcoma of the vertebral column, *Skeletal Radiol* 33:506–513, 2004.

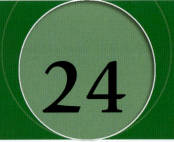

24 Metastatic Disease of the Cervical Spine

Justin E. Bird and Rex A.W. Marco

CHAPTER PREVIEW

Chapter Synopsis	The spine is the most common site of metastatic disease involving bone. The cervical spine is less often affected by metastatic disease, yet metastasis still occurs with a greater frequency per year than do primary bone sarcomas. Metastatic cervical spine disease presents unique challenges, and optimal care requires a multidisciplinary team approach. The purpose of this chapter is to discuss the pathophysiology, clinical presentation, diagnosis, and management considerations.
Important Points	The spine is the most common site of metastatic disease involving bone.
	Optimal care of the patient with metastatic cervical spine disease requires a multidisciplinary team approach.
	Goals of management should be to prevent irreversible damage, confirm the diagnosis of metastatic disease, and develop an individualized management plan.
	Biopsy, either needle or open, should be carefully planned to maximize the chance of confirming a tissue diagnosis while reducing the risk of contaminating the surrounding normal tissue.
	Treatment of metastatic disease of the cervical spine varies based on pathologic features of the primary tumor, location, level of disease, and patient-specific factors.

Cancer has consistently been a leading cause of death in the developed world and, by most predictions, has now become *the* leading cause of death worldwide. Carcinomas arising from lung, breast, prostate, and thyroid are by far the most common types of cancer, with more than 1.5 million new cases in the United States annually. Ten to thirty percent of those patients present with symptomatic metastases to bone.[1] Sarcomas involving bone are less common and comprise approximately 2000 new cases per year.

The spine is the most common site of metastatic disease involving bone. Most spine metastases occur in the thoracic and lumbar spine. The cervical spine is less often affected by metastatic disease, yet metastasis still occurs with a greater frequency per year than do primary bone sarcomas.

Metastatic cervical spine disease presents unique challenges to both the patients fighting their malignant diseases and the medical professionals involved in their care. Optimal care of the patient with metastatic disease of the cervical spine requires a multidisciplinary team that includes physicians specializing in both spinal surgery and oncology, medical oncologists, radiation

oncologists, interventional radiologists, pathologists, therapists, nutritionists, and skilled nursing staff. All these individuals are critical in (1) identifying the unique challenges metastatic spine disease presents and (2) developing a comprehensive treatment plan that addresses all the necessary issues to give the patient the best possible functional outcome.

The approach to the patient with a pathologic lesion in the cervical spine should be systematic, with three basic points in mind: (1) prevent irreversible damage in the acute setting, (2) confirm the diagnosis of metastatic disease, (3) and develop an individualized treatment plan based on the personality of the patient and the specific features of the disease (Fig. 24-1).

First, the clinician must determine the acuity of the patient's symptoms and the possibility for rapid decline. This determination helps the clinician determine whether prompt care is warranted, thereby superseding other basic principles that guide care in the oncologic patient. When an emergency arises, prompt medical and surgical treatment should be initiated to stabilize the patient while at the same time minimizing future complications that may affect the definitive management of the patient.

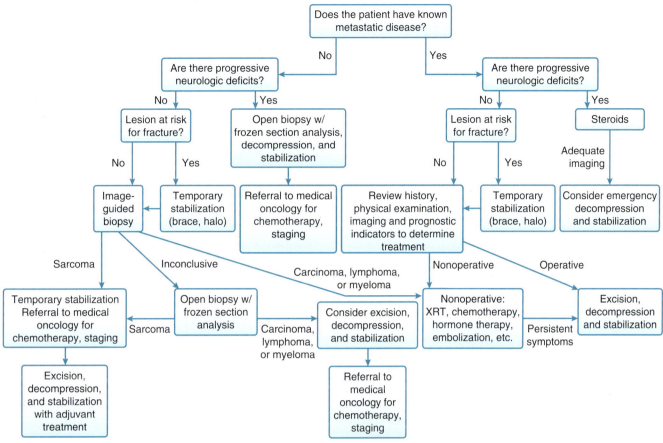

FIGURE 24-1 Algorithm for surgical management of pathologic lesions in the cervical spine.

Second, the clinician must determine whether the lesion is a metastatic lesion. Imaging should be obtained to localize all areas of disease. Does the patient have a known primary tumor? Are multiple lesions present, or is this a solitary lesion? Is the lesion anatomically and radiologically consistent with metastatic disease? The imaging results can often help the clinician make a radiologic diagnosis of metastatic disease; occasionally however, radiologic findings are equivocal, and further steps must be taken. If the lesion cannot be firmly attributed to metastatic disease, then the clinician is obligated to obtain tissue to make the diagnosis.

The biopsy should adhere to firm principles that limit contamination of vital structures anatomically associated with the lesion. A core needle biopsy usually provides diagnostic tissue without the potential destabilizing consequences of an open biopsy requiring laminectomy or corpectomy. A needle biopsy also minimizes contamination of surrounding tissue when compared with an open biopsy. If the results of a needle biopsy are nondiagnostic, then an open biopsy should be performed. The open biopsy must be well planned and coordinated with a pathologist so that a firm pathologic decision can be made and the appropriate intraoperative procedures can be performed.

Third, the definitive management plan must consider the patient's overall health, prognosis, ability to withstand invasive procedures, and personal goals and expectations. Clear and realistic expectations must be defined and related to the patient. Counseling regarding planned treatments and possible complications should be comprehensive and involve as many members of the family and health care team as possible, under the direction of a team leader.

Pathophysiology

The term *metastasis* was first introduced in 1829 by Joseph Récamier when he differentiated primary bone and soft tissue "sarcomas" from lesions that arose in bone secondarily from another site, "metastasis." His description of metastasis was preceded by Astley Cooper's reporting in 1818 of several cases of "tumors of a similar kind forming other parts of the body . . . and in organs of the greatest importance to life." Such early observations have inspired years of investigation by brilliant, dedicated people, yet the exact mechanism by which tumors spread from one organ to another is, frankly, not well understood.

Similarly, the reason that the spine is the most common site of metastatic disease is unknown. Bidirectional blood flow through Batson valveless venous channels may explain to some degree the tendency for metastasis to occur with such frequency in the spine.[2] Several such theories exist; however, none of them can fully explain the observed phenomena. The most reasonable explanation for metastatic deposits in the spine is likely multifactorial, involving both mechanical and biologic factors.[3]

Once the tumor has metastasized to bone, the effects of the tumor on bone can vary. The subsequent progression of disease is related to the aggressiveness of the tumor, the level of the lesion within the cervical spine, the location of the lesion within the vertebral body, and the association of the lesion with anatomic structures. Tumor growth cannot occur within the vertebral body without displacing or destroying that which previously exists. The tumor cells accomplish this by activating osteoclasts, which then resorb bone, thereby allowing further growth of the tumor while undermining the structural integrity of the spine.[4]

The loss of the structural integrity of the cervical spine has serious ramifications. Locally, the collapse of the vertebral body may lead to significant kyphotic deformity. The deformity can cause, alone or in the presence of extruded tumor, compression on the neural structures resulting in progressive and permanent neurologic dysfunction. Tumor can also compress the vertebral or spinal arteries and lead to ischemic complications.

Disease Level and Location

The cervical spine is composed of seven vertebrae, three biomechanically distinct regions, and two junctions. The posterior half of the vertebral body is most likely affected early, and disease in this location may be related to vascular transmission of tumor from the primary site.[5] As tumor progresses and cortical bone is destroyed, the anterior half of the vertebral body, as well as areas dense in cortical bone such as the pedicles, lateral masses, and transverse processes, is affected.[5]

The upper cervical region (C1 and C2) functions as a distinct unit and, when considered with its occipital articulation, forms the basis of the occipitocervical junction. The middle cervical region (C3 to C6) is the most common region affected by metastatic disease. It is responsible for the lordotic sagittal alignment and does not contain a transitional zone. The last cervical segment (C7), together with the upper thoracic vertebrae (T1 and T2), forms the cervicothoracic junction.

The location and the level of the lesion affect not only the patient's symptoms, but also the indication for invasive treatments and their approaches. The spacious spinal canal and thick ligaments in the upper cervical region make spinal cord compression and neurologic deficits uncommon; mechanical instability and pain predominate.[6] Recalcitrant pain and instability are indications for surgical treatment.

In the midcervical region, spinal cord compromise is more common, and patients often present with pain and myelopathy. Sagittal imbalance may occur, leading to a disabling kyphotic posture.

The normal transition from lordosis of the midcervical spine to kyphosis of the thoracic spine occurs at the cervicothoracic junction. This region is normally under high stress. When the structural support is disrupted by tumoral progression, it results in a high rate of myelopathy secondary to exacerbation of the kyphotic stresses and a relative small spinal canal size.

Clinical Presentation

Most patients with spinal metastases present in the sixth decade with pain, although incidental lesions are found approximately 11% of the time.[5] Pain is often nonmechanical and worse at rest. Difficulty sleeping may be reported. Destructive lesions in the C2 spinous process may disrupt the tension band effect of the paraspinal ligaments and musculature and cause the patient to report a progressive feeling of head heaviness and an inability to hold the head upright without assistance.[1] Neurologic dysfunction occurs in 5% to 10% of patients, and patients may report burning pain, weakness, and fine motor and gait disturbances.[1]

Diagnostic Considerations

Plain radiographs should be obtained routinely, yet they all too often fail to demonstrate pathologic lesions of the spine clearly. However, radiographs can demonstrate instability related to a pathologic lesion. When lesions are, in fact, noted on radiographs, a significant amount of bony destruction has already occurred. Relatively normal disk spaces are commonly noted. When a pathologic lesion of the cervical spine is seen on radiographs, it warrants additional imaging. A skeletal survey should be obtained to determine whether lesions are also present in the appendicular skeleton.[5]

In contrast to plain radiography, bone scintigraphy is a valuable screening tool and can identify an affected area within the cervical spine many months earlier than plain radiography. Although bone scintigraphy can highlight areas of high bone turnover, it does not provide enough information to differentiate among the various pathologic conditions that may cause high bone turnover (e.g., tumor, infection, fracture). Bone scintigraphy is also unable to identify lesions caused by tumors with extremely high osteoclastic activity, as seen in some patients with aggressive tumors such as myeloma, lymphoma, and renal cell carcinoma.

When clinical or radiologic suspicion exists, more sensitive imaging studies should be obtained, such as computed tomography (CT) and magnetic resonance imaging (MRI) scans. A CT scan is particularly valuable in demonstrating the degree of bone destruction and the remaining microarchitecture. MRI scans should be obtained with and without gadolinium contrast enhancement to determine the degree of uptake and the relative activity of the lesion. MRI is particularly valuable in identifying the extent of the tumor and the involvement of associated anatomic structures. The utility of positron emission tomography is still unclear; however, it may help identify lesions with activity within the cervical spine that may otherwise be missed on routine imaging.

Both the surgeon and the radiologist should perform a coordinated evaluation of the lesion with these modalities. This diagnostic information not only is critical in making a radiologic diagnosis but also provides invaluable information for the surgeon and pathologist at the time of biopsy.

Management

The care of any patient should be based on both the histologic diagnosis and the overall condition of the patient (i.e., age, comorbidities, functional status, goals, motivation, and support systems). The ideal physician is (1) knowledgeable about the pathologic process, (2) considerate regarding the numerous factors that affect prognosis, and (3) facile in guiding the patient through the ordeal in a way that minimizes both physical and psychosocial complications.

The overall management of a patient with a pathologic lesion in the spine is complex. An algorithm for the evaluation of such a patient is provided in Figure 24-1. The following two questions must immediately be asked once a patient with a cervical lesion is encountered: (1) Does this patient have known, tissue-supported metastatic disease? and (2) Does the patient have progressive neurologic dysfunction?

A patient with known metastatic disease without progressive neurologic dysfunction can be approached using a relatively simple management strategy with goals to reduce pain, limit local tumor progression, and prevent progressive deformity. The management strategy is more complex when a patient presents with a lesion without documented metastatic disease, has a known carcinoma and now presents with a solitary bone lesion, or presents with progressive neurologic dysfunction. The management of these patients must be carefully considered. The goals of treatment should be to relieve pressure from the compressed neurologic structures, obtain a tissue diagnosis in a manner that limits contamination to nearby structures, and stabilize the spine.

Biopsy

The biopsy of a lesion in the cervical spine is of utmost importance, and a delicate approach is required. A balance must be struck to perform the least invasive procedure possible while obtaining enough tissue to make the diagnosis. At present, with the advent of image-guided techniques, this procedure can often be performed by closed methods using fine-needle aspiration or core needle biopsy. When image-guided techniques are not feasible, an open biopsy should be performed. Again, great care and consideration must be taken to obtain the tissue in a way that limits contamination.

An open biopsy should be performed with an experienced musculoskeletal pathologist available to carry out a frozen section to make intraoperative decisions whether (1) enough tissue has been obtained for diagnosis and (2) the lesion represents carcinoma, lymphoma, myeloma, sarcoma, or infection. If the lesion represents a sarcoma based on frozen section analysis, a staged surgical plan may be prudent. Confirmed metastatic carcinoma may be treated accordingly, with the goals of removing as much local tumor as possible and stabilizing the remaining anatomy. Additional tissue should always be sent for permanent analysis whenever frozen section techniques are used. Lesions located completely within the spinous process or lamina may be treated with an excisional biopsy.

The information gained by the biopsy is vital and helps guide treatment plans and expectations. Tumor-specific

biology determines in large part whether the patient can expect to live months or years. Patients with favorable primary tumors such as breast carcinoma and multiple myeloma have reported mean survival times of approximately 1 to 2 years compared with patients with unfavorable primary tumor types such as lung and gastrointestinal carcinoma, which have reported mean survival times of less than 4 months.[7-9] Individual prognoses vary significantly; however, the clinician can only gather prognostic clues once a tumor-type specific diagnosis has been made.

Nonoperative Treatment Modalities

The treatment of metastatic disease of the cervical spine varies based on the primary tumor biology, the location and level of disease, and patient-specific factors with respect to comorbidities, personal treatment goals, and life expectancy. Carcinomas variably respond to a wide array of treatments including steroids, hormone therapy, radiation, cryoablation, embolization, radiofrequency ablation, and chemotherapy.

Steroids are commonly used in patients with spinal cord compression secondary to metastatic spine disease and may have both analgesic and treatment effects. However, when a biopsy is indicated, steroids should be held until after the biopsy has been performed because their oncolytic effect on tumors such as lymphoma and myeloma may result in a nondiagnostic biopsy result.

Radiation therapy may be used as a palliative measure to reduce pain and control local disease.[10] Radiation is most appropriate as a treatment when the patient has not previously received radiation therapy and presents with significant neck pain without evidence of spinal instability, progressive neurologic compromise, or progressive deformity. Radiation therapy is not curative but may be used alone or in conjunction with other treatment modalities such as surgery to control the disease and prolong life.[11] Radiation therapy does carry a degree of risk, and significant numbers of patients may develop pain, difficulty swallowing, burns, spinal cord injury, and postoperative wound problems. The judicious use of radiation therapy is recommended and should be performed by experienced radiation oncologists.

Breast and prostate carcinoma may be particularly responsive to hormonal therapy. Vascular tumors such as renal cell carcinomas may require embolization before surgical intervention and may even be controlled with serial embolizations. Lymphoma and myeloma are often treated with chemotherapy; however, radiation therapy has been shown to be an effective palliative treatment even in patients with spinal instability (Fig. 24-2).[12] Cryoablation and radiofrequency ablation may be used to gain local disease control in some situations.

Operative Management

Although most patients with metastases to the cervical spine can be treated without surgical intervention, surgery can provide the best means of removing the tumor burden, ameliorating pain, and stabilizing the cervical spine for some patients. A healthy patient with cervical metastases from a relatively radioresistant tumor who demonstrates physiologic spinal instability is an ideal

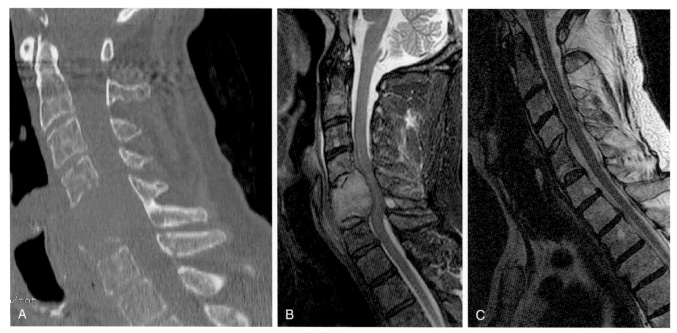

FIGURE 24-2 A 65-year-old woman with multiple myeloma involving C5 and C6 was neurologically intact. Sagittal computed tomography scan (**A**) and T2-weighted magnetic resonance imaging (MRI) (**B**) were performed. The patient elected to proceed with nonoperative treatment with halo immobilization, chemotherapy, and radiation therapy. Sagittal T2-weighted MRI (**C**) obtained 1 month after instituting nonoperative therapy demonstrates resolution of the spinal cord compression.

candidate for surgical treatment (Fig. 24-3).[12a] White and Panjabi defined physiologic instability of the spine as the development of one of the following criteria under normal physiologic loading: (1) progressive neurologic dysfunction, (2) progressive deformity, and (3) pain recalcitrant to medical treatment. The surgeon must carefully weigh the risk-to-benefit profile and the patient's predicted survival.

Tokuhashi and colleagues developed a scoring system for prognosis in patients with metastatic spine tumors that is based on six parameters ranging from general health condition to neurologic status to primary tumor type.[13] Enkaoua and associates reported a median survival of 5.3 months for patients with a Tokuhashi score of 7 or lower versus a median survival of 23.6 months for those with a Tokuhashi score of 8 or higher.[14] Primary tumors arising from the lung or kidney, low performance status, and unresectable organ metastases have been reported to be significantly associated with poor survival.[9] These data may help both the patient and the surgeon decide whether to proceed with surgical intervention.

Once the decision has been made to undergo surgical treatment, the surgeon must decide the best surgical procedure to perform. Decompression with reconstruction is the most common form of surgical treatment for metastatic cervical spine disease. However, Fehlings and associates reported on the lack of a single level 1 study in the literature to help guide decision making in patients with metastatic disease of the cervical spine.[15] The available studies do suggest that junctional location of the tumor and the presence of collapse and kyphotic deformity positively influence the majority of spine surgeons to stabilize the spine. Additionally, Fehlings and colleagues concluded that (1) posterior approaches are favored for

occiput-C2 (C0 to C2) disease, (2) anterior techniques are recommended to manage subaxial disease (C3 to C7), and (3) either an anterior or a posterior approach can be used at the cervicothoracic junction (C7 to T1). These investigators also recommended the use of combined approaches in the setting of circumferential disease and compromised bone quality.

Metastatic disease involving the C1 and C2 levels does not usually require tumor removal. Most patients with C1 or C2 involvement can be treated nonoperatively with radiation therapy and a cervical orthosis. Halo vest immobilization is considered for patients with a prolonged life expectancy who present with upper cervical instability from relatively radiosensitive tumors such as myeloma and lymphoma. However, patients with upper cervical spine metastases who remain healthy yet who demonstrate physiologic spinal instability despite appropriate nonoperative treatment usually benefit from occipital cervical fusion and instrumentation.[16]

Patients with subaxial tumor involvement who meet criteria for surgical intervention usually benefit from corpectomy. Once the tumor has been surgically removed and the neural components decompressed, the normal alignment must be restored, the defect reconstructed, and the construct stabilized. Reconstruction may include the use of cages and grafts, although fusion of the grafts may be difficult to obtain, given the limited healing potential of a patient with metastatic cervical spine disease who may have undergone treatments such as radiation and chemotherapy preoperatively or will do so postoperatively.

In some cases, methylmethacrylate is an alternative to grafting and can provide a solid construct.[17] This technique is most useful in patients with very limited life

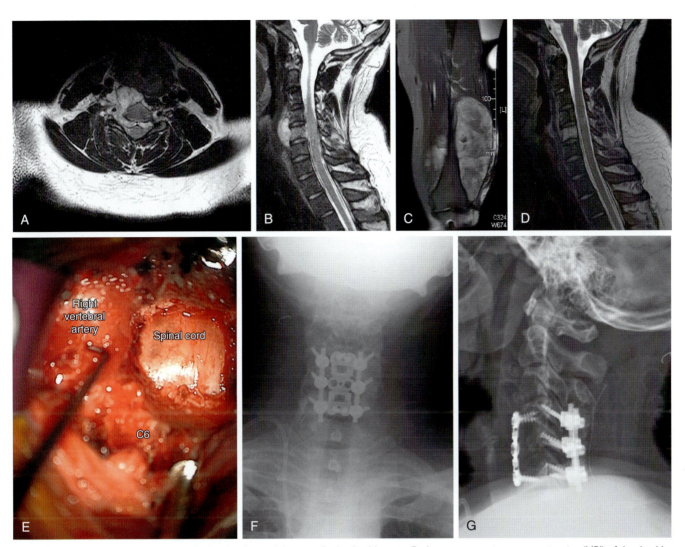

FIGURE 24-3   A 36-year-old man presented with a 3-month history of right shoulder pain. Findings on magnetic resonance imaging (MRI) of the shoulder were normal. However, a C5 lesion with spinal cord compression was noted on axial and sagittal T2-weighted MRI (**A** and **B**). A biopsy was obtained and confirmed the diagnosis of myxoid liposarcoma. Further examination of the patient revealed an inordinately large left thigh. **C,** MRI of the left thigh demonstrated the primary site of the tumor. The patient underwent neoadjuvant chemotherapy followed by a distal femur resection and replacement. **D,** Repeat MRI revealed a marked decrease in tumor burden in C5. The patient desired to proceed with an intralesional excision (**E,** intraoperative microscopic photogram), followed by anterior and posterior spinal fusion and instrumentation (**F** and **G**), to minimize the likelihood of local tumor recurrence.

expectancy. Patients with vertebral body involvement of C3 may benefit from anterior and posterior stabilization because anterior fixation into the base of C2 is usually suboptimal as a result of the narrow vertebral body of C2. Specialized plates with a midline, single screw into the base of C2 and two screw holes into the C4 vertebral body can provide reasonable anterior fixation. However, posterior instrumentation may be prudent for many of these patients. Anterior and posterior instrumentation is also prudent for most patients who undergo corpectomy at C7, to minimize instrumentation failure related to the increased stress at the cervicothoracic junction.

In general, the use of these techniques in the proper patient population can yield satisfactory results, with significant improvements in ambulatory status and pain relief.[18] Despite these reports, the complication rate of the surgical treatment of metastatic cervical spine disease can be high even when procedures are performed by the most experienced and dutiful surgeons.

Complications

Wound complications, infections, tumor recurrence, injuries to critical structures (dura, neural components, viscera, or major blood vessels), pulmonary complications, blindness, thromboembolic disease, hardware failure, and persistent pain have all been observed. The surgical team must be vigilant with respect to these unfortunate developments. The prompt and judicious treatment of such complications should decrease the patient's long-term morbidity.[19]

Conclusions

Metastatic disease of the cervical spine is a challenging problem and is occurring with greater frequency. A multidisciplinary approach led by physicians trained in both spine and oncologic principles will ultimately lead to improved outcomes.

REFERENCES

1. Phillips E, Levine A: Metastatic lesions of the upper cervical spine, *Spine (Phila Pa 1976)* 14:1071–1077, 1989.
2. Batson O: The Role of vertebral veins in metastatic processes, *Ann Intern Med* 16:38–45, 1942.
3. Jenis GJ, Dunn EJ, An HS: Metastatic disease of the cervical spine, *Clin Orthop Relat Res*(359)89–103, 1999.
4. Clohisy DR, Ramnaraine ML: Osteoclasts are required for bone tumors to grow and destroy bone, *J Orthop Res* 16:660–666, 1998.
5. Rao S, Davis R: Cervical spine metastases. In Cervical Spine Research Society, editor: *The cervical spine*, ed 3, Philadelphia, 1998, Lippincott-Raven, pp 603–619.
6. Kato Y, Itoh T, Kubota M: Clinical evaluation of Luque's segmental spinal instrumentation for upper cervical metastases, *J Orthop Sci* 8:148–154, 2003.
7. Pointillart V, Vital JM, Salmi R, et al.: Survival prognostic factors and clinical outcomes in patients with spinal metastases, *J Cancer Res Clin Oncol* 137:849–856, 2011.
8. Wibmer C, Leithner A, Hofman G, et al.: Survival analysis of 254 patients after manifestation of spinal metastases: evaluation of seven preoperative scoring systems, *Spine (Phila Pa 1976)* 36:1977–1986, 2011.
9. Yamashita T, Siemionow KB, Mroz TE, et al.: A prospective analysis of prognostic factors in patients with spinal metastases: use of the revised Tokuhashi score, *Spine (Phila Pa 1976)* 36:910–917, 2011.
10. Maranzano E, Latini P: Effectiveness of radiation therapy without surgery in metastatic spinal cord compression: final results from a prospective trial, *Int J Radiat Oncol Biol Phys* 32:959–967, 1995.
11. Patchell RA, Tibbs PA, Regine WF, et al.: Direct decompressive surgical resection in the treatment of spinal cord compression caused by metastatic cancer: a randomized trial, *Lancet* 366:643–648, 2005.
12. Rao G, Ha SC, Chakrabarti I, et al.: Multiple myeloma of the cervical spine: treatment strategies for pain and spinal instability, *J Neurosurg Spine* 5:140–145, 2006.
12a. White AA, Panjabi MM: Clinical biomechanics of the spine: ed 2, Lippincott; 1990.
13. Tokuhashi Y, Matsuzaki H, Toriyama S, et al.: Scoring system for the preoperative evaluation of metastatic spine tumor prognosis, *Spine (Phila Pa 1976)* 15:1110–1113, 1990.
14. Enkaoua EA, Doursounian L, Chatellier G, et al.: Vertebral metastases: a critical appreciation of the perioperative prognostic Tokuhashi score in a series of 71 cases, *Spine (Phila Pa 1976)* 22:2293–2298, 1997.
15. Fehlings MG, David KS, Vialle L, et al.: Decision making in the surgical treatment of cervical spine metastases, *Spine (Phila Pa 1976)* 34(Suppl):S108–S117, 2009.
16. Nockels RP, Shaffrey CI, Kanter AS, et al.: Occipitocervical fusion with rigid internal fixation: long-term follow-up data in 69 patients, *J Neurosurg Spine* 7:117–123, 2007.
17. Miller DJ, Lang FF, Wals GL, et al.: Coaxial double-lumen methylmethacrylate reconstruction in the anterior cervical and upper thoracic spine after tumor resection, *J Neurosurg* 92(Suppl):181–190, 2000.
18. Sundaresan N, Rothman A, Manhart K, Kelliher K: Surgery for solitary metastases of the spine: rationale and results of treatment, *Spine (Phila Pa 1976)* 27:1802–1806, 2002.
19. Marco RA, An HS: Complications of surgical and medical care, anticipation and management. In McLain RF, editor: *Cancer in the spine*, Totowa, NJ, 2006, Humana Press, pp 323–336.

Infections of the Cervical Spine 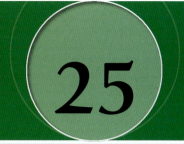 25

Casey C. Bachison and Jeffrey S. Fischgrund

CHAPTER PREVIEW

Chapter Synopsis	Infections of the cervical spine account for less than 10% of all spine infections, but they are the source of 27% of all neurologic deficits associated with an infectious process. The classification of cervical infections includes diskitis and osteomyelitis. This chapter discusses pyogenic, granulomatous, and postoperative infections of the cervical spine
Important Points	Vertebral osteomyelitis and diskitis comprise a spectrum of disease, and one rarely exists without the other.
	Infections of the cervical spine are more likely to lead to neurologic complications.
	Staphylococcus species is the most common cause of pyogenic hematogenous cervical spine infections, and methicillin-sensitive *Staphylococcus aureus* (MSSA) is the most common species.
	Methicillin-resistant *S. aureus* (MRSA) species are on the rise.
	Delayed diagnosis of cervical infections is common because of the nonspecific nature of the symptoms.
	Obtaining a tissue diagnosis to confirm the presence of cervical osteodiskitis and for directing therapy is vital; if possible, the use of antibiotics should be avoided before biopsy, except in patients with sepsis.
	The goals of treatment include establishing a diagnosis, preserving neurologic function, relieving pain, maintaining or correcting deformity, and eradicating the infection.
	Postoperative infections are uncommon in the cervical spine, and the incidence appears to be higher after posterior cervical spine procedures than after anterior cervical procedures.
Video	Video 25-1: Application of Wound Vacuum-Assisted Closure

Infection of the cervical spine accounts for less than 10% of all spine infections, but it is the source of 27% of all neurologic deficits associated with an infectious process. The classification of cervical infections includes diskitis and osteomyelitis and is identical to the system used in the thoracic and lumbar spine. Multiple factors can be used to classify spine infection, including the pathogen, method of inoculation, anatomic location, and duration of infection.[1,2] The most common types of spinal infections are hematogenous bacterial infection, epidural abscess, and postoperative wound infection.[3] Table 25-1 provides classification methods. This chapter discusses pyogenic, granulomatous and postoperative infections of the cervical spine.

Pyogenic Hematogenous Cervical Spine Infection

Demographics, Etiology, and Epidemiology

Hadjipavlou and colleagues described pyogenic spine infection as a spectrum of disease comprising spondylitis, diskitis, spondylodiskitis, pyogenic facet arthropathy, and epidural abscess.[1] Of these disorders, more than 95% manifest as spondylodiskitis. Hematogenous pyogenic vertebral osteomyelitis in the cervical spine represents 6% of all cases of vertebral osteomyelitis.[4] Vertebral pyogenic osteomyelitis is two to three times more common in male patients than in female patients. The rising numbers of patients with immunosuppression, whether from human immunodeficiency virus infection, chronic disease, or steroid use, along with intravenous drug abuse and an aging population, are increasing the prevalence of pyogenic infections. Multiple studies evaluating potential risk factors concluded that a current active infection at any site in the body is the leading risk factor for the development of pyogenic vertebral osteomyelitis.[1,5,6] Recent urinary tract infection was the most common concurrent infection (28%), followed by soft tissue infection and respiratory tract infection, respectively.[5,6] Box 25-1 contains a list of risk factors.

Staphylococcus species has been isolated as the causative pathogen in 50% to 80% of cases.[1,6] Methicillin-sensitive *Staphylococcus aureus* (MSSA) accounts for greater than 36% of the *Staphylococcus* species isolated, but the incidence of methicillin-resistant *S. aureus* (MRSA) is on the rise (6.8%). *Streptococcus* species were isolated from 19% of culture specimens, whereas gram-negative bacteria were found in approximately 14%. *Pseudomonas* and *Escherichia coli* are the most commonly isolated gram-negative bacteria at 3.9% and 2.9%, respectively. Investigators found that 24% to 40% of cultures were unable to isolate a causative organism.[1,7]

Pathogenesis

Vertebral osteomyelitis and diskitis were once viewed and treated as two distinct pathologic entities.[8] More recent studies suggested, however, that these two infectious processes comprise a spectrum of disease, with one rarely existing without the other.[1] The vascular supply to the intervertebral disk is robust at birth. This hypervascular blood supply allows pathogens direct access to the nucleus pulposus in children, as manifested in the increased incidence of isolated diskitis seen in the pediatric population.[9] Pediatric diskitis occurs most commonly in the lumbar spine but is seldom seen in the cervical spine.[9] With age, the vascularity of the intervertebral disk is obliterated, and isolated diskitis is rarely seen in the adult population (only 1% of all cases of spinal infection).[1] In adults, the pathogenesis of spondylodiskitis begins with seeding of the vertebral metaphysis near the vertebral end plate.

The inflammatory cascade instigated by the infectious process upregulates osteoclastic destruction of bone and enzymatic degeneration of the intervertebral disk.[10] Pain and neurologic deficits develop as the destruction of the spine leads to instability, protrusion of intervertebral disks, and development of kyphosis across the affected segment. Invasion of the epidural space by pus or granulation tissue may cause direct compression of neurologic elements. Ischemic damage to neural tissue may also result from septic thrombosis or inflammatory infiltration of the dura.[6,8,10]

Hematogenous seeding of the cervical spine also occurs in the pathogenesis of postinfectious cervical osteomyelitis of the atlantoaxial articulation or upper subaxial spine.[11] This condition, known as Grisel syndrome, is most common in patients less than 30 years old who have had a recent or active upper respiratory infection.[10] It may also result from otolaryngologic procedures.[12,13] The atlantoaxial articulation is directly seeded by the pharyngovertebral venous plexus that allows upper respiratory pathogens direct access to the upper cervical spine. Periodontoid inflammation of the C1-C2 articulation leads to attenuation of the transverse ligament, pain, rotatory subluxation, torticollis, and atlantoaxial instability. Most patients recover with immobilization and treatment of the underlying infection.

Diagnosis

History and Physical Presentation

Neck pain and back pain are the primary symptoms in 92% of patients presenting with spondylodiskitis.[6] The presentation may be acute, subacute, or chronic.[8,14] Delayed diagnosis of cervical infection is common as a result of the nonspecific nature of the symptoms. More than 50% of patients present with a history of symptoms lasting longer than 3 months. Sapico and Montgomerie reported that 15% of patients presented with atypical symptoms such as chest and abdominal pain, dysphasia, and headaches.[6] Patients may experience low-grade fever, chills, night sweats, fatigue, malaise, or decreased appetite. Only half of patients presenting with cervical infections experience fevers, and individuals with acute infections lasting less than 3 weeks are more likely to have fever.

Physical findings in patients with cervical spondylodiskitis are limited. The most universal findings are tenderness to palpation, muscle spasm, and decreased range of motion. When patients present with signs of

Table 25-1	Classification of Spinal Infection
Region	Cervical
	Thoracic
	Lumbar
Pathogen	Pyogenic (bacterial)
	Granulomatous (tuberculosis or fungal)
	Parasitic (echinococcosis)
Location within the spinal elements (Had)	Diskitis (isolated to the intervertebral disk)
	Spondylitis (isolated to the vertebral body)
	Spondylodiskitis (involving the vertebral body and intervertebral disk)
	Pyogenic facet arthropathy (isolated to the facet joints; very rare)
	Epidural abscess (infection within the spinal canal)
Duration	Acute (<6 wk)
	Subacute (6 wk-3 mo)
	Chronic (>3 mo)

BOX 25-1   Risk Factors for Hematogenous Pyogenic Vertebral Osteomyelitis

- Infection in another part of body (greatest risk factor)
- Intravenous drug abuse
- Smoking
- Diabetes
- Liver disease
- Older age in men
- End-stage renal disease
- Malignant disease
- HIV infection
- Ankylosing spondylitis
- Trauma

Data from Hadjipavlou AG, Mader JT, Necessary JT, Muffoletto AJ: Hematogenous pyogenic spinal infections and their surgical management. *Spine (Phila Pa 1976)* 25:1668, 2000; and Sapico FL, Montgomerie JZ: Pyogenic vertebral osteomyelitis: report of nine cases and review of the literature. *Rev Infect Dis* 1:754-776, 1979.

HIV, Human immunodeficiency virus.

radiculopathy or myelopathy, an associated epidural abscess or neurologic compression should be suspected.

Laboratory Evaluation

Laboratory workup for cervical infection should consist of a complete blood count (CBC) with differential, erythrocyte sedimentation rate (ESR), and C-reactive protein (CRP). In addition, urine and blood cultures with Gram stain should be obtained. Sapico and Montgomerie reported leukocytosis in 50% of patients with cervical infections.[6] In the same study the ESR was elevated in almost all cases (92%). CRP is sensitive and is a more specific inflammatory marker than the white blood cell count or ESR. Spine and joint replacement literature has shown CRP to be useful in the diagnosis and treatment of infection.[15-17]

CRP levels increase within 6 hours of the onset of an infection or inflammatory process. The CRP doubles every 8 hours and peaks at 3 to 5 days.[18] As the infection or inflammatory process resolves, CRP drops precipitously, having a half-life of 24 to 48 hours. With resolution of an inflammatory process or infection the CRP returns to normal within 10 days.

ESR peaks at 5 to 7 days and remains elevated for more than 3 weeks after resolution. Thelander and Larsson studied the trends of CRP and ESR after routine spinal surgical procedures. These investigators found that CRP returned to baseline levels in 5 to 14 days.[19] Elevation in CRP after this time should raise concerns for spinal infection. With the exception of a positive culture or biopsy result, CRP is the presumably the most informative laboratory test in the diagnosis and treatment of cervical infection. Results of blood cultures are positive in 24% to 59% of cases.

Imaging Studies

Multiple imaging modalities exist, and each has advantages and disadvantages in the evaluation of spondylodiskitis. Plain radiographs are inexpensive and easily obtained in the clinical setting; however, they cannot detect infection before it has caused significant damage to the intervertebral disk and vertebral end plate. Plain radiographs are the ideal studies for assessment of cervical alignment, and they aid in the detection of cervical deformity.

Computed tomography (CT) is an excellent modality to visualize the bony integrity of the spine. The true extent of bone destruction caused by spondylodiskitis can be evaluated with a CT scan, and an operative plan can be made accordingly (Fig. 25-1, *A* and *B*).

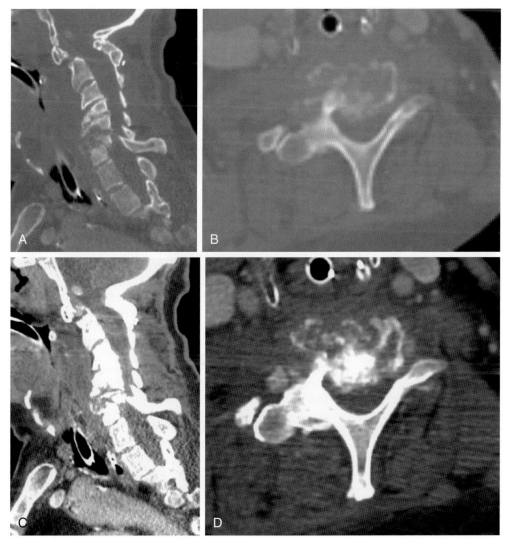

FIGURE 25-1 Parasagittal (**A**) and axial (**B**) computed tomography (CT) scan of a 58-year-old man who developed spontaneous osteodiskitis with bony destruction of the C5 and C6 vertebral bodies with segmental kyphosis. Although it is not as detailed as magnetic resonance imaging, "soft tissue" windowing on these parasagittal (**C**) and axial (**D**) CT scans can provide some additional information about the presence of an abscess associated with the osteodiskitis. (Courtesy Francis H. Shen, MD.)

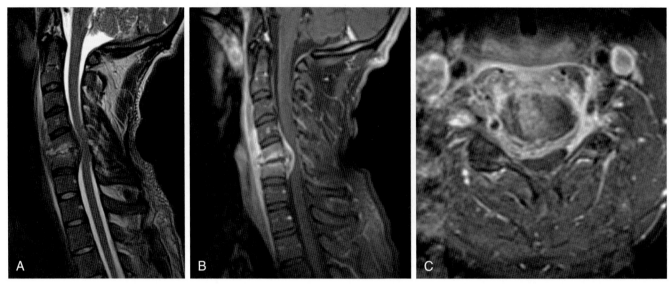

FIGURE 25-2   **A,** T2-weighted sagittal magnetic resonance imaging (MRI) demonstrates changes seen in a patient with presumed osteodiskitis. Notice the increased signal intensity within the C5-C6 intervertebral disk space with associated end plate changes on both sides of the disk space. T1-weighted sagittal (**B**) and axial (**C**) MRI with gadolinium demonstrates the rim enhancement and characteristic findings associated with a large epidural abscess and soft tissue component associated with the osteodiskitis. (Courtesy Francis H. Shen, MD.)

Paravertebral abscesses can also be visualized with CT imaging (Fig. 25-1, *C* and *D*). Not uncommonly, patients have medical conditions such as cardiac stents, cerebral aneurysm clips, or automated internal cardiac defibrillators (AICD) that preclude them from obtaining a magnetic resonance imaging (MRI) scan. In these patients, CT scan following myelography can be helpful in the evaluation of the spinal canal and areas of neural compression. However, myelography may be contraindicated in cases of suspected epidural abscess, and puncture should not be performed in the area of a suspected abscess.

Early detection of spondylodiskitis is possible with radionuclide studies. They also provide imaging of the entire body with localization of multiple foci of infection, which occur in 4% of cases. MRI is the modality of choice for evaluation of spondylodiskitis. The accuracy, sensitivity, and specificity of MRI are superior to those of any other imaging method. MRI provides detailed anatomic information about the disk, vertebral body, and surrounding soft tissues (Fig. 25-2). Eismont noted some degree of neurologic deficit in 80% of patients with cervical osteomyelitis, and MRI can also help identify the site and extent of compression. A comparison of imaging characteristics is provided in Table 25-2.

Biopsy

Open biopsy is the gold standard for the definitive diagnosis of cervical osteomyelitis and osteodiskitis. Many patients are treated initially with nonsurgical interventions. Percutaneous needle aspiration of the infected disk space has increased in popularity as a means of avoiding an open surgical procedure in patients who can otherwise be treated with antibiotics and bracing. Needle biopsy can be performed safely in the cervical spine (Fig. 25-3). Perronne and associates reported that percutaneous needle aspiration resulted in bacteriologic diagnosis in 74% of cases.[5]

A drawback to the use of percutaneous needle biopsy is the risk of false-negative or nondiagnostic results. The use of antibiotics before biopsy increases the likelihood of a false-negative result. Open biopsy is performed when needle biopsy fails to produce a positive result. In the setting of cervical instability or neurologic deficit, open biopsy is performed as part of the definitive procedure. Regardless of the biopsy method, whether percutaneous or open, antibiotics should be held until a positive culture result is obtained. Exceptions to this rule include patients with clinical signs of sepsis, cases of pediatric diskitis, which occur rarely in the cervical spine, and patients with a clinical presentation consistent with vertebral osteomyelitis whose blood culture has produced a positive result.[20]

Management

In multiple, well-authored publications, Kim and Currier outlined the goals of treatment for vertebral osteomyelitis. The goals of treatment are to (1) establish tissue and bacteriologic diagnosis, (2) prevent or reverse neurologic deficit, (3) relieve pain, (4) establish or maintain spinal stability, (5) correct symptomatic spinal deformity, (6) eradicate infection, and (7) prevent relapses.[10,20] When these goals can be met with antibiotic chemotherapy and bracing, no need exists for surgical intervention. However, the high rate of secondary epidural abscess and neurologic compromise associated with osteomyelitis of the cervical spine should raise the vigilance of the treating physician and lower the threshold for surgical intervention.

Medical (Nonsurgical) Management

In the absence of neurologic deficit, abscess, or instability, cervical osteomyelitis can be treated with immobilization and appropriate antibiotic therapy. Antibiotic therapy should be pathogen specific, based on the results of positive cultures and specificities. As previously stated in the discussion of biopsies, antibiotics should be held until a pathogen is isolated. Patients requiring broad-spectrum

Table 25-2 Characteristics of Available Imaging Modalities (Currier)

	Time Frame	Imaging Characteristics	Advantages	Disadvantages
Radiograph	2-4 wk	Disk space narrowing Abnormal prevertebral soft tissue contour	Accuracy 74% Lowest cost	Delay between disease progression and ability to
	3-6 wk	End plate irregularities Destructive changes in anterior vertebral body	Ease of obtaining in clinic Best evaluation of overall cervical alignment or deformity	visualize changes Poor ability to differentiate pyogenic and nonpyogenic infection
	>6 wk	Reactive bone formation Fracture or collapse Kyphosis Involvement of adjacent segment (79%)		
CT scan	<2 wk	Extent of bone destruction Formation of soft tissue abscesses (anteriorly) Ability to visualize spinal canal Postmyelogram CT when MRI is contraindicated	Lower cost than nuclear scans and MRI Aid to differentiating infection from neoplasm (neoplasm may be blastic and/or involve posterior elements)	Limited visualization of soft tissue detail
Nuclear scans Technetium Gallium SPECT Indium	Early (gallium is earliest)	Scan of entire body showing multiple foci of infection (present in 4%)	Accuracy 85% Early detection of infection Gallium scan resolving with infection; ability to follow response to treatment SPECT scan allowing three-dimensional localization	Technetium elevation for months; inability to follow treatment Indium scan not helpful in the evaluation of spondylodiskitis; accuracy 31%
MRI with gadolinium	Early (equivalent to gallium)	Multiplanar anatomic information characterizing extent of infection and tumor Visualization of location and extent of abscess Visualization of neural elements	Modality of choice Early diagnosis of infection Delineation of infection from tumor Sensitivity 96% Specificity 93% Accuracy 94%	High cost Limited availability Persistent changes after clinical resolution of infection Need for tissue biopsy

CT, Computed tomography; *MRI,* magnetic resonance imaging; *SPECT,* single-photon emission computed tomography.

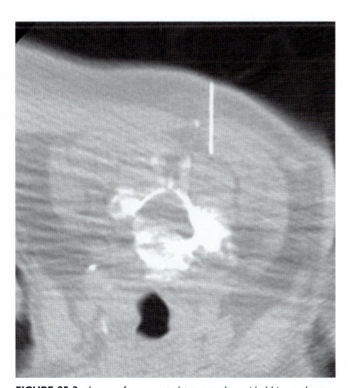

FIGURE 25-3 Image of a computed tomography–guided biopsy demonstrating the trajectory of the biopsy needle entering the posterior paraspinous musculature directed toward the infected facet joint in a 34-year-old woman with a history of intravenous drug use. (*Courtesy Francis H. Shen, MD.*)

empiric antibiotic treatment before pathogen isolation (i.e., patients with sepsis and neurologic deficit) generally would benefit from early surgical débridement in which an open biopsy can be performed.

Patients with clinical evidence of cervical osteomyelitis but negative culture results after open biopsy should be treated with a full course of broad-spectrum antibiotics. Initially, broad-spectrum antibiotics with coverage of both gram-positive and gram-negative bacteria should be chosen. Vancomycin is recommended for coverage of MRSA, and a third-generation cephalosporin is ideal for coverage of gram-negative bacteria. As results of cultures and sensitivity tests are obtained, the antibiotic coverage can be narrowed to target the isolated pathogen more specifically. Newer antibiotics have become available with specificity for coverage of drug-resistant bacteria. Quinupristin-dalfopristin, linezolid, and daptomycin all have activity against drug-resistant bacteria including MRSA, vancomycin-resistant *S. aureus* (VRSA), and vancomycin-resistant enterococcus (VRE).[21]

A 6-week course of intravenous antibiotics has become the standard protocol for treatment of vertebral osteomyelitis in North America. Early studies of vertebral osteomyelitis showed good results with therapy for 4 weeks or longer.[6] Shorter courses resulted in high recurrence rates. Conventionally, the ESR has been used as a guide to follow the resolution of vertebral osteomyelitis, with the value dropping to one half to two thirds the pretherapy level by completion of antimicrobial therapy. More recently, however, CRP has become a more useful laboratory test in the evaluation of adequate antibiotic treatment. Patients with elevated inflammatory markers at completion of a full course of antibiotics should undergo repeat biopsy and another course of pathogen-directed antibiotic treatment.[15]

Immobilization of the cervical spine provides support to the bony vertebral column, prevents deformity, and allows soft tissue recovery. Below the axis, a rigid cervical collar provides adequate immobilization of the cervical spine. Lesions of the cervicothoracic junction require a collar with a thoracic extension. Conventionally, a halo vest has been advocated for lesions involving the upper cervical spine and for cases with extensive multilevel involvement. More recent studies suggest that significant morbidity is associated with the use of a halo vest. Minor complications include pin loosening, localized infection, periorbital edema, superficial pressure sores, and unsightly scars. Major complications include pin penetration through the skull, osteomyelitis, subdural abscess, nerve palsies, fracture, overdistraction, and persistent instability.[22-24]

Young patients with an upper cervical infection may tolerate halo vest immobilization better than older patients. Majercik and colleagues showed that in older patients, mortality rates were higher in patients treated with a halo vest than in those treated with surgical procedures or a rigid cervical collar.[23] In most cases, external bracing is sufficient and is better tolerated.[20] Bracing is recommended for patients with destruction of more than 50% of the vertebra. The duration of brace wear is 3 to 4 months.

Surgical Management

Surgical intervention is typically reserved for patients with persistent infection despite appropriate medical management, gross spinal instability, progressive cervical deformity, and neurologic deficits. An open biopsy may be needed if percutaneous aspiration fails to produce a bacteriologic diagnosis.

The hallmark of surgical intervention is thorough débridement of infected tissues and abscesses followed by early stabilization. Spondylodiskitis of the cervical spine is approached anteriorly in most cases. The anterior approach provides direct access to the infected tissue and allows for thorough débridement of disk and bone. The débridement should be carried down to healthy bone at the superior and inferior extent of the involved segments. In cases of epidural abscess, the posterior longitudinal ligament can be excised for complete decompression of the spinal canal. The anterior approach to the cervical spine also facilitates placement of structural grafts and anterior instrumentation at the time of the initial procedure. Studies showed rapid improvement in neurologic deficits, decreased kyphosis, eradication of infection, and bony fusion in patients treated with single-stage anterior procedures.[25] Iliac crest autograft, fibular autograft, allograft struts, and titanium mesh cages have all been used successfully in the treatment of cervical spondylodiskitis.[7,26,27]

To date, no single graft material has proved superior to the others. Some controversy still exists with regard to the use of metal implants and allograft bone in the setting of active infection. However, studies suggest that use of these

materials does not impede the resolution of infection or inhibit bony fusion after thorough débridement has taken place.[25,27,28] Titanium implants may be resistant to the formation of bacterial glycocalyx, thus preventing adhesion of biofilm on the implant surface (Fig. 25-4).

Surgical débridement of the upper cervical spine can be accomplished by transoral drainage or through a high anterior approach. In patients with significant loss of bony stability, consideration should be given to concomitant posterior arthrodesis.

The posterior approach for cervical spine infection is indicated for cases of isolated pyogenic facet arthropathy or a posteriorly located epidural abscess. Cervical laminectomy performed without adequate anterior column débridement and stabilization often leads to kyphosis and neurologic deterioration.[29] Posterior stabilization performed as a second-stage procedure following anterior decompression and strut grafting may be judicious in patients who would otherwise require halo vest immobilization.

Outcomes

The outcome following treatment of cervical spondylodiskitis is influenced by the type of infection and by the

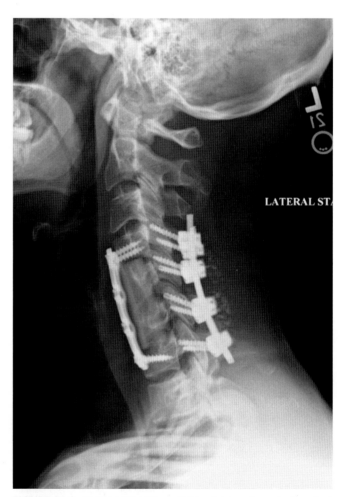

FIGURE 25-4 Postoperative 10-month lateral plain radiograph of a patient after multilevel corpectomy and circumferential reconstruction with allograft fibular strut and long-term intravenous and oral antibiotics. Notice the incorporation of strut graft. (Courtesy Francis H. Shen, MD.)

degree of neurologic compromise before treatment. The results in patients with cervical osteomyelitis treated with anterior débridement, structural grafting, and stabilization followed by a complete course of parenteral antibiotics are favorable. Numerous studies have shown reversal or improvement of neurologic deficits, eradication of infection, improvement in preoperative deformity, and development of bony fusion.[7,25,27,28] Relapse of infection occurs in up to 25% of cases but is much less common when antibiotics are administered for more than 4 weeks. A study evaluating patients who present with paralysis found that old age, a more cephalad level of infection, diabetes, and rheumatoid arthritis increase the risk of irreversible paralysis after cervical osteomyelitis.[29] Almost all patients treated nonoperatively for cervical osteomyelitis develop spontaneous fusion after resolution of their infection.

Nonpyogenic "Granulomatous" Cervical Osteomyelitis

Nonpyogenic vertebral osteomyelitis is caused by bacteria, fungi, and spirochetes that incite a granulomatous immune response in the human body (see Chapter 26). The most notable of these pathogens is *Mycobacterium tuberculosis*. *Mycobacterium*, *Actinomyces*, and *Nocardia* belong to the common order Actinomycetales, and each of these species causes granulomatous infection of the spine. The clinical presentation, workup, and surgical management of osteomyelitis caused by all granulomatous pathogens are similar to those of tuberculosis (see Chapter 26, which discusses the evaluation and treatment of tuberculosis in detail).

Postoperative Infection

Demographics, Etiology, and Epidemiology

Postoperative infection after cervical spinal surgery occurs infrequently. However, certain techniques and predisposing factors increase the risk of developing such an infection. Box 25-2 contains a list of risk factors for postoperative infection.

Postoperative infection after anterior (Smith-Robinson) approach to the cervical spine is uncommon, occurring in 0% to 2% of cases.[30,31] The risk of infection increases significantly with the addition of instrumentation in the thoracolumbar spine. In contrast, placement of instrumentation in the anterior cervical spine increases the rate of postoperative infection only slightly.

The rate of postoperative infection following posterior cervical surgical procedures is considerably higher than after surgical procedures of the anterior neck and ranges from 0% to 18%.[10,32] Postoperative infection can occur as a result of open surgical interventions, percutaneous procedures such as epidural steroid injections, and diskography or as a late complication of surgical instrumentation, as is the case with esophageal erosion.[33,34]

Diagnosis

The presentation of postoperative cervical spine infection typically occurs 7 or more days after the index surgical procedure. The patient generally presents with increasing neck pain and tenderness. The signs are those typical of any infection and include erythema, swelling, drainage, fever, and wound breakdown. The infection may be superficial, deep, or both. In the case of an isolated deep (subfascial) infection, the typical signs may not be present, and the index of suspicion should be high in patients with unexplained increase in neck pain or decreased range of motion. The presence of a new neurologic deficit should raise concern for nerve root or epidural involvement, and appropriate imaging should be obtained immediately.

As with pyogenic hematogenous vertebral osteomyelitis, the ESR and CRP assays are good indicators of postoperative infection. These inflammatory markers are typically elevated following the index surgical procedures, and an elevated ESR or CRP is not as specific for acute infection in the postoperative period. The CRP value returns to normal levels much more quickly than does the ESR, and CRP has become the standard for evaluation of acute infection. CRP levels peak on postoperative day 2 and normalize within 5 to 14 days. ESR levels peak at day 5 and remain elevated for up to 40 days.

When postoperative infection is suspected, antibiotics should be held until a biopsy can be obtained, generally at the time of débridement. Preoperative cultures of wound drainage are often contaminated, and the results are misleading. In the case of suspected diskitis following a surgical procedure, a percutaneous needle biopsy should be obtained if the superficial tissues appear uninfected.

Management

Management of postoperative infections begins with prophylaxis at the index procedure. Preoperative antibiotics administered 30 to 60 minutes before the incision is made reduce postoperative infection by 60%. Using two pair of gloves, limiting operating room traffic, and handling tissue carefully with intermittent release of self-retaining spinal retractors have been shown to decrease the rate of postoperative wound infection.[35] Postoperative use of antibiotics for 24 to 48 hours is considered the standard

---

BOX 25-2	Risk Factors for Postoperative Cervical Spine Infection

Preoperative Risk Factors	Intraoperative Risk Factors
• Age >60 yr	• Blood transfusion
• Diabetes	• Posterior approach
• Malnutrition	• Rheumatoid arthritis
• Obesity	• Down syndrome
• ASA score ≥3	• Allograft use*
• Elevated glucose levels	• Instrumentation*
• Traumatic cervical injury	• Duration of surgical procedure*
• Smoking	
• Use of corticosteroids	
• Immunosuppression	
• Prior external beam radiation treatment	

ASA, American Society of Anesthesiologists.
*Trended toward increased risk of infection without reaching statistical significance.

of care by most physicians, although this practice has not been substantiated in peer-reviewed literature.

Medical Management

Patients with evidence of superficial wound infection or cellulitis who have no clinical evidence of abscess or fluid collection may be treated with a trial of oral antibiotics. A gram-positive skin pathogen such as *S. aureus* is generally the offending bacterium, and antibiotic coverage should target this organism.

Surgical Management

The treatment of postoperative wound infection involves aggressive irrigation and débridement of the infected wound. A titrated approach to irrigation and débridement may be used when it is unclear whether the infection is isolated to the superficial tissues or extends to the deep subfascial portion of the wound. This approach involves débridement of the superficial wound with exploration of the fascial closure. If a breach is found, the débridement continues to the deep wound. If no breach is encountered, the superficial wound can be closed over a drain. Many surgeons prefer to débride both portions of the wound to avoid future return to the operating suite. Intraoperative cultures should be taken and sent for speciation of the inciting pathogen. Broad-spectrum antibiotics are initiated in the operating room following intraoperative cultures. A more appropriate antibiotic is chosen when results of cultures and specificity tests have returned from the laboratory. During débridement of postoperative cervical infection, the implants and bone graft should be left in place because they provide stability to the cervical spine.[36,37] In cases of loose or broken implants, the instrumentation can be removed or replaced. Removal of all stabilizing implants at the time of irrigation and débridement may slow or inhibit recovery.

Following débridement, the wound is closed in layers over drains in a primary fashion. When primary closure is not possible, the wound can be treated with packing and delayed closure, or a vacuum-assisted dressing may be applied to assist in wound reapproximation. Ploumis and associates used vacuum-assisted closure to treated 79 patients with deep wound infection. The wounds of 87% of these patients were closed at an average of 7 days. All but 2 patients had complete closure of the wound without removal of implants at 1 year[38,39] (Video 25-1, Application of Wound Vacuum-Assisted Closure).

REFERENCES

1. Hadjipavlou AG, Mader JT, Necessary JT, Muffoletto AJ: Hematogenous pyogenic spinal infections and their surgical management, *Spine (Phila Pa 1976)* 25:1668, 2000.
2. Vaccaro A, editor: *Core knowledge in orthopaedics: spine,* St. Louis, 2005, Mosby.
3. Tay BK-B, Deckey J, Hu SS: Spinal Infections, *J Am Acad Orthop Surg* 10:188–197, 2002.
4. Malawski SK, Lukawski S: Pyogenic infection of the spine, *Clin Orthop Relat Res* (272): 58, 1991.
5. Perronne C, Saba J, Behloul Z, et al.: Pyogenic and tuberculous spondylodiskitis (vertebral osteomyelitis) in 80 adult patients, *Clin Infect Dis* 19:746–750, 1994.
6. Sapico FL, Montgomerie JZ: Pyogenic vertebral osteomyelitis: report of nine cases and review of the literature, *Rev Infect Dis* 1:754–776, 1979.
7. Emery SE, Chan DP, Woodward HR: Treatment of hematogenous pyogenic vertebral osteomyelitis with anterior debridement and primary bone grafting, *Spine (Phila Pa 1976)* 14:284, 1989.
8. Kemp HB, Jackson JW, Jeremiah JD, Hall AJ: Pyogenic infections occurring primarily in intervertebral discs, *J Bone Joint Surg Br* 55:698, 1973.
9. Fernandez M, Carrol CL, Baker CJ: Discitis and vertebral osteomyelitis in children: an 18-year review, *Pediatrics* 105:1299, 2000.
10. Currier BL, Kim CW, Heller JG, Eismont FJ: Cervical spine infections. In Clark CR, Benzel EC, editors: *The cervical spine,* Philadelphia, 2004, Lippincott Williams & Wilkins.
11. Parke WW, Rothman RH, Brown MD: The pharyngovertebral veins: an anatomical rationale for Grisel's syndrome, *J Bone Joint Surg Am* 66:568–574, 1984.
12. Patel A, Madigan L, Poelstra K, et al.: Acute cervical osteomyelitis and prevertebral abscess after routine tonsillectomy, *Spine J* 8:827–830, 2008.
13. Samuel D, Thomas DM, Tierney PA, Patel KS: Atlanto-axial subluxation (Grisel's syndrome) following otolaryngological diseases and procedures, *J Laryngol Otol* 109:1005–1009, 1995.
14. Kulowski J: Pyogenic osteomyelitis of the spine: an analysis and discussion of 102 cases, *J Bone Joint Surg* 18:343, 1936.
15. Larsson S, Thelander U, Friberg S: C-reactive protein (CRP) levels after elective orthopedic surgery, *Clin Orthop Relat Res* (275): 237–242, 1992.
16. Parvizi J, Suh D-H, Jafari SM, et al.: Aseptic loosening of total hip arthroplasty: infection always should be ruled out, *Clin Orthop Relat Res* 469:1401–1405, 2011.
17. Schulitz KP, Assheuer J: Discitis after procedures on the intervertebral disc, *Spine (Phila Pa 1976)* 19:1172–1177, 1994.
18. Jaye DL, Waites KB: Clinical applications of C-reactive protein in pediatrics, *Pediatr Infect Dis J* 16:735–746, 1997. quiz 746–747.
19. Thelander U, Larsson S: Quantitation of C-reactive protein levels and erythrocyte sedimentation rate after spinal surgery, *Spine (Phila Pa 1976)* 17:400–404, 1992.
20. Kim CW, Currier BL, Eismont FJ: Infections of the spine. In Herkowitz HN, Garfin SR, Eismont FJ, et al.: *Rothman-Simeone the spine,* Philadelphia, 2011, Saunders, pp 1513–1570.
21. Brodke DS, Fassett DR: Infections of the spine. In Spivak JM, Connolly PJ, editors: *Orthopaedic knowledge update: spine 3, ed 3,* Rosemont, Ill, 2006, American Academy of Orthopaedic Surgeons, pp 367–375.
22. Hayes VM, Silber JS, Siddiqi FN, et al.: Complications of halo fixation of the cervical spine, *Am J Orthop* 34:271–276, 2005.
23. Majercik S, Tashjian RZ, Biffl WL, et al.: Halo vest immobilization in the elderly: a death sentence?, *J Trauma* 59:350–356, 2005. discussion 356-358.
24. Ray A, Iyer RV, King AT: Cerebral abscess as a delayed complication of halo fixation, *Acta Neurochir (Wien)* 148:1015–1016, 2006.
25. Rezai AR, Woo HH, Errico TJ, Cooper PR: Contemporary management of spinal osteomyelitis, *Neurosurgery* 44:1018–1025, 1999. discussion 1025–1026.
26. Graziano GP, Sidhu KS: Salvage reconstruction in acute and late sequelae from pyogenic thoracolumbar infection, *J Spinal Disord* 6:199–207, 1993.
27. Korovessis P, Petsinis G, Koureas G, et al.: One-stage combined surgery with mesh cages for treatment of septic spondylitis, *Clin Orthop Relat Res* 444:51–59, 2006.
28. Kuklo TR, Potter BK, Bell RS, et al.: Single-stage treatment of pyogenic spinal infection with titanium mesh cages, *J Spinal Disord* 19:376–382, 2006.
29. Eismont F, Bohlman H, Soni P, et al.: Pyogenic and fungal vertebral osteomyelitis with paralysis, *J Bone Joint Surg Am* 65:19–29, 1983.
30. McAfee P, Cassidy JR, Davis RF, et al.: Fusion of the occiput to the upper cervical spine: a review of 37 cases, *Spine (Phila Pa 1976)* 16(Suppl):S490, 1991.
31. Weinstein MA, McCabe JP, Cammisa FP Jr: Postoperative spinal wound infection: a review of 2,391 consecutive index procedures, *J Spinal Disord* 13:422, 2000.
32. Weiland DJ, McAfee PC: Posterior cervical fusion with triple-wire strut graft technique: one hundred consecutive patients, *J Spinal Disord* 4:15–21, 1991.
33. Connor PM, Darden BV: Cervical discography complications and clinical efficacy, *Spine (Phila Pa 1976)* 18:2035, 1993.

34. Smith MD, Bolesta MJ: Esophageal perforation after anterior cervical plate fixation: a report of two cases, *J Spinal Disord* 5:357, 1992.

35. Polk HC, Simpson CJ, Simmons BP, Alexander JW: Guidelines for prevention of surgical wound infection, *Arch Surg* 118: 1213–1217, 1983.

36. Gepstein R, Eismont FJ: Postoperative spine infections. In Garfin SR, editor: *Complications of spine surgery,* Baltimore, 1989, Williams & Wilkins, pp 302–322.

37. Lonstein J, Winter R, Moe J, Gaines D: Wound infection with Harrington instrumentation and spine fusion for scoliosis, *Clin Orthop Relat Res* (96): 222, 1973.

38. Ploumis A, Mehbod AA, Dressel TD, et al.: Therapy of spinal wound infections using vacuum-assisted wound closure: risk factors leading to resistance to treatment, *J Spinal Disord* 21:320–323, 2008.

39. Yuan-Innes MJ, Temple CLF, Lacey MS: Vacuum-assisted wound closure: a new approach to spinal wounds with exposed hardware, *Spine (Phila Pa 1976)* 26:E1, 2001.

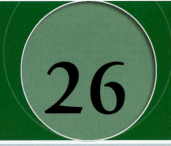

26

Tuberculosis of the Cervical Spine

S. Rajasekaran

CHAPTER PREVIEW

Chapter Synopsis   Tuberculosis (TB) continues to be a global health care challenge. The increased susceptibility to coinfection in the presence of human immunodeficiency virus infection and the emergence of drug-resistant strains have led to a higher burden of the disease worldwide. Although cervical spine involvement is relatively uncommon, it can be an important cause of instability of the craniovertebral junction and atlantoaxial and subaxial cervical spine that can result in severe neurologic deficit and even sudden death secondary to acute cervicomedullary compression.

Important Points   TB continues to be a global health care challenge, with a prevalence of 14 million cases and 9.4 million new cases detected every year.

A high index of suspicion is necessary because symptoms of early TB involvement of the cervical spine are typically nonspecific.

Unlike pyogenic infections, TB frequently manifests with a large associated paraspinous abscess, and the development of late spinal deformity can be common.

Multidrug chemotherapy remains a vital component of both the surgical and nonsurgical management of the patient with spinal TB.

Surgical management of TB should take into consideration involvement of the atlantoaxial or subaxial spine and the presence or absence of basilar invagination.

Tuberculosis (TB) continues to be a global health care challenge, with a prevalence of 14 million cases and 9.4 million new cases detected every year.[1] The increased susceptibility to coinfection in the presence of human immunodeficiency virus infection (HIV) and the emergence of drug resistant strains have led to a higher burden of the disease worldwide.

Of the patients with TB, 10% to 15% have involvement of the musculoskeletal system, and spinal infections account for nearly half of these cases. Cervical spine involvement is relatively uncommon and accounts for only 10% of all cases of spinal TB. C1 and C2 involvement is rare, with an incidence of only 1%. However, the importance of cervical TB lies in its potential to cause of instability of the craniovertebral junction and of the atlantoaxial and subaxial cervical spine that can result in severe neurologic deficit and even sudden death secondary to acute cervicomedullary compression.[2,3]

Pathogenesis

Unlike the other regions of the spine where spread of infection is hematogenous, bone involvement in the cervical spine TB is usually secondary to direct spread from retropharyngeal lymph nodes. The infection spreads from the retropharyngeal tissues to involve the bone and ligamentous stabilizers and results in instability and deformity.[4] Vertebral body involvement is common in the cervical spine, whereas in thoracic and thoracolumbar TB paradiskal involvement predominates.

In early disease of the upper cervical spine, the diagnosis is usually delayed until an advanced stage because of the nonspecific nature of symptoms and paucity of findings in plain radiographs. In the C1-C2 complex, the lateral masses of atlas are involved in 72% and the dens in 62% of the patients.[2,3] Destruction of bony elements of C1 and C2 can lead to dangerous instability and rotatory deformities of the craniovertebral junction (Fig. 26-1). The intervertebral disks are relatively resistant to TB because of their avascular nature and low oxygen tension and hence may remain intact even in the presence of severe bone destruction. In the subaxial spine, and especially in children, destruction of an entire vertebral body is common, and it leads to cervical kyphotic deformity and instability with a potential threat to the spinal cord. Effective antitubercular chemotherapy along

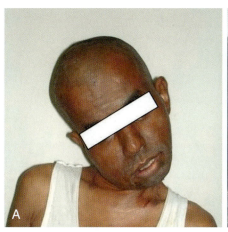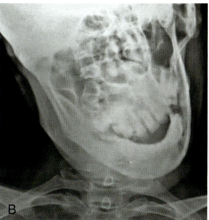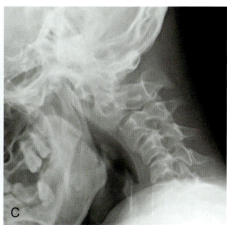

FIGURE 26-1 **A** to **C,** Tuberculosis infection with unilateral destruction of the lateral mass of atlas. The patient developed severe rotatory subluxation and deformity over a period of a few weeks.

with traction or immobilization results in healing in early stages, whereas surgical intervention may be necessary in advanced disease associated with severe neurologic deficit, deformity, or instability.

Pathology

TB is caused by bacilli of *Mycobacterium* genus, and *Mycobacterium tuberculosis* is responsible for most human infections. The bacilli possess a cell wall rich in mycolic acid, which is impervious to the Gram stain. This bacilli have acid-fast properties on Ziehl-Neelsen staining, hence the name acid-fast bacilli. The organism is an obligate aerobe and has affinity for tissues with high oxygen tension.

Under the microscope, the lesions produce a typical picture in which the tubercle bacilli are engulfed by mononuclear cells, which then coalesce to form epithelioid cells. The epithelioid cells are then encircled by lymphocytes to form the tuberculous granuloma (Fig. 26-2). Caseating necrosis develops in the center of this granuloma. As the inflammatory process progresses, the extent of bone destruction and liquefaction increases to form an abscess, which is a collection of caseous material, bony sequestra, serum, and polymorphonuclear leukocytes with scant tubercular bacilli. The abscess may be confined to the prevertebral space, or it can track along the tissue planes to distant locations such as the anterior or posterior triangle of neck or in the axilla and along the brachial plexus sheath. Here the usual hallmarks of an acute inflammation of an abscess are absent, thus earning the name "cold abscess."[5]

Neurologic deficit in spinal TB results from mechanical compression of the spinal cord, direct dural infiltration, or ischemia of the spinal cord secondary to vascular thrombosis.[6] The incidence of neurologic deficit in cervical TB varies widely between the upper and lower cervical spine. The spinal cord occupies only one third of the spinal canal at the level of C1 and C2, and the free space available makes neurologic deficit uncommon. Neurologic deficit is observed only with extensive destruction and large abscesses, which may result in atlantoaxial dislocation or

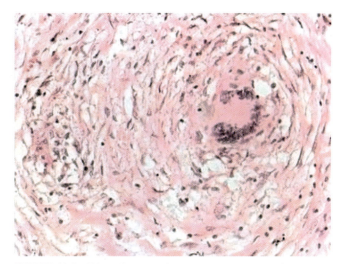

FIGURE 26-2 Tuberculous granuloma is an accumulation of epithelioid macrophages arranged in small clusters or nodular collections surrounded by a fibroblastic rim punctuated by lymphocytes. Some of the macrophages form giant cells. A central area of caseating necrosis is characteristically seen.

basilar invagination with cervicomedullary compression causing quadriplegia, respiratory compromise, and even sudden death.[7] The space available for the spinal cord is much less in the subaxial cervical spine, and hence lesions of this region are associated more commonly with early onset of neurologic deficit (Fig. 26-3).

The age of the patient influences the clinical presentation and long-term outcome. In children less than 10 years old, the fulcrum of cervical spine motion is at the C2-C3 disk level because of the relatively large size of the child's head. The increased mechanical stress makes the upper cervical spine a common location of TB in this age group. Younger children also have increased ligamentous laxity, poor muscle control, and horizontally oriented facets that predispose them to extensive destruction of growth plates, collapse, and severe kyphosis. Larger abscess formation and multiple-level involvement of the cervical region are also observed in the younger age group.[8,9] By the age of 10 years, the facets become vertical, and the fulcrum of movement is shifted to the

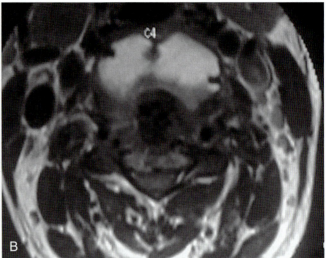

FIGURE 26-3 In the subaxial cervical spine, neural compression is early because of the limited space available for the spinal cord at this level. Sagittal (**A**) and axial (**B**) T2-weighted magnetic resonance images in a case of C4 tuberculosis with myelopathy. The compression results from a combination of abscess, sequestrated fragments, granulation tissue, and retropulsion of the diseased vertebra.

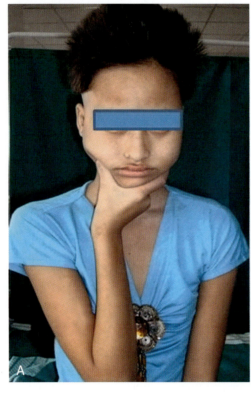

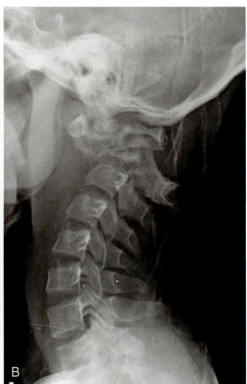

FIGURE 26-4 Extensive destruction of the C2 vertebral body with destruction of the odontoid that resulted in severe instability. **A,** The patient was unable to sit without supporting the chin with her hand. **B,** The lateral radiograph shows a large prevertebral soft tissue shadow in the upper cervical spine along with severe bone destruction.

midcervical spine, thereby making this region more susceptible in patients more than 10 years old. The propensity for large abscess formation and kyphotic deformity is also lower in adults.

Clinical Features

The usual presenting symptoms of cervical spine TB are pain and restriction of movements of the neck. Occipital headache can be a presenting symptom in craniovertebral TB. Constitutional symptoms of fever, loss of weight, and appetite are also common but can be absent in patients who are well nourished and who have good immunity. Early lesions, especially of the upper cervical spine, can

easily be missed because the clinical symptoms are nonspecific and changes in plain radiographs may appear late. Suspicion of infection must prompt investigations with computed tomography (CT) or magnetic resonance imaging (MRI) scans, which will reveal the diagnosis very early.

Late diagnosis leads to destruction of bone with subsequent instability and deformity. The patient frequently supports the chin with hands to alleviate pain and to stabilize the cervical spine (Fig. 26-4). Torticollis may also be present and may reflect sternocleidomastoid spasm or lateral mass destruction of atlas with instability.

Rarely, the presenting feature of cervical TB can be swelling in the neck secondary to cold abscess. The features of cold abscess vary with the site of tracking of the

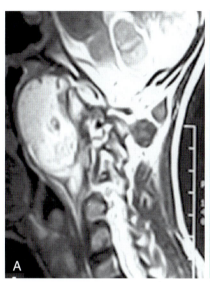
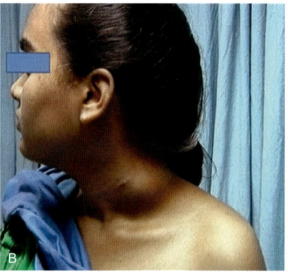

FIGURE 26-5 A, Lesions of the upper cervical spine can manifest with a large retropharyngeal abscess. These abscesses can manifest acutely with difficulties in respiration and swallowing. **B,** Clinical photograph of a patient with a tuberculous infection of C6 and C7 who presented with a cold abscess in the posterior triangle of the neck.

pus. The pus from the upper cervical region may manifest as a retropharyngeal abscess or as swelling in the posterior triangle of the neck, or it may spread beneath the prevertebral fascia into the mediastinum. Large retropharyngeal abscesses can manifest with dysphagia, dyspnea, and dysphonia (Fig. 26-5, A).

In severe cases, cervical TB may also result in respiratory stridor, referred to as Millar asthma. Pus from the subaxial cervical spine may also track along the deep cervical fascia to appear in the anterior triangle of the neck, sternocleidomastoid, or trapezius. It can also manifest as swelling in the supraclavicular fossa, axilla, or elbow by gravitating along the brachial plexus (Fig. 26-5, B). Concomitant cervical lymphadenopathy with or without draining sinuses may also be observed in some cases. Rarely, cervical TB may manifest with an isolated kyphotic deformity causing minimal clinical symptoms.

Neurologic Symptoms

Neurologic symptoms of varying degrees are seen in nearly 25% of patients with TB of the cervical spine. In the active phase of the disease, granulation tissue, pus, and other debris can compress the spinal cord (see Fig. 26-3). Although the reported incidence of spinal cord compression noted on MRI in craniovertebral TB is 42%, the incidence of neurologic deficit is only 15% to 20%.[10] Instability or deformity of the involved vertebrae can cause neural compression both in the active phase and in the healed phase.

Symptoms of spinal cord compression include altered gait pattern, spasticity, weakness, and paresthesias of extremities with loss of bowel and bladder control. Sudden death has also been reported following atlantoaxial instability and cervicomedullary compression secondary to upper cervical TB.[11] Vertebral and basilar arterial thrombosis resulting in lower cranial nerve deficits, monoplegia, and hemiplegia has also been reported following cervical TB.[4]

Clinical Findings

Clinical examination reveals tenderness of the affected cervical segments and torticollis with associated paracervical muscle spasm. All the movements of the neck are severely restricted by pain and spasm. Rarely, kyphotic deformity can be visualized with a palpable knuckle or gibbus. In patients with compression of the cervical spinal cord, upper motor neuron signs of exaggerated reflexes, extensor plantar response, spasticity, and clonus can be elicited. Gait should be carefully analyzed to document subtle signs of unsteadiness that may be the only sign of cord compression. A careful neurologic evaluation must be performed to document the power of the muscles of both upper and lower limbs, with evaluation of the bowel and bladder. Respiratory and abdominal examinations should be done to detect any other focus of infection.

Imaging

Plain Radiographs

In the very early stages, an increased prevertebral soft tissue shadow in the lateral radiographs without any bony destruction may give the first indication of cervical TB (Fig. 26-6).[12] Changes of disk space narrowing and blurring of end plates are visible only after a delay of 2 to 3 weeks after the onset of infection. Radiologic evidence of bony destruction is visible only after the lesion involves at least 50% of the vertebral body. Based on the radiologic location of the tuberculous focus, the lesions are classified as paradiskal, central, anterior, and appendicular (Fig. 26-7). Central and whole body lesions are more common in children and rapidly lead to deformity.

Erosion of atlas, body of the axis, occipital condyles, or the odontoid can lead to atlantoaxial dislocation and severe instability. Destruction of vertebral bodies in the subaxial cervical spine results in a visible kyphotic deformity of the neck. A scalloped appearance of the anterior margin of the vertebral bodies can be seen when two adjacent vertebral bodies are infected, thus skipping the

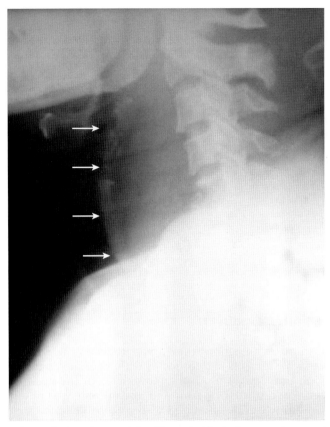

FIGURE 26-6 Infection of the C5 vertebral body showing only minimal bony erosion on the anterior cortex but a large prevertebral soft tissue shadow (*arrows*) indicating the presence of tuberculous infection.

intervening avascular disk by extension of infection under the anterior longitudinal ligament. With progression of deformity, the horizontal orientation of facet joints can quickly lead to an unstable spine with subluxation or dislocation of facet joints. Paravertebral calcifications of the abscess may rarely be observed in chronic tubercular infections.

Computed Tomography

CT scan delineates the bony anatomy in detail and shows the bony destruction earlier than radiographs (Fig. 26-8). Although not as effective as MRI, CT scans can also identify the extent of paravertebral abscess and soft tissue shadows to a certain extent. Bilateral paravertebral abscess with calcifications and fragmented osteolytic lesions with bony fragments within soft tissues are pathognomonic of TB. CT scans, however, can provide excellent details of the integrity of the facet joints, pedicles, and laminae, which are important in deciding the timing and nature of surgical intervention. Axial CT cuts may miss early end plate destruction, and multiplanar reconstructions are necessary to identify early lesions. Contrast-enhanced CT scans better delineate the abscess walls and infected granulation tissues. An important additional benefit of CT is to identify the best location for CT-guided biopsy of the lesion.[13]

Magnetic Resonance Imaging

MRI provides excellent soft tissue detail and is highly sensitive in showing the early signal intensity changes in the bone marrow and spinal cord so that appropriate treatment can be instituted earlier.[14] The

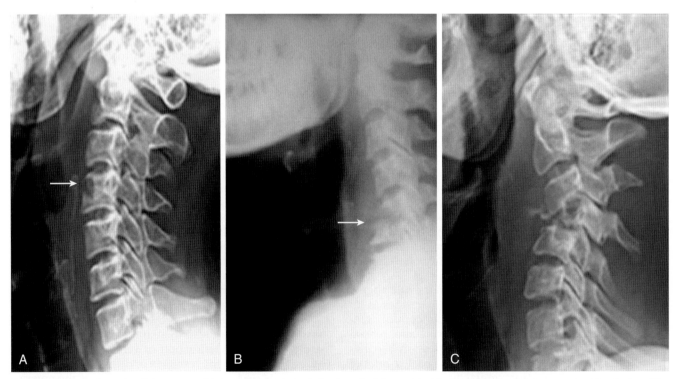

FIGURE 26-7 Radiographs of three types of lesions. **A,** An anterior lesion (*arrow*) of the vertebral body of C4. The disk spaces are not involved, and the vertebral body has not collapsed. **B,** Typical paradiskal type of destruction (*arrow*) of C5 and C6. **C,** A central and complete lesion of the C4 vertebra with acute kyphotic collapse. The increased prevertebral soft tissue shadow is a common feature of all these lesions.

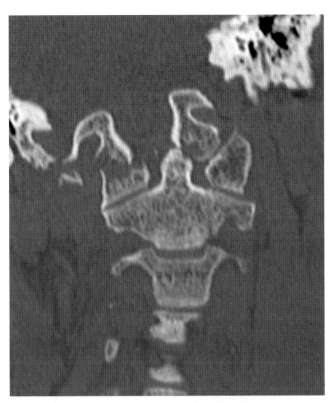

FIGURE 26-8 Computed tomography scan of C1 and C2 shows the destruction of right lateral mass of C1 and the occipital condyle. The patient had severe nuchal pain for more than 3 months, and the diagnosis was delayed because the initial plain radiographs did not show the lesion.

earliest MRI changes include decreased signal intensity in T1-weighted images and increased signal changes in T2-weighted images as a result of bone marrow edema. Early reduction in the height of the disk space is noted, although primary involvement of the disks typically occurs late. Subligamentous extension of infection to the adjacent vertebrae, mainly anteriorly, is commonly observed.

MRI can also provide information on the cause of the neurologic deficits. It can help identify mechanical compression by the abscess, granulation tissue, bony fragments, instability, and basilar impression. Intrinsic signal changes within the spinal cord can be clearly visualized and help direct appropriate treatment to improve the chances of neurologic recovery. In particular, MRI can be useful in identifying TB in uncommon sites, such as the craniovertebral and cervicodorsal junction, where other investigatory modalities can be difficult to interpret. Basilar invagination, extent of paraspinal abscess, intradural disease, and atlantoaxial dislocation with compression of the spinal cord are other disorders that are often better delineated by MRI (Fig. 26-9). The reported sensitivity, specificity, and accuracy of MRI in diagnosing TB are 96%, 92%, and 94%, respectively.[15]

A multilocular, calcified abscess in the retropharyngeal and paraspinal region with a thick, irregular enhancing rim and associated bony fragmentation is characteristic of TB. Intraosseous, paravertebral, and epidural abscesses are clearly visualized by fat-suppressed, gadolinium

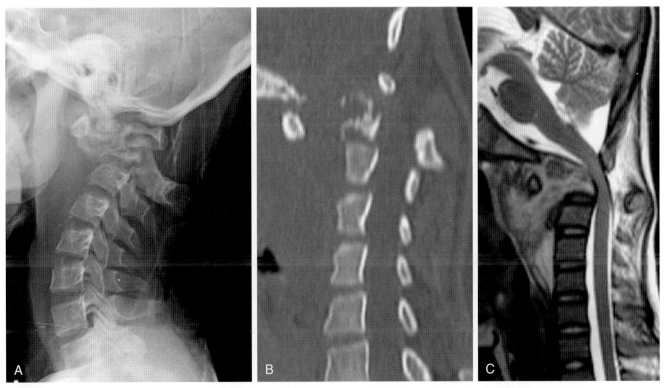

FIGURE 26-9 **A** and **B,** Plain radiography and computed tomography are not helpful for identifying the pathoanatomy of the neural structures, as shown in this case of atlantoaxial tuberculosis with basilar invagination. **C,** Magnetic resonance imaging helps to visualize the neural anatomy and compression clearly.

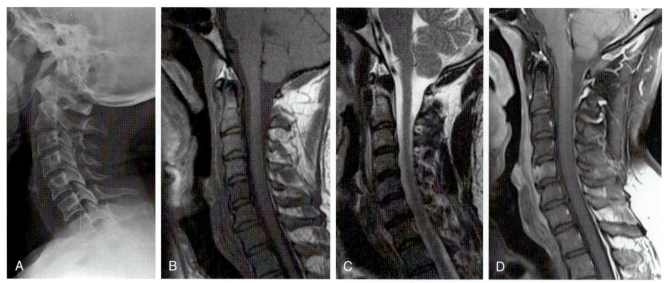

FIGURE 26-10   Contrast-enhanced magnetic resonance imaging (MRI) can detect early tubercular lesions. **A,** The plain radiograph of a 30-year-old man who presented with severe neck pain is unremarkable. **B** and **C,** T1- and T2-weighted MRI images are unable to delineate any disease. **D,** Fat-suppressed gadolinium-enhanced images show features of an early tubercular spondylitic lesion in the C5 body.

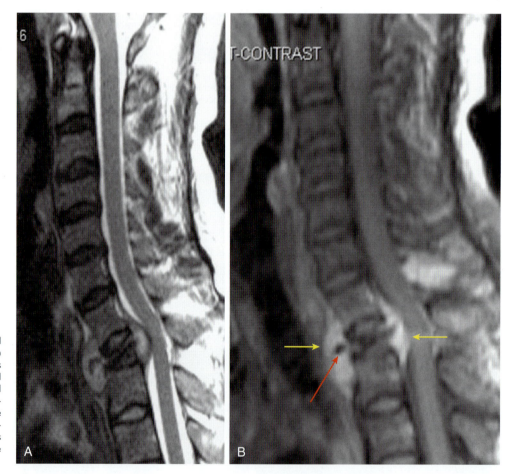

FIGURE 26-11   Contrast-enhanced magnetic resonance imaging (MRI) can differentiate between abscess and granulation tissue. **A,** T2-weighted MRI shows epidural and prevertebral soft tissue at the cervicodorsal junction. **B,** Gadolinium-enhanced image shows uniform enhancement of granulation tissue (*yellow arrows*), whereas abscesses are seen as clefts within the tissue (rim enhancing; *red arrow*).

contrast-enhanced MRI (Figs. 26-10 and 26-11). Contrast-enhanced MRI can also help in differentiating granulation tissue, which shows homogeneous enhancement, from abscess, which has only rim enhancement.

Progressive healing of the lesion and its response to treatment can be documented by follow-up MRI scans. Early signs of healing include increased signal intensity in T1-weighted sequences resulting from the replacement of infected bone by normal fatty marrow. However, the radiologic signs in MRI have a lag period of 6 months when compared with clinical signs of healing. MR angiography may be needed in patients with severe destruction of the upper cervical spine to delineate the vertebral arteries before surgical intervention.

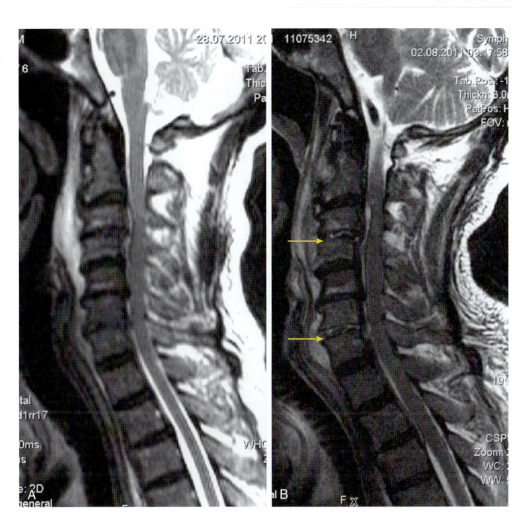

FIGURE 26-12 In pyogenic spondylodiskitis, early and rapid destruction of intervertebral disks occurs, as shown in this case of C3-C4 and C6-C7 infection. **A,** Prevertebral and epidural collection at C2 to C6 without significant changes in the disk space. **B,** T2-weighted image a week later when the symptoms worsened shows high signal intensity in the C3-C4 and C6-C7 intervertebral disks (*arrows*) suggestive of destruction.

Differential Diagnosis

Other diseases with similar clinical and radiographic features include pyogenic spondylodiskitis, fungal infections, rheumatoid arthritis, brucellosis, and tumors such as chordoma and lymphoma. The characteristic paraspinal and anterior epidural abscess differentiates TB from most other conditions. Rheumatoid arthritis with pannus formation and erosion of upper cervical spine and associated dislocation can mimic TB. However, adjacent soft tissue involvement and extension are commonly observed in TB, whereas multiple-level vertebral involvement is common in rheumatoid arthritis. Brucellosis is associated with systemic features of arthralgia and fever. A characteristic abscess as seen in TB is also less common. Fungal infections such as blastomycosis and aspergillosis are differentiated from TB by their decreased signal intensities in both T1- and T2-weighted MRI sequences as a result of the presence of fungal hyphae. Pyogenic spondylodiskitis can be differentiated from TB to a certain extent by the early involvement of disk, hyperintensity within the disk space in T2-weighted images, and loss of intranuclear cleft (Fig. 26-12). The extent of bony destruction and paraspinal abscess formation is relatively larger in TB when compared with pyogenic spondylodiskitis.

A conclusive diagnosis cannot be achieved from radiologic features alone, and the importance of a biopsy leading to a confirmed tissue diagnosis whenever doubt exists cannot be overemphasized.

Biopsy

In spite of characteristic radiologic features, the cornerstone of the diagnosis of TB is the identification of tubercular granulomas in the histopathologic examination of tissue specimen (see Fig. 26-2). Biopsy can be performed percutaneously using wide-bore Jamshidi needles because fine-needle aspiration rarely gives adequate material for histopathologic examination or culture. Lesions located in the anterior aspect of C1 and C2 can be approached by the transoral route. CT- or fluoroscopically guided percutaneous biopsy can be obtained through the anterolateral approach for lesions between C3 and C7.[16] However, because of the presence of vital neurovascular structures in the anterior aspect of the neck, some surgeons advocate an open biopsy through the standard Southwick-Robinson approach. In the presence of instability or neurologic deficit, the definitive procedure can also be performed at the same stage. The specimen should also be sent for drug susceptibility testing so that appropriate drug therapy can be instituted. This is especially important in regions where multidrug-resistant TB is common.

Management

The goals of management of cervical TB include disease cure with minimal residual deformity and the prevention or reversal of any neurologic deficit. Appropriate and adequate chemotherapy remains the cornerstone of treatment even when surgical procedures are performed. Effective antitubercular chemotherapy has made conservative treatment eminently possible in the early stages of the disease. Surgical intervention is favored in patients at risk for instability, deformity, or neurologic deficit. Surgical treatment also allows early mobilization and reduces the need for bracing.[17]

Chemotherapy

The principles of chemotherapy are the same in patients treated conservatively or surgically. Multidrug chemotherapy for a duration of 6 to 9 months is needed for the chemotherapy to be effective and to prevent the emergence of drug resistance. Short-term chemotherapy is very effective, and chemotherapy is extended beyond 9 months only in exceptional circumstances. The World Health Organization guidelines (2010) recommended 2 months of an intensive phase with a combination of four drugs (isoniazid, rifampicin, ethambutol, and pyrazinamide), followed by a 4-month continuation phase with two drugs (isoniazid and rifampicin)[18,19] (Table 26-1).

Nonoperative Management

All cases of cervical TB without instability, deformity and neurologic deficit with or without minimal bony destruction can be managed conservatively with chemotherapy, rest, and appropriate bracing (Fig. 26-13). Even large paravertebral abscesses and osseous lesions without instability can heal completely with chemotherapy alone[20] (Fig. 26-14). Cervical spine traction can reduce pain and relieve muscle spasm in the early stage of the disease. It may also be used to reduce the subluxation/dislocation and restore spinal alignment.[21]

Table 26-1 Recommended Doses of First-Line Antituberculosis Drugs for Adults

| Drug | Dose for Daily Regimen | | Dose for Three Times per Week Regimen | |
	Dose and Range (mg/kg body weight)	Maximum (mg)	Dose and Range (mg/kg body weight)	Daily Maximum (mg)
Isoniazid	5 (4-6)	300	10 (8-12)	900
Rifampicin	10 (8-12)	600	10 (8-12)	600
Pyrazinamide	25 (20-30)	—	35 (30-40)	—
Ethambutol	15 (15-20)	—	30 (25-35)	—
Streptomycin	15 (12-18)	—	25 (25-30)	1500

*Patients who are more than 60 years old may not be able to tolerate more than 500 to 750 mg daily, so some guidelines recommend reduction of the dose to 10 mg/kg daily in patients in this age group. Patients weighing less than 50 kg may not tolerate doses higher than 500 to 750 mg daily.[19]

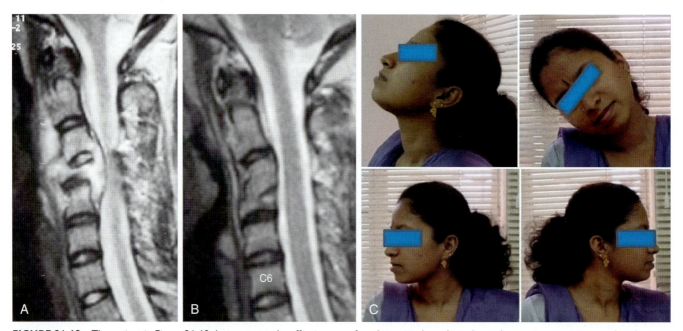

FIGURE 26-13 The patient in Figure 26-12 demonstrates the effectiveness of modern antituberculous chemotherapy in restoring normal neck movements. **A,** Extensive destruction of C4 with epidural abscess and spinal cord compression. The patient had normal neurologic findings and was treated conservatively with antituberculous therapy. **B,** Magnetic resonance imaging 6 months after treatment shows complete resolution of the abscess and good healing of bone without any major kyphosis. **C,** The patient had an excellent recovery with normal neck movements. (Courtesy Dr. Shekhar Y. Bhojraj.)

Surgical Management

Indications

Although chemotherapy achieves disease clearance, it cannot arrest instability and the development and progression of deformity. Chemotherapy may not be successful in certain patients with neurologic deficit caused by mechanical conditions such as retropulsed bony fragments and pathologic dislocation.

Surgical intervention in cervical TB may be required in the following circumstances:

1. Acute onset and severe neurologic deficit
2. Cervical kyphotic deformity following destruction of an entire vertebral body and resulting in impending spinal cord compromise secondary to the internal gibbus
3. Presence of instability in the form of subluxation or dislocation in the cervical spine that threatens the spinal cord
4. Large retropharyngeal abscess producing pressure symptoms in the form of dyspnea, dysphagia, or dysphonia
5. Lack of clinical and radiologic improvement after chemotherapy for 6 to 8 weeks
6. Need to obtain a tissue specimen in patients with an inconclusive CT-guided biopsy
7. Need for early mobilization in patients at risk for complications associated with prolonged immobilization

The primary goals of surgical intervention include thorough débridement of the infected tissues, bony fragments, and disk material to achieve adequate decompression of the spinal cord and reconstruction of the cervical column. Reconstruction may be achieved with autografts or titanium cages with additional stabilization to protect the graft and maintain or restore alignment. Surgical management depends on the location of the disease. Surgical options depend on whether the site of involvement is atlantoaxial TB or subaxial cervical spine TB and whether basilar invagination is present.

Atlantoaxial (C1-C2) Tuberculosis

C1-C2 TB in patients without instability and spinal cord compression can be managed nonoperatively with chemotherapy, bracing, and rest. The brace should rigidly immobilize all movements of the cervical spine and should support the chin and occiput cranially and cervicodorsal junction caudally. Periodical radiologic supervision to rule out subluxation or instability is needed.

It was traditionally believed that a period of chemotherapy for 3 weeks was necessary before elective surgery to avoid wound-healing complications. However, the author's experience is that this is not necessary because good wound healing and uneventful progress can be obtained if thorough débridement is performed and chemotherapy is started immediately postoperatively. Preoperative chemotherapy may also sterilize the infective focus and interfere with culture tests that may be necessary to determine drug sensitivity. The nutritional status of the patient is very important, and adequate care must be given in this area to obtain good results.

When atlantoaxial dislocation or subluxation is present without neurologic deficit, the dislocation should be reduced with preliminary traction. After achieving reduction, posterior C1-C2 fusion should be performed (Fig. 26-15). In the presence of severe or progressive neurologic deficit, decompression and alignment can be achieved during the surgical procedure. In the presence of severe instability or destruction of C1 and C2 bodies, occipitocervical fusion may be necessary[22] (Fig. 26-16). Anterior decompression through a transoral or retropharyngeal approach may be rarely necessary if the patient has persistent features of spinal cord compression

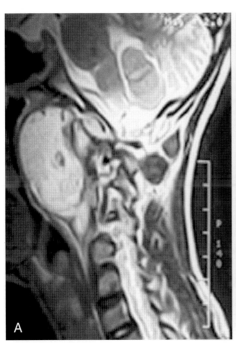
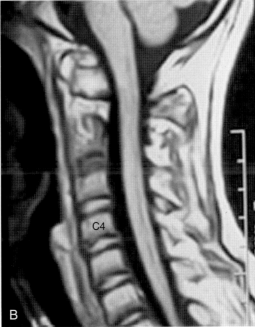

FIGURE 26-14 A, This patient presented with a large retropharyngeal abscess secondary to tuberculosis of the upper cervical spine. **B,** The lesion resolved completely with antitubercular chemotherapy.

anteriorly. In patients with healed irreducible C1-C2 dislocation with persistent anterior spinal cord compression following traction, first-stage anterior decompression (odontoidectomy) followed by posterior C1-C2 fusion is performed. This procedure is performed in a single stage or in a staged fashion, depending on the patient's condition and the experience of the surgical team.

Subaxial Cervical Tuberculosis

Subaxial cervical lesions in patients with normal lordosis and normal neurologic findings can be treated conservatively with a brace. Partial destruction of a single vertebra is not a major concern in the cervical region because of the presence of inherent lordosis, which may protect against a major kyphotic collapse. However, patients must

be carefully followed, given that the cervical facet joints are horizontally oriented, thus predisposing to segmental kyphotic deformity that may require surgical correction.[23]

In most cases of chronic cervical TB, correction of preoperative deformity can be achieved by traction. This can be followed by thorough anterior débridement of the lesion through the standard Southwick-Robinson approach. Débridement may involve corpectomy with diskectomy, and the resultant gap is usually filled with a tricortical iliac crest graft firmly wedged between the end plates. Additional instrumentation can be safely done without fear of aggravating the disease (Fig. 26-17). Titanium implants are preferred for a variety of reasons. They have less tendency to form a biofilm that harbors and protects bacteria. These implants also allow postoperative

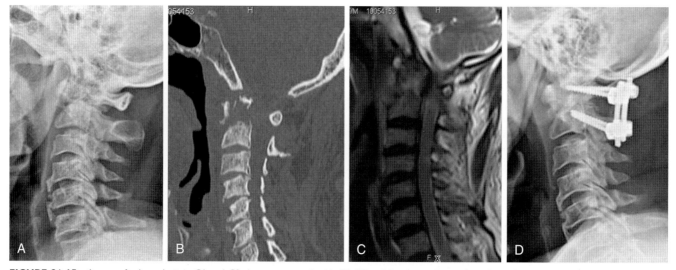

FIGURE 26-15 A case of tuberculosis in C1 and C2 that was treated with C1-C2 stabilization and antituberculous chemotherapy. Plain radiographs (**A**), computed tomography (**B**), and magnetic resonance imaging (**C**) demonstrate destruction of odontoid with maintenance of spinal alignment. **D,** Postoperative radiograph after C1-C2 stabilization.

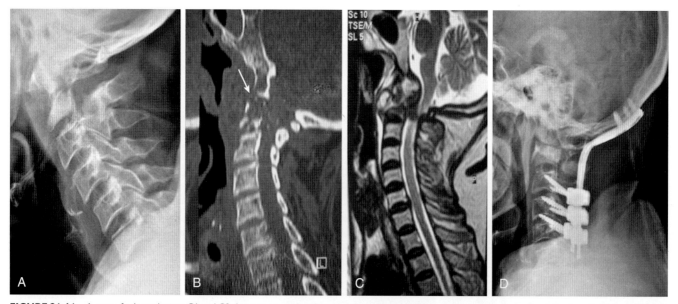

FIGURE 26-16 A case of tuberculosis in C1 and C2 that was treated with occipitocervical stabilization and antituberculous chemotherapy. **A,** Plain radiograph shows destruction of the odontoid. **B,** Computed tomography image showing involvement of the odontoid and the anterior arch of the atlas. **C,** Magnetic resonance image showing destruction of the atlantoaxial articulation with epidural soft tissue compressing spinal cord. **D,** Plain radiograph following occipitocervical fusion.

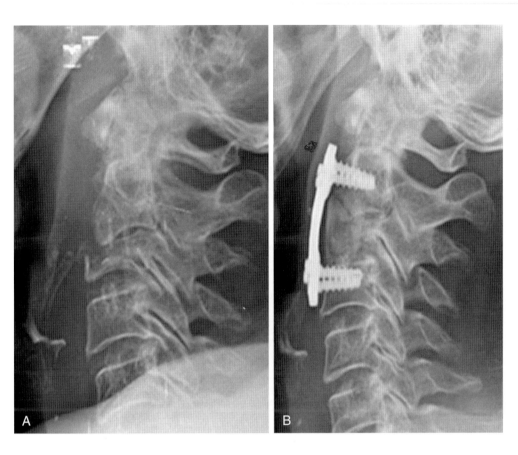

FIGURE 26-17 A, Extensive destruction of C3 vertebra secondary to tuberculous involvement leading to severe pain and disability. **B,** The patient underwent corpectomy of C3 and reconstruction with tricortical iliac crest graft and titanium plates and screws.

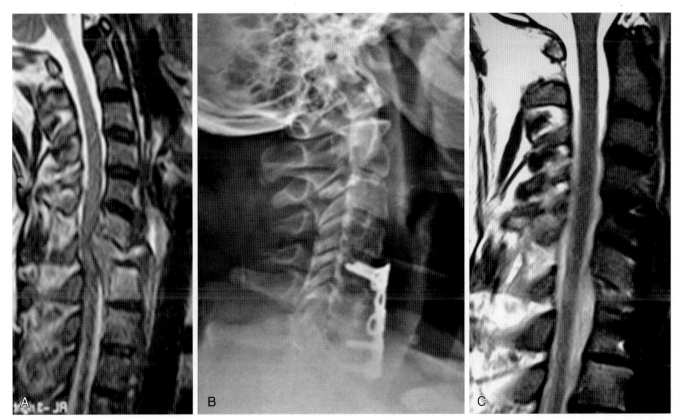

FIGURE 26-18 A case of C6 and C7 spondylodiskitis with compressive myelopathy. **A,** Preoperative imaging shows C7 bony destruction, kyphosis, and spinal cord compression resulting from infected debris. **B** and **C,** Eighteen months after surgical débridement, fusion with anterior plating, and antitubercular chemotherapy, the lesion has healed well with bony union. Clinically, myelopathic signs had completely resolved.

imaging studies because of their minimal interference with image quality (Fig. 26-18). Although generally anterior surgical procedures are adequate, concomitant posterior stabilization may be necessary in patients with severe destruction of vertebral bodies requiring long grafts and in patients with multiple-level infections, involvement of all three columns, poor bone stock, and osteoporosis that compromises the strength of an isolated anterior fixation.

Basilar Invagination

Tuberculous destruction of the lateral masses of atlas or occipital condyles results in cranial settling that leads to basilar invagination and cervicomedullary compression by the vertically displaced odontoid. Reduction of the odontoid is attempted preoperatively by traction; after achieving reduction, the segment is stabilized with instrumented posterior occipitocervical fusion. When reduction is not achieved, a combined approach in the form of anterior odontoidectomy and decompression of cervicomedullary junction followed by posterior occipitocervical fusion may be needed.

Role of Posterior Surgical Procedures

Posterior surgical procedures are usually performed as adjuncts to anterior surgical procedures. An isolated posterior surgical procedure for an anterior lesion in TB is usually contraindicated because it does not address the anterior lesion and also compromises the stability provided by the retained normal posterior structures.

The indications for posterior surgical procedures in cervical TB include the following:

1. Neurologic deficit secondary to a posterior epidural abscess or granuloma
2. Isolated posterior element TB with spinal cord compression and neurologic deficit
3. As adjuncts to anterior surgical procedures in tuberculous involvement of all three columns of the spine
4. When the stability of the stand-alone anterior fixation constructs is in doubt, as in cases of extensive bony destruction, osteoporosis, and multiple-level involvement compromising fixation strength.

Posterior stabilization with pedicle screws or lateral mass screws and rods should always be performed following laminectomy and decompression of the cord.

Conclusions

Although cervical TB constitutes only 10% of cases of spinal TB, early diagnosis and management are necessary to prevent the potential risks of instability and neurologic deficit. Patients with minimal bony destruction without deformity, instability, or neurologic deficit can be managed nonoperatively by adequate chemotherapy and bracing. Chemotherapy is important in achieving disease cure in patients who are treated conservatively, as well as in those treated surgically. Hence, the patient's compliance with uninterrupted chemotherapy must be emphasized. Surgical intervention is necessary in patients with instability, deformity, severe bony destruction, and neurologic deficit. The current trend is toward operative management to enable early return to activities and to facilitate fusion.

REFERENCES

1. World Health Organization: *Global tuberculosis control, WHO report*, Geneva, 2010, World Health Organization.
2. Hsu LC, Leong JC: Tuberculosis of the lower cervical spine (C2 to C7), *J Bone Joint Surg Br* 66:1–5, 1984.
3. Kim NH, Lee HM, Suh JS: Magnetic resonance imaging for the diagnosis of tuberculous spondylitis, *Spine (Phila Pa 1976)* 19:2451–2455, 1994.
4. Monhindra S, Gupta KS, Mohindra S, et al.: Unusual presentations of craniovertebral junction tuberculosis: a report of 2 cases and literature review, *Surg Neurol* 66:94–99, 2006.
5. Anderson WA: *Pathology*, ed 7, St. Louis, ????, Mosby, pp 1112–1114.
6. Watson Jones R: Spontaneous hyperaemic dislocation of the atlas, *Lancet* 25:586, 1932.
7. Arora S, Sabat D, Maini L, et al.: The results of nonoperative treatment of craniovertebral junction tuberculosis: a review of twenty-six cases, *J Bone Joint Surg Am* 93:540–547, 2011.
8. Govender S, Ramnarain A, Danaviah S: Cervical spine tuberculosis in children, *Clin Orthop Relat Res* 46:78–85, 2007.
9. Banks GM, Transfeldt EE: Biomechanics—clinical applications. In Weinstein SL, editor: *The pediatric spine: principles and practice*, New York, 1994, Raven, pp 110–120.
10. Tuli SM: Tuberculosis of the craniovertebral region, *Clin Orthop Relat Res* (104):209–212, 1974.
11. Kotil K, Dabayarak S, Alan S: Craniovertebral junction Pott's disease, *Br J Neurosurg* 18:49–55, 2004.
12. Lifeso R: Atlantoaxial tuberculosis in adults, *J Bone Joint Surg Br* 69:183–187, 1987.
13. Stoker DJ, Kissin CM: Percutaneous vertebral biopsy: a review of 135 cases, *Clin Radiol* 36:569–577, 1985.
14. Hsu LC, Leong JC: Tuberculosis of the lower cervical spine (C2 to C7), *J Bone Joint Surg Br* 66:1–5, 1984.
15. Modic MT, Feiglin DH, Piraino DW, et al.: Vertebral osteomyelitis: assessment using MR, *Radiology* 157:157–166, 1985.
16. Nourbakhsh A, Grady JJ, Garges KJ: Percutaneous spine biopsy: a meta-analysis, *J Bone Joint Surg Am* 90:1722–1725, 2008.
17. Jain AK, Kumar S, Tuli SM: Tuberculosis of spine (C1 to D4), *Spinal Cord* 37:362–369, 1999.
18. World Health Organization: *Treatment of tuberculosis: guidelines*, Geneva, 2010, World Health Organization, p 30.
19. World Health Organization: WHO model formulary. http://apps.who.int/medicinedocs/documents/s16879e/s16879e.pdf, 2008 Accessed April 16, 2014.
20. Jain AK, Jena A, Dhammi IK: Correlation of clinical course with magnetic resonance imaging in tuberculous myelopathy, *Neurol India* 48:132–139, 2000.
21. Tuli SM: Differential diagnosis. In Tuli SM, editor: *Tuberculosis of the skeletal system*, New Delhi, 1997, Jaypee Publications, pp 206–269.
22. Arunkumar MJ, Rajshekhar V: Outcome in neurologically impaired patients with craniovertebral junction tuberculosis: results of combined anteroposterior surgery, *J Neurosurg* 97:166–171, 2002.
23. Moon MS, Moon JL, Kim SS, et al.: Treatment of tuberculosis of the cervical spine: operative versus nonoperative, *Clin Orthop Relat Res*(460)67–77, 2007.

Rheumatoid Arthritis of the Cervical Spine

27

Nader S. Dahdaleh, James A. Stadler III, Arnold H. Menezes, and Richard G. Fessler

CHAPTER PREVIEW

Chapter Synopsis	Rheumatoid arthritis is a chronic autoimmune inflammatory polyarthritis that often involves the joints of the upper and subaxial cervical spine. The common spinal manifestations include atlantoaxial subluxation, rheumatoid basilar invagination, and subaxial subluxation.
Important Points	Selection of the appropriate approach, technique, and construct depends on the severity of symptoms and preoperative reducibility of the subluxation or basilar invagination, or both.
Clinical and Surgical Pearls	Because this disease preferentially affects the upper cervical spine, knowledge of the neurovascular anatomy at the craniocervical region that often is disrupted is key to successful surgical management, feasibility, and selection of the appropriate surgical construct.
Clinical and Surgical Pitfalls	Assessment of bone quality should not be overlooked in patients with rheumatoid arthritis, and efforts should be made to optimize bone health by using a multidisciplinary strategy.

Rheumatoid arthritis is a chronic autoimmune inflammatory polyarthritis of the peripheral joints. It often involves the joints of the upper and subaxial cervical spine and has a variety of pathologic entities and a spectrum of clinical presentations. The introduction of disease-modifying antirheumatic drugs (DMARDs) and of agents that block tumor necrosis factor-α (TNF-α) altered the natural history of the disease by preserving the integrity and function of the joints.[1] Thus, the incidence and severity of rheumatic spinal disorders encountered by most spine surgeons have decreased since the 1990s.

In-depth knowledge of the pathophysiology, natural history, and management of the spinal disorders that result from this chronic disease is important and facilitates decision making when treating these disorders, which can be challenging and complex. Involvement of the cervical spine in patients with rheumatoid arthritis is also associated with higher morbidity and mortality than is similar cervical spine involvement in patients who do not have rheumatoid arthritis.[2] The goal of this chapter is to describe the pathophysiology and clinical presentation of patients with rheumatoid arthritis–related involvement of the cervical spine, more specifically atlantoaxial subluxation, occipitoatlantoaxial impaction, and subaxial subluxation.

Pathophysiology

Approximately one fourth of patients with rheumatoid arthritis will have at least radiographic involvement of the cervical spine, mainly the upper cervical spine.[3] The synovial joints between the transverse atlantal ligament and the odontoid process, the alar ligament, and the joints between the anterior arch of the atlas and the odontoid are frequently affected. With chronic inflammation, the transverse ligament weakens and eventually ruptures. Decalcification also takes place and erodes the odontoid. This process results in various degrees of atlantoaxial subluxation.[4]

The atlanto-occipital and atlantoaxial joints can also be affected. With destruction and collapse of these joints and lateral atlantal masses, the odontoid process telescopes rostrally, with resulting occipitoatlantoaxial impaction or basilar invagination. Subaxially, the facet joints can be involved, leading to variable degrees of subaxial subluxations and deformity. However, because of the presence of intervertebral disks, which are spared in this inflammatory process, subaxial subluxation is usually a late manifestation of the disease.[3]

Presentation

Although the occurrence of radiographic evidence of disease as atlantoaxial subluxation in asymptomatic patients is common, the most frequent presenting symptom is pain. It is usually a combination of occipital and neck pain that either is caused by mechanical instability or is radicular, as a result of compression of C1 and C2 nerves. A positive Sharp-Purser test is a clicking sensation in extension that results with spontaneous reduction of atlantoaxial subluxation.

Neurologic manifestations are less common and are caused by mechanical neurovascular compression on the cervical spine and cervicomedullary junction. Patients may present with cervical myelopathy manifesting as gait dystaxia, hand clumsiness, and difficulty with dexterity. Objective findings of myelopathy include weakness, hyperreflexia, and positive Hoffmann, Babinski, and Lhermitte signs. Cruciate paralysis and even sudden death from respiratory arrest have also been reported.[5] The deep tendon reflex may not be elicited because of appendicular joint destruction.

Clinical Entities

Atlantoaxial subluxation, occipitoatlantoaxial impaction, and subaxial subluxation can occur separately or in combination in patients with rheumatoid arthritis.

Atlantoaxial Subluxation

Anterior subluxation of the atlas on the axis results from weakening and disruption of the transverse ligament following joint inflammation around it. The subluxation can be anterior, posterior, lateral, or rotatory. This disorder is diagnosed with plain radiography as an increased anterior atlantodens interval, as well as a decreased posterior atlantodens interval in flexion (Fig. 27-1). An anterior atlantodens interval greater than 5 mm is diagnostic. A posterior atlantodens interval of less than 14 mm is more predictive of neurologic deficit.[6] Patients can be symptomatic or can present with neck pain and later with neurologic deficits, depending on the degree of spinal cord compression.

Patients with symptomatic instability are generally managed with operative stabilization. If the subluxation is reducible, a posterior approach and fixation are used (Figs. 27-2 and 27-3). This fixation is achieved with semirigid constructs, such as Brooks and Gallie wiring, or rigid constructs with the use of transarticular C1-C2 screws (Fig. 27-4) or C1 lateral mass screws and either C2 pars interarticularis/pedicle screws (Fig. 27-5) or C2 translaminar screws. Occipitocervical fusion may be considered in this patient population (Fig. 27-6), given the increased risk of craniocervical settling. When the subluxation is not reducible or when it is associated with anterior pannus compressing the upper cervical spine, anterior release of odontoid is generally required before posterior fusion.

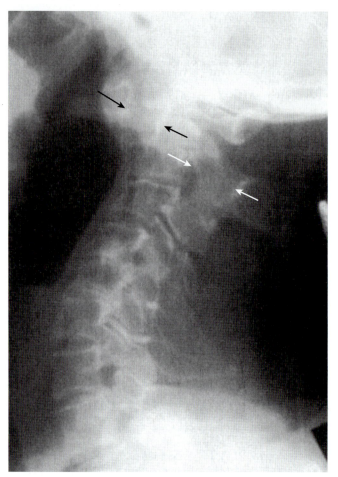

FIGURE 27-1 Lateral radiograph demonstrating the anterior (*black arrows*) and posterior (*white arrows*) atlantodens interval. (From Shen FH, Samartzis, D, Jenis LG, An HS: Rheumatoid arthritis: evaluation and surgical management of the cervical spine. *Spine J* 4:689-700, 2004.)

Occipitoatlantoaxial Impaction (Basilar Invagination)

With disease progression, the atlanto-occipital and atlantoaxial joints and lateral masses are destroyed, resulting in cranial migration of the odontoid process and hence "settling" and rheumatoid basilar invagination (Fig. 27-7). This condition leads to variable degrees of neurovascular cervicomedullary compression. The corresponding symptoms are similarly variable, ranging from pain to potential serious and disastrous neurologic consequences.

Basilar invagination can be diagnosed in various ways (Fig. 27-8). Normally, the odontoid process should lie below the McRae line, which connects the basion to the opisthion; basilar invagination is diagnosed when the odontoid tip crosses this line. The McGregor line connects the posterior hard palate to the opisthion. Basilar invagination occurs when the odontoid tip lies 4.5 mm above the McGregor line. When plain radiographs do not adequately display the anatomy for accurate measurements, the Ranawat and the Redlund-Johnell methods can be used.[4,7] These craniometric measurements were useful before the magnetic resonance imaging (MRI) era. Multiplanar computed tomography and MRI studies that delineate the bony and the neurovascular anatomy, respectively, should always be used during the workup because they also facilitate the diagnosis.

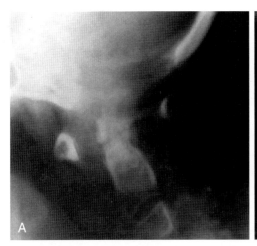
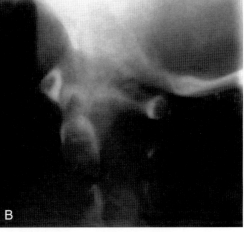

FIGURE 27-2 A 20-year-old woman with a history of rheumatoid arthritis, and a known C1-C2 subluxation for 3 years, presented with quadriparesis of 3 months' duration. **A** and **B,** Radiographs demonstrating C1-C2 reducible subluxation.

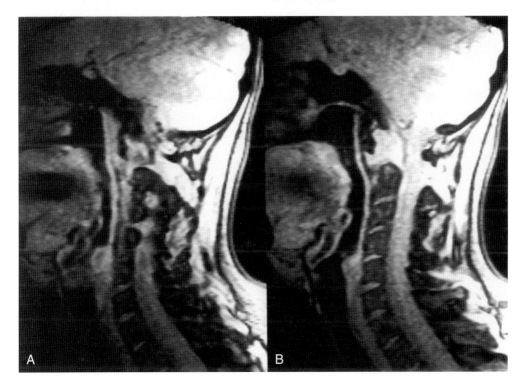

FIGURE 27-3 Composite T2-weighted magnetic resonance imaging in the parasagittal (**A**) and sagittal (**B**) plane of the same patient as in Figure 27-2 demonstrating active pannus from the occiput to C2.

When patients are symptomatic, when radiographic evidence of instability is present, or when the degree of compression of cervicomedullary junction is severe, surgical intervention is indicated. Assessment of the cervicomedullary angle (CMA) on sagittal MRI images can be helpful. Increasing migration of the dens into the foramen magnum results in a more acute CMA (normal CMA > 135 degrees), as well as increasing compression of the medulla and brainstem (Fig. 27-9).

The approach depends on the ability to achieve reduction preoperatively.[8,9] A sagittal T2-weighted MRI scan in flexion and extension is helpful in determining the extent or lack thereof of reduction. Often, preoperative traction can also be used in achieving reduction and is successful in 75% or 80% of the cases. When reduction occurs, dorsal occipitocervical fusion, with or without suboccipital decompression, is sufficient. This can be achieved in various ways; an occipital plate combined with a C1-C2 rod and screw construct is the most biomechanically

rigid. When the invagination is not reducible, transoral resection of the odontoid/pannus should precede dorsal occipitocervical fusion (Figs. 27-10 to 27-12).

Subaxial Subluxation

Subaxial kyphotic deformities and subluxations can result from inflammation and destruction of the synovially lined facet joints (Fig. 27-13). These conditions can be determined by lateral plain radiography demonstrating more than 4 mm or 20% listhesis of vertebral body diameter.[10] Flexion and extension dynamic radiographs are important to determine the presence and extent of radiographic stability. Symptomatic subluxations, instability, and subluxation with a sagittal spinal canal diameter of less than 14 mm are generally thresholds for surgical intervention.[4] Whenever possible, surgical stabilization and fusion should include the most distal subluxed level, which on occasion may require extension into the thoracic spine. Anterior only, posterior

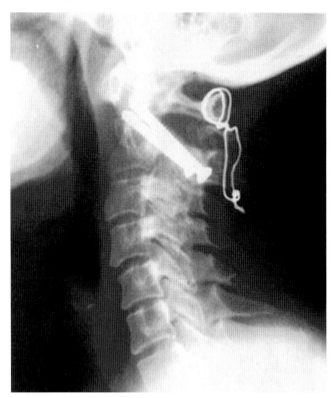

FIGURE 27-4 Postoperative lateral radiograph illustrating C1-C2 transarticular screw fixation with interspinous wiring. (From Shen FH, Samartzis, D, Jenis LG, An HS: Rheumatoid arthritis: evaluation and surgical management of the cervical spine. *Spine J* 4:689-700, 2004.)

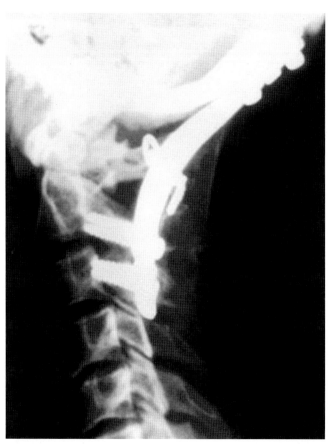

FIGURE 27-6 Postoperative lateral radiograph demonstrating posterior occipitocervical plate-screw fixation. (From Shen FH, Samartzis, D, Jenis LG, An HS: Rheumatoid arthritis: evaluation and surgical management of the cervical spine. *Spine J* 4:689-700, 2004.)

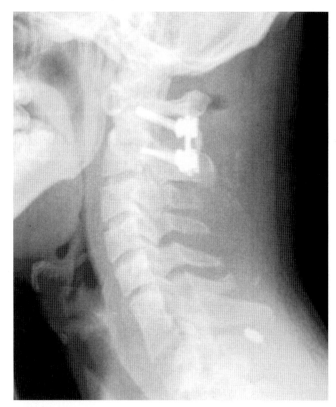

FIGURE 27-5 Postoperative lateral radiograph illustrating a C1 lateral mass and C2 pars interarticularis screws. (From Shen FH, Samartzis, D, Jenis LG, An HS: Rheumatoid arthritis: evaluation and surgical management of the cervical spine. *Spine J* 4:689-700, 2004.)

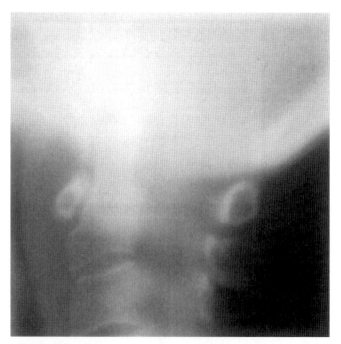

FIGURE 27-7 Sagittal tomography demonstrating cranial settling with superior migration of the odontoid process into the foramen magnum. (Modified from Shen FH, Samartzis, D, Jenis LG, An HS: Rheumatoid arthritis: evaluation and surgical management of the cervical spine. *Spine J* 4:689-700, 2004.)

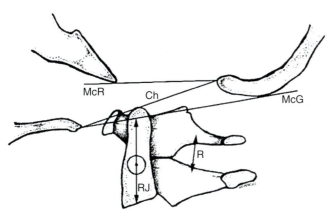

FIGURE 27-8 Lateral illustration of the upper cervical spine and lower occiput depicting radiographic measurement criteria to determine cranial settling. The McRae line (McR) is drawn from the basion to the posterior aspect of the foramen magnum. Projection of the odontoid above this line is considered abnormal. The Chamberlain line (Ch) is depicted as the line from the posterior region of the hard palate to the posterior lip of the foramen magnum. The McGregor line (McG) represents the margin between the posterior margin of the hard palate and the most caudal aspect of the occiput. The Ranawat line (R), measured along the long axis of the odontoid, is measured from the sclerotic ring of C2 to the transverse axis of the atlas. As cranial settling increases, this distance becomes shorter. The Redlund-Johnell (RJ) occipitoatlantoaxial index of cranial settling is measured by the distance from the McGregor to the sagittal midpoint at the base of the axis. (From Shen FH, Samartzis, D, Jenis LG, An HS: Rheumatoid arthritis: evaluation and surgical management of the cervical spine. *Spine J* 4:689-700, 2004.)

only, or combined approaches are used as surgical options, depending on a variety of factors including radiographic appearance and the surgeon's preference.

Conclusions

Involvement of the cervical spine often follows the peripheral joints in patients with rheumatoid arthritis. Awareness of the various pathologic processes that can affect the upper and cervical spine cannot be overemphasized.

A role exists for conservative management using soft or rigid collars, orthoses, and physical therapy in early stages of the disease when the symptoms are mild. Most clinicians agree that surgical intervention is indicated with progression of symptoms, including pain and neurologic deficit. The patient's preoperative neurologic state plays a role in determining outcome and prognosis and overall survival.[2,11]

The challenges in managing patients with rheumatoid arthritis go beyond the operative approach and surgical plan. These patients often have other medical comorbidities and are taking steroids and immunosuppressive medications that can affect bone quality and impede wound healing. A multidisciplinary approach is key in achieving successful treatments while minimizing potential serious complications.

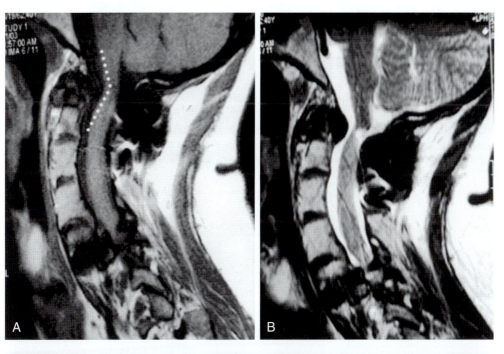

FIGURE 27-9 Cervicomedullary angle. **A** and **B,** Magnetic resonance images of a patient with myelopathic rheumatoid arthritis with a cervicomedullary angle measuring 130 degrees (*dotted white line* in **A**). Notice the effect of progressive cranial settling combined with an increasing retroodental pannus on the craniocervical junction. (From Shen FH, Samartzis, D, Jenis LG, An HS: Rheumatoid arthritis: evaluation and surgical management of the cervical spine. *Spine J* 4:689-700, 2004.)

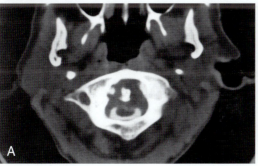
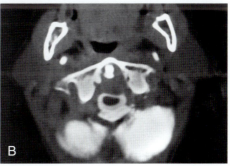

FIGURE 27-10 Flexion computed tomography (CT) myelogram. **A,** Note the odontoid position and pannus with cervicomedullary junction compression in a patient with rheumatoid arthritis. **B,** With an extension CT myelogram, the pannus is still present, thus demonstrating irreducibility of the mass.

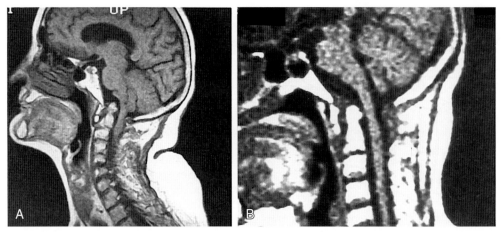

FIGURE 27-11 **A,** Basilar invagination in a patient with rheumatoid arthritis before traction. **B,** The lesion is reduced following traction.

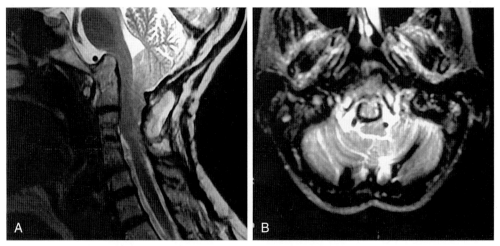

FIGURE 27-12 This 54-year-old patient with rheumatoid arthritis who previously underwent occipital-C2-C3 dorsal fusion in situ, presented with quadriparesis after a fall. **A,** Sagittal T2-weighted magnetic resonance imaging (MRI) shows the odontoid at the pontomedullary junction. **B,** Axial T2-weighted MRI 2 cm above the foramen magnum. Note the odontoid tip against the medulla and vertebral vessels.

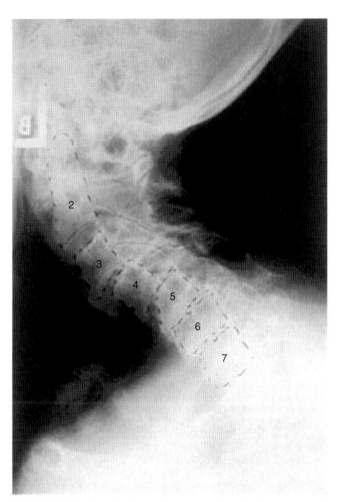

FIGURE 27-13 Lateral radiograph demonstrating subaxial subluxation of the cervical spine at multiple levels that resulted in a classic "stairstep" deformity. (Modified from Shen FH, Samartzis, D, Jenis LG, An HS: Rheumatoid arthritis: evaluation and surgical management of the cervical spine. *Spine J* 4:689-700, 2004.)

REFERENCES

1. Kauppi MJ, Neva MH, Laiho K, et al.: Rheumatoid atlantoaxial subluxation can be prevented by intensive use of traditional disease modifying antirheumatic drugs, *J Rheumatol* 36:273–278, 2009.
2. Paus AC, Steen H, Roislien J, et al.: High mortality rate in rheumatoid arthritis with subluxation of the cervical spine: a cohort study of operated and nonoperated patients, *Spine (Phila Pa 1976)* 33:2278–2283, 2008.
3. Rawlins BA, Girardi FP, Boachie-Adjei O: Rheumatoid arthritis of the cervical spine, *Rheum Dis Clin North Am* 24:55–65, 1998.
4. Kim DH, Hilibrand AS: Rheumatoid arthritis in the cervical spine, *J Am Acad Orthop Surg* 13:463–474, 2005.
5. Zeidman SM, Ducker TB: Rheumatoid arthritis: neuroanatomy, compression, and grading of deficits, *Spine (Phila Pa 1976)* 19:2259–2266, 1994.
6. Boden SD, Dodge LD, Bohlman HH, Rechtine GR: Rheumatoid arthritis of the cervical spine: a long-term analysis with predictors of paralysis and recovery, *J Bone Joint Surg Am* 75:1282–1297, 1993.
7. Ranawat CS, O'Leary P, Pellicci P, et al.: Cervical spine fusion in rheumatoid arthritis, *J Bone Joint Surg Am* 61:1003–1010, 1979.
8. Menezes AH, VanGilder JC: Transoral-transpharyngeal approach to the anterior craniocervical junction: ten-year experience with 72 patients, *J Neurosurg* 69:895–903, 1988.
9. Menezes AH, VanGilder JC, Clark CR, el-Khoury G: Odontoid upward migration in rheumatoid arthritis: an analysis of 45 patients with "cranial settling," *J Neurosurg* 63:500–509, 1985.
10. Yonezawa T, Tsuji H, Matsui H, Hirano N: Subaxial lesions in rheumatoid arthritis: radiographic factors suggestive of lower cervical myelopathy, *Spine (Phila Pa 1976)* 20:208–215, 1995.
11. Casey AT, Crockard HA, Geddes JF, Stevens J: Vertical translocation: the enigma of the disappearing atlantodens interval in patients with myelopathy and rheumatoid arthritis. Part I. Clinical, radiological, and neuropathological features, *J Neurosurg* 87:856–862, 1997.

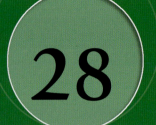

28 Ankylosing Spondylitis of the Cervical Spine

Brian C. Werner, Eric Feuchtbaum, Francis H. Shen, and Dino Samartzis

CHAPTER PREVIEW

Chapter Synopsis	Ankylosing spondylitis (AS) is a disease of unknown origin that is characterized by inflammation of the axial skeleton. It affects the cervical spine in many patients in the late stages of the disease. Cervical spine involvement invariably leads to kyphotic deformity, which can cause severe functional impairment and can also predispose patients to cervical spine fractures. Several diagnostic and treatment strategies are available for early and late manifestations of AS, including surgical options for nontraumatic deformity correction and fracture management. The purpose of this chapter is to discuss the epidemiology, evaluation, management, and complications associated with operative and nonoperative treatment of patients with AS of the cervical spine.
Important Points	AS typically affects young men, beginning in the sacroiliac joints and moving proximally to the cervical spine in the later stages of the disease.
	Nonoperative management options include physical therapy, nonsteroidal antiinflammatory drugs, and disease-modifying agents such as anti–tumor necrosis factor-α medications.
	Cervical spine fractures are frequent and can have devastating complications requiring strict spine precautions and advanced imaging of the entire spine before surgical intervention.
	Nontraumatic cervical spine deformity (chin-on-chest) can be debilitating and can require cervical extension osteotomy in selected patients.

Ankylosing spondylitis (AS) is a seronegative spondyloarthropathy of unknown cause characterized by inflammation of the axial skeleton. It typically affects the sacroiliac joints at early stages in the disease, which is followed by enthesopathy of the paravertebral joints and disk spaces of the spine. Left untreated, this condition causes early fusion of the paravertebral zygapophyseal joints and intervertebral disk spaces leading to the "bamboo spine" that characterizes the disease, hyperkyphotic posture, and compromised sagittal balance. These deformities can lead to severe functional impairment and can also predispose patients to traumatic spinal injury.

Several diagnostic and treatment strategies are available for early and late manifestations of AS, including medical therapy and operative management for late deformity correction. Similarly, diagnostic and management approaches are established for managing traumatic spinal column injuries and their complications. The ankylosed cervical spine presents a unique set of challenges, in addition to those listed earlier, because of the characteristic chin-on-chest deformity that results from

the hyperkyphotic spine.[1-6] The purpose of this chapter is to discuss the epidemiology, evaluation, management, and complications associated with operative and nonoperative treatment of patients with AS of the cervical spine.

Epidemiology

AS typically affects young adults, most commonly male patients (3:1) in their second to fourth decade of life. The estimated prevalence of AS in the United States is 197 in 100,000 adults, with a range of 68 to 210 in 100,000 adults reported worldwide. Adequate evidence indicates that the incidence of AS has remained stable and is estimated to be 7.3 in 100,000 person-years in the United States.[7-9] Up to 20% of those patients diagnosed with AS have a positive family history of the disease, and 80% to 95% are human leukocyte antigen (HLA)-B27 positive. In the general population, however, AS is likely to develop in only 1% to 2% of HLA-B27–positive adults. No studies have specifically investigated the epidemiology of cervical spine involvement in AS.

Etiology

The true cause of AS is still undetermined, and genetic and environmental factors likely play significant roles in the etiology of the disease. Although the direct involvement of HLA-B27 in the pathogenesis of the disease is well established, not all individuals who are HLA-B27 positive develop AS, and several other theories have emerged. In addition to the well-established genetic basis of the disease, which includes HLA-B27 and numerous other genes, researchers have postulated the contribution of the immune system to the disease and have investigated the possibility of an autoimmune component to the disorder. Additionally, other theories implicate autoimmune responses to specific bacterial antigens as a potential environmental cause of the disease, by noting the elevated levels of antibodies to *Klebsiella pneumoniae* and *Escherichia coli* in patients with AS. The true etiology, however, is undoubtedly multifactorial and remains a subject of considerable research and debate.[7-9]

Pathophysiology

The hallmark pathologic features of AS include inflammation of the axial joints and large peripheral joints, accompanied by bony destruction. Fibrous tissue and inflammatory cell infiltrates invade the bone adjacent to entheseal attachments. The new bone that forms in response to this process leads to ankylosis of the affected joints. In the spine, subsequent loss of motion secondary to this ankylosis leads to syndesmophyte formation and the radiographic bamboo spine characteristic of AS.[2,8-10]

All regions of the spine can be affected by the disease process, and although inflammation typically ascends the spine, the cervical spine can be involved first, and the disease may skip vertebral segments. Two major factors inherent to the disease process are integral to understanding the effect of AS on the cervical spine: altered vertebral bone composition and altered spine biomechanics. The combination of these factors leads to deformity and results in the observed increased incidence and prevalence of vertebral fractures in AS, as well as the increased associated risks of such fractures.

Altered Vertebral Bone Composition

The prevalence of osteoporosis or clinically significant low bone mineral density (BMD) in patients with AS is reported to be up to 62% in the literature. This number surprisingly underestimates the true trabecular bone loss resulting from spurious increases in BMD caused by syndesmophyte formation and ligament ossification in AS. Furthermore, conventional assessments of BMD such as dual-energy x-ray absorption yield falsely normal results for the same reasons. Men with AS lose bone at a rate of 2.2% annually, with a 2.9% annual loss of total body calcium, compared with an annual loss of total body calcium of only 0.7% in men who are more than 50 years old who do not have AS.[7-9]

Osteoporosis associated with AS leads to a higher rate of vertebral fractures, as well as a higher risk of vertebral fracture from significantly lower-energy mechanisms secondary to altered bone biology. Unfortunately, the true cause of osteoporosis in AS remains unknown. Studies suggest a multifactorial etiology, with phases of enhanced bone resorption or reduced bone deposition at inflammatory sites early in the disease, paralleled by inflammatory cytokine mediation and altered hormonal influences. With progressive AS, the patient has continued demineralization of the axial skeleton that contributes significantly to progressive deformity and an increased rate of vertebral fractures.

Altered Spine Biomechanics

The ankylosed spine loses flexibility and becomes increasingly kyphotic. This condition is caused by the generalized paravertebral ossification that bridges primarily the small vertebral joints, the costotransverse joints, and the sacroiliac joints. Although ossification of the ligamentous structures occurs in patients with AS, this does not provide extraneous support to the spine. The spine in AS loses its elasticity, and this causes it to behave in a manner similar to that of long bones. The resulting rigid, kyphotic deformity produces a long, fused lever arm that places patients at a high risk of spinal fractures after minor or negligible trauma and of multiple spinal fractures in a single traumatic event.[11]

Clinical History, Workup, and Physical Examination

Clinically significant disease progression of AS usually begins in adolescence and young adulthood. Symptoms rarely first manifest after the age of 40 years. The most common initial presenting symptoms of AS are low back pain and stiffness; however, mechanical low back pain must be differentiated from the inflammatory pain associated with AS. In the early phases of disease, the lower back pain has an insidious onset, is unilateral, and is poorly localized to the deep gluteal region. Later, the pain localizes to the sacroiliac joints, where direct pressure may elicit discomfort. Eventually, the pain becomes continuous and bilateral and encompasses the entire lumbar region. The lumbar pain becomes associated with stiffness that is characteristically worse in the morning, often waking the patient from the latter half of sleep. Disease progression in the lumbar spine is characterized by an increasing loss of mobility and normal lordosis.

As the diseases progresses to the thoracic spine, patients may report pleuritic chest pain as a result of enthesopathy of the costosternal and manubriosternal joints. This pain is also exacerbated by sudden movements such as coughing or sneezing. In addition, ankylosis of the thoracic spine results in mild to moderate reductions in chest expansion that can be observed early in the disease. Eventually, the thoracic spine becomes increasingly kyphotic, and chest expansion is significantly limited. Breathing becomes progressively more difficult for the patient who relies heavily on diaphragmatic contraction for respiration. As the cervical spine becomes involved, the patient reports neck pain and limited range of motion, specifically loss of flexion and extension. Ankylosis of the cervical spine results in significant neck stiffness, an increased chin-brow angle, and the characteristic chin-on-chest deformity (Fig. 28-1).

Laboratory Workup

Routine blood tests for inflammatory markers such as the erythrocyte sedimentation rate (ESR) and C-reactive protein (CRP) are not reliable indicators of AS. Although nearly 75% of patients may have elevated ESR and CRP, levels have not been shown to correlate with severity of the disease. Of patients with spinal disease alone, 38% and 45% of patients have elevations of ESR and CRP, respectively. Other laboratory tests may demonstrate mild microcytic anemia, mild elevations in alkaline phosphatase and serum immunoglobulin A, and decreased lipid levels, most notably high-density lipoprotein.[7-10]

Rheumatoid factor and HLA-B27 are also routinely checked when AS is suspected as a diagnosis, and in most cases of confirmed AS, testing results for rheumatoid factor are negative and for HLA-B27 are positive, although variations in these results should not eliminate AS from the differential diagnosis.

Radiologic Imaging

The most common changes on plain radiographs are seen in the axial skeleton, specifically the diskovertebral, costovertebral, costotransverse, and apophyseal joints. Changes in the sacroiliac joints are the most notable radiographically, although many patients have been described to have active disease without this finding. Eventually, sclerosis becomes the most prominent feature radiographically as fibrosis, calcification, bridging, and ossification occur.[9,10,12-15]

Inflammatory changes of the vertebral body result from erosions and sclerosis. A cycle of osteitis and repair causes squaring of vertebral bodies, which is followed by ossification of the annulus fibrosis and adjacent vertebral ligaments. This combination of inflammatory changes can lead to nearly complete fusion of the spine, referred to as bamboo spine. These same changes notable in the lumbar spine also occur in the cervical spine. Erosions and sclerosis in the cervical spine lead to osteoporosis and inflammatory changes of the diskovertebral, apophyseal, and costovertebral joints, the atlantoaxial articulation with and without subluxation, and the posterior ligamentous attachment (Fig. 28-2).

Plain radiography remains the initial imaging study to evaluate patients with inflammatory back and neck pain; however, it lacks the sensitivity to demonstrate active inflammation.[6,14,15] Magnetic resonance imaging (MRI) is the study of choice to visualize inflammation of the spinal column, which is most notably found at the vertebrae, intervertebral disk, facet joints, pedicles, and transverse processes. Computed tomography (CT) is superior

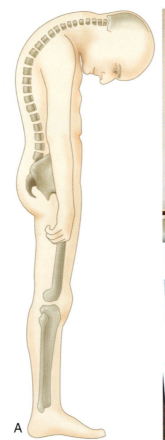
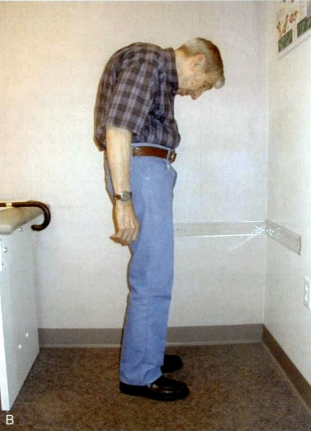

FIGURE 28-1 Drawing (**A**) and photograph (**B**) of a patient with ankylosing spondylitis with the characteristic "chin-on-chest" deformity resulting from extreme cervical kyphosis. This deformity can lead to devastating disability, including the inability to look straight ahead (loss of horizontal gaze) or lie flat at night. (Modified from Simmons ED: Spinal deformities in ankylosing spondylitis. In Shen FH, Shaffrey CI, editors: *Arthritis and arthroplasty: the spine,* Philadelphia, 2010,.Saunders.)

A   B

to MRI for visualizing bone; however, MRI can provide dynamic imaging measurement, as well as better imaging of cartilaginous structures. MRI is also far superior to CT for imaging of the sacroiliac joint.[16]

Fracture identification is particularly difficult in patients with AS. Fractures must be sought in a patient with AS who presents with spinal axial pain or spinal cord injury following trauma. Before the advent of MRI, the diagnosis of vertebral fractures as a complication of long-standing AS was considered very difficult. Plain radiographs may demonstrate fractures, especially of the anterior elements, but because of osteoporosis, ossification of ligamentous structures, and the complicated osseous deformities associated with AS, plain radiographs are frequently challenging to interpret or falsely thought to be negative. Concomitant spinal injuries (e.g., lumbar spine injuries in suspected cervical spine fracture) are common in patients with AS as a result of lever-arm biomechanics, as already discussed; therefore, many authors recommend routine CT and MRI of the entire spine whenever a fracture is suspected.[1,2,5,6,12,14-16] (Fig. 28-3).

Nonoperative Management

Physical therapy including exercise has been proven effective in managing the pain and stiffness associated with AS in the short term. Controlled trials demonstrated that supervised group therapy is superior to individual therapy in terms of reduction of symptomatic pain and stiffness, although individual therapy is better than no therapy. The optimal regimen of physical therapy includes a combination of inpatient physical therapy and spa treatments followed by weekly supervised outpatient group physical therapy.

The use of nonsteroidal antiinflammatory drugs (NSAIDs) has long been established as an effective method to decrease pain and stiffness while increasing spinal mobility. No single NSAID has proven to have the most optimal efficacy, and therefore many different agents are used. Consideration of cyclooxygenase-2 inhibitors should be given for individuals with risk factors for gastrointestinal morbidity. Randomized controlled trials demonstrated that continuous use of NSAIDs, as opposed to on-demand use, is better for slowing the radiographic progression of disease.

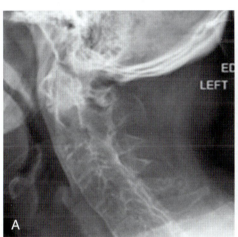
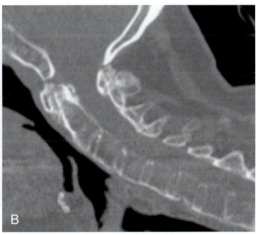

FIGURE 28-2 Lateral plain radiograph (**A**) and sagittal computed tomography scan (**B**) of the cervical spine of a 70-year-old patient with ankylosing spondylitis. Note the diffuse osteopenia, ankylosis of the facet joints throughout the cervical spine, and symmetric flowing syndesmophytes consistent with the disease.

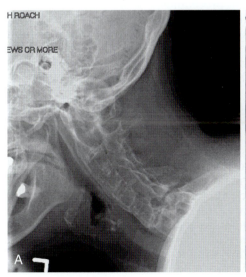
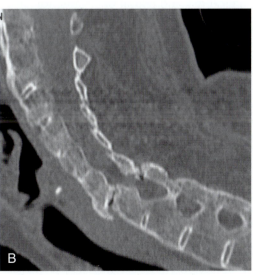

FIGURE 28-3 Lateral plain radiograph (**A**) and computed tomography scan (**B**) of a 60-year-old woman with ankylosing spondylitis and neck pain following a ground-level fall several months before presentation. The radiographs demonstrate a three-column fracture extending through the disk and posterior elements at C6 and C7 in a completely ankylosed cervical spine. Sclerosis along the posterior portion of the fracture line indicates likely chronicity.

One of the major advances in the treatment of AS has been development of anti–tumor necrosis factor-α (anti–TNF-α) medications. The basis of their use for AS is the finding of TNF-α receptors in biopsy samples of the sacroiliac joints of patients with AS, as well as the reproduction of sacroiliitis in mice overexpressing TNF-α. Anti–TNF-α drugs have been validated in a clinical trial in which patients were noted to have short-term improvements in disease activity, function, and quality of life. Three TNF-α antagonists have been approved for use: infliximab, etanercept, and adalimumab. Their use is recommended when any of the following are present: a definitive diagnosis of AS, the presence of the disease for at least 4 weeks, refractory disease (failure of two types of NSAIDs in a 3-month period), failure of local corticosteroid use, failure of sulfasalazine use in patients with peripheral AS, and the absence of contraindications to anti–TNF-α use. These medications have been proven to be disease-modifying agents; however, their long-term safety and efficacy are still being evaluated.[7-9]

Management of Traumatic Injury

The treatment of vertebral fractures in patients with AS differs greatly from that of the general population as a result of poor bone quality, altered spine biomechanics, inherent instability of the fractures, and high risk of neurologic sequelae. Protected transfers are absolutely mandatory for patients with AS, given the risk of spinal cord compression and devastating neurologic sequelae. Surgical treatment is generally indicated because of the inherent instability of the fractures and frequent neurologic deficits; however, nonoperative management has been successfully employed in very selected instances.

Nonoperative Management

A thorough meta-analysis of all available literature on treatment and complications of spinal fractures in AS was published by Westerveld and colleagues in 2009.[17] These investigators found that conservative management was pursued in 46% of patients with AS who had spine fractures; however, the main reasons for nonsurgical management were unacceptably high surgical risk and refusal of surgical management by patients. Most of the vertebral fractures in this review were located in the cervical spine (81%); thus, the most common conservative treatments were cervical collar and cervical traction. The investigators further noted that surgical treatment seemed to lead to neurologic improvement and a decrease in overall complication rate in more patients with AS than did conservative treatment both in the posttreatment phase and at follow-up.[17]

Aside from these cases in which high surgical risk or other patient-related factors preclude surgical treatment, nonoperative care for patients with AS who have unstable spinal fractures is not ideal in terms of neurologic and spinal stability. Patients with AS have an inordinately high rate of complications following cervical traction and cervicothoracic bracing, including skin ulcerations and pulmonary complications. Furthermore, the presence of any neurologic deficit, persistent dislocation, or bony fragments within the spinal canal warrants strong consideration for operative stabilization.[11]

Operative Management

Approximately half of spinal fractures in patients with AS reported in the literature are treated operatively, and the current trend is toward an even higher percentage of operative intervention. Compelling reasons for operative intervention reported frequently are secondary deterioration of neurologic status, unstable fracture configuration, and the presence of an epidural hematoma. Furthermore, in patients with AS who present with immediate neurologic deficits after spinal fracture, operative intervention results in no progression of the deficit in 59% of patients and improvement of the deficit at follow-up in 27% of patients.[3,8,17-21]

The location of the fracture influences the surgical approach and plan. Most operatively stabilized fractures in patients with AS, regardless of location, are treated through a posterior approach. This approach allows the surgeon to recreate the preexisting alignment of the spine, confer stability to the injured segment, and complete decompression of the neural elements if necessary.

The same three surgical approaches used for patients who do not have AS are available for fixation of cervical spine fractures in patients with AS: anterior fixation alone, posterior fixation alone, and combined anterior-posterior fixation. Reports in the literature support each of these approaches in the patient with AS depending on fracture pattern, albeit mostly in case reports and series.[3,17-20]

Approximately 15% of operatively managed cervical spine fractures in patients with AS are treated with anterior fixation alone. Published case reports have demonstrated reasonable success with this approach for fracture management. In most cases, however, three-column instability is present; posterior instability and ruptured posterior ligaments are often not detectable on plain radiography. Providing anterior stability alone has often led to implant loosening resulting from stress forces from the posterior part of the spine. Failure rates of an initial anterior approach surgical procedure have been reported to be has high as 50%, thus causing many surgeons to abandon this approach as a surgical option. Furthermore, anterior surgical procedures can be particularly difficult in this patient population because of the associated chin-on-chest deformity. In this disabling manifestation of AS, cervical hyperkyphosis causes the patient's chin nearly to touch the chest and thereby leads to a narrow window for surgical approach and extremely challenging intubation.[17]

The posterior approach, a more widely used and described approach to fracture fixation in AS, is reported to be used in approximately 50% of operatively managed patients. Numerous case reports and series have been published demonstrating successful management of cervical spine fractures in AS by using posterior fixation alone. The major argument for the use of posterior fixation alone in patients with AS is the biomechanical advantage that multisegmented posterior fixation with autologous cancellous bone graft offers over combined anterior-posterior fixation with wires, plates, or screws. Although numerous reports document the success of

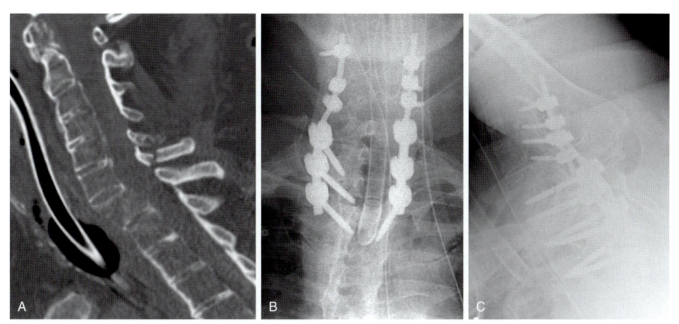

FIGURE 28-4 A 47-year-old man with ankylosing spondylitis fell during transfer and sustained immediate tetraparesis of his upper and lower extremities. Sagittal computed tomography scan (**A**) demonstrates a fracture through the C6 spinous process, through the facet joints at C6 to C7, and completely through the C7 vertebral body both anteriorly and posteriorly. Given the instability of the fracture and neurologic deficits, the patient was taken for emergency posterior spinal fusion with iliac crest bone graft from C4 to T3 (**B** and **C**).

circumferential fixation in this patient population, poor bone stock and the rigid, long lever-arm noted in patients with AS cause short plates, screws, and wires to yield poor constructs that lead to screw loosening and back-out. Posterior fixation alone adequately addresses the altered biomechanical forces associated with an AS spine and avoids potential complications associated with a more challenging combined anterior-posterior approach[17,22] (Fig. 28-4).

Combined anterior-posterior fixation is the final operative approach for the management of cervical spine fractures in patients with AS and is used in approximately 25% of cases.[17,20] Although it is not as popular as posterior-alone fixation for the reasons discussed earlier, it still has significant utility, especially for correction of fixed deformity at the same time as fracture fixation. As with other surgical methods, numerous published case reports have demonstrated reasonable outcomes. Supporters of combined anterior-posterior fixation argue that fractures usually occur at a point in the cervical spine that is completely stiff, which usually results in a displaced unstable injury. Accordingly, the presence of a gap in the anterior column places excessive loads on the posterior instrumentation. The addition of an anterior construct theoretically acts as a load-sharing device. Additionally, the fused ill-defined posterior elements may result in difficulty in localizing the anatomic landmarks, and the osteopenic nature of the bone may render single-approach fixation suboptimal.

The choice of approach and fixation is ultimately at the surgeons' discretion, but it should take into careful account the fracture location and deformity present. Anterior-alone procedures seem to be associated with higher failure rates, and thus posterior-alone or combined anterior-posterior fixation should be considered.

Surgical Correction of Cervical Deformity

Progressive increases in cervical and thoracic kyphosis, coupled with a loss of normal lumbar lordosis and impaired motion of the hips, lead to a stooped posture and significant functional impairment in patients with AS. Further progression of these deformities can lead to incapacitating symptoms such as the inability to look straight ahead (chin-on-chest deformity) or the inability to lie flat in bed at night. Although correction of this deformity involves consideration of all involved joints including the hips, surgical intervention may be indicated for cervical deformity that has significantly affected the patient's daily life.

Correction of deformity at the level of the cervical spine is indicated in patients with AS who have maintained sagittal balance, or who have regained sagittal balance through deformity correction elsewhere, but who have persistent kyphotic deformity that impairs forward vision or functionality or interferes with daily activities, hygiene, or swallowing. The nature of the deformity, the complexity of the underlying disease, and the limited treatment options make management of cervical flexion deformity a challenging problem. Surgical correction of cervical kyphosis is available but is technically demanding and carries the potential risk of devastating neurologic injury; thus, the risks and benefits must be carefully weighed preoperatively.

Urist first described the use of cervical extension osteotomy for the treatment of fixed cervical kyphotic deformity ("chin-on-chest" deformity) in AS, a technique he adapted from Smith-Peterson and colleagues. His technique involved removing a posterior wedge of bone from C7 with subsequent gradual extension of the head and

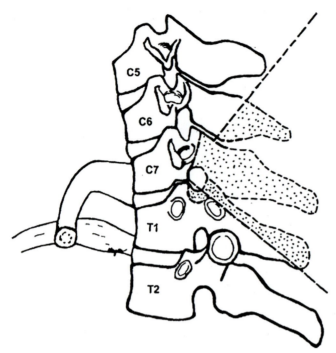

FIGURE 28-5 Cervical extension osteotomy for the correction of cervical deformity in ankylosing spondylitis as described by Urist and Simmons. The entire posterior arch of C7 with the inferior portion of C6 and the superior portion of T1 are removed, and then the osteotomy is closed. (From Simmons ED, DiStefano RJ, Zheng Y, Simmons EH. Thirty-six years' experience of cervical extension osteotomy in ankylosing spondylitis: techniques and outcomes. *Spine (Phila Pa 1976)* 31:3006-3012, 2006.)

neck to "close" the osteotomy defect and achieve sagittal correction (Fig. 28-5). The advantage of this operation is that it can be performed using local anesthesia with the patient awake to facilitate neurologic monitoring during the reduction and thereby avoid the potential hazards of intubation. The center of the level of correction is C7 to T1 because of the relative width of the spinal canal at this level and the relative mobility of the cervical spinal cord and nerve roots compared with other levels. Although modifications of anesthesia, instrumentation, and neuromonitoring have been developed, the original description of the procedure remains the standard treatment for cervical flexion deformity in AS.

Patients with AS may also present with instability, including subluxation of C1 and C2 leading to kyphotic deformity. In these patients, a period of halo traction must be used as treatment before surgical arthrodesis to restore accurate alignment of the spinal canal.

Complications and Hazards

AS is a challenging disease; similarly, both the nonoperative treatment and the operative management of the disease and its sequelae present unique challenges and risks of complications. Published complication rates of spine fractures in patients with AS are high in most series, ranging from 50% to 84%. These complications are reported at equally high rates in both conservatively and operatively managed cohorts. Reported complications include

general complications such as postoperative wound infections, deep venous thrombosis, pneumonia, and respiratory insufficiency. More unique complications specific to the population with AS also occur with notable frequency, including epidural hematoma and aortic dissection. The clinician must be aware of the higher complication rate and the notably higher mortality rate associated with spine fractures in patients with AS in the emergency, conservative, or operative treatment of these injuries, and this higher potential for complications should be factored into decision making.[2,4,12,14,17,23,24]

Surgical correction of nontraumatic fixed flexion deformity of the cervical spine also has a higher risk of complications in patients with AS than in the general population. Reviews of literature report an approximately 3% risk of spinal cord injury with cervical extension osteotomy, a 4% risk of death in the postoperative period, and a 19% risk of peripheral nerve injury. Other reported complications with cervical extension osteotomy include postoperative dysphagia and pseudarthrosis.

Conclusions

AS is a disease of unknown cause characterized by inflammation of the axial skeleton. It affects the cervical spine in many patients in the late stages of the disease. Cervical spine involvement invariably leads to kyphotic deformity, which can cause severe functional impairment and can also predispose patients to cervical spine fractures and traumatic spine injury.

Several diagnostic and treatment strategies are available for early and late manifestations of AS, including medical therapy and operative management for late deformity correction. Similarly, diagnostic and management approaches are established for managing traumatic spinal column injuries and their complications. Unfortunately, complications are frequent in this disease and result in high mortality rates. However, if practitioners are appropriately educated regarding the medical and surgical management of patients with AS and are cognizant of the complications related to the transport, transfer, and positioning of these patients, good outcomes can be achieved.

REFERENCES

1. Carnell J, Fahimi J, Wills CP: Cervical spine fracture in ankylosing spondylitis, *West J Emerg Med* 10:267, 2009.
2. Caron T, Bransford R, Nguyen Q, et al.: Spine fractures in patients with ankylosing spinal disorders, *Spine (Phila Pa 1976)* 35: E458–E464, 2010.
3. Cooper PR, Cohen A, Rosiello A, Koslow M: Posterior stabilization of cervical spine fractures and subluxations using plates and screws, *Neurosurgery* 23:300–306, 1988.
4. Einsiedel T, Schmelz A, Arand M, et al.: Injuries of the cervical spine in patients with ankylosing spondylitis: experience at two trauma centers, *J Neurosurg Spine* 5:33–45, 2006.
5. Kaneko T, Koyanagi I, Murakami T, Houkin K: Fracture of the cervical spine in ankylosing spondylitis: a case report, *No Shinkei Geka* 38:839–843, 2010. [in Japanese].
6. Murray GC, Persellin RH: Cervical fracture complicating ankylosing spondylitis: a report of eight cases and review of the literature, *Am J Med* 70:1033–1041, 1981.

7. Feldtkeller E, Vosse D, Geusens P, van der Linden S: Prevalence and annual incidence of vertebral fractures in patients with ankylosing spondylitis, *Rheumatol Int* 26:234–239, 2006.
8. Fordham S, Lloyd G: Clinical management of injured patients with ankylosing spondylitis, *BMJ* 339:b2568, 2009.
9. Gran JT, Husby G: Clinical, epidemiologic, and therapeutic aspects of ankylosing spondylitis, *Curr Opin Rheumatol* 10: 292–298, 1998.
10. Kanter AS, Wang MY, Mummaneni PV: A treatment algorithm for the management of cervical spine fractures and deformity in patients with ankylosing spondylitis, *Neurosurg Focus* 24:E11, 2008.
11. Shen FH, Samartzis D: Successful nonoperative treatment of a three-column thoracic fracture in a patient with ankylosing spondylitis: existence and clinical significance of the fourth column of the spine, *Spine (Phila Pa 1976)* 32:E423–E427, 2007.
12. de Peretti F, Hovorka I, Aboulker C, et al.: Fracture of the spine, spinal epidural haematoma and spondylitis: report of one case and review of the literature, *Eur Spine J* 1:244–248, 1993.
13. Hadjicostas PT, Tsirogianni AK, Soucacos PN, Thielemann FW: Odontoid fracture in severe ankylosing spondylitic patient, *Injury* 41:231–234, 2010.
14. Harrop JS, Sharan A, Anderson G, et al.: Failure of standard imaging to detect a cervical fracture in a patient with ankylosing spondylitis, *Spine (Phila Pa 1976)* 30:E417–E419, 2005.
15. Lee HS, Kim TH, Yun HR, et al.: Radiologic changes of cervical spine in ankylosing spondylitis, *Clin Rheumatol* 20:262–266, 2001.
16. Campagna R, Pessis E, Feydy A, et al.: Fractures of the ankylosed spine: MDCT and MRI with emphasis on individual anatomic spinal structures, *AJR Am J Roentgenol* 192:987–995, 2009.
17. Westerveld LA, Verlaan JJ, Oner FC: Spinal fractures in patients with ankylosing spinal disorders: a systematic review of the literature on treatment, neurological status and complications, *Eur Spine J* 18:145–156, 2009.
18. Cornefjord M, Alemany M, Olerud C: Posterior fixation of subaxial cervical spine fractures in patients with ankylosing spondylitis, *Eur Spine J* 14:401–408, 2005.
19. Lange U, Pape HC, Bastian L, Krettek C: Operative management of cervical spine injuries in patients with Bechterew's disease, *Unfallchirurg* 108:63–68, 2005. [in German].
20. Liao CC, Chen LR: Anterior and posterior fixation of a cervical fracture induced by chiropractic spinal manipulation in ankylosing spondylitis: a case report, *J Trauma* 63:E90–E94, 2007.
21. Shen FH, Samartzis D: Surgical management of lower cervical spine fracture in ankylosing spondylitis, *J Trauma* 61:1005–1009, 2006.
22. El Masry M.A., Badawy W.S., Chan D.: Combined anterior and posterior stabilisation for treating an unstable cervical spine fracture in a patient with long standing ankylosing spondylitis, *Injury* 35:1064–1067, 2004.
23. Clarke A, James S, Ahuja SL: Ankylosing spondylitis: inadvertent application of a rigid collar after cervical fracture, leading to neurological complications and death, *Acta Orthop Belg* 76:413–415, 2010.
24. Nahed BV, Walcott BP, Ortman AJ, et al.: Interval, acute onset airway obstruction associated with a fracture of the C4 vertebra in a patient with ankylosing spondylitis, *J Clin Neurosci* 17: 1085–1088, 2010.

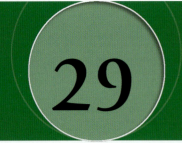

29

Syringomyelia

Ulrich Batzdorf

CHAPTER PREVIEW

Chapter Synopsis   Partial obstruction of the subarachnoid space can be identified as the underlying cause of syringomyelia in almost all patients: tonsillar descent causes this in Chiari malformation–related syringomyelia, and arachnoid webs or scars are the most common causes in patients with primary spinal syringomyelia. Relief of obstruction forms the basis of the preferred surgical treatment and is generally possible for Chiari malformation–related syringomyelia and in some patients with primary spinal syringomyelia. When this is not possible or when decompression of the subarachnoid space has failed, syrinx cavity fluid diversion by shunting becomes necessary. Even in successfully treated patients, the syringomyelic cavity may only diminish in size and not collapse completely. Resolution of symptoms is related in part to the patient's age, as well as to the severity and duration of symptoms preoperatively.

Important Points   The surgeon must ascertain that the patient has true syringomyelia, not hydromyelia.

The surgeon must perform adequate decompression of the foramen magnum in patients with Chiari malformation–related syringomyelia, to restore unobstructed continuity of the cranial and spinal subarachnoid space.

The level and extent of spinal subarachnoid space narrowing must be identified in patients with primary spinal syringomyelia by whatever diagnostic means are necessary.

The surgeon must recognize that limb atrophy, especially hand atrophy, profound sensory loss, and dysesthetic pain are unlikely to show significant change even after successful reduction in syrinx size.

Syringomyelia is best defined as a confluent collection of fluid within the spinal cord. The fluid closely resembles or is identical to cerebrospinal fluid (CSF). As such, the clinician must distinguish syringomyelia from spinal cord edema, a condition in which the increased tissue fluid is not identified as confluent but is interstitial, and from tumor-associated cysts. The fluid in tumor cysts generally has higher protein content than CSF, and it may also have other tumor-related constituents. Most importantly, the treatment of tumor cysts is quite different from that of syringomyelia.

Classification

Both from the diagnostic point of view and with respect to treatment planning, it is useful to classify syringomyelia as follows:

1. Syringomyelia related to abnormalities at the foramen magnum

Tonsillar descent (Chiari malformation); arachnoid veil with fourth ventricle outlet obstruction
2. Primary spinal syringomyelia
   a. Posttraumatic, including postsurgical
   b. Postinflammatory: infection, neoplastic meningitis
   c. Related to abnormalities of the arachnoid: arachnoid cysts, presumably developmental in origin
   d. Related to focal structural lesions narrowing the subarachnoid space
      (1) Tumor
      (2) Disk
   e. Idiopathic

Two other conditions must be noted when considering a classification of syringomyelia: presyrinx and hydromyelia. *Presyrinx* is defined on the basis of imaging technology as a focal area of spinal cord edema often adjacent to a confluent syrinx cavity. A mechanism of fluid accumulation similar or identical to that postulated for syringomyelia is considered the basis of the presyrinx state. The potential for progression of such tissue fluid accumulation over time to form a confluent cavity is the reason for the designation of the presyrinx state.

Hydromyelia, which is also defined as a confluent CSF cavity within the spinal cord, is considered a remnant of the central canal of the spinal cord, which is a normal structure in embryogenesis. It has a characteristic imaging appearance, fusiform in the longitudinal axis and round and central within the spinal cord on axial images (Figs. 29-1 and 29-2). The spinal cord is generally not expanded by these small, slitlike cavities, which are not associated with symptoms and are not considered pathologic entities. When these findings are present in adults, they generally do not change over time. Hydromyelia is not uncommonly encountered in children, but involution of the central canal occurs most rapidly during the first 10 years of life.[1]

The rostro-caudal extent of the syrinx cavity must be considered. Syrinx cavities may be confined to one region of the spinal cord, such as cervical or thoracic, or they may involve both these areas. Cavities may also extend through the entire length of the spinal cord, a condition often referred to as holocord syringomyelia.

These various entities are discussed in the following sections.

Pathophysiology

A general understanding of the formation of syringomyelic cavities is very important to a consideration of treatment principles and therapeutic options.

Formation

The mechanism of formation of syrinx cavities associated with Chiari malformations has been studied more extensively than has that of other types of syringomyelia. The theory that syrinx cavities fill from the fourth ventricle is of historical interest and has mostly been abandoned, largely because such a communication cannot be demonstrated by modern imaging studies in most patients with Chiari malformation–related syringomyelia. Progressive enlargement of a syringomyelic cavity frequently occurs even in the absence of such a communication.

The concept proposed by Oldfield and colleagues is that the pulsatile action of the cerebellar tonsils acts like a piston on an essentially enclosed CSF compartment, the spinal subarachnoid space below the tonsils.[2] Severe constriction of the subarachnoid space by the cerebellar tonsils within the dura and bony confines at the level of the foramen magnum prevents wide dispersion of the fluid pressure wave. This piston-like action is postulated to force fluid into the spinal cord parenchyma along the Virchow-Robin (V-R) spaces, and the fluid ultimately coalesces to form a confluent cavity. Investigators have suggested that the presence of a segment of the residual central canal within the spinal cord may favor the coalescence of fluid migrating along the V-R spaces.[3] Arteriolar pulsations along the V-R spaces appear to aid in propelling the fluid centrally, but the work by Bilston, Brodbelt, Stoodley, and Fletcher also makes it clear that the mechanism for fluid accumulation within the spinal cord is likely to be far more complex.[4,5]

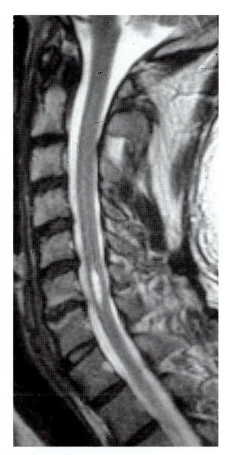

FIGURE 29-1 Sagittal T2-weighted magnetic resonance imaging showing a typical fusiform, slitlike hydromyelic cavity in the cervical spinal cord. Note the fine linear rostral extension.

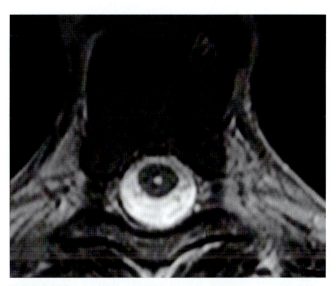

FIGURE 29-2 Axial T2-weighted magnetic resonance imaging of a hydromyelic cavity, round and central within the spinal cord.

Current treatment of Chiari malformation–related syringomyelia is based on the premise that reducing the piston-like action of the cerebellar tonsils on the spinal subarachnoid space will inactivate the filling mechanism of the syringomyelic cavity. This treatment is accomplished by (1) enlarging the subarachnoid space at the level of the foramen magnum so that the subarachnoid space of the posterior fossa is in unobstructed continuity with the spinal subarachnoid space[6] and (2) by reducing the size of the cerebellar tonsils to diminish their effectiveness as pistons acting on the spinal subarachnoid fluid.[7] Although the technical aspects of treatment vary widely among surgeons, depending on the patient's age group (pediatric versus adult) and other considerations, the syrinx cavities generally respond well to treatment based on these principles. Long-standing cavities and cavities in older patients are less likely to undergo complete collapse.

The formation of primary spinal syringomyelia can be considered analogous to that described for Chiari malformation–related syringomyelia, with an arachnoid barrier fulfilling the same role as the cerebellar tonsils in producing an incomplete but significant obstruction of the spinal subarachnoid space.[8,9] This can be most clearly visualized when one considers an arachnoid band or web, presumably but not necessarily developmental in origin, stretching across the subarachnoid space to form an arachnoid cyst. Such a web would then propagate the pulsatile pressure wave of the CSF to the subarachnoid fluid compartment just caudal to the web, which behaves as an enclosed fluid compartment. The reason that such pulse waves still exert significant pressure on the CSF is that compartmentalization of the spinal subarachnoid space by the web reduces the size of the compliance reservoir as compared with the intact subarachnoid space. A different mechanism may apply in some patients with trauma to the spinal cord. Trauma can result in focal tissue disruption within the spinal cord, thus permitting more direct entry of fluid into the cord tissue. A cavity, once established, may extend, as discussed later.

An arachnoid cyst and web comprise the simplest and most straightforward example of a focal obstruction of the spinal subarachnoid space.[10] Traumatic scars following spinal injury may also be focal, but because of the crushing nature of many such injuries, as well as associated subarachnoid bleeding that promotes scar formation, the rostrocaudal extent of subarachnoid scarring may be much greater and may extend over several vertebral levels. Scarring can occur ventral or dorsal to the spinal cord, it may be circumferential, or it may develop as a combination of these distributions. Scar tissue tends to thicken over time, perhaps because it is exposed to the continuous pulsations of CSF, and this may explain the time interval between spinal injury and the development of syringomyelia. It is not uncommon for years to elapse between injury and symptoms of syringomyelia. A strict correlation may not necessarily exist between the severity of spinal injury and the development of a syrinx cavity.

Postinflammatory syringomyelia may have an even more complex distribution of scar formation. When scarring follows meningitis, it obviously can take place throughout the spinal subarachnoid space. The same can be said of scarring that may follow spontaneous subarachnoid hemorrhage or neoplastic meningitis, even when this disorder has been treated successfully. Of infectious organisms, some, such as the tubercle bacillus, seem to evoke a much stronger scar tissue response than do other acute bacterial or viral infections.

Tumors, whether or not they are accompanied by a true tumor cyst, may compress the subarachnoid space and thereby set the stage for similar development of syringomyelia. Not uncommonly, a spinal cord tumor may have both a true cyst containing somewhat proteinaceous fluid and a syrinx cavity. Syringomyelia has been reported to form in relation to disk protrusion,[11] with the disk acting similarly to narrow the subarachnoid space.

Progression

A large, fluid-filled cavity within the spinal cord is exposed to complex dynamic forces that may propel the fluid rostrally, caudally, or in both directions, thereby contributing to the rostrocaudal enlargement of the syrinx cavity over time. Williams particularly studied the role of distention of spinal epidural veins (Batson plexus) in propelling the fluid cavity within the spinal cord, dissecting through the spinal cord, and enlarging the cavity.[12] Alterations in CSF pressure may contribute by externally compressing the spinal cord containing a cyst and thus extending the syrinx caudally.[9] Dural compliance may also play a role in this process. The presence of a potential space between rests of ependymal cells, or even a distinct residual central canal, may facilitate rostrocaudal enlargement of a syrinx cavity.

The treatment of primary spinal syringomyelia consequently is also predicated on removing the partial obstruction of the subarachnoid space and thereby allowing the CSF pressure wave to be propagated along the length of the spinal canal. This acts to inactivate the force driving fluid into the spinal cord. Only when such an approach is technically not feasible must other fluid diversion strategies be considered.

Preoperative Considerations

Clinical Presentation

The clinical manifestations of syringomyelia are varied and relate, in part, to the underlying pathogenesis. Thus, patients with syringomyelia related to Chiari malformation and similar abnormalities may have symptoms of partial CSF obstruction at the foramen magnum, symptoms related to compression of the brainstem by the descended and impacted cerebellar tonsils, and symptoms resulting from the associated syringomyelia. The last type of symptoms also may vary, depending on the anatomic level of the syrinx cavity.[3]

Only the most commonly encountered symptoms are listed here. They may be categorized as follows:

a. Symptoms resulting from partial obstruction of CSF flow at the foramen magnum
   Tussive headaches and other strain-related activities
b. Symptoms resulting from direct brainstem compression
   Swallowing difficulty
   Voice changes
   Nystagmus
   Balance problems
   Sleep apnea

c. Symptoms related to syringomyelia
  Sensory loss, which classically involves the upper limbs, but may extend further down
  Upper extremity weakness
  Hand and upper extremity atrophy
  Gait impairment
  Spasticity of lower extremities
  Bowel and bladder control problems
  Dysesthetic pain

Symptoms in patients with primary spinal syringomyelia most commonly fall into category c, but they may vary to some degree, depending on the underlying origin. In types of syringomyelia related to scarring of the arachnoid, a significant time interval may occur between the insult (i.e., trauma, infection, subarachnoid hemorrhage) and the development of symptoms related to syringomyelia. In patients with posttraumatic syringomyelia, the clinical presentation often is a mixture of symptoms and signs attributable to the spine and spinal cord injury and symptoms related to the development of the syrinx cavity. The time interval between injury and recognition of symptoms may be measured in years and is sometimes masked by neurologic deficit resulting directly from the injury, such as paraplegia. In such patients, the first manifestation of the presence of syringomyelia may be a subtle ascent of an existing sensory level.

Findings on examination related to syringomyelia are essentially findings of spinal cord dysfunction. They include motor findings of weakness and atrophy, long tract signs such as spasticity, and findings of sensory deficit, which may or may not be asymmetric. Asymmetry of neurologic deficit is sometimes seen, and the Brown-Séquard syndrome is a classic example.

Postinflammatory syringomyelia tends to be quite extensive in rostrocaudal extent, and dysesthetic pain often is an early and dominant symptom. Symptoms and signs of cauda equina arachnoid scarring would not be unexpected in some of these patients.

Diagnostic Evaluation

Syringomyelia Related to Chiari Malformation

Magnetic resonance imaging (MRI) is the most widely used imaging modality to detect syringomyelia associated with Chiari malformations. The obvious advantage of MRI is that it is noninvasive and causes no disturbance of CSF dynamics. Depending on the particular case series, tonsillar descent is accompanied by true syrinx formation in approximately half of adult patients with Chiari malformation, but the relationship between severity of tonsillar descent and development of a syrinx cavity is not linear.[7] Syringomyelia may also develop as a result of posterior fossa abnormalities other than tonsillar descent, such as outlet obstruction of the fourth ventricle or an arachnoid membrane at the level of the foramen magnum. T2-weighted MRI images, which highlight the fluid spaces including the cisterns surrounding the base of the cerebellum as well as the fluid in the syrinx cavity, tend to exaggerate the size of the fluid compartments, whereas T1-weighted images are anatomically more precise. It is uncommon to see cystic spinal cord tumors in combination with tonsillar descent, but such coincidental findings do occur and justify the use of a gadolinium contrast–enhanced study to rule out tumor in selected cases in which the presence of a tumor may be suspected.

Imaging of the brain is important in patients with Chiari malformation to determine whether they have coexisting hydrocephalus or a mass lesion and to assess the particular architecture of the posterior fossa that may be critical in determining the optimal surgical procedure for a particular patient. Although the midsagittal image presents a classic view of the descended tonsils, often with an associated "medullary beak" resulting from long-term compression, the axial image at the level of the foramen magnum is also very important. It often shows distortion of the lower brainstem at the cervicomedullary junction by the tonsils, with obliteration of the subarachnoid space between the brainstem and the tonsils. Asymmetric descent of the tonsils is frequently identified. Cardiac gated CSF flow studies are particularly helpful in sorting out borderline cases in which the tonsils may be somewhat low in position but not clearly pointed or peglike as a result of chronic pressure. When cardiac gated flow studies demonstrate the presence of a normal CSF flow pattern dorsal to the tonsils and the lower cerebellum, tonsillar descent is not likely to be the underlying factor responsible for development of the syringomyelic cavity. Constructive interference with steady-state MRI sequences may help to define obstructive disease that is not otherwise recognized.[13]

Primary Spinal Syringomyelia

MRI is currently also the most widely used imaging modality for the diagnosis of primary spinal syringomyelia. T1-weighted images demonstrate the intramedullary fluid-filled cavity. A study with intravenously administered contrast medium (gadolinium) is frequently necessary to rule out the presence of an associated spinal cord tumor. This is particularly true when the patient has no evidence of tonsillar descent. T2-weighted images may show the presence of an arachnoid web near the lower end of the syrinx cavity, a capability improved by use of the high-resolution T2 sequence scan, which is very useful in demonstrating fine anatomic details, such as septa, in the subarachnoid space.[13] Cardiac gated flow studies, such as those used to study CSF flow at the level of the foramen magnum, have not been widely available for exclusively spinal studies because overlying vertebral bone interferes with imaging the flow patterns of CSF around the spinal cord.

The configuration of the syrinx cavity, particularly when the caudal end looks blunt, may suggest obstructive subarachnoid pathology, such as a web[10] (Fig. 29-3). In such cases, consideration should be given to performing a myelogram, followed by a thin-section computed tomography scan of the region of interest. Such a study may give a very clear delineation of obstructive arachnoid disease and may indicate the precise level for a surgical approach (Fig. 29-4). Performing myelography through a C1-C2 puncture, rather than by the lumbar route, has the advantage of allowing pooling of contrast material at the level of the web. This pooling may not occur when contrast material is introduced by the lumbar route in situations in which the obstructive subarachnoid membrane may act as a one-way valve.

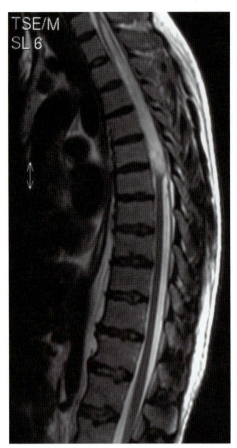

FIGURE 29-3 T2-weighted magnetic resonance imaging showing the characteristic blunt end of the subarachnoid space, indicative of an arachnoid web.

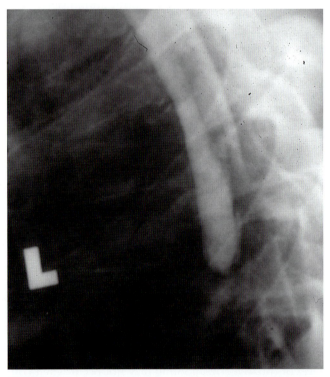

FIGURE 29-4 Posttraumatic syringomyelia. Myelogram, performed by high cervical (C1-C2) puncture, shows the subarachnoid block to flow of contrast and confirms the nature and vertebral level of the arachnoid obstruction.

A potential area of communication between the syrinx and the subarachnoid space, which can exist particularly in posttraumatic syringomyelia, may be very difficult to demonstrate on imaging studies unless immediate filling of the syrinx cavity occurs at the time of myelography. Occasionally, it is desirable to introduce contrast material from both the C1-C2 route and the lumbar route to bracket the area of arachnoid adhesions causing obstruction, a very important consideration in surgical planning for the patient.

Septations within the syrinx cavity are not uncommonly seen and may be important if shunting of the syrinx cavity is a consideration. This is particularly true if the septation is present in the longitudinal axis of the spinal cord, inasmuch as shunting of one of two (or more) parallel cavities that are not in communication with each other may result in expansion of the remaining unshunted cavity or cavities.

Indications and Contraindications to Surgical Therapy

Syringomyelia Related to Chiari Malformation

Indications for treatment of syringomyelia in association with a Chiari malformation are relatively clear. Most surgeons favor foramen magnum decompression if syringomyelia is present. The only caution is not to mistake hydromyelia for true syringomyelia and recommend surgical decompression on this basis. Hydromyelic cavities have a typical appearance, as described earlier, and one would not expect to see symptoms as listed in the earlier section on clinical presentation or findings of myelopathy in association with hydromyelia. Progressive enlargement of a syrinx cavity on imaging studies over a period of time also favors surgical intervention.

Primary Spinal Syringomyelia

Indications for surgical intervention in this group of patients are perhaps not as clear as in the group of patients with Chiari malformation. Progressive neurologic deficit, including ascent of an existing sensory level and development of new motor deficits including gait difficulty, which may be manifested as impaired balance, would indicate the need for surgical treatment. Limb atrophy, unless recently progressive, is unlikely to be reversible in an adult and as such should not be the sole indication for surgical treatment. The presence of dysesthetic pain as an indication for surgical intervention also is more questionable because such pain does not respond well to surgical decompression and in many instances is better managed with medication. Progressive enlargement of a syrinx cavity on sequential studies obtained over time also favors surgical intervention.

Surgical Technique

Syringomyelia Related to Chiari Malformation

The treatment of syringomyelia related to tonsillar descent or other obstructive disorders at the level of the foramen magnum is directed at the obstructive disorder. Oral acetazolamide has been used in a few patients who are not candidates for surgery, but in general the approach to this type of syringomyelia is posterior fossa decompression with reestablishment of a continuous cranial and spinal subarachnoid space at the level of the foramen magnum. Many variations on the specific technique employed are available, depending on the patient's age, the severity of tonsillar descent, and the surgeon's preference, as well as whether the planned procedure is the first procedure for the patient or is a reoperation for persistent or recurrent symptoms. The procedures may be listed in order of complexity:

1. Craniectomy with enlargement of the foramen magnum, with or without C1 laminectomy
2. Number 1 plus removal of the outer layer of the dura
3. Number 1 plus opening of the dura over the cerebellar tonsils and upper cervical spinal cord, thus leaving the arachnoid intact
4. Numbers 1 and 3, with placement of a dural patch graft over the intact arachnoid
5. Numbers 1 and 3, opening of the arachnoid, followed by placement of a dural patch graft
6. Numbers 1, 3, and 5, reduction of the cerebellar tonsils, followed by number 5.
7. Numbers 1 and 6, followed by placement of a titanium plate over the decompression site

Patients with basilar invagination or associated instability may require a different approach, which may include craniocervical stabilization, with or without transoral odontoid resection.

The patient is positioned prone on the operating table, with the head and neck secured with a skeletal clamp. The size of the craniectomy should be sufficient to expose the cerebellar tonsils yet leave adequate bony support for the cerebellar hemispheres. A helpful technique is to estimate the amount of bone to be removed from the edge of the foramen magnum by measurement, using preoperative MRI. Removal of more than 20 mm of bone from the edge of the foramen magnum is rarely necessary, and a smaller amount of bone removal is common in the author's experience. The width of the craniectomy is usually 20 to 25 mm. Violation of the atlanto-occipital joint should be avoided.

Procedures most commonly used today are bony decompression only (number 1 in the previous list), duraplasty over the intact arachnoid (number 4), duraplasty after opening the arachnoid (number 5), and duraplasty after some form of reduction of the cerebellar tonsils or other maneuvers to open the arachnoid spaces (number 6). The end point of any of these procedures should be the establishment of unobstructed CSF flow at the level of the foramen magnum, with construction of a significant subtonsillar CSF cistern.[6,7] The less invasive procedures are appropriately employed more commonly in pediatric practice. The greater elasticity of the dura, as well as the mechanical qualities of cerebellar tonsillar tissue in infants and small children, may account for satisfactory outcomes with simpler surgical procedures, such as numbers 1, 2 and 3 in the previous list.

The material chosen for duraplasty also varies widely and includes synthetic dural substitutes, bovine pericardium, autologous local fascia, and autologous pericranium. Synthetic materials are used together with autologous tissue by the author and some other surgeons. The author uses autologous pericranium lined with polytetrafluoroethylene dural substitute for the duraplasty. A Valsalva maneuver is performed on the patient to ascertain that a watertight dural closure has been obtained, and the suture line is covered with fibrin sealant and collagen sponge. CSF leakage is to be avoided. It may result in pseudomeningocele formation and may thereby interfere with syrinx reduction.

Although the author recognizes the desirability of performing a simpler procedure, particularly in small children, his experience, which is limited to adult practice, favors the more comprehensive procedure.[7] The author routinely performs C1 cervical laminectomy and suboccipital craniectomy and, with few exceptions, opens the dura and arachnoid and reduces the cerebellar tonsils (Figs. 29-5 and 29-6). Procedures that do not include direct inspection of the outlet of the fourth ventricle by opening the arachnoid risk leaving the underlying disease in place. The negative aspects of performing a later second surgical procedure through the same incision include potential problems with wound healing, not to mention the discomfort for the patient. The absence of any demonstrable side effects attributable to reduction of the cerebellar tonsils leads the author to favor this additional step in the treatment of most patients. Reduction of the cerebellar tonsils by application of a low setting of bipolar current

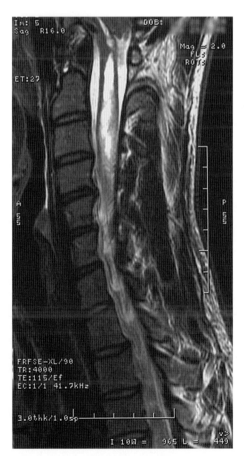

FIGURE 29-5 Preoperative T2-weighted magnetic resonance imaging of a patient with Chiari malformation and syringomyelia.

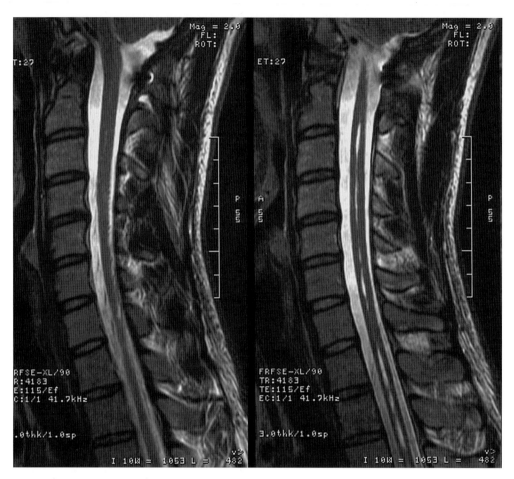

FIGURE 29-6 Same patient as in Figure 29-5 (adjacent sagittal images) after he underwent posterior fossa decompression with reduction of cerebellar tonsils and duraplasty as described. Note the relatively large subtonsillar and retrotonsillar cerebrospinal fluid cisterns and the significant reduction in the size of the syrinx cavity.

to the pial surface of the cerebellar tonsils is well tolerated. Current is applied particularly to the medial, dorsal, and caudal aspect of the tonsils, thus leaving the pia intact. This procedure assists greatly in creating a sizable cisterna magna. In rare instances, when chronic compression has made the cerebellar tonsils very gliotic, they do not shrink with the application of bipolar current. In such instances, the author makes a small incision over the dorsal aspect of the pia over each tonsil and performs subpial resection of tissue by using the ultrasonic aspirator. After hemostasis is obtained, the pia is reapproximated with a figure-of-eight suture using 8-0 suture material.

Primary Spinal Syringomyelia

The most important steps in planning a surgical procedure for patients with primary spinal syringomyelia are to define the area and vertebral level of subarachnoid space constriction or blockage and to establish whether the adherence of the arachnoid extends over only a short distance or over many vertebral levels. The diagnostic tools to help in this determination are discussed earlier.

When the subarachnoid obstruction is very focal, as in a patient with an arachnoid cyst, laminectomy or laminoplasty over the area of abnormality with resection of accessible portions of the arachnoid cyst wall is the best approach.[10] The abnormal membrane can usually be defined clearly, but the introduction of a drop of indigo carmine through a very fine (27- or 29-gauge) needle into the rostral subarachnoid space once the dura has been opened may help to define the block. Resection of more

than the dorsal web and its lateral extensions is not necessary, and this procedure that does not require manipulation of the spinal cord. Resection of the ventral portion of the membrane, when present, is generally not attempted. Primary dural closure is often feasible in patients who have an arachnoid cyst as the basis of their syringomyelia.

Focal posttraumatic arachnoid scars may lend themselves to a very similar approach, but the author would be more inclined to perform expansile duraplasty after resection of arachnoid scar in such cases. Klekamp and Samii recommended attaching the suture line of the duraplasty to the muscle wall above the level of the lamina, thereby expanding the subarachnoid space and preventing collapse of the graft onto the spinal cord.[14]

For patients with syringomyelia whose subarachnoid adhesions are so extensive that they preclude resection, or in whom resection of scar with or without duraplasty has been attempted but has failed to result in significant reduction of the syrinx cavity and related symptoms, diversion of CSF must be considered (Figs. 29-7 and 29-8). For such patients, current practice is to shunt the syrinx cavity into the peritoneal cavity, into the pleural cavity, or into the spinal subarachnoid space. The laminectomy and myelotomy should be performed near the caudal end of the syrinx cavity. Hemilaminectomy often suffices. Hemilaminectomy, particularly with preservation of the interspinous ligament, reduces the likelihood of postoperative spinal deformity, a potential risk when surgical procedures are performed near a junctional area of the spine (i.e., cervicothoracic).

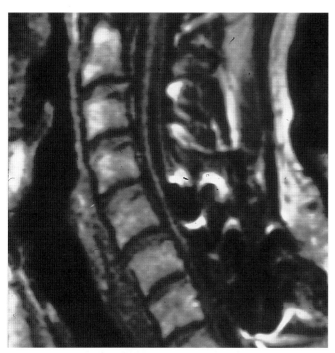

FIGURE 29-7 Posttraumatic cervical syringomyelia. T1-weighted magnetic resonance imaging.

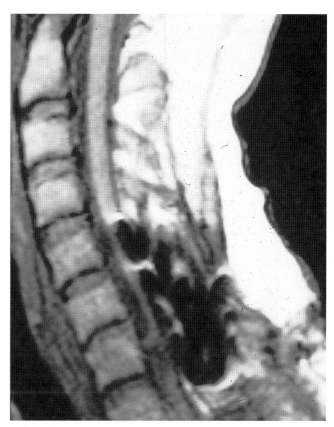

FIGURE 29-8 Same patient as in Figure 29-7, following placement of a syringopleural shunt. T1-weighted magnetic resonance imaging.

The decision to perform a midline myelotomy or a myelotomy through a thinned-out portion of the spinal cord lateral to the midline depends in part on the neurologic state of the patient. Some surgeons prefer a lateral entry point in patients with preexisting significant sensory impairment on the premise that the myelotomy will then not cause new neurologic deficits. The midline may be readily definable, but it is sometimes obscured by distention of the spinal cord. Introducing a thin shunt catheter with multiple perforations for a distance of at least 1 cm is preferable. Very long catheters may fold on themselves within the syrinx cavity and thereby occlude.

Placing the distal end of the shunt catheter into the intact spinal subarachnoid space, rather than into an extraspinal location, has advantages, and this is the author's preference unless reason exists to assume that a problem with resorption of CSF from the subarachnoid space would occur. Iwasaki and associates advocated placing the distal end of the drainage catheter anterior to the dentate ligament in the exposed area.[15] The catheter must be anchored to the dura with a small suture. Placement of the catheter into an extraspinal location necessitates a second incision and may raise questions of postural effects on drainage that are avoided with intraspinal positioning. Pleural shunting has the advantage of permitting the patient to be kept in the prone position on the operating table. Shunting into the peritoneal cavity requires that the patient be on his or her side for the laminectomy or else necessitates repositioning of the patient on the table, a maneuver that is cumbersome and adds to the risks of contamination. In all instances, except in patients with communication of a posttraumatic syrinx with the subarachnoid space, a shunt valve need not be placed into a syringomyelic shunt system.

A select group of high-risk patients with syringomyelia consists of those with arachnoid obstructive disease at high cervical levels.[16] Resection of scar tissue from the spinal cord or other manipulation of the high cervical spinal cord may pose a risk of respiratory dysfunction. For these patients, the author has recommended shunts from the rostral subarachnoid space, rather than from the syrinx cavity, into an extraspinal location (i.e., the pleural or peritoneal cavity), as previously described by Vengsarkar and colleagues.[17] All these patients require a valve in line with the shunt system. Reducing pulsatility and perhaps also pressure of this high cervical subarachnoid compartment forms the physiologic basis for this procedure.

Strictest adherence to surgical asepsis is essential in syrinx shunt operations. Infections, particularly if associated with meningitis, may cause significant morbidity. Watertight dural closure is essential. A high incidence of shunt failure is a major disadvantage of this form of treatment.[18,19] It is inherent in most shunt systems that the walls of the syrinx cavity may collapse around the openings of the shunt tubing within the syrinx cavity and thereby prevent the shunt from working. Fortunately, this does not happen in all patients, but in a sufficiently high percentage that patients must be forewarned.

Because of early recognition of posttraumatic kyphotic deformities of the spine and their surgical correction, fewer such patients have been seen in recent years. However, ventral compression of the subarachnoid space as a result of trauma can result in focal subarachnoid space

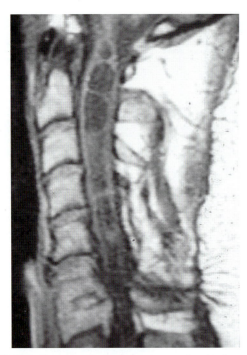

FIGURE 29-9 Posttraumatic cervical syringomyelia with fracture of C6 and C7. T1-weighted magnetic resonance imaging.

narrowing and thus lead to syringomyelia. Treatment of these patients requires surgical decompression of the ventral aspect of the spinal canal (Figs. 29-9 and 29-10), and it usually also requires segmental spinal fusion.

Results

Syringomyelia Related to Chiari Malformation

Collapse of the syrinx cavity is the desired outcome of posterior fossa decompression, but it is less likely to occur in adults than in children and in patients with long-standing distended syrinx cavities. Widening of the subarachnoid space alongside the syrinx cavity may be an early indication of decreased filling of the cavity, and reduction in size may take place over the course of months following the decompression. In the author's own experience, reduction of the syrinx cavity was seen in more than 80% of patients.[7] Other investigators have reported similar results.[13,20]

Primary Spinal Syringomyelia

The best results, in terms of syrinx collapse, have been seen in patients with focal arachnoid cysts and syringomyelia associated with spinal cord tumors.[8] The least satisfactory results in terms of symptomatic improvement have been seen in patients with postinflammatory syringomyelia, but these patients are also more likely to have significant dysesthetic pain, a recalcitrant symptom. Shunting, with shunt revision, is not uncommon in this group of patients, as well as in patients with posttraumatic syringomyelia. The author's overall experience with almost 100 patients with primary spinal syringomyelia was that 36% required reoperation, 31% stabilized, 14% improved, and 17% became worse.[8]

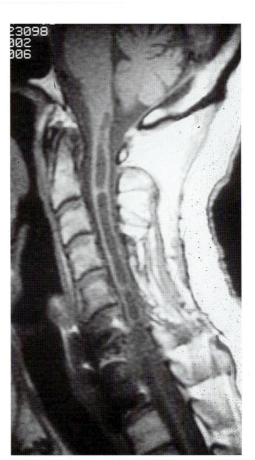

FIGURE 29-10 Same patient as in Figure 29-9, following anterior cervical decompression and fusion. T1-weighted magnetic resonance imaging. Note the reduction in size of the syrinx cavity.

REFERENCES

1. Yasui K, Hashizume Y, Yoshida M, et al.: Age-related morphologic changes of the central canal of the human spinal cord, *Acta Neuropathol (Berl)* 97:253–259, 1999.
2. Oldfield EH, Muraszko K, Shawker TH, Patronas NJ: Pathophysiology of syringomyelia associated with Chiari I malformation of the cerebellar tonsils, *J Neurosurg* 80:3–15, 1994.
3. Milhorat TH, Capocelli AL, Anzil AP, et al.: Pathological basis of spinal cord cavitation in syringomyelia: analysis of 105 autopsy cases, *J Neurosurg* 82:802–812, 1995.
4. Bilston LE, Stoodley MA, Fletcher DF: The influence of the relative timing of arterial and subarachnoid space pulse waves on spinal perivascular cerebrospinal fluid flow as a possible factor in syrinx development, *J Neurosurg* 112:808–813, 2012.
5. Brodbelt A, Stoodley M: CSF pathways: a review, *Br J Neurosurg* 21:510–520, 2007.
6. Sahuquillo J, Rubio E, Poca MA, et al.: Posterior-fossa reconstruction: a surgical technique for the treatment of Chiari malformation and Chiari I/syringomyelia complex: preliminary results and magnetic resonance imaging quantitative assessment of hindbrain migration, *Neurosurgery* 35:874–885, 1994.
7. Batzdorf U, McArthur DL, Bentson JR: Surgical treatment of Chiari malformation with and without syringomyelia: experience with 177 adult patients, *J Neurosurg* 118:232–242, 2013.
8. Batzdorf U: Primary spinal syringomyelia, *J Neurosurg Spine* 3:429–435, 2005.
9. Heiss JD, Snyder K, Peterson MM, et al.: Pathophysiology of primary spinal syringomyelia, *J Neurosurg Spine* 17:367–380, 2012.
10. Holly LT, Batzdorf U: Syringomyelia associated with intradural arachnoid cysts, *J Neurosurg Spine* 5:111–116, 2006.
11. Kaden B, Cedzich C, Schultheiss R, et al.: Disappearance of syringomyelia following resection of extramedullary lesion, *Acta Neurochir (Wien)* 123:211–213, 1993.

12. Williams B: On the pathogenesis of syringomyelia: a review, *J R Soc Med* 73:798–806, 1980.
13. Klekamp J: Treatment of posttraumatic syringomyelia, *J Neurosurg Spine* 17:199–211, 2012.
14. Klekamp J, Samii M: *Syringomyelia: diagnosis and treatment*, Heidelberg, 2002, Springer.
15. Iwasaki Y, Koyanagi I, Hida K, et al.: Syringo-subarachnoid shunt for syringomyelia using hemilaminectomy, *Br J Neurosurg* 13:41–45, 1999.
16. Lam S, Batzdorf U, Bergsneider M: Thecal shunt placement for obstructive primary syringomyelia, *J Neurosurg Spine* 9:581–588, 2008.
17. Vengsarkar US, Panchal VG, Tripathi PD, et al.: Percutaneous thecoperitoneal shunt for syringomyelia: report of three cases, *J Neurosurg* 74:827–831, 1991.
18. Klekamp J, Batzdorf U, Samii M, Bothe HW: Treatment of syringomyelia associated with arachnoid scarring caused by arachnoiditis or trauma, *J Neurosurg* 86:233–240, 1997.
19. Sgouros S, Williams B: A critical appraisal of drainage in syringomyelia, *J Neurosurg* 82:1–10, 1995.
20. Klekamp J: Treatment of syringomyelia related to nontraumatic arachnoid pathologies of the spinal canal, *Neurosurgery* 72:376–389, 2013.

SECTION 5

Surgical Techniques

Anterior Cervical Diskectomy and Fusion

30

Adam S. Wilson, Dino Samartzis, and Francis H. Shen

CHAPTER PREVIEW

Chapter Synopsis	Anterior cervical diskectomy and fusion (ACDF) comprises a common procedure used to treat cervical radiculopathy and cervical myelopathy. Excellent results can be achieved through careful patient selection and operative technique, which allows for reliable decompressiosn of the neuroforamen and the spinal canal for anterior cervical disease.
Important Points	The ACDF procedure is indicated for treatment of degenerative changes of the cervical spine resulting in central and neuroforaminal stenosis.
	This procedure is used in treatment of radicular and myelopathic symptoms that are refractory to nonoperative management.
	The ACDF procedure is not a reliable surgical option for the management of axial neck pain secondary to degenerative disk disease.
	Anterior cervical plating provides increased stability to the construct in the immediate postoperative period and may increase fusion rates in multilevel ACDF procedures.
Clinical and Surgical Pearls	The correct intervertebral level should be identified intraoperatively before proceeding with further surgical steps.
	Removal of the anterior lip of the inferior end plate of the superior vertebral body allows for significantly improved visualization of the intervertebral disk space.
	Posterior longitudinal ligament resection may be required if a sequestered disk fragment is present, but it is not absolutely indicated in all cases.
	Careful sizing and placement of graft are crucial to final results.
Clinical and Surgical Pitfalls	An intraoperative radiograph should be used to confirm the correct level before proceeding with diskectomy.
	Excessive bone removal should be avoided during end plate preparation to reduce the risk of graft settling.
	During foraminotomy, the Kerrison rongeur should maintain contact with the uncinate process to avoid nerve root and vertebral artery injury.
	Careful plate selection should be performed to allow for adequate screw placement while making sure not to impinge on adjacent intervertebral disk levels.
Video	Video 30-1: Anterior Cervical Diskectomy and Fusion

Cervical spondylosis refers to age-related degenerative changes of the cervical spine that are seen throughout the entire adult population. Most of these changes are asymptomatic; however, when they are symptomatic, they manifest as axial neck pain, radiculopathy of the upper extremity, or cervical myelopathy. These symptom complexes can be caused by a variety of degenerative changes. These changes include disk degeneration, disk herniation, facet arthrosis, and osteophytic spur formation. Degenerative changes within cervical disks are most often a result of desiccation of the disk, which leads to a cycle of progressive degenerative changes that can result in compression of neural structures and cause radiculopathy, myelopathy if the spinal cord is compressed, or a combination of both as in myeloradiculopathy.

Anterior cervical diskectomy and fusion (ACDF) are frequently used for treatment of cervical degenerative disease. The ACDF procedure is used to decompress an exiting nerve root to treat radicular symptoms, and it is also used for treatment of cervical myelopathy if the compressive disorder is anterior to the spinal cord. The ACDF procedure is performed through an anterior cervical approach that is described in further detail in Chapter 3. This chapter discusses preoperative considerations, surgical technique, and postoperative care related to ACDF.

Preoperative Considerations

History

A careful history and physical examination should be performed on any patient presenting with neck or arm pain. Patients frequently present with axial neck pain; however, axial neck pain secondary to degenerative disk disease alone is typically not an indication for surgery. However, patients also frequently present with radicular symptoms. These symptoms include burning or radiating pain extending distally in the affected arm, typically in a specific nerve root distribution, although occasionally the symptoms may not always follow a specific dermatomal pattern. In addition to pain, patients can also present with paresthesia and, less commonly, motor weakness in the affected extremity. These symptoms can frequently be exacerbated by specific head positions, such as the neck in extension with rotation toward the affected extremity (Spurling sign).

The clinician must also attempt to elicit any myelopathic symptoms. Frequently, the patient must be questioned specifically regarding myelopathic symptoms because he or she may not relate them to the presenting complaint. Patients should be questioned about changes in their handwriting, or difficulty with fine motor coordination of the fingers in the affected extremity. Asking a patient whether he or she has noticed any difficulty handling change or keys can often elicit a history of this symptom. Patients must also be questioned about any difficulty with walking or balance. A patient may have noted significant difficulty with balance but may not provide this information unless questioned because the presenting complaint is neck or arm pain.

Physical Examination

A complete and thorough neuromuscular examination should focus not only on the extremity from which the patient's symptoms and signs stem but also the asymptomatic extremity. This information provides a valuable comparison for all aspects of the examination. Moreover, neurologic findings may be normal in many patients with radicular pain.

The motor examination should focus on all muscle groups of the upper extremities. The examination should be performed sequentially, with specific comparisons with the asymptomatic extremity. Asymmetric motor weakness along with the specific location of sensory changes can help localize the level of the possible disease. Additionally, deep tendon reflexes should be tested and compared with the asymptomatic extremity. Specifically, the biceps, brachioradialis, and triceps reflexes should be tested. Changes in deep tendon reflexes with radiculopathy often show asymmetric decrease in deep tendon reflexes specific to the site of compression. Alternatively, a myelopathic patient may have hyperactive deep tendon reflexes, possibly accompanied by Hoffmann sign and sustained clonus. The presence of pathologic reflexes should raise the suspicion of an upper motor neuron lesion.

Imaging

Preoperative imaging is a crucial part of both the workup of a patient with radicular or myelopathic symptoms and for preoperative planning. Plain radiographs are typically the initial study of choice and should include standing anteroposterior and lateral radiographs, along with lateral flexion and extension films. These images are of limited value in evaluating possible neural compression, but they provide valuable information about overall spinal alignment, stability, and the presence of bony disease.

If advanced imaging is desired, then magnetic resonance imaging (MRI) is the modality of choice. Among other things, the MRI provides excellent imaging of the neural elements, surrounding soft tissue structures, the intervertebral disks, and the vertebral artery (Fig. 30-1). In the presence of stenosis, MRI allows for localization of the compressive structure and assessment for evidence of myelomalacia or spinal cord edema (Fig. 30-2). If the patient is unable to undergo MRI, or if assessment for bony compression is required, then computed tomography (CT) myelography is the next imaging modality of choice. This method provides good resolution of both neural elements and bony structures (Fig. 30-3).

Differential Diagnosis

Thorough history, physical examination, and imaging typically help determine whether the disorder is most likely cervical. However, a list of differential diagnoses should include, among other things, cervical radiculopathy, cervical myelopathy, brachial plexus injury, complex regional pain syndrome, thoracic outlet syndrome, inflammatory arthropathy, shoulder disease, peripheral nerve compression (cubital tunnel syndrome or carpal tunnel syndrome), multiple sclerosis, diabetic neuropathy, stroke, syringomyelia, Guillain-Barré syndrome, normal-pressure hydrocephalus, and spinal cord tumor. In selective cases, the use of electromyography and nerve conduction studies can also help to assist in determining the source of the disorder.

Nonoperative Management

An initial course of nonoperative management should be considered on initial presentation of a patient with cervical radiculopathy. The natural history in the majority of

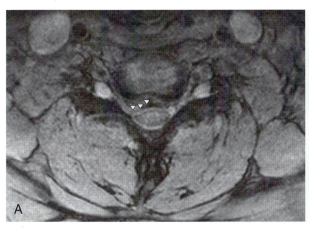
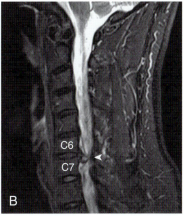

FIGURE 30-1 Axial (**A**) and parasagittal (**B**) T2-weighted magnetic resonance imaging demonstrating a large paracentral right-sided C6-7 herniated cervical disk (*arrowheads*).

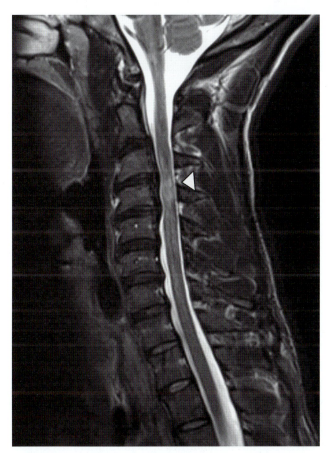

FIGURE 30-2 Sagittal T2-weighted magnetic resonance imaging demonstrated cervical stenosis with spinal cord signal change (*arrowhead*).

patients with cervical radiculopathy is spontaneous resolution, or at least significant improvement with nonoperative management. Nonoperative management should include physical therapy, antiinflammatory medications, judicious use of pain medications, and possibly epidural steroid injections.

Indications for Anterior Cervical Diskectomy and Fusion

A patient with a radiculopathy should be considered for surgical intervention if his or her symptoms fail to improve after a course of nonoperative management and if advanced imaging demonstrates neural compression in the neural foramen or the anterior spinal canal. In addition to patients who resist nonoperative management, surgery may also be considered for patients with progressive weakness or instability evident on dynamic imaging. Finally, patients with progressive myelopathic symptoms should be considered candidates for surgery. The location of the specific patient's disorder will determine whether the ACDF technique is appropriate or whether a posterior procedure would be more beneficial.

Contraindications to Anterior Cervical Diskectomy and Fusion

In the patient with anterior cervical disease and persistent or progressive symptoms localized to the level of the intervertebral disk, few absolute contraindications to ACDF exist. Certainly, in patients with lesions behind the vertebral body, or posterior compressive disorders, an ACDF procedure will not relieve the offending lesion. In these cases, anterior cervical corpectomy and/or a posterior cervical procedure, respectively, should be considered.

In addition, careful preoperative planning should be performed in a patient who has any known anatomic anomalies (specifically of the vertebral arteries) or a history of previous anterior cervical surgical procedures. Previous surgical treatments can lead to a much more difficult approach with less definitive anatomic planes or altered anatomy. Preoperative evaluation by an otolaryngologist using either direct or indirect laryngoscopy for assessment of the vocal cords for recurrent laryngeal nerve function should be considered preoperatively for an anterior approach in a revision ACDF procedure or in a patient who has had other anterior neck operations.

Other considerations include patients with multilevel cervical disease who may require four or more ACDF procedures and/or patients with ossification of the posterior longitudinal ligament (OPLL). In these patients, the increased risk of pseudarthroses and dural tears may make multilevel corpectomies or a posteriorly based surgical procedure, or both, more attractive alternatives.

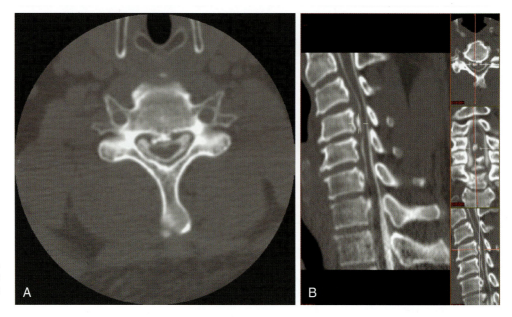

FIGURE 30-3 Axial (**A**) and para-sagittal (**B**) computed tomography scan demonstrating ossification of the posterior longitudinal ligament.

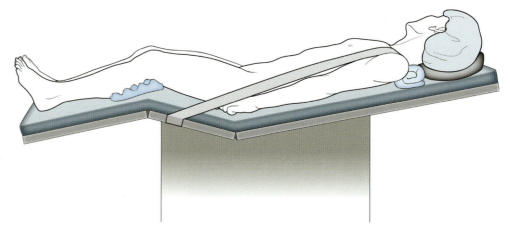

FIGURE 30-4 Supine positioning for anterior cervical diskectomy and fusion. The shoulders are taped with downward traction to ensure improved intraoperative imaging of the cervical spine. (From Miller MD, Chhabra AB, Hurwitz S, et al, editors: *Orthopaedic surgical approaches,* Philadelphia, 2008, Saunders, p 232.)

Surgical Technique

Anesthesia and Positioning

A patient undergoing an ACDF procedure should receive general anesthesia with endotracheal intubation administered by an anesthesiologist familiar with and comfortable with ACDF surgery. The endotracheal tube should be taped at the corner of the mouth opposite the side of the planned approach. The patient is typically positioned supine on a radiolucent operating table. A bump or gel roll is placed under the scapulae with the occiput on a foam or gel doughnut to prevent any sources of pressure. The cervical spine should be placed in extension, as tolerated on preoperative examination, with the head rotated away from the side of approach. Manipulation of the cervical spine should be done with extreme caution in patients with myelopathy because hyperextension of the cervical spine can exacerbate the disorder. The patient's arms should be tucked at the sides, and the shoulders should be taped with downward traction to ensure the best visualization and ability to obtain intraoperative imaging (Fig. 30-4).

Approach

The anterior approach to the cervical spine and relevant anatomic landmarks and anatomy are discussed in Chapter 3. Knowledge of these approaches is critical to providing adequate visualization of the appropriate level, as well as avoiding anatomic structures in the neck.

Surgical Anatomy

The anterior longitudinal ligament traverses the anterior surface of the vertebral bodies. The ligament widens as it travels caudally and is intimately associated with the intervertebral disks, as well as the vertebral end plates.

The posterior longitudinal ligament (PLL) is composed of a smooth dense group of fibers that runs along the posterior surface of the vertebral bodies within the spinal canal. OPLL or bulging of the PLL can lead to spinal canal stenosis and spinal cord compression. The PLL is thicker centrally and thins as it spreads laterally to its attachments to the uncinate processes.

Intervertebral disks are composed of an outer annulus fibrosis and an inner gelatinous nucleus pulposus. The disks are intimately attached to the subchondral bone

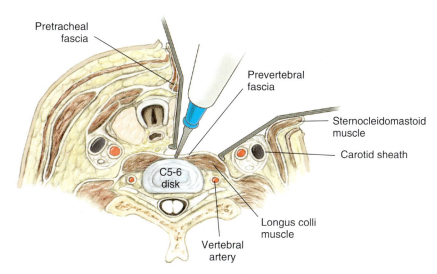

Pretracheal fascia

Prevertebral fascia

Sternocleidomastoid muscle

Carotid sheath

C5-6 disk

Longus colli muscle

Vertebral artery

FIGURE 30-5 Handheld retractors are placed during the exposure. The sternocleidomastoid muscle and the carotid sheath are retracted laterally, whereas the tracheoesophageal structures and strap muscles are retracted medially. The prevertebral fascia overlying the anterior vertebral body is exposed and divided. (From Miller MD, Chhabra AB, Hurwitz S, et al, editors: *Orthopaedic surgical approaches*, Philadelphia, 2008, Saunders, p 239.)

of both the superior and inferior vertebral bodies. The intervertebral disks are, however, not attached to the outermost cortical rim of the end plates, and this configuration provides an area where osteophytic spurs may more readily form.

The uncovertebral joints are important bony landmarks during an ACDF operation and provide the lateral border of the "safe zone" during the procedure. The surgeon must always remain oriented to the location of the uncinate process. This is also a location where spurs commonly arise, thus leading to impingement of the exiting nerve roots where they enter the foramen.

The vertebral arteries may be intimately opposed to, and run along, the medial aspect of the uncinate process. Care must be taken to avoid injury to the vertebral arteries. In addition, the preoperative imaging should be examined carefully for recognition of any aberrant course of the vertebral arteries.

During decompression, care must also be taken to avoid injury to the cervical spinal nerve roots. The nerve roots are divided into the dorsal and ventral roots. The ventral root is located just dorsal to the uncovertebral joint, whereas the dorsal root is just ventral to the superior articular facet. The nerve roots leave the spinal cord, and canal, at roughly a 45-degree angle ventrolaterally. This is very important when performing osteophyte resection from the uncovertebral joint. The surgeon must hug the posterior aspect of the uncinate process during foraminotomy.

Surgical Steps of Anterior Cervical Diskectomy and Fusion

Various methods are available for ACDF. The authors prefer using the Smith-Robinson technique, which is described here.

Once the approach to the anterior cervical spine is completed, the correct intervertebral level must be identified. This can be done by palpation of anterior osteophytes that have been identified on careful examination of the preoperative imaging. Although this method is possible, current recommendations from the North American Spine Society suggest using intraoperative imaging to verify the level.[1-4] The use of specially designed cervical

markers or a spinal needle can enable the surgeon to achieve this goal. The authors prefer using a spinal needle with two 90-degree angles placed in it. Shaping the spinal needle in this fashion prevents plunging of the needle, which can have disastrous effects. Care should be taken to identify the correct level as accurately as possible before insertion of a needle into the intervertebral disk because studies have shown that disk levels that are marked with a needle are three times as likely to develop degenerative changes in the future.[4]

Once the correct level is identified and confirmed, the prevertebral fascia over the anterior vertebral body is divided (Fig. 30-5). This technique allows visualization of the longus colli muscles. These muscles should be elevated medially to laterally using blunt dissection. Care should be taken to make sure that the self-retaining retractors are placed deep to the longus colli muscle to maintain the exposure. Placement superficial to the longus colli muscle places the sympathetic chain at risk and may lead to development of Horner syndrome postoperatively (Fig. 30-6).

After the vertebral body and disk are completely exposed, the anterior lip of the inferior end plate of the superior vertebral body should be removed using a high-speed burr, rongeur, or Kerrison rongeur. Removal of this lip allows the surgeon a direct line of sight into the posterior disk space during diskectomy and permits proper visualization for foraminotomy and PLL resection should they be desired. Additionally, this technique allows optimal placement and fit of the graft.

Next, the diskectomy should be performed. The anterior longitudinal ligament and the anterior portion of the annulus should be incised with a number 15 scalpel blade (Fig. 30-7). The blade should be held such that it never faces the carotid artery during insertion or removal from the wound. Following incision of the annulus, the superficial portion of the disk is removed using a pituitary rongeur. No instrument should ever be forced into the disk space if it does not enter it easily. Disk material and cartilaginous end plates should then be removed using a combination of small straight and angle curets. During diskectomy, it is extremely important to identify the orientation of the uncinate process, which defines the lateral border of the safe zone. If a curet (or other instrument) is placed lateral to this border, the risk of vertebral artery laceration is greatly increased.

Distraction pins or intervertebral spreaders may then be placed to facilitate removal of the posterior half of the disk. This method allows for greater disk space mobilization. If intervertebral spreaders are used, they should be placed laterally against the uncus. If distraction pins are used, they should be located within the vertebral bodies with placement in the superior vertebral body slightly superior to the middle of the vertebral body to facilitate

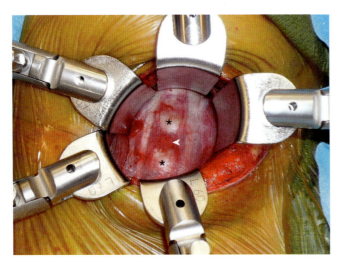

FIGURE 30-6 Intraoperative photograph demonstrating the approach to the anterior cervical spine. The longus colli muscles have been elevated bilaterally, and the retractors are placed deep to the longus colli. The intervertebral disk (*asterisks*) and the vertebral bodies (*arrowhead*) are noted as the "hills and valleys," respectively. (Modified from Miller MD, Chhabra AB, Hurwitz S, et al, editors: *Orthopaedic surgical approaches*, Philadelphia, 2008, Saunders, p 239.)

preparation of the end plate. Frequently, the inferior end plate of the superior vertebral body requires more preparation as a result of its concave shape. Excessively intervertebral disk space distraction and placement of too large a graft should be avoided because of the risk for postoperative neck pain secondary to facet impingement. If the patient has significant spinal cord compression, distraction should not be applied until after compression is relieved, to avoid further tenting of the spinal cord over the area of compression.

A combination of pituitary rongeur and small curets should be used to remove the remainder of disk material. All cartilaginous material should be removed from the end plates. The surgeon should maintain a working angle parallel to the disk space. The final result of a completed diskectomy should allow visualization of the bony end plates, PLL, and uncinate processes.

Once visualized, the PLL should be inspected for any defects through which disk material may have extruded. The presence of a sequestered disk fragment is an indication for PLL resection. When PLL resection is indicated, the PLL should be inspected with a nerve hook or a microcuret to identify any tears within the PLL. Once a tear or plane is identified within the PLL, a 2-mm Kerrison rongeur should be used to create a window in the PLL that is large enough to visualize the dura and remove any free disk fragments from the spinal canal. Whether PLL resection is beneficial in every case is debatable. Resection of the PLL on the side of compression is frequently done, especially if disk extrusion is present. Alternatively, if no sequestered disk fragments are present, adequate decompression can most likely be achieved without removing the PLL.

Although controversial, anterior foraminotomy may be necessary in selected cases. Frequently, appropriate neuroforaminal height can be achieved through indirect

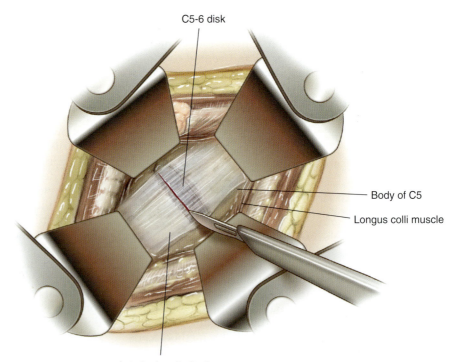

C5-6 disk

Body of C5

Longus colli muscle

Anterior longitudinal ligament

FIGURE 30-7 Annulotomy is performed with a number 15 scalpel blade, and diskectomy is performed in standard fashion. (From Miller MD, Chhabra AB, Hurwitz S, et al, editors: *Orthopaedic surgical approaches*, Philadelphia, 2008, Saunders, p 241.)

distraction with restoration of the intervertebral disk height (Fig. 30-8). As mentioned earlier, care should be taken not to overdistract the disk space. Graft size can be accurately estimated from preoperative lateral radiographs, with the graft height being 2 or 3 mm greater than the height of the diseased disk space. In addition, the height of the intervertebral disk space of the adjacent superior and inferior level can help as well, although in many patients these levels can be degenerative and collapsed as well.[5] If foraminotomy is considered, performing it before PLL resection may provide some protection of the neural elements.

Once diskectomy is completed, the posterior uncinate can be directly visualized. Foraminotomy is more easily performed with the surgeon standing on the contralateral to the symptomatic side, to allow for better visualization and reach toward the area of work. The medial portion of the uncinate can be thinned using a high-speed burr. The liberal use of irrigation when using a burr decreases the likelihood of thermal injury to any neural elements. Following thinning of the uncinate, a 1- or 2-mm Kerrison rongeur should easily fit into the foramen. The Kerrison rongeur and microcurets can then be used to remove any remaining osteophytes and decompress the foramen laterally. It is very important during foraminotomy to remember the trajectory of the exiting nerve root. An instrument should never blindly be placed into the foramen. Additionally, it is critical that the surgeon keep all instruments firmly up against the uncinate process while working within the foramen. Foraminotomy is considered complete when a nerve hook can be freely passed into the foramen anterior to the exiting nerve root.

At this point, it is necessary to prepare the end plates adequately. Again, the inferior end plate of the superior vertebral body usually has a concave shape, which requires greater preparation. The superior end plate of the inferior vertebral body tends to be flatter and requires less work. At both end plates, it is important not to remove too much end plate, which can weaken the cortex and predispose the graft to subside. The end plates can be prepared using a combination of high-speed burr and curets. The resulting space should be rectangular to provide maximal bony contact with the graft. The height of the rectangle should approximately match the largest height of the intervertebral space, which is usually seen at the center of the disk

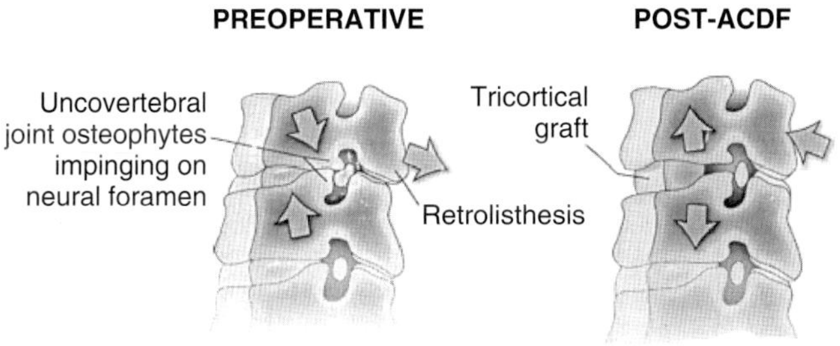

space. End plates should be decorticated to reveal bleeding bone, to maximize the likelihood of successful fusion.

The graft size must then be determined. Graft size can often be accurately estimated from preoperative lateral radiographs, with the graft height 2 or 3 mm greater than the height of the diseased disk space and the depth of the graft 2 to 3 mm less that the disk space. Graft height should ultimately be determined intraoperatively by using commercially available sizers. Sizers should be gently tamped into place using a mallet with the disk space under gentle distraction. A trial should fit snugly while disk space is distracted. If one size trial is too large but the next size down is too small, slight additional decortication should be performed to allow the larger size to be placed comfortably. Once size is determined, the graft can be placed. The authors prefer the use of commercially prepared cortical allograft, but tricortical autograft can be obtained from the iliac crest as well.

The graft should be placed with the disk space slightly distracted. Care should be taken to remove any anterior osteophytes, and the graft should be tamped to 2 mm posterior to the anterior edge of the end plates and should sit approximately 4 mm anterior to the dura to prevent impingement of the spinal canal. At this point, distraction should be released. Stability of the graft should then be tested using a right-angled probe.

Although a single-level ACDF procedure can be performed without instrumentation, the authors prefer the use of a plate on the anterior vertebral body surface. The plate provides additional stability and decreases motion during the period before development of a solid fusion mass. In addition, the plate prevents anterior translation of the graft postoperatively. Plate size should be determined after graft placement. The plate must be long enough to allow for screw placement in both the superior and inferior vertebral bodies, but not so long that it causes impingement of adjacent disk spaces. Too long a plate can quickly lead to adjacent-level disease.

Plates come in a variety of designs, each with benefits and drawbacks. Plate selection largely depends on the surgeon's preference, experience, and comfort level and is beyond the scope of this chapter. Once the proper plate has been selected, the plate should be contoured to match the natural lordosis of the cervical spine. The plate should be positioned so that it is centered on the disk space in both the inferosuperior plane and the coronal plane. Screws should then be placed, angled laterally to medially to reduce the risk of vertebral artery injury. Most vertebral bodies can accommodate 14- to 16-mm screws. Screw position and length should be selected such that screws do not violate the adjacent disk spaces.

See Video 30-1.

Multilevel Anterior Cervical Diskectomy and Fusion

Multilevel ACDF procedures are frequently performed. If a multilevel ACDF procedure is planned, each disk space should be decompressed, and the graft should be placed sequentially. If it is not performed sequentially, an imbalance of the grafts and disk spaces frequently results. Moreover, ACDF procedure of up to three levels may be performed safely without instrumentation; however, the

PREOPERATIVE   **POST-ACDF**

Uncovertebral joint osteophytes impinging on neural foramen

Tricortical graft

Retrolisthesis

FIGURE 30-8 Uncovertebral decompression can be performed either directly or indirectly. During indirect decompression, the neuroforaminal height can be restored through vertebral realignment and neuroforaminal distraction. (From Shen FH, Samartzis D, Khanna N, et al. Comparison of clinical and radiographic outcome in instrumented anterior cervical discectomy and fusion with or without direct uncovertebral joint decompression. *Spine J* 4: 629-635, 2004.)

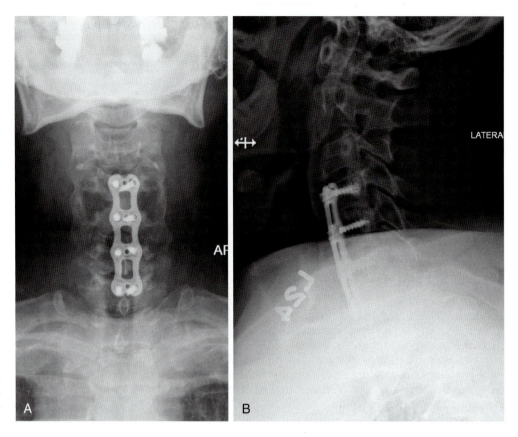

FIGURE 30-9 Anteroposterior (**A**) and lateral (**B**) postoperative radiographs of instrumented multilevel anterior cervical diskectomy and fusion.

authors strongly recommend the use of plating for all multilevel ACDF surgical procedures (Fig. 30-9).

Postoperative Care

Postoperative bracing using a cervical collar is widely debated among spine surgeons. Many surgeons routinely use a cervical collar for 4 to 6 weeks postoperatively. If plating is not used, a cervical collar for this period is strongly recommended. The authors use plates in almost all our ACDF procedures and do not routinely use a cervical collar. The authors believe that, when using a plate, the construct provides adequate stability that the morbidities associated with cervical collars are not warranted.

The authors also routinely leave a drain in place at the end of the surgical procedure. The drain is placed in the retropharyngeal space to prevent postoperative hematoma formation. In most cases, the drain is removed the morning after the surgical procedure.

The patient's diet may be advanced postoperatively as tolerated. Most patients experience some degree of dysphagia following ACDF, and this should be used as a guide for the rate of diet advancement. Some surgeons advocate cold drinks and ice cream in the immediate postoperative period because they believe that this regimen may reduce swelling and limit the degree of dysphagia.[6]

Complications

As stated earlier, almost all patients experience some degree of dysphagia following ACDF. In most patients, the degree of dysphagia is not clinically significant and improves within 3 week postoperatively. Chronic dysphagia is uncommon, occurring in approximately 4% of patients.[6]

Dysphonia is noted in some patients postoperatively. In most patients, this is also caused by postsurgical swelling and quickly resolves; in some patients, however, the surgeon should consider the possibility of nerve injury. The superior laryngeal nerve innervates the cricothyroid muscle and provides supraglottic sensation. Injury to the superior laryngeal nerve can lead to aspiration, along with difficulty with high pitches.[6-9] The recurrent laryngeal nerve innervates the muscles that abduct the vocal cords. Injury to the recurrent laryngeal nerve often manifests as hoarseness and can lead to airway obstruction.[7-9]

If autograft is used from the iliac crest, patients can experience morbidity at this site. This includes long-term pain at the site of harvest, as well as injury to the femoral cutaneous nerve.[9-12]

If a drain is not placed during closure, patients may develop a postoperative hematoma. If the hematoma becomes clinically significant, some patients will require reexploration and hematoma evacuation.

Pseudarthrosis is a frequently discussed complication in all of spine surgery. Most cervical pseudarthroses are asymptomatic and therefore do not require additional intervention. If pseudarthrosis is determined to be the source of recurrent or unrelieved symptoms, it may be treated with a revision ACDF procedure or with posterior cervical spine fusion.[8,13,14]

Adjacent segment disease is believed to be a result of increased mechanical strain placed on adjacent intervertebral disks following diskectomy and fusion. Approximately 3% of patients will develop adjacent segment disease.

Esophageal injuries are rare but result in a significantly increased infection risk, as well as a prolonged postoperative course.

Spinal cord injury and nerve root injury are the most feared complications of ACDF. Once neural injury occurs, it is likely permanent, and very little can be done to salvage nerve function reliably. If neuromonitoring is used intraoperatively, stopping any current surgical activity and returning all structures to their resting positions should immediately address any changes in signals. Spinal cord injury and nerve root injury can be devastating and should be avoided at all costs.

Results

Numerous studies have demonstrated that more than 90% of patients experience relief of symptoms following ACDF when radiculopathy is the preoperative diagnosis.[15-20] Myelopathic patients also are reported to have excellent results, although the response to decompression may depend more on the duration of compression than it does in radiculopathy.[1,17] In the case of axial neck pain, results are more variable, and this pain should not be the primary indication for performing ACDF. Patients should be informed preoperatively that the main goal of ACDF is to improve radicular or myelopathic symptoms, not axial neck pain. Isolated axial neck pain does not reliably improve following ACDF and thus is not frequently used alone as a surgical indication.

Conclusions

In summary, the ACDF procedure is a common surgical procedure performed for treatment of cervical radiculopathy and cervical myelopathy. It is indicated for surgical treatment of degenerative changes of the cervical spine resulting in central or foraminal stenosis. The ACDF procedure is not a reliable treatment for axial neck pain from degenerative disk disease, but it has been shown to provide reliable decompression of the neuroforamen and spinal canal in patients with anterior cervical disease.

Proper surgical technique is important when performing ACDF. The correct intervertebral level should be confirmed using fluoroscopy before proceeding with decompression. Care should be taken in removing an appropriate amount of the end plates for sufficient visualization during decompression; however, excess bone removal should be avoided, to prevent graft settling. Extreme caution should be taken during foraminotomy to avoid injury to both the exiting nerve root and the vertebral artery. Finally, plate selection should be correct because anterior plating has been shown to increase stability of the construct and may increase fusion rates, especially in multilevel ACDF.

REFERENCES

1. Silber JS, Albert TJ: Anterior approaches for the surgical treatment of multilevel cervical spondylotic myelopathy, *Curr Opin Orthop* 12:231–237, 2001.
2. Palit M, Schofferman J, Goldthwaite N, et al.: Anterior discectomy and fusion for the management of neck pain, *Spine (Phila Pa 1976)* 24:2224–2228, 1999.
3. Brigham CD, Tsahakis PJ: Anterior cervical foraminotomy and fusions: surgical techniques and results, *Spine (Phila Pa 1976)* 20:766, 1995.
4. Macnab I: Complications of anterior cervical fusion, *Orthop Rev* 1:29, 1972.
5. Shen FH, Samartzis D, Khanna N, et al.: Comparison of clinical and radiographic outcome in instrumented anterior cervical discectomy and fusion with or without direct uncovertebral joint decompression, *Spine J* 4:629–635, 2004.
6. Frempong-Boadu A, Houten JK, Osborn B, et al.: Swallowing and speech dysfunction in patients undergoing anterior cervical discectomy and fusion, *J Spinal Disord Tech* 15:362, 2002.
7. Dimopolous VG, Chung I, Lee GP, et al.: Quantitative estimation of recurrent laryngeal nerve irritation by employing spontaneous intraoperative electromyographic monitoring during anterior discectomy and fusion, *J Spinal Disord Tech* 22:1–9, 2009.
8. Samartzis D, Shen FH, Matthews DK, et al.: Comparison of allograft to autograft in multilevel anterior cervical discectomy and fusion with rigid plate fixation, *Spine J* 3:451–459, 2003.
9. Haller JM, Iwanik M, Shen FH: Clinically relevant anatomy of recurrent laryngeal nerve, *Spine (Phila Pa 1976)* 37:97–100, 2012.
10. Haller JM, Iwanik M, Shen FH: Clinically relevant anatomy of high anterior cervical approach, *Spine (Phila Pa 1976)* 36: 2116–2121, 2011.
11. Samartzis D, Shen FH: What's your call? Postoperative iliac-crest avulsion fracture, *CMAJ* 29(175):475–476, 2006.
12. Shen FH, Samartzis D, An HS: Cell technologies for spinal fusion, *Spine J* 5(Suppl):231S–239S, 2005.
13. Samartzis D, Shen FH, Goldberg EJ, et al.: Is autograft the gold standard in achieving radiographic fusion in one-level anterior cervical discectomy and fusion with rigid anterior plate fixation? *Spine (Phila Pa 1976)* 30:1756–1761, 2005.
14. Samartzis D, Shen FH, Lyon C, et al.: Does rigid instrumentation increase the fusion rate in one-level anterior cervical discectomy and fusion? *Spine J* 4:636–643, 2004.
15. Smith GW, Robinson RA: The treatment of certain cervical spine disorders by anterior removal of the intervertebral disc and interbody fusion, *J Bone Joint Surg Am* 40:607, 1958.
16. Bohlman HH, Emery SE, Goodfellow DB, Jones PK: Robinson anterior cervical discectomy and arthrodesis for cervical radiculopathy: long-term follow-up of one hundred and twenty-two patients, *J Bone Joint Surg Am* 75:1298–1307, 1993.
17. Chin KR, Ozuna R: Options in the surgical treatment of cervical spondylotic myelopathy, *Curr Opin Orthop* 11:151–157, 2000.
18. Xie J, Hurlburt RJ: Discectomy versus discectomy with fusion versus discectomy with fusion and instrumentation: a prospective randomized study, *Neurosurgery* 61:107–117, 2007.
19. Kiefapfel H, Koller M, Hinder D, et al.: Integrated outcome assessment after anterior cervical discectomy and fusion, *Spine (Phila Pa 1976)* 29:2501–2509, 2004.
20. Robinson RA, Smith GW: Anterolateral cervical disc removal and interbody fusion for cervical disc syndrome, *Bull Johns Hopkins Hosp* 96:223, 1955.

31

Anterior Cervical Corpectomy and Fusion and Hybrid Techniques

Rahul Basho and Jeffrey C. Wang

CHAPTER PREVIEW

Chapter Synopsis

Surgical decompression of the neural elements is of paramount importance in all spinal procedures, especially those of cervical myelopathy. Neural compression at the level of the disk space can be addressed by performing anterior cervical diskectomy and fusion. When the compression occurs posterior to the disk spaces, corpectomy is typically necessary. Multilevel corpectomies can result in mechanical instability, and therefore posterior stabilization is required. A novel hybrid technique that consists of a combination of corpectomies with diskectomies has been used to avoid the morbidity associated with posterior stabilization. The goal of this chapter is to provide a detailed description of this novel technique and the standard corpectomy, indications for these procedures, and perioperative concerns.

Important Points

A detailed history and physical examination should be performed and correlated with radiographs and advanced imaging studies to identify myelopathic patients.

Indications for these techniques include symptomatic myelopathy with multilevel spinal cord compression posterior to the vertebral bodies.

Contraindications include posterior compressive disease in patients with lordotic cervical alignment.

Magnetic resonance imaging (MRI) is the advanced imaging modality of choice. It allows visualization of spinal cord signal change seen in myelopathic patients. Computed tomography myelogram is an option for patients who cannot undergo MRI; it may also provide additional information about osteophytes and ossification of the posterior longitudinal ligament (OPLL).

Clinical and Surgical Pearls

Preoperative imaging should be carefully studied for anatomic variations, such as an anomalous course of the vertebral artery.

The uncinate processes should be clearly defined during exposure because this allows the surgeon to define the midpoint of the vertebral body. Straying off center can result in an eccentric corpectomy.

Preoperative planning should include evaluation of the width of the vertebral body and knowledge of available cage sizes.

Clinical and Surgical Pitfalls

OPLL should be identified preoperatively to minimize the likelihood of a dural tear during the corpectomy.

Neural compression posterior to the vertebral body cannot be addressed by cervical diskectomy.

Inadequate or incomplete decompression should be avoided, regardless of the surgical approach selected.

The anterior approach to the cervical spine is used to address neural compression resulting from tumor, infection, trauma, or degenerative disease. Addressing ventral compression of the spinal cord from behind the vertebral body typically requires corpectomy.[1] A thorough history and physical examination are always necessary; however, their importance cannot be underscored enough in patients with cervical myelopathy. Subtle findings of declining manual dexterity and balance difficulty should be screened for during both history taking and examination because the presence of myelopathy can dramatically alter treatment. These findings should be correlated with advanced imaging studies, of which magnetic resonance imaging (MRI) remains the gold standard. In patients in whom MRI is contraindicated, a computed tomography (CT) myelogram should be ordered. In addition to visualizing the neural elements, CT myelograms allow a more detailed evaluation of bony anatomy and spondylosis in the cervical spine.

Alleviating the compressive lesions from the spinal cord is of paramount importance in cervical myelopathy. When these lesions occur posterior to the disk spaces, simply performing anterior cervical diskectomy and fusion (ACDF) at the diseased levels is sufficient. However, when these lesions occur posterior to the vertebral body, corpectomy is necessary. Multilevel corpectomies can result in iatrogenic instability within the cervical spine and therefore have historically required supplemental posterior fixation. In selected cases, a hybrid technique that combines diskectomies with multilevel corpectomies can be performed to avoid the morbidity of posterior fixation.[2] The goal of this chapter is to provide a detailed account of the surgical techniques and perioperative considerations for both anterior cervical corpectomy and hybrid techniques.

Preoperative Considerations

The classic signs and symptoms of cervical myelopathy should be elicited when obtaining a detailed patient history. Neck and arm pain may be present, but myelopathic patients with minimal to no pain may also be encountered. Typical symptoms include numbness and tingling in the hands or arms, decreased strength, diminished dexterity and coordination, and balance difficulty. Questions should center on tasks that require fine motor movements; patients will report difficulty buttoning buttons and picking up coins off the floor, and their handwriting may worsen.[1]

Certain physical examination findings are indicative of cervical myelopathy and should be routinely evaluated. Flexion-extension radiographs of the neck may reproduce pain or electric shocks down the arms and back (Lhermitte sign). Strength and light touch in the upper extremities may or may not be normal. However, a careful monofilament examination of the palmar digits can reveal subtle impairment. Other physical examination findings suggestive of upper motor neuron disease include hyperreflexia, inverted radial reflex, Hoffmann sign, clonus, and Babinski sign. Tandem gait evaluation should be performed to assess coordination and balance.[3]

Imaging studies should consist of anteroposterior, lateral, flexion, and extension views of the cervical spine (Fig. 31-1). Sagittal and coronal alignment, as well as any dynamic instability, should be noted. MRI studies allow evaluation of the disks, spinal cord, nerve roots, and ligamentous structures. Compression of the spinal cord can lead to edema within the substance of the spinal cord itself that manifests as a hyperintense signal on T2-weighted images. In addition to the substance of the spinal cord, the vertebral arteries should be carefully evaluated on the MRI images. The vertebral artery most commonly enters the foramen transversarium at C6, but variability exists. Even when the vertebral artery resides within the foramen, it may take a medial course into the vertebral body; serious consequences can result if this is not identified preoperatively, and corpectomy is performed at that level.[4,5]

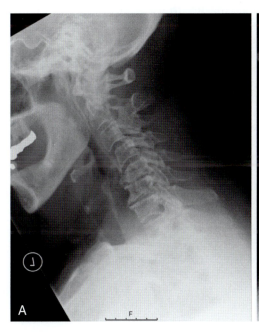
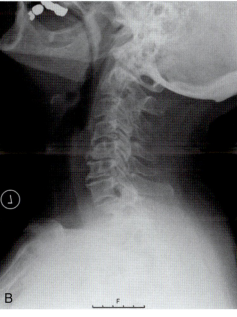

FIGURE 31-1 Preoperative flexion (**A**) and extension (**B**) radiographs show multilevel spondylosis from C3 to C7. The extension view shows that the patient's alignment does correct into lordosis.

MRI remains the imaging modality of choice; additional information can be gleaned from a CT scan with or without a myelogram. A more detailed depiction of the bony anatomy can be appreciated, and in revision procedures, previous fusions can be assessed. Regardless of the imaging modality selected, the surgeon must be able to extrapolate a three-dimensional understanding of the neural compression from two-dimensional images. This understanding allows the surgeon to determine whether diskectomy, corpectomy, or a hybrid approach is appropriate.

Surgical Considerations

Adequate decompression can be achieved from either an anterior or a posterior approach, depending on the patient's alignment and direction of compression.[6] Kyphosis that does not correct in extension typically requires an anterior approach. In the kyphotic spine, performing posterior decompression for anterior compressive disease does not allow posterior migration of the spinal cord. The patient will continue to be symptomatic from the neural compression postoperatively.

Neural compression that occurs posterior to the disk spaces can be easily addressed with ACDF. Compression that occurs posterior to the disk spaces may require corpectomy. Extruded disk fragments located posterior to the vertebral body, but near the disk space, can sometimes be removed with a ball-tipped micro-nerve hook. However, if the extruded fragment cannot be removed in this manner, corpectomy becomes necessary. In the setting of ossification of the posterior longitudinal ligament, less ambiguity exists. Compression posterior to the vertebral bodies requires corpectomy to be addressed anteriorly. For multilevel ACDF procedures, corpectomy can reduce the number of healing surfaces and can potentially improve fusion rates.[7] Multiple corpectomies, however, can destabilize the spine because of the long lever arms involved. Patients in whom such constructs are contemplated should be considered for a hybrid construct. In this construct, segmental fixation is placed within the intervening retained vertebral bodies to increase construct stability and preclude the need for posterior fixation.

A previous anterior surgical procedure is a relative contraindication to a secondary anterior procedure. Performing the approach through the contralateral side allows the surgeon to avoid scar and work through native tissue planes. However, the competence of the recurrent laryngeal nerve and vocal cords must be assessed preoperatively by direct or indirect laryngoscopy. Injury to the recurrent laryngeal nerve on the previously operated side should dissuade one from approaching the cervical spine from the contralateral side because this may lead to bilateral vocal cord paralysis.

Surgical Technique

Anesthesia and Positioning

During the patient's initial visit, the surgeon should assess for reproduction of symptoms with extension of the neck.

Although extension can assist with exposure and visualization, the degree of stenosis may limit the amount of extension the patient can tolerate. In these situations, a neutral neck position must be maintained until the decompression is completed.

Standard positioning involves placing a roll between the shoulder blades to allow for extension of the neck. The shoulders are taped inferiorly to aid in radiographic visualization of the lower cervical segments. The head may also be taped in position to prevent any rotation during the surgical procedure. A marking pen should be used to demarcate the sternal notch, a useful landmark for the midline. Drapes should encompass as wide a field as possible, to give the surgeon a better understanding of the patient's overall positioning and alignment.

Neuromonitoring protocols depend on the patient, surgeon, and institution and should be individualized accordingly. The authors' preference is to use both motor-evoked potentials (MEPs) and somatosensory-evoked potentials (SSEPs) during surgical procedures. Communication with the anesthesia team is paramount because inhaled agents and paralytic drugs must be avoided. After prepositioning baseline values are obtained, the patient's head and neck are extended, and the shoulders are taped inferiorly. MEPs and SSEPs are then retested to ensure no deviation from baseline.[8,9]

Surgical Landmarks and Incisions

Palpation of the patient's cervical spine can reveal anatomic landmarks that assist in localization of the incision: the hyoid bone located at C3, the thyroid cartilage at C4 to C5, and the cricoid cartilage at C6. The authors' preference is to mark the skin, under fluoroscopic guidance, to ensure ideal placement of the incision. A transverse incision is typically used and is placed within a skin crease to give a favorable cosmetic result. A well-positioned transverse skin incision in a thin patient can give access to four disk spaces within the cervical spine.

Approach and Exposure

It is the authors' practice to use a left-sided approach to the cervical spine because of the more consistent course of the recurrent laryngeal nerve. Careful development of the tissue planes above and below the platysma greatly assists in soft tissue mobilization and exposure. The esophagus and trachea are retracted medially and the carotid sheath and its contents laterally. The prevertebral fascia is then encountered, with the longus colli muscles on either side laterally. The fascia is split in a longitudinal fashion, to expose the anterior longitudinal ligament. A metallic marker is used to confirm the correct level, and then electrocautery is used to expose the central portion of the vertebral bodies. The exposure is taken out laterally to the level of the uncinates bilaterally. Bleeding may be encountered from the undersurface of the longus colli as the exposure is taken out laterally. This bleeding can be controlled with a procoagulant agent and surgical patties. Extensive osteophyte formation may be encountered and can obscure the disk spaces and uncinate joints; these osteophytes can be removed with a rongeur. Self-retaining retractors are then placed with the blades under the longus colli.

Corpectomy

The exposure should clearly reveal the disk spaces above and below the vertebral body of interest. Complete diskectomies are performed above and below this vertebra by using a combination of curets, Kerrison rongeurs, and a high-speed burr. Caspar distraction pins are typically used to facilitate the decompression. Once both diskectomies have been performed, a high-speed burr is used to make two longitudinal troughs in line with the uncinate joints two thirds of the way through the vertebral body. The central bone between the troughs is removed with a rongeur and is saved. The high-speed burr is then used to thin the posterior wall of the vertebral body until it is transparent. The posterior longitudinal ligament is released at the disk spaces above and below the vertebral body of interest. The intervening ligament is then lifted and removed en bloc, thus completing the corpectomy and decompression.

Corpectomy Reconstruction

Reconstruction of the corpectomy defect can be performed with either an artificial cage or an allograft strut. Polyetheretherketone (PEEK) and metallic cages are commonly used artificial options (Fig. 31-2). PEEK cages have the advantage of being radiolucent and therefore allowing visualization of the fusion mass on radiographs and CT scans. Metallic cages range from the classic Harm cage to expandable options. Regardless of which cage is selected, it must be carefully sized and appropriately positioned to optimize the chance of solid fusion. An anterior cervical plate is then applied to add stability to the construct and to reduce the risk of cage migration.

Hybrid Constructs

When performing a hybrid construct consisting of ACDF adjacent to corpectomy, the authors perform ACDF first. Once the diskectomy and decompression are performed, the appropriately sized graft is selected. Multiple options are available, including allograft, tricortical autograft, and PEEK. The authors do not use autograft because of donor site morbidity and prefer PEEK cages filled with demineralized bone matrix. After placement of the cage, the corpectomy is performed in the aforementioned manner. Table 31-1 shows literature review results of the aforementioned constructs.

Considerations for Supplemental Posterior Instrumentation and Fusion

The addition of supplemental posterior fixation is the final point that must be considered when performing multilevel anterior decompressions and fusions. The authors' standard practice is to perform supplemental posterior fixation when more than three levels are addressed anteriorly. Regardless of the number of levels involved, poor bone quality or tenuous anterior fixation should be supplemented posteriorly. A construct consisting of lateral mass screws with connecting rods is used. Allograft bone is placed over the decorticated lamina and, because of the large surface area available for healing, typically results in excellent fusion rates. Lateral mass screws are inserted from C3 through C7; if the C7 lateral mass is too diminutive, the construct is extended to T1, where the pedicles are large enough to accept screws easily.

Postoperative Considerations

Postoperatively, patients are typically admitted to a monitored hospital floor with 24-hour observation to mitigate the risk of postoperative swelling that may result in airway compromise. If the operation lasted more than 5 hours or if excessive bleeding is encountered, the authors' standard practice is to keep the patient intubated overnight. Patients are kept in a cervical collar for 4 weeks postoperatively and are then weaned from the collar as they begin physical therapy. Prolonged use of the cervical collar may

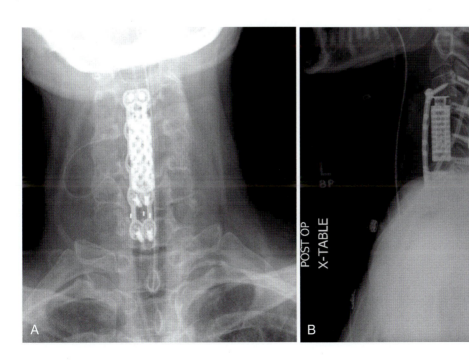

FIGURE 31-2 A and **B**, Complete C4 and C5 corpectomies, metallic cage placement, and supplemental posterior fixation was performed in this patient. Note the hybrid construct anteriorly with polyetheretherketone cage placement at the C6-C7 interspace. Because of the number of levels involved, posterior fixation was necessary despite the use of a hybrid construct anteriorly.

Table 31-1 Cervical Corpectomy Outcomes

Authors, Year	Number of Patients	Procedure	Mean Patient Age in Year (Range)	Mean Follow-up (Range)	Fusion Rate (%)	Results
Yan et al, 2011[10]	75	Cervical corpectomy with cage-plate reconstruction	73 (67-79)	28 mo (24-32 mo)	100	JOA and VAS scores improved in all patients, 8.6 to 15.3 and 7.2 to 1.5, respectively
Sevki et al, 2004[11]	26	Cervical corpectomy with cage-plate reconstruction	64.9 (55-74)	2.8 yr (6 mo-5 yr)	100	Nurick and JOA scores improved, 3.5 to 2 and 7 to 11, respectively
Wei-bing et al, 2009[2]	20	Hybrid fusion corpectomy with cage-plate and stand-alone ACDF	58.75 (48-68)	20 mo (18-24 mo)	100	JOA improved from 12.55 to 15.45
Oh et al, 2009[12]	17	One-level corpectomy with cage-plate reconstruction	55.12 (28-77)	27.33 mo (12-63 mo)	100	JOA and arm VAS scores improved, 13.38 to 14.72 and 5.63 to 2.63, respectively: no improvement noted in neck VAS, 3.69 to 3.63
Ikenaga et al, 2006[13]	31	Four-level corpectomy with autograft fibular strut using Shikata grafting technique[14]	60 (29-77)	10-14 yr (mean not specified, range 10-14 yr)	91	JOA scores improved from 10.9 to 14.0; no significant complications but 10% rate of graft site pain

ACDF, Anterior cervical diskectomy and fusion; *JOA,* Japanese Orthopaedic Association; *VAS,* Visual Analog Scale

be necessary in patients with poor bone quality, but it can result in atrophy of the cervical paraspinal musculature. Patients are followed up radiographically at 2 weeks and then at 6 weeks with anteroposterior and lateral radiographs. Flexion and extension radiographs are obtained at 3 months, 6 months, and 1 year postoperatively.

Complications

The risks and potential complications from multilevel anterior surgeries are significant and must be discussed in detail with patients preoperatively. The most commonly encountered complications are those inherent in the anterior approach. Injury to the esophagus, vertebral arteries, recurrent and superior laryngeal nerves, and spinal cord all can occur.[2,11-14] Prolonged operative times with excessive retraction can cause immediate postoperative complications such as dysphagia, as well as injury to the cervical sympathetic plexus resulting in Horner syndrome. If the dysphagia precludes oral intake for up to 5 postoperative days, either a feeding tube or a percutaneous enterogastric tube is placed. By carefully reviewing preoperative imaging studies and having a detailed plan, the surgeon can reduce operative time and mitigate the occurrence of many of the aforementioned complications.

REFERENCES

1. Bohlman HH, Emery SE: The pathophysiology of cervical spondylosis and myelopathy, *Spine (Phila Pa 1976)* 13:843–846, 1988.
2. Wei-bing X, Wun-Jer S, Gang L, et al.: Reconstructive techniques study after anterior decompression of multilevel cervical spondylotic myelopathy, *J Spinal Disord Tech* 22:511–515, 2009.
3. Chiles BW 3rd, Leonard MA, Choudhri HF, Cooper PR: Cervical spondylotic myelopathy: patterns of neurological deficit and recovery after anterior cervical decompression, *Neurosurgery* 44:762–769, 1999. discussion 769–770.
4. Curylo LJ, Mason HC, Bohlman HH, Yoo JU: Tortuous course of the vertebral artery and anterior cervical decompression: a cadaveric and clinical case study, *Spine (Phila Pa 1976)* 25:2860–2864, 2000.
5. Eskander MS, Connolly PJ, Eskander JP, Brooks DD: Injury of an aberrant vertebral artery during a routine corpectomy: a case report and literature review, *Spinal Cord* 47:773–775, 2009.
6. Yonenobu K, Fuji T, Ono K, et al.: Choice of surgical treatment for multisegmental cervical spondylotic myelopathy, *Spine (Phila Pa 1976)* 10:710–716, 1985.
7. Wang JC, McDonough PW, Endow KK, Delamarter RB: A comparison of fusion rates between single-level cervical corpectomy and two-level discectomy and fusion, *J Spinal Disord* 14:222–225, 2001.
8. Smith PN, Balzer JR, Khan MH, et al.: Intraoperative somatosensory evoked potential monitoring during anterior cervical discectomy and fusion in nonmyelopathic patients: a review of 1,039 cases, *Spine J* 7:83–87, 2007.
9. Khan MH, Smith PN, Balzer JR, et al.: Intraoperative somatosensory evoked potential monitoring during cervical spine corpectomy surgery: experience with 508 cases, *Spine (Phila Pa 1976)* 31:E105–E113, 2006.
10. Yan D, Wang Z, Deng S, et al.: Anterior corpectomy and reconstruction with titanium mesh cage and dynamic cervical plate for cervical spondylotic myelopathy in elderly osteoporosis patients, *Arch Orthop Trauma Surg* 131:1369–1374, 2011.
11. Sevki K, Mehmet T, Ufuk T, et al.: Results of surgical treatment for degenerative cervical myelopathy: anterior cervical corpectomy and stabilization, *Spine (Phila Pa 1976)* 29:2493–2500, 2004.
12. Oh MC, Zhang HY, Park JY, Kim KS: Two-level anterior cervical discectomy versus one-level corpectomy in cervical spondylotic myelopathy, *Spine (Phila Pa 1976)* 34:692–696, 2009.
13. Ikenaga M, Shikata J, Tanaka C: Long-term results over 10 years of anterior corpectomy and fusion for multilevel cervical myelopathy, *Spine (Phila Pa 1976)* 31:1568–1574, 2006. discussion 1575.
14. Ikenaga M, Shikata J, Tanaka C: Anterior corpectomy and fusion with fibular strut grafts for multilevel cervical myelopathy, *J Neurosurg Spine* 3:79–85, 2005.

Cervical Disk Arthroplasty

32

Rick C. Sasso and M. David Mitchell

CHAPTER PREVIEW

Chapter Synopsis	The ability for cervical total disk arthroplasty (TDA) to treat specific cervical spine disorders while maintaining cervical motion is now feasible. Although unclear, it appears that cervical TDA may be an effective alternative to anterior cervical diskectomy and fusion (ACDF) for the management of cervical myelopathy or radiculopathy, or both, in selective cases. Careful patient selection and surgical technique are vital to maintaining good patient outcomes. Concerns and challenges regarding proper patient selection, developing effective salvage procedures, and managing implant wear-related disease remain. Long-term outcome studies should continue to provide answers to many of these questions. The purpose of this chapter is to review the indications, contraindications, surgical techniques, complications, and results of cervical TDA.
Important Points	Cervical TDA is indicated for patients with single-level disease that is causing cervical radiculopathy or myelopathy, or both. One TDA design has received approval for two-level placement.
	Cervical TDA is not indicated for diskogenic neck pain.
	Careful attention to patient selection remains vital for maintaining favorable patient outcomes.
	In selected cases, cervical TDA may be an effective alternative to ACDF and is designed to maintain motion at the disk space.
	Early short-term results suggest that cervical TDA may be equivalent to ACDF in terms of neck disability index and visual analog scores.
	The ability of cervical TDA to prevent adjacent segment disease is not yet conclusively proven.
	Patients scheduled for cervical TDA should be informed preoperatively of the possibility for conversion from TDA to ACDF, depending on intraoperative findings.
Clinical and Surgical Pearls	The patient is placed in a position that encourages cervical lordosis, but the surgeon must remember that excessive lordosis may exacerbate myelopathy.
	Performance of adequate neurologic decompression relieves the patient of symptoms before end plate preparation.
	The anteroposterior (AP) fluoroscopic view is key to proper positioning of the cervical TDA. The spinous process is oriented equidistant between the pedicles on the AP radiograph.
	The sagittal fluoroscopic view is checked during trials to ensure proper lordotic alignment.
Clinical and Surgical Pitfalls	Lack of meticulous hemostasis has been implicated in the formation of heterotopic ossification.
	Overdistraction of the disk space may create facet pain.
	Placing the disk prosthesis off center and not fitting the disk completely in the medial lateral orientation can adversely affect outcomes.
	Implant malpositioning and improper sizing can be reduced by careful intraoperative trials and the use of fluoroscopy.

The most common surgical procedure for the treatment of cervical disk disease resulting in radiculopathy or myelopathy is the combination of anterior cervical diskectomy and fusion (ACDF).[1] Although it is effective for relieving symptoms of neural compression, questions still remain about the effect of cervical fusion on cervical biomechanics and subsequent adjacent segment disease. Therefore, the main goal for the development of a cervical total disk arthroplasty (TDA) system is to preserve motion while maintaining spinal stability to minimize adjacent segment disease.[2] Other advantages of TDA over other conventional surgical procedures may include quicker return to activities of daily living and improved acceptance by patients. Other motion-preserving procedures such as cervical laminoplasty and anterior and posterior cervical foraminotomies are discussed elsewhere in the textbook.

The history of current cervical TDA can be linked back to the development of lumbar spine arthroplasty systems. The original purpose for the development of lumbar TDA was to address lumbar axial diskogenic pain while providing the benefit of motion preservation. In selected cases, when conservative measures have failed, lumbar TDA may be of benefit in the management of lumbar degenerative disk disease. Since their development, the lumbar disk systems have been extensively studied biomechanically. However, as lumbar TDA has become more extensively used and investigated, several questions remain unanswered, including questions about in vivo wear rates, revision strategies, and payer acceptance.[3]

Several differences exist between cervical and lumbar TDA systems, however. Biomechanically, the load demand on TDA in the cervical spine is less than in the lumbar spine. Furthermore, identifying acceptable motion of the instantaneous axis of rotation may be more important and position sensitive in cervical TDA design in comparison with lumbar TDA. Perhaps most fundamentally different is that the indication for cervical TDA is the management of radiculopathy and myelopathy and not axial diskogenic pain, in contrast to the indication for lumbar disk arthroplasty.[4] Therefore, as for all surgical procedures, the best results of cervical TDA require careful patient selection and precise surgical technique.

Indications and Contraindications

Currently, cervical TDA is indicated and approved in the United States, depending on the implant selected for patients with single-level or two-level disease causing cervical radiculopathy or myelopathy, or both. Unlike in lumbar arthroplasty, cervical diskogenic pain is not an indication.

Patients should be evaluated with a minimum of a cervical spine radiographic series including flexion and extension views to assess for radiographic evidence of instability. Magnetic resonance imaging should be obtained to help confirm the surgical level and to correlate with the clinical examination. In some cases, a computed tomography scan may also be of benefit to determine the extent of facet arthropathy and cervical spondylosis and the presence or absence of ossification of the posterior

---

BOX 32-1   Contraindications to Total Disk Arthroplasty

Cervical instability
>11 degrees of angulation
>3 mm of segmental translation
Multilevel disease
Radiographic evidence of severe facet joint degeneration
Radiographic evidence of severe osteoarthritis with loss of normal disk space height >80%
"Hard disk" disease
Lack of motion of target disk space on preoperative radiographs
Postlaminectomy status with kyphotic deformity
Osteoporosis
Metabolic bone disease
Rheumatoid arthritis, ankylosing spondylitis
Ossification of the posterior longitudinal ligament or diffuse hyperostosis
Infection (past or present)
Malignant disease
Known hypersensitivity to cobalt, chromium, molybdenum, titanium, or polyethylene
Traumatic injury
Pregnancy or possible pregnancy within 3 years of implantation

From Pickett G, Sekhon L, Sears WR, Duggal N: Complications with cervical arthroplasty. *J Neurosurg Spine* 4:98-105, 2006.

---

longitudinal ligament. A bone mineral density scan may help in assessing patients with suspected osteoporosis.

Although several contraindications to placement of cervical TDA exist, particular attention should be paid to both clinical and radiographic evidence of moderate to severe facet arthropathy. The presence of facet arthropathy is believed to be a contraindication to cervical TDA because motion preservation at the operated level may aggravate or even result in pain within the arthritic facet joints. Other contradictions include cervical instability, osteoporosis, and a history of cervical spine infections. A complete list of contraindications is listed in Box 32-1.[5]

Therefore, careful review of the indications for and contraindications to placement of cervical TDA reveals that most patients have limited degenerative problems and are physiologically younger than patients typically undergoing ACDF. Regardless, all patients selected for cervical TDA should be informed preoperatively that if intraoperative findings dictate, the TDA procedure may have to be converted to ACDF.

Surgical Technique

Surgical Approach and Exposure

The surgical approach and exposure for implantation of cervical TDA are analogous to the approach used for ACDF. The patient is positioned supine on the operating room table, with the patient's head placed in a doughnut holder to help reduce motion. A small towel is placed under the shoulders to allow for cervical lordosis. Intraoperative radiographs should confirm that the spine is in a lordotic position. Taping of the shoulders is also recommended to allow for better visualization of the intraoperative cervical spine radiographs (Fig. 32-1).

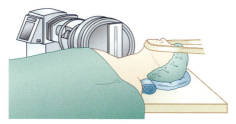

FIGURE 32-1 Careful patient positioning during placement of cervical arthroplasty is vital to maintain physiologic lordosis without creating hyperlordosis in the cervical spine. This goal can be facilitated by placement of a towel roll under the cervical spine. In addition, obtaining clear intraoperative images in both the anteroposterior and lateral views is essential. Taping of the patient's shoulders before sterile draping can help assist in obtaining adequate images. Newer techniques do not routinely require traction as demonstrated in this schematic. (Courtesy Rick Sasso, MD, Indianapolis, Ind.)

The standard Smith-Robinson approach is performed from either the right or the left side. In most cases, the standard horizontal ACDF incision may have to be extended across the midline toward the contralateral side to achieve adequate exposure to allow for proper centering of the instrumentation. The authors prefer to expose the platysma in a longitudinal fashion, thus freeing it from the overlying subcutaneous tissue, and then splitting the platysma longitudinally and developing the plane between the sternocleidomastoid and the strap muscles. Care is taken to control hemostasis at all times because postoperative heterotopic bone may be related to the presence of a hematoma and thus may diminish disk motion.[6-8] The proper cervical level is confirmed radiographically. This surgical exposure should allow for determination of the exact coronal center point of the disk being addressed.

The longus colli muscles are carefully elevated off the anterior cervical spine, and the blade retractors are placed under the longus colli muscles bilaterally. Pin distractors are placed in the vertebral bodies above and below the disk to be removed. The involved disk is then removed along with the posterior longitudinal ligament. Removal of the posterior longitudinal ligament allows for proper sizing of the components and prevents posterior tethering of the motion segment. Resection of the posterior longitudinal ligament is also frequently needed to decompress the segmental disorder adequately. Identification of the uncovertebral joints bilaterally aids in the identification of the anatomic midline.

Placement of Cervical Total Disk Arthroplasty

Because the primary indication for cervical TDA remains persistent radiculopathy or myelopathy, or both, the surgeon should address the underlying pathologic features at the disk level. Therefore, symmetric partial resections of the uncovertebral joints are performed as necessary. The uncovertebral joints are believed to be necessary for biomechanical stability, and preservation of nonoffending portions should be maintained. Once diskectomy and bony resections are complete, distraction pins can be placed into the intervertebral disk space as necessary to ensure that end plates are parallel. If necessary, any other offending degenerative osteophytes are removed (Fig. 32-2).

Lordotic sagittal cervical alignment is then again confirmed radiographically before end plate preparation.

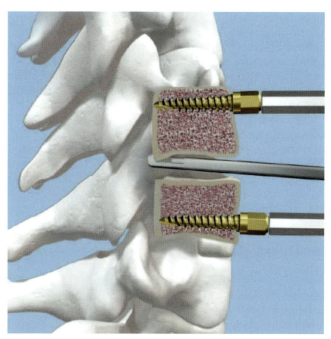

FIGURE 32-2 Schematic demonstrating resection of bony osteophytes. Whenever possible, bony end plates should be preserved, and the cartilaginous end plates should be removed. The uncinate processes should be preserved; however, foraminotomies and posterior osteophytes can be resected as necessary to complete the bony decompression and to ensure proper placement of the subsequent trials and final implant. Also notice placement of the distraction pins confirming parallel preparation of the vertebral end plates.

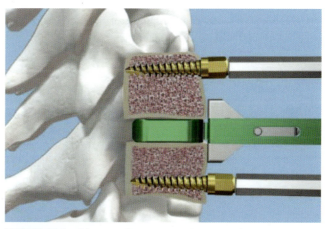

FIGURE 32-3 Schematic demonstrating placement of a trial to help determine appropriate implant size. Typically, trial height should be selected to match the normal adjacent disk heights. The use of lateral radiographs helps assess the appropriate size.

This is a critical step necessary for ensuring proper alignment of the prosthesis. Preparation of the end plates varies with the type of cervical TDA, but it is typically performed with the manufacturer's specialized instruments. Typically, the cartilaginous end plates are removed, but the subchondral bone is preserved to reduce the risk of implant subsidence.

Initial implant sizing is approximated by preoperative templating, but the actual size is always determined by the insertion of disk trials at the time of the surgical procedure. Trials are sequentially selected to recreate the normal disk height and allow for optimum medial to lateral coverage on the vertebral end plates (Fig. 32-3). The goal in medial to lateral sizing is to place the implant on the cortical rim of the vertebral body and not solely onto the softer cancellous bone in the middle of the vertebral body. The use of intraoperative fluoroscopy during these trials allows for proper orientation in the coronal and sagittal planes. The depth of the implant is determined by the type of implant and the corresponding sizing guides.

The disk space is reinspected after the trials to ensure that adequate neural decompression has been completed, and the final implant is inserted. The coronal and sagittal alignments are checked fluoroscopically before final implant fixation. The wound is checked for hemostasis as the retractors are removed, and the wound is closed in standard fashion (Box 32-2).[9]

Postoperative Care

Postoperatively, the cervical spine is not immobilized, and nonsteroidal antiinflammatory drugs are given for a few weeks to reduce the chance of heterotopic bone ossification. Admission to the hospital may be elected but is not mandatory. Postoperative radiographs may be taken to compare with radiographs taken at subsequent

BOX 32-2 Surgical Technique

Positioning of the patient in a normal, lordotic position (avoid intraoperative kyphosis)
Full decompression of neural structures
Preparation of end plates based on instrumentation or techniques of the selected arthroplasty device (do not violate end plate integrity)
Choice of correct implant size
Correct positioning of implant (based on technical specifics of the selected device)
Conversion to anterior cervical diskectomy and fusion if unable to implant device "successfully"

From Mummaneni P, Robinson J, Haid RW: Cervical arthroplasty with the PRESTIGE LP cervical disc. *Neurosurgery* 60(ONS Suppl 2):310-315, 2007.

follow-up (Fig. 32-4). Patients are not restricted from ordinary activities.

Complications

As with any anterior cervical procedure, general surgical complications include dysphagia, transient unilateral vocal cord paralysis, retropharyngeal hematoma, esophageal perforation, and spinal cord, nerve root, and dural injury and infections.

Implant-specific complications include subsidence and implant migration into the vertebral body. Heterotopic bone after cervical TDA has been described in the literature. The formation of heterotopic bone is undesirable in a procedure developed to help maintain motion of a cervical spine segment. Prolonged use of nonsteroidal antiinflammatory drugs should be minimized in most cases, to allow for implant fusion to the vertebral body.

Implant delay in fusing to the vertebral surfaces in TDA may occur and may result in neck pain or device migration.[10] These findings may require early or late conversion to ACDF. To help avoid these complications, the end plates must be carefully prepared for bony ingrowth with preservation of the end plate subchondral cortical bone. The more severe bony destruction resulting in device removal may result in anterior corpectomy and posterior fusion.

Osteoporosis, which could result in implant subsidence or migration, should be evaluated in all patients who have risk factors for this condition and evaluated with a bone density test if indicated. Severe osteoporosis is a contraindication to TDA and presents a challenge to ACDF. Osteoblastic pharmaceutical agents show some promise in decreasing this problem.

Implant failure secondary to wear continues to be an evolving area of interest and research. Currently, the in vivo wear rate is believed to be very low, and the osteolysis seen in major synovial joints (hips and knees) has not been observed. The cervical disk (uncovertebral) joint is not considered a synovial joint.

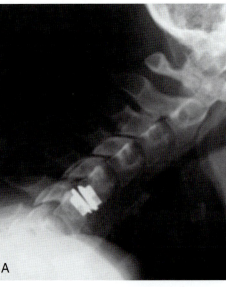
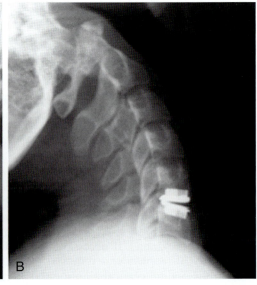

FIGURE 32-4 Postoperative flexion (**A**) and extension (**B**) lateral radiographs of The PRODISC-C device. The device retains motion at the index surgical level in this patient, who was successfully treated with an arthroplasty at C5-C6. (Copyright Synthes Spine, Paoli, Pa., with permission.)

A

B

Clinical Trial Findings

Studies indicated that both ACDF and cervical TDA produced significant improvement in all clinical parameters, with a trend toward greater improvement in the neck disability index (NDI) and neck visual analog scale (VAS) in the cervical TDA group.[2]

Anderson and Rouleau reported reoperation rates after 2 years of follow-up in 1229 patients enrolled in a prospective clinical study of cervical TDA that used ACDF as a control.[11] The reoperation rate in the TDA group was 2.9% and in the ACDF group was 4.8%. This finding suggests that adjacent segment disease may be decreased by TDA. Results of newer 7-year studies confirmed these findings.[12]

Conclusions

Cervical TDA can now be used to treat specific types of cervical spine disease and to maintain cervical motion. Early short-term results suggested that cervical TDA may be equivalent to ACDF in terms of NDI and VAS scores. However, the ability of cervical TDA to prevent adjacent segment disease is probable but not yet proven conclusively. Evolving concerns and challenges regarding proper patient selection, development of effective salvage procedures, and management of implant wear-related disease remains. Long-term outcome studies should continue to provide answers to many of these concerns. Although unclear, it appears that cervical TDA may be an effective alternative to ACDF for the management of cervical myelopathy or radiculopathy, or both, and in selected cases may be the preferred treatment in patients with degenerative cervical spine disease. The clinical follow-up interval for patients undergoing TDA should be most likely be longer than for the patients having traditional ACDF, to observe for any possible device-related events.[10]

REFERENCES

1. Sasso R, Smucker J, Hacker J, et al.: Clinical outcomes of BRYAN cervical disc arthroplasty: a prospective, randomized, controlled multicenter trial with a 24-month follow-up, *J Spinal Disord Tech* 20:481–491, 2007.
2. Goffin J, Geusens E, Vantomme N, et al.: Long term follow-up after interbody fusion of the cervical spine, *J Spinal Disord Tech* 17:79–85, 2004.
3. German J, Foley K: Disc arthroplasty in the management of the painful lumbar motion segment, *Spine (Phila Pa 1976)* 30(Suppl):S60–S67, 2005.
4. Anderson P, Sasso R, Rouleau JP, et al.: The BRYAN cervical disc: wear properties and early clinical results, *Spine J* 4(Suppl): 303S–309S, 2004.
5. Pickett G, Sekhon L, Sears WR, Duggal N: Complications with cervical arthroplasty, *J Neurosurg Spine* 4:98–105, 2006.
6. Mehren C, Suchomel P, Grochulla F, et al.: Heterotopic ossification in total cervical artificial disc replacement, *Spine (Phila Pa 1976)* 31:2802–2806, 2006.
7. Leung C, Casey A, Goffin J, et al.: Clinical significance of heterotopic ossification in cervical disc replacement: a prospective multicenter clinical trial, *Neurosurgery* 57:759–763, 2005.
8. Goffin J: Complications of cervical disc arthroplasty, *Semin Spine Surg* 18:87–98, 2006.
9. Mummaneni P, Robinson J, Haid RW: Cervical arthroplasty with the PRESTIGE LP cervical disc, *Neurosurgery* 60(ONS Suppl 2): 310–315, 2002.
10. Hacker F, Babcock R, Hacker R: Very late complications of cervical arthroplasty of two controlled randomized prospective studies from a single investigator site, *Spine (Phila Pa 1976)* 38:2223–2226, 2013.
11. Anderson P, Rouleau J: Intervertebral disc arthroplasty, *Spine (Phila Pa 1976)* 29:2779–2786, 2004.
12. Tryanelis V, Mummaneni P, Burkus K, Haid R: Clinical and radiographic analysis of an artificial cervical disc: seven-year clinical and radiographic outcome from a prospective randomized controlled clinical trial. Paper number 5. Presented at the 41st annual meeting of the Cervical Spine Research Society, Los Angeles, CA December 5–7, 2013.

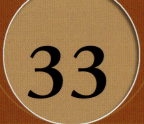

33 Anterior Cervical Foraminotomy

Sang-Ho Lee and Jun Seok Bae

CHAPTER PREVIEW

Chapter Synopsis	This chapter describes in detail the surgical techniques and merits of transcorporeal anterior cervical microforaminotomy for cervical radiculopathy. This procedure involves a modification of the previous anterior microforaminotomy in terms of its medial starting point and tunneling on the upper vertebral body.
Important Points	Transcorporeal anterior cervical microforaminotomy allows for direct decompression of the cervical nerve root while preserving the uncovertebral joint and intervertebral disk integrity and avoiding injury to the vertebral artery and cervical sympathetic chain.
	Indications include cervical radiculopathy secondary to compression anterior or medial to the cervical nerve root.
	Contraindications include bilateral foraminal stenosis, predominant axial neck pain, signs suggestive of infection, mechanical instability, and cervical myelopathy.
Clinical and Surgical Pearls	Foraminal magnetic resonance imaging and reconstructed computed tomography images perpendicular to the cervical foramen can help identify and define the foraminal disease.
	Typically, the anterior cervical exposure to the upper vertebral body and affected disk space is approached from the side corresponding to the radiculopathy.
	The longus colli muscle is dissected from its medial border. The starting point for microscopic drilling is just lateral to the medial margin of the longus colli muscle at the midvertebral body level heading toward the posterior tip of the uncinate process.
	In the case of spondylotic foraminal stenosis, the ideal decompression is limited by the upper and lower pedicle and full lateral bony decompression to the transverse foramen.
	In the case of soft disk herniation, the surgeon must excise the posterior longitudinal ligament to explore for any residual free fragments penetrating the ligament.
Clinical and Surgical Pitfalls	Care should be taken not to violate the upper vertebral end plate because that can result in late intervertebral disk collapse and narrowing.
	Uncertainty of the sagittal orientation tends to bring about more caudally directed drilling. Usually, a 15-degree caudal angle on the sagittal plane is appropriate.
	Tilting the patient to the proper angle can place the desired drill hole perpendicular to the ground in both the sagittal and axial planes.
	In the case of the extruded disk, a careful search for additional extruded fragments must be performed if intraoperative findings do not confirm preoperative imaging results.

Cervical radiculopathy is mainly caused by anterior cervical disorders, including cervical disk herniation and uncovertebral osteophytes. Smith and Robinson and Cloward established the anterior approach to treat the cervical spine.[1,2] In 1968, Verbiest reported using the anterolateral approach for cervical foraminal stenosis,[3] and in 1976, Hakuba introduced the transuncodiskal approach.[4] In 1996, Jho reported transuncal microforaminotomy, which was similar to the Hakuba technique but simpler, preserving the disk.[5] Choi and colleagues proposed a modification of upper vertebral transcorporeal anterior cervical microforaminotomy (ACF), which starts with a drill hole at a relatively medial position compared with the previous technique.[6] This newer concept of transcorporeal ACF offers direct decompression of the cervical nerve root while preserving the uncovertebral joint and intervertebral disk integrity and avoiding injury to the vertebral artery and the cervical sympathetic chain. The goal of this chapter is to review the preoperative and postoperative considerations, surgical technique, complications, and results of ACF procedures.

Preoperative Considerations

Eligible patients are those with persistent unilateral cervical radiculopathy and pain unresponsive to conservative treatment for longer than 6 weeks. If patients continue to have severe radicular symptoms not alleviated by opioids or have profound motor deficits, consideration for earlier operative intervention is indicated. Physical examination that shows a positive Spurling sign and weakness or sensory loss in a corresponding pain dermatome secondary to cervical radiculopathy can be expected. However, examination findings consistent with myelopathy, such as a positive Lhermitte sign or Hoffmann sign, are considered contraindications to ACF.

The required preoperative imaging study includes oblique and dynamic flexion and extension lateral radiographs, magnetic resonance imaging (MRI), and computed tomography (CT) scan. Foraminal MRI, which consists of axial MRI images obtained perpendicular to the cervical foramen, is also helpful in evaluating foraminal disorders. The extension of disk herniation or osteophytes, calcification and migration of disks, and location and variation of the vertebral artery in the transverse foramen should be checked in preparation for the operation. Axial CT scan and sagittal CT reconstruction images are useful in determining the location of the drill hole and for measuring the transcorporeal trajectory.

ACF is indicated when the history and examination confirm persistent unilateral radiculopathy that correlates with preoperative imaging studies demonstrating posterolateral disk herniation or uncovertebral osteophytes that compress the cervical nerve root anteriorly. In patients with multilevel disease or vague symptoms, electrophysiologic study, including nerve conduction velocity and electromyography, may help confirm the diagnosis. Multilevel foraminal stenosis and disk herniation are not often present and also can be indications for ACF (Fig. 33-1).

Bilateral foraminal stenosis, predominant axial neck pain, signs suggestive of infection, instability, and the presence of myelopathy are contraindications to ACF. Unilateral foraminal decompression performed in the presence of bilateral foraminal stenosis may aggravate the development of radiculopathy on the contralateral side. Axial neck pain secondary to degenerative cervical disk disease is also a contraindication to ACF. Anterior cervical diskectomy and fusion (ACDF) may be an option in patients who are not candidates for ACF.

Surgical Technique

The patient is placed supine, with the neck in an extended position. General anesthesia is used. Both shoulders are slightly pulled caudally and are maintained by adhesive tape to help improve intraoperative radiographic visualization. The level of the intended skin incision can be confirmed on the lateral radiograph and should be centered on the upper portion of the vertebral body of interest.

The surgical approach is made on the affected side. After preparation and draping, a 3-cm transverse skin incision along the skin crease is made. Because the trajectory of the drill hole is in the cranial-to-caudal direction, the skin incision should be centered on the upper portion of the vertebral body. The fascial plane just medial to the carotid sheath is sharply incised and bluntly dissected to the anterior surface of the vertebral body. After identifying the midline, the surgeon opens the prevertebral fascia layer longitudinally and detaches the longus colli muscle from its medial margin to the lateral margin of the uncovertebral joint.

Identifying the lateral margin of the uncovertebral joint and vertebral body is important to help determine the starting point of the drill hole. Unlike in ACDF or transuncal anterior foraminotomy, the upper vertebral body and affected disk space must be exposed, and the lower vertebral body does not need to be exposed for transcorporeal ACF. Self-retaining Casper retractors (Aesculap, Tuttlingen, Germany) are applied under the longus colli muscle laterally and the tracheoesophageal complex medially (Fig. 33-2). Cranial-to-caudal retraction is not usually necessary if subfascial dissection is sufficient; however, in the patient with thick neck muscles, a narrow retractor is applied for craniocaudal retraction.

To confirm the accurate level, an 18-gauge needle is inserted at the expected point of the drill hole on the upper vertebral body (Fig. 33-3). The needle must be inserted perpendicular to the anterior surface of the vertebral body. This placement helps to confirm the level of vertebral body exposure and also guides the direction of the drill hole compared with the vertical position of the needle. The entry point is at the midbody level (or 4 to 6 mm above the lower border of the exposed vertebra), just lateral to the medial margin of the longus colli muscle (Figs. 33-4 and 33-5). This starting point is relatively more medial compared with earlier described techniques. The transuncal ACF first reported by Jho was to preserve the motion segment and to accomplish adequate anatomic decompression of the spinal canal anteriorly in the transverse and longitudinal axis, as well as the ipsilateral foramen. However, with this technique, the vertebral artery may be exposed and endangered because the hole is drilled at the most lateral portion of the vertebral body.

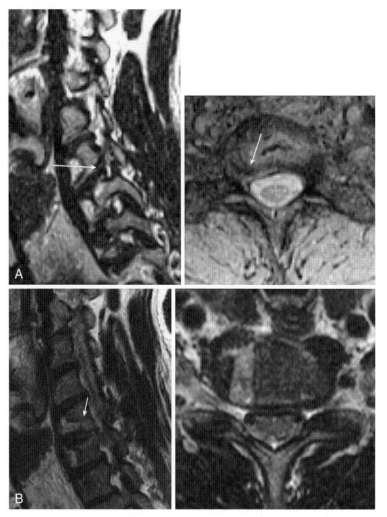

FIGURE 33-1 **A**, Preoperative cervical magnetic resonance imaging (MRI) shows foraminal disk herniation at the C6-C7 level compressing the right C7 nerve root (*arrows*). **B**, Postoperative MRI shows complete removal of the herniated disk fragment and decompression of the C6-C7 neural foramen (*arrow*).

Transverse cutting of the longus colli muscle may risk injury to the cervical sympathetic chain leading to the development of Horner syndrome. When the entire uncinate process is removed, intervertebral space narrowing occurs, even when the disk is preserved as much as possible. Modification of the upper vertebral transcorporeal ACF, as proposed by Choi and colleagues,[6] which starts with a drill hole at the level of medial border of the longus colli muscles, is a relatively medial position compared with the previous techniques. With this technique, the adequate foraminal decompression is achieved by removing the posterolateral disk tissue and the uncinate osteophyte while reducing the risk of vertebral artery or sympathetic chain injury.

At this point, an operative microscope is placed, and the drill hole is created using a high-speed drill (Black Max, Anspach, Palm Beach Gardens, Fla.). The target point of the drill hole is the posterior uncovertebral joint, at the anterior wall of the cervical neural foramen (Fig. 33-6). A 6-mm drill hole is made obliquely in a medial-to-lateral and cranial-to-caudal direction. Care should be taken not to violate the upper vertebral end plate during creation of the transcorporeal tunnel.

The authors use a 4-mm diamond burr to start the drill hole and change to a 3-mm burr for better visualization and finer drilling. Usually, the trajectory is greater than 20 mm, and the routine diamond burr tip is less than 20 mm, so the diameter of the drill hole must be expanded up to 6 mm to drill more deeply in the foramen. In other words, unless the drill goes deep inside the drill hole, it has little chance to injure the neural structure, as long as the trajectory remains in the right direction.

Before widening of the drill hole and bringing the drill down to the posterior uncovertebral joint, the authors take care not to violate the end plate and remain in the right trajectory. Subsequently, the authors may need to change the drilling burr to a longer one, but being careful to avoid any tremor of the drill. When the drilling reaches the posterior margin, the posterolateral margin of the disk space is encountered (Fig. 33-7). To expose the neural foramen, the posterior drill hole can be widened carefully at the posterior tip of the uncinate process (Fig. 33-8). The posterior longitudinal ligament protects the neural structure during drilling close to the posterior cortical bone.

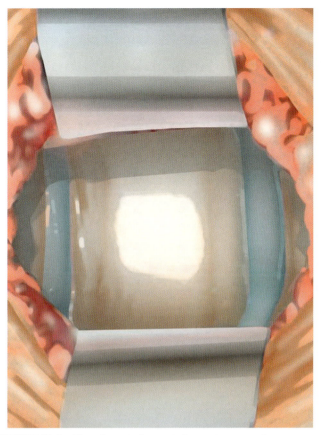

FIGURE 33-2 This schematic drawing indicates the appropriate exposure for anterior aspect of the cervical spine. The longus colli muscle is detached from the medial margin to expose the lateral margin of uncovertebral joint. The upper vertebral body and affected disk space are exposed with a self-retaining Casper retractor.

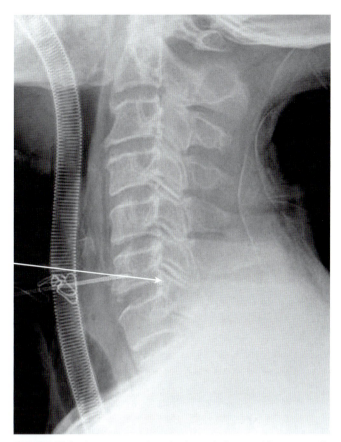

FIGURE 33-3 Intraoperative lateral radiograph shows an 18-gauge needle inserted at the C6 vertebral body during transcorporeal anterior cervical microforaminotomy at the C6 vertebral body. The needle is inserted perpendicularly into the corresponding vertebral body, and the appropriate trajectory for the drill hole (*arrow*) is approximately 15 degrees in the craniocaudal direction compared with the needle from the same point where the needle is inserted.

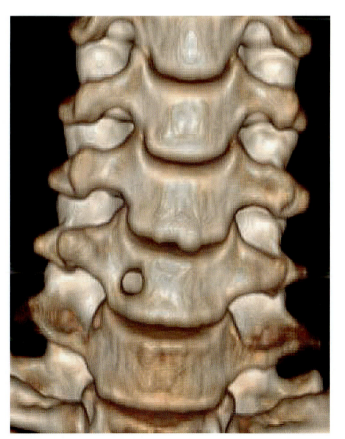

FIGURE 33-4 Postoperative follow-up three-dimensional computed tomography scan shows the exact location of the drill hole on the vertebral body.

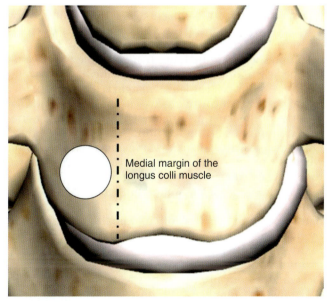

FIGURE 33-5 Anterior view of the entry point of the drill hole. This point is at the midbody level just lateral to the medial margin of the longus colli muscle.

Medial margin of the longus colli muscle

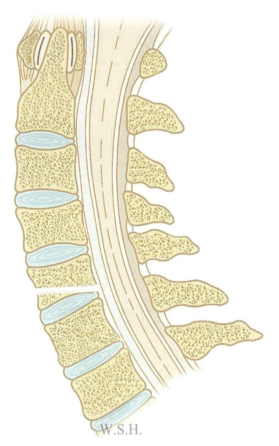

FIGURE 33-6 Lateral view of the trajectory of the drill hole. The target point of the drill hole is the posteroinferior margin of the upper vertebral body.

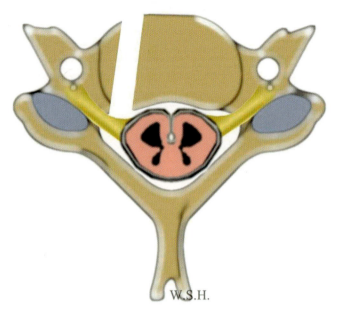

FIGURE 33-7 Schematic drawing demonstrating transcorporeal anterior cervical microforaminotomy. Initial drilling is made from the anterior vertebral body to the posterior uncovertebral joint at the affected level.

Once the posterior cortical bone of the upper and lower vertebral body becomes thin enough, it can be trimmed by a 1-mm Kerrison punch (Fig. 33-9). For adequate decompression, the cranial and caudal margin of foraminal decompression is at the lower margin of the upper vertebral pedicle and the upper margin of the lower vertebral pedicle, respectively. The lateral margin is the lateral border of the posterior uncinate process. To preserve the normal integrity of the anterior vertebral column, the uncovertebral joint must be kept intact during the entire procedure. Only the posterior margin of the uncovertebral joint, where the hypertrophied osteophyte compresses the nerve root, is removed for foraminal decompression.

Care should be taken not to injure the vertebral artery while removing the lateral margin of the posterior uncinate process in the case of foraminal stenosis caused by uncovertebral hypertrophy. To avoid vertebral artery injury, the posterior longitudinal ligament should be maintained intact, and the punch should be kept in contact with the bony prominence to avoid bites deep within the transverse foramen. The uncovertebral spondylotic spur that compressed the nerve root is removed by steps; however, in the case of cervical spondylotic foraminal stenosis, removal of the posterior longitudinal ligament is not mandatory.

As the drill hole moves closer to the posterior margin, bone bleeding may be encountered, and this can easily be controlled by bone wax. Epidural bleeding after removal of the posterior cortical bone and posterior longitudinal ligament is controlled by Avitene (Bard Davol, Warwick, R.I.), thrombin-soaked Gelfoam (Upjohn, Kalamazoo, Mich.), or FLOSEAL (Fusion Medical Technologies, Mountain View, Calif.). Bipolar coagulation can be used for some epidural bleeding from definite bleeding vessels, as occurs during removal of the posterior longitudinal ligament.

In the case of soft disk herniation, ruptured disk fragments are encountered after drilling of the posterior medial neural foramen (Fig. 33-10). The herniated disk fragments can be removed with pituitary forceps. Frequently, ruptured disk fragments penetrate the posterior longitudinal ligament. To ensure that no residual disk fragments remain behind, careful exploration under the posterior longitudinal ligament is needed after removing the ligament with a Kerrison punch (Fig. 33-11). If the fragment is not a single piece but multiple pieces, the surgeon must anticipate the number of fragments preoperatively and match the actual fragments with this expected number. When the actual number of fragments is not found, meticulous exploration with a probe will frequently yield more disk fragments.

After full decompression of the nerve root, pulsation and anterior shifting of the posterior displaced nerve root are observed. Shim and associates applied the transcorporeal approach for disk herniation at the C2-C3 level.[7] These investigators made an entry point from the C3 vertebral body and extended the hole cranioposteriorly to the superoposterior border of the C3 end plate. The ruptured disk located at the midline of C2-C3 was then removed.

The authors do not fill the bony tunnel with Gelfoam or bone chips. The remaining hole acts as drainage for epidural hemorrhage to prevent epidural hematoma. In addition, new bone formation at the drilled hole is observed during follow-up (Fig. 33-12). After meticulous hemostasis, the wound is closed layer by layer, with one Jackson-Pratt drain left behind.

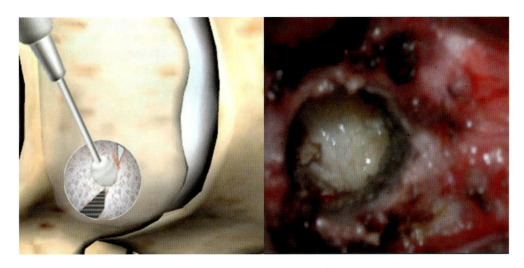

FIGURE 33-8   To expose the neural foramen, careful drilling at the posterior tip of the uncinate process and the posterior cortical bone of the upper and lower vertebral body is performed.

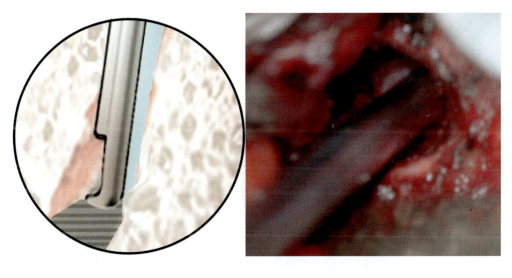

FIGURE 33-9   After thinning of the posterior cortical bone, the bone can be trimmed with a 1-mm Kerrison punch.

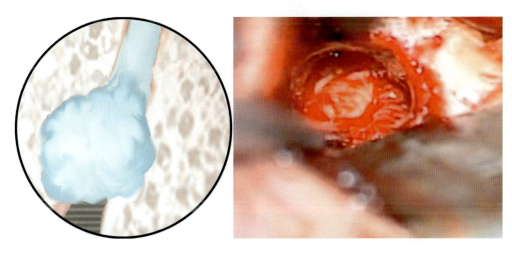

FIGURE 33-10   A ruptured disk fragment may be visible.

Image-Guided Anterior Cervical Microforaminotomy

For a safe, precise, and minimally invasive procedure, the authors have applied image-guided surgical techniques to ACF. The patient is placed in the supine position and is under general anesthesia. After preparation and draping of the patient, the authors make arrangements for computer-assisted spinal surgery under the O-arm (Medtronic Navigation, Louisville, Colo.) and the StealthStation TREON system (Medtronic Navigation) (Fig. 33-13). The intended skin incision level is identified with the help of spinal navigation on the affected side, and a 2.5-cm transverse skin incision is made along the skin crease. A tubular retractor can be applied for an even more minimal incision. After the prevertebral facial incision and blunt finger dissection are completed, the tubular retractor is positioned to expose the adequate portion that is superior to the affected level and the medial portion of the corresponding uncinate process without violation of the longus colli muscle. The drilling and decompression technique that follows is not different from the technique

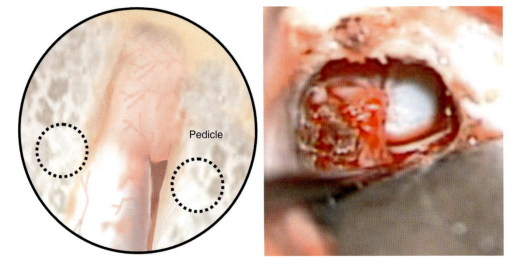

FIGURE 33-11 The posterior longitudinal ligament is removed to confirm decompression of the nerve root. Removal of the posterior longitudinal ligament may not be necessary in the case of spondylotic foraminal stenosis.

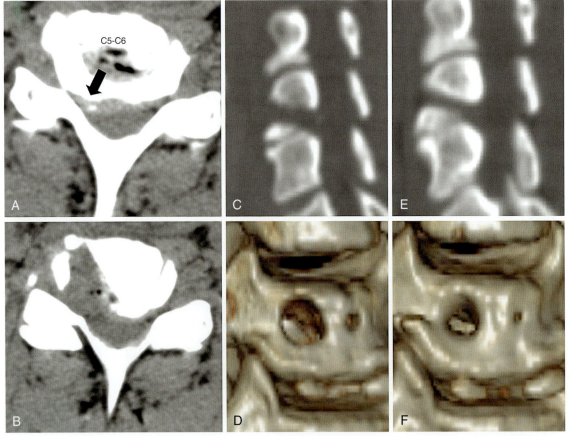

FIGURE 33-12 Anterior cervical microforaminotomy was performed for spondylotic foraminal stenosis at the right C5-C6 level (**A,** *arrow*). Immediate postoperative axial, sagittal, and three-dimensional reconstructed computed tomography (CT) scans showing complete decompression (**B**) and the position of the drill hole (**C** and **D**). Thirty-month follow-up sagittal and three-dimensional reconstructed CT scans showing new bone formation at the drilled hole (**E** and **F**).

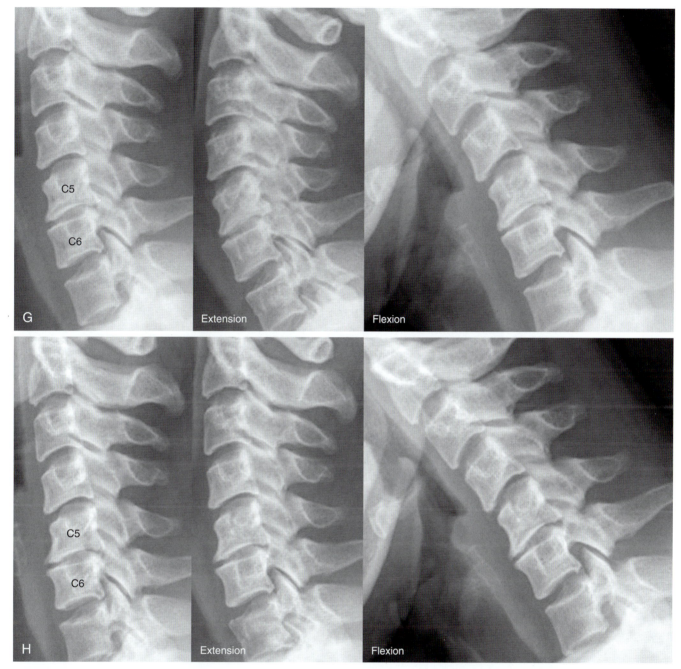

FIGURE 33-12, cont'd   Comparison of preoperative (**G**) and 30-month follow-up dynamic radiographs (**H**) showing no instability and preservation of intervertebral disk integrity.

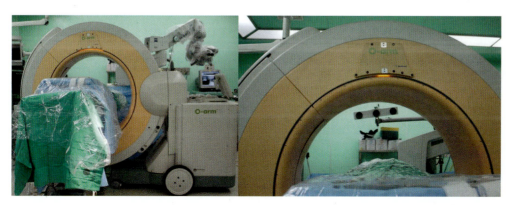

FIGURE 33-13 Operation room setting showing the navigation camera and O-arm, which are used for intraoperative computed tomography scanning. The operative field is draped with a sterile plastic sheet. (Courtesy Medtronic Navigation, Louisville, Colo.)

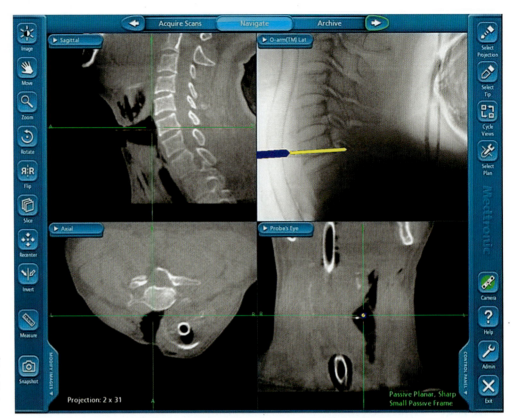

FIGURE 33-14 Screen capture of a navigation monitor showing the accurate vertebral level and the correct trajectory. (Courtesy Medtronic Navigation, Louisville, Colo.)

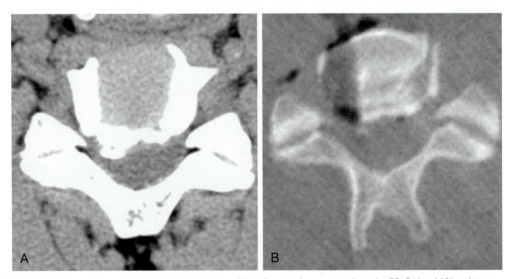

FIGURE 33-15 Preoperative computed tomography scan showing spondylotic foraminal stenosis at the right C5-C6 level (**A**) and intraoperative O-arm scanning to confirm that the foraminal decompression is adequate (**B**).

previously described. With a navigation system, surgeons can confirm the accurate disk space level and the appropriate trajectory during drilling, to avoid violation of the end plate and the medial wall of the transverse foramen (Fig. 33-14).

After sufficient decompression, then, the authors check the intraoperative O-arm scans to verify whether the vertebral tunnel is consistent with preoperative planning and that foraminal decompression is adequate (Fig. 33-15). Using an intraoperative O-arm–based navigation system and tubular retractor, Kim and colleagues reported a decrease in the size of the skin incision and drill hole.[8] Because it

gives intraoperative real-time feedback, image-guided surgery allows the surgeon to check the depth and trajectory of the drill hole. Considering the small operative field and drill hole, the navigation system is an effective and safe method.

Postoperative Considerations

The patient is placed in a soft cervical collar immediately after the surgical procedure and should be able to ambulate as soon as he or she recovers from anesthesia. In the authors' practice, postoperative intravenous antibiotics are given for 3 days and are changed to oral antibiotics for 4 days. An antiinflammatory medication, mild muscle relaxant, and analgesics are prescribed in the immediate postoperative period. The patient is discharged after removal of the wound drain at approximately the third postoperative day. Depending on the number of levels involved, the patient is asked to wear a soft collar for 2 to 4 weeks.

Complications

Theoretically, various complications may accompany ACF, related to anterior cervical exposure, such as postoperative hematoma, recurrent laryngeal nerve injury, and dysphagia, which can be minimized by meticulous surgical technique. For transuncal ACF, vertebral artery injury and sympathetic chain injury causing Horner syndrome are possible complications. Jho reported that 2 of 104 patients treated by transuncal ACF experienced transient Horner syndrome, 1 patient experienced transient hemiparesis, and another patient experienced diskitis resulting in spontaneous bone fusion.[9] Sung and Lee reported a case of disk space collapse after transuncal ACF.[10] The present technique, transcorporeal ACF, is relatively safer because of its more medial starting point than previous techniques. Choi and colleagues reported transient tingling sensation or numbness in the ipsilateral limb in 3 of 30 patients treated by transcorporeal ACF.[11] Kim and associates reported that transient dysphagia occurred in only 2 of 8 patients after transcorporeal ACF using O-arm–guided intraoperative navigation.[8]

Results

Although some differences exist among surgical methods for ACF, the clinical results reported are generally good. Jho and colleagues reported a series of 104 patients treated by transuncal ACF in which 99% excellent or good results and functional anatomic features were preserved for 99% of the patients.[9] Johnson and co-workers reported a series of 21 patients treated by the same technique described by Jho and associates, in which 91% of the patients experienced improvement of radicular pain and 9% experienced improvement of persistent radicular pain, thus necessitating further surgical intervention.[12] Saringer and colleagues reported a series of 16 patients treated by modified ACF using the MED system, which preserved a thin lateral cortical wall of uncinate process, in which all patients showed improvement in radicular pain, motor weakness, and sensory deficit after the procedure.[13] Choi and co-workers reported a series of 30 patients treated by transcorporeal ACF in which all patients experienced significant improvement of symptoms.[6,11]

REFERENCES

1. Smith GW, Robinson RA: The treatment of certain cervical-spine disorders by anterior removal of the intervertebral disc and interbody fusion, *J Bone Joint Surg Am* 40:607–624, 1958.
2. Cloward RB: The anterior approach for removal of ruptured cervical disks, *J Neurosurg* 15:602–617, 1958.
3. Verbiest H: A lateral approach to the cervical spine: technique and indications, *J Neurosurg* 28:191–203, 1968.
4. Hakuba A: Trans-unco-discal approach: a combined anterior and lateral approach to cervical discs, *J Neurosurg* 45:284–291, 1976.
5. Jho HD: Microsurgical anterior cervical foraminotomy for radiculopathy: a new approach to cervical disc herniation, *J Neurosurg* 84:155–160, 1996.
6. Choi G, Lee SH, Bhanot A, et al.: Modified transcorporeal anterior cervical microforaminotomy for cervical radiculopathy: a technical note and early results, *Eur Spine J* 16:1387–1393, 2007.
7. Shim CS, Jung TG, Lee SH: Transcorporeal approach for disc herniation at the C2-C3 level: a technical case report, *J Spinal Disord Tech* 22, 2009. 4594–4562.
8. Kim JS, Eun SS, Prada N, et al.: Modified transcorporeal anterior cervical microforaminotomy assisted by O-arm–based navigation: a technical case report, *Eur Spine J* 20(Suppl 2):S147–S152, 2011.
9. Jho HD, Kim WK, Kim MH: Anterior microforaminotomy for treatment of cervical radiculopathy. Part 1, Disc-preserving "functional cervical disc surgery," *Neurosurgery* 51(Suppl):S46–S53, 2002.
10. Sung YS, Lee SH: Microsurgical anterior cervical foraminotomy: less invasive technique, *Rachis* 9:303–308, 1997.
11. Choi G, Arbatti NJ, Modi HN, et al.: Transcorporeal tunnel approach for unilateral cervical radiculopathy: a 2-year follow-up review and results, *Minim Invasive Neurosurg* 53:127–131, 2010.
12. Johnson JP, Filler AG, McBride DQ, Batzdorf U: Anterior cervical foraminotomy for unilateral radicular disease, *Spine (Phila Pa 1976)* 25:905–909, 2000.
13. Saringer WF, Reddy B, Nobauer-Huhmann I, et al.: Endoscopic anterior cervical foraminotomy for unilateral radiculopathy: anatomical morphometric analysis and preliminary clinical experience, *J Neurosurg* 98:171–180, 2003.

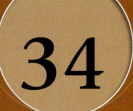

34 Laminectomy and Fusion

Gabriel Liu and Hee Kit Wong

CHAPTER PREVIEW

Chapter Synopsis	Symptomatic cervical myelopathy from multilevel spinal cord compression in older patients is an increasing clinical problem. Multilevel anterior cervical surgical procedures carry significant morbidity. The posterior cervical approach reduces surgical morbidity. Although laminoplasty is often the surgical procedure of choice, laminectomy with spinal fusion and instrumentation is indicated in older patients who have significant neck pain and a K-line–negative or kyphotic cervical spine. This chapter describes the surgical indications for, contraindications to, pitfalls in, and tips for the successful execution of laminectomy and spinal fusion with instrumentation.
Important Points	Laminectomy and spinal fusion with instrumentation are indicated in patients who have three or more intervertebral disk levels of spinal cord compression and significant neck pain, spinal instability, and a K-line–negative or kyphotic cervical spine.
	Laminectomy and spinal fusion are indicated in patients presenting with cervical myelopathic symptoms, including clumsy hands and unsteady gait.
	Lateral mass screw placement is the surgical fixation technique of choice when compared with cervical pedicle screw fixation in most patients with cervical spondylotic myelopathy and ossification of the posterior longitudinal ligament.
	Facet fusion is an important technique to ensure fusion in patients undergoing laminectomy and spinal fusion.
	The surgeon must ensure that cervical lordosis can be achieved before laminectomy, instrumentation, and fusion.
Surgical Pearls	To reduce the risk of junctional kyphosis, the surgeon should avoid muscle dissection at the C2 and C7 spinous processes by performing domelike osteotomy at C3 and partial cephalad C7 laminectomy.
	Removing the lamina en bloc instead of in pieces may reduce the risk of spinal cord injury by minimizing the frequency that the Kerrison rongeur is inserted into the stenotic spinal canal.
	When creating the gutter at the lamina-facet junction, the surgeon should angle the burr tip medially toward the lamina away from the facet to ensure a clean lamina cut.
	A number 4 Penfield instrument can be used to dissect the dural adhesion carefully from the undersurface of the lamina during en bloc removal of the lamina.
Surgical Pitfalls	During prone positioning, adequate space between the patient's face and the Mayfield clamp must be ensured to avoid facial compression by the clamp.
	Overzealous use of shoulder tapes to depress the patient's shoulders to improve the C6 to T1 fluoroscopic spinal image should be avoided because it may cause postoperative rotator cuff injury and brachial plexus injury.
	Recoil of the lamina can occur during the en bloc resection, with resulting iatrogenic spinal cord injury.
	Potential dynamic infolding of the posterior cervical muscle or postlaminectomy membrane into the spinal cord may result in postoperative spinal cord compression.
	Prophylactic bilateral posterior C4-C5 foraminotomies performed together with laminectomy and spinal fusion may reduce postoperative C5 palsy occurrence.

Surgical intervention is indicated in patients with symptomatic cervical myelopathy resulting from spinal cord compression. Direct anterior multilevel cervical decompression and spinal fusion with instrumentation carry significant surgical morbidity.[1,2] To avoid these anterior surgical complications, indirect multilevel posterior surgical decompression techniques were developed.[3] Posterior decompression allows the spinal cord to migrate posteriorly away from the offending anterior spinal cord lesions.

Multilevel laminectomies without spinal fusion and instrumentation should be avoided because they may result in postoperative kyphotic spinal deformity. Motion-preserving laminoplasty is often the technique of choice in the posterior cervical surgical approach; however, it is contraindicated in patients with a painful kyphotic spine or K-line–negative spinal alignment.[4] Multilevel laminectomies and spinal fusion with instrumentation eliminate the micromotion of the kyphotic spine and have better postoperative clinical outcomes than does laminoplasty in patients with K-line–negative alignment.[5] This chapter describes the surgical indications for, contraindications to, pitfalls in, and tips for the successful execution of laminectomy and spinal fusion with instrumentation. All laminectomy and spinal fusion techniques described in this chapter refer to laminectomy and spinal fusion with instrumentation.

Preoperative Considerations

Cervical laminectomy with fusion is a surgical technique designed for patients presenting with three or more levels of spinal cord compression associated with spinal instability resulting from various clinical conditions ranging from cervical spondylotic myelopathy (CSM), to cervical trauma to spinal metastasis.[6] In general, these patients present with cervical canal stenosis with spinal cord compression, resulting in a clinical diagnosis of cervical myelopathy. The patient typically reports "clumsy hands" symptoms that cause difficulties in writing or performing fine motor skill activities. The patient also reports an unsteady gait or even frequent falls. Clinical examinations often reveal findings of upper motor neuron lesions and long tract signs. Of these myelopathic signs, Lhermitte sign, bilateral Hoffmann sign, inverted radial reflex, inability to complete a finger grip-and-release test (20 times in 10 seconds), positive Romberg test result, and failure to perform tandem gait are the most representative of cervical myelopathy.[1,2,7]

Radiologic imaging to confirm the diagnosis of cervical myelopathy and for surgical planning includes radiographs, magnetic resonance imaging (MRI), and computed tomography scans. Anteroposterior and lateral upright radiographs assess cervical spinal alignment, which is essential for surgical approach planning. Flexion and extension lateral cervical spine radiographs exclude segmental spinal instability and confirm cervical lordosis in the extension film. MRI is the gold standard for the diagnosis of cervical canal stenosis and its pathologic features. Computed tomography is indicated to confirm the diagnosis of ossification posterior longitudinal ligament (OPLL) and ossification of the yellow ligament.

Controversies exist between the anterior cervical approach and the posterior cervical approach in the surgical treatment of cervical myelopathy.[2,3,6,7] The principle of the posterior cervical approach is based on the indirect spinal cord decompression method. Posterior decompression and expansion of the spinal canal diameter allow the spinal cord to migrate posteriorly away from the offending anterior spinal cord lesion and result in indirect spinal cord decompression without direct removal of the anterior spinal cord lesion.

The success of the posterior cervical approach depends on the sagittal alignment of the cervical spine, and this approach is contraindicated in patients with a grossly kyphotic cervical spine.[8] Various investigators have reported that the appropriate cervical sagittal alignment for the posterior surgical cervical approach ranges from less than 10 degrees of kyphosis to neutral sagittal alignment. Rao and colleagues suggested that the posterior approach is indicated if cervical lordosis is present in the lateral extension cervical radiograph.[7]

Fujiyoshi and associates used a novel K-line concept, in which the K-line was defined as a line that connects the midpoints of the spinal canal at C2 and C7 in the sagittal view.[4] OPLL that did not extend posterior to the K-line was described as K-line positive, and OPLL that extended past the K-line was termed K-line negative. The observed outcome of laminoplasty was better in K-line–positive patients.[4] In a follow-up study, Fujiyoshi and co-workers further reported that laminectomy and fusion resulted in a better outcome than did laminoplasty in patients with K-line–negative OPLL.[5] Taniyama and colleagues validated the K-line concept in patients with CSM.[9]

In general, the authors prefer the laminoplasty technique for the posterior cervical surgical approach.[9] However, laminoplasty is not without limitations. Liu and colleagues described the following reasons for the revision of laminoplasty procedures: significant axial neck pain, segmental kyphosis, and anterior spinal cord compression of more than 50% of the spinal canal.[8] The authors' current indications for laminectomy and fusion with instrumentation are in older patients, with three of more levels of spinal cord compression from conditions such as OPLL or ossification of the yellow ligament, who have K-line–negative sagittal alignment and significant axial neck pain.

Surgical Technique

Anesthesia and Positioning

The patient, who is under general anesthesia, is positioned for a standard posterior cervical approach with the use of a radiolucent Mayfield clamp. Spinal cord monitoring using somatosensory-evoked potentials (SSEPs) and transcranial motor-evoked potentials (MEPs), with attention to placement of the deltoid electrode to detect C5 palsy, should be considered.

Adequate space between the patient's face and the Mayfield clamp must be ensured to avoid facial compression by the clamp. The patient's head, neck, and upper torso should be elevated above the level of the patient's heart through reverse Trendelenburg positioning to reduce intraoperative spinal and epidural bleeding. Overzealous use of shoulder tapes to depress the patient's shoulders to improve on the C6 to T1 fluoroscopic spinal image should be avoided because it may cause postoperative rotator cuff and brachial plexus injury (see Fig. 4-1).

Cervical lordosis is typically ensured preoperatively with the use of flexion and extension radiographs. Careful gentle manipulation of the Mayfield clamp under fluoroscopy guidance before laminectomy, instrumentation, and fusion may be considered. However, this can be a concern in patients with severe stenosis in whom extension before decompression can result in spinal cord compression. In general, because most cervical cord compression requiring surgical treatment occurs between C3 and C6 to C7, placement of the cervical spine in normal lordotic alignment is of no significant concern except when the planned spinal fusion will include the occipitocervical junction or the cervicothoracic junction.

A kyphotic or hyperlordotic occipitocervical junction may cause postoperative dysphagia and dysphonia. Care should be taken to match the preoperative erect sagittal occipito-C2 angle (an angle between the McGregor line and the line parallel to the base of the C2 body) with fluoroscopic images after occipitocervical fusion, to reduce postoperative complications. Avoiding cervicothoracic fusion in a patient with hyperlordotic or hyperextended alignment will reduce the patient's postoperative distress resulting from an inability to see the feet during ambulation and when attending to genital hygiene.

Surgical Landmarks and Incisions

The surgical field is isolated using 3M Steri-Drape 1000 (3M, St. Paul, Minn.), from the external occipital protuberance to the spine of the scapula (see Fig. 4-1). Sterile scrub using povidone-iodine (Betadine) and removed with isopropyl alcohol is performed before definite surgical cleansing using povidone-iodine and surgical draping. This may reduce postoperative wound infection.

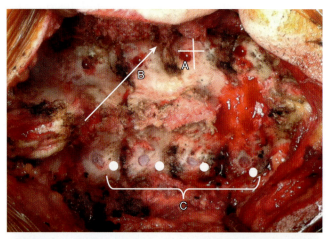

FIGURE 34-1 Surgical dissection exposes the lateral border of the lateral masses from C3 to C6. The lateral mass screw entry point is located just off the center (*A*) of the lateral mass, in the inferior medial quadrant. *B* shows the trajectory of the lateral mass screw. At the pilot hole, the tip of the screw drill bit aims toward the superior lateral corner of the index lateral mass, whereas the handle of the drill bit rests on top of the spinous process of the lateral mass. *C* compares the location of the cervical pedicle screw entry points (*white dots*) with their corresponding lateral mass screw entry points.

The surgical incision is marked out by a straight line connecting the external occipital protuberance to the spinous process of C7 or T1. The extent of the surgical incision can be identified by fluoroscopy or by intraoperative palpation of C2 spinous process, which is the first palpable spinous process.

Meticulous midline dissection along the white median raphe minimizes bleeding and allows better preservation of surgical planes for wound closure. The median raphe can be identified and dissected effectively as follows. In one hand, the surgeon holds a self-retraining retractor to actively spread apart the paraspinal muscle. This places even tension on the muscles to help expose the midline raphe. In the other hand, the surgeon holds the diathermy device to dissect the raphe down to the spinous process.

Unnecessary muscle dissection beyond the intended spinal levels for decompression should be avoided, and when possible, the muscle insertions at C2 and C7 spinous processes should be preserved. Takeuchi and associates compared the axial neck pain after C4-C6 laminoplasty with C3 laminectomy and conventional C3-C7 laminoplasty.[10] These investigators found that preserving the semispinalis cervicis muscle attachment to the C2 spinous process (which is more often damaged in C3 laminoplasty than in C3 laminectomy) reduces postoperative neck pain and stiffness.[10] Similarly, Hosono and co-workers found that preserving the trapezius muscle insertion at the C7 spinous process reduces postoperative axial neck pain.[11]

Because most cases of cervical canal stenosis with spinal cord compression arise from the C3 to the C6 to C7 spinal region, the authors prefer to perform laminectomies extending from lower C3 to upper C7. The C3 lamina is undercut, much like the C2 dome osteotomy, resulting in the preservation of the C2-C3 interspinous ligaments and the muscle attachments at the C2 spinous process.[8] Upper C7 laminectomy is performed without disturbing the trapezius muscle insertion at the C7 spinous process. Spinal fusion and instrumentation are then performed from C3 to C7.

Spinal Instrumentation

Lateral Mass Screw Insertion

Spinal instrumentation is required for spinal stabilization to avoid postlaminectomy kyphosis, and it allows for spinal fusion. Screws holes are prepared before the laminectomy to avoid the loss of surgical anatomy required for screw insertion should laminectomy be performed first. Currently, two types of spinal instrumentation are available: lateral mass screw fixation[1] and cervical pedicle screw fixation.[1,12] In general, the authors prefer the use of lateral mass screws as the spinal fixation method of choice in most of degenerative cervical conditions including CSM and OPLL. Lateral mass screw insertion is quick, safe, and easily reproducible, and it provides adequate posterior spinal column stabilization in patients without anterior column disruption.

Various lateral mass screw insertion techniques have been described. The authors prefer the lateral mass screw entry point to be located just inferior and medial to the center of the lateral mass (Fig. 34-1). This can be done first by visualizing an imaginary cross ("+") placed at the center of the lateral mass. Next, the lateral mass screw entry point is located just medial and inferior to the center of this imaginary "+". This places the starting point slightly within the inferomedial quadrant of the lateral mass. A burr is used to create a pilot hole at the lateral mass screw entry point for better anchorage of the screw drill bit. At the pilot hole, the screw trajectory is formed by aiming the tip of the screw drill bit toward the superior lateral corner of the index lateral mass while resting the shaft of the drill bit on top of the corresponding the spinous process of the vertebrae caudal to the index lateral mass screw hole.

The pilot hole is deepened and drilled using a 2.4-mm diameter electrically driven drill bit, with the drill bit length set at its minimum possible length of 10 mm. This safety precaution limits screw passage advancement beyond a 10-mm depth from the screw hole entry point, to avoid unexpected neurovascular injury. The integrity of the screw hole is checked using a ball-tip thin metal wire, "the feeler," to ensure that no bony cortical breach of the medial, lateral, superior, inferior, and anterior bony walls of the screw hole has occurred.

The screw hole is examined for a sudden spurt of arterial blood from vertebral artery damage and of clear cerebrospinal fluid leakage from spinal nerve damage before the screw hole is deepened by further drilling. If arterial bleeding or a cerebrospinal fluid leak is found, further drilling the screw hole should be aborted. The drill bit length is then reset; it is increased 2 mm at a time, and the screw hole is deepened 2 mm at each drilling. The "feeler" is used to examine the screw hole after each cycle of drilling. The final screw length is determined by identifying the perforation or near perforation of the anterior wall of the screw hole by the drill bit with the "feeler," and this location marks the maximum screw length that can be used.

The lateral mass screw length varies depending on each spinal segment's anatomic variability. A 3.5- or 4-mm diameter titanium polyaxial screw with a minimum screw length of 14 mm is preferred. Once the screw hole preparation is completed and the appropriate screw length is determined, bone wax is applied to seal off the screw hole before the laminectomy is performed. Early insertion of the lateral mass screws will obscure the lamina and can make performing the laminectomy difficult.

Cervical Pedicle Screw Insertion

Cervical pedicle screw fixation is indicated in patients with spinal instability requiring three-column spinal stabilization. The routine use of cervical pedicle screw fixation in stable degenerative disease is not required. The use of cervical pedicle screws is indicated in patients with spinal fractures, especially patients with conditions such as ankylosing spondylitis or diffuse idiopathic skeletal hyperostosis or those requiring kyphotic spine correction.[12] Iatrogenic foraminal stenosis resulting in new radiculopathies after the conversion of cervical kyphosis to lordosis when using the pedicle screw system is a potential concern. The surgical technique for cervical pedicle screw insertion is challenging.

The authors prefer to use the original cervical pedicle screw insertion technique described by Abumi and colleagues and the subaxial cervical pedicle screw entry point location described by Rao and associates (see Fig. 34-1).[12,13] The accuracy of the cervical pedicle screw entry point can further be enhanced by using Yukawa cervical pedicle axis views on fluoroscopy[14] (Fig. 34-2). Once the pilot hole is formed, a crater is created around the hole. A small, angled curet is used for curettage of the medial pedicle wall. A cervical pedicle awl is then held at 40 to 50 degrees medially angled to the lateral mass and is advanced slowly in the anteroposterior direction following the sagittal cervical spine image under fluoroscopic guidance. A pedicle probe "feeler" is used to check the integrity of the pedicle screw hole.

In general, a 3.5-mm diameter titanium polyaxial screw with screw length of 24 to 26 mm is used. Cervical pedicle screws can be inserted before the laminectomy and will not affect the laminectomy procedure because the screw entry point is located more laterally away from the lamina than that of the lateral mass screw (Fig. 34-3).

Laminectomy

Laminectomy is performed under the direct vision of an operating microscope (Fig. 34-4). The use of a surgical

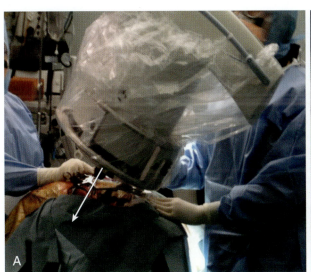

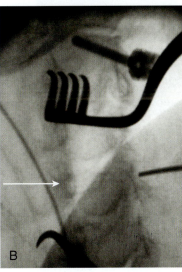

FIGURE 34-2 A, The fluoroscopy position to create the pedicle axis view described by Yukawa and associates.[14] The C-arm is rotated 35 to 55 degrees from the vertical axis to locate the round cervical pedicle image (*arrow*). **B,** The bird's-eye cervical pedicle fluoroscopic image (*arrow*).

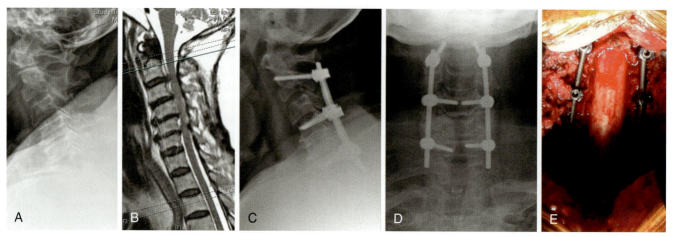

FIGURE 34-3 A 70-year-old man presented with posttraumatic cervical spinal cord compression with reduced cervical kyphosis. Preoperative cervical spine radiograph (**A**) and magnetic resonance imaging (**B**). **C** and **D**, C2, C4, and C6 pedicle screw fixation after C2 dome osteotomy and C3 to C6 laminectomies. **E**, Intraoperative image of C2 dome osteotomy with C3 to C6 laminectomies using C2, C4, and C6 pedicle screw fixation and fusion.

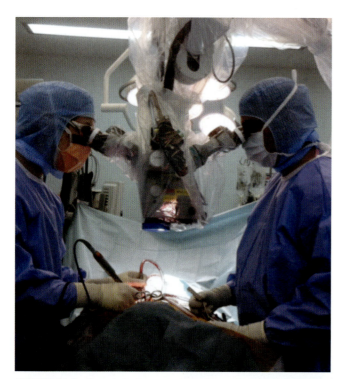

FIGURE 34-4 A surgical microscope is used to perform the laminectomy. Direct vision of the surgical field under magnification reduces iatrogenic dural injuries and gives better control of hemostasis.

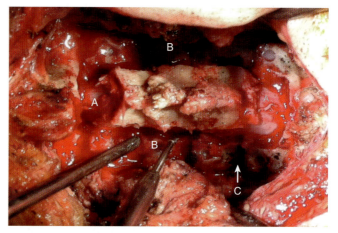

FIGURE 34-5 *A* shows en bloc removal of the ligamentum flavum at the interlaminar levels above and below the laminectomies. A 3-mm MH Midas Rex MR7 high-speed pneumatic burr (Medtronic, Minneapolis, Minn.) is used to create a gutter at the lamina-facet junction at both side of the laminectomy (*B*). The lamina is removed en bloc after careful dissection of the dural adhesion on the undersurface of the lamina with a number 4 Penfield instrument. The lamina is morselized and used as local bone graft. Each facet joint is decorticated using the burr and is packed with local bone graft for facet fusion before instrumentation (*C*).

microscope should be strongly considered for this surgical procedure. The microscope allows clear vision of the surgical field under magnification to reduce iatrogenic dura injury and to improve hemostasis and finer control of the bony aspects of the procedure.

A bone rongeur is used to remove the interspinous ligaments at the interlaminar levels above and below the laminectomies (Fig. 34-5, *A*). With a short, ball-tip nerve hook used to create a plane between the ligamentum flavum and the dura, a 1- to 2-mm Kerrison rongeur is then used to remove the flavum and expose the dura. The authors prefer to perform the laminectomies in an en bloc manner. The lamina is removed in one piece instead

of in pieces with the Kerrison rongeur, and by minimizing the use of the Kerrison rongeur between the lamina and the spinal cord in a stenotic environment, this reduces spinal cord injury.

To perform the en bloc laminectomy, two lamina gutters are created on both sides of the lamina at the lamina-facet junction. A 30-mm MH Midas Rex MR7 high-speed pneumatic burr (Medtronic, Minneapolis, Minn.) is used to create the gutter at the lamina-facet junction (Fig. 34-5, *B*). The burr tip is angled medially toward the lamina and perpendicular to it. This burr trajectory ensures a clean cut at the lamina-facet junction. Care should be taken not to angle the burr tip vertically down toward the lamina and the facet because this cuts into the facet and the lateral mass and results in an undefined lamina cut (Fig. 34-6).

Each lamina is thickest at its cephalad and caudal ends. Therefore the authors recommend that additional

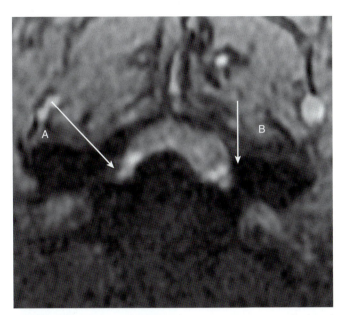

FIGURE 34-6 *A* shows the correct burr trajectory to create the lateral gutter for the laminectomy. The burr tip is angled medially and perpendicular to the lamina. *B* shows the incorrect burr trajectory to create the lateral gutter for the laminectomy. The burr tip is angled vertically down toward the lamina and the facet. This trajectory cuts into the facet and the lateral mass and results in an undefined lamina cut.

attention be given to first burring out the tricortical ends of the lamina. Frequently, this can help reduce some of the difficulties encountered when attempting to remove the lamina en bloc. This surgical step also helps the surgeon mentally to align each lamina cut and allows an overall straight gutter cut. The burr is then used first to remove the white outer table of the lamina, then deeper to remove the red cancellous bone, and finally to thin out, without breaking, the whitish-gray inner table of the lamina. This sequence avoids traumatic burr injury to the nerve roots. Copious normal saline irrigation through a syringe at the burr tip is recommended to remove the bone dust for clear vision during the gutter cut, to reduce heat-induced nerve root injury by the burr, and to lessen any potential traumatic nerve injury should the burr tip breach the inner table.

A ball-tip nerve hook is used to dissect the epidural veins away from the inner table of the lamina and the flavum at the gutter. The inner table and the flavum are then cut by a 1-mm Kerrison rongeur. This maneuver reduces troublesome bleeding from the epidural vein. The epidural veins often become hyperemic in the setting of acute posttraumatic spinal cord injury; a hemostatic matrix sealant agent (FLOSEAL; Baxter, Deerfield, Ill.) and a cell saver to recycle the blood are useful in managing the intraoperative blood loss. When epidural bleeding at the gutter becomes difficult to control, the authors notice that the bleeding often subsides with the reduction of epidural pressure on quick completion of the laminectomy.

After the gutter cut is completed on one side of the lamina, the gutter cut at the lamina-facet junction is commenced on the opposite side of the lamina. Instead of using the Kerrison rongeur to cut the inner table of the lamina and induce epidural bleeding, the inner table of the second lamina gutter can be gently fractured off in a controlled osteoclastic manner by slowly lifting up the

lamina from the side of the gutter that was completely cut open. A large, angled curet is placed under the lamina at the gutter where the inner table was cut open. As the angled curet is lifted up under the cut lamina, the surgeon can use his or her thumb to push the spinous process gently away from the curet to fracture off the inner table of the lamina at the opposite gutter. A number 4 Penfield instrument is used to dissect the dural adhesion carefully from the undersurface of the lamina, and the entire lamina is removed in an en bloc fashion. At all times, the surgeon must keep the angled curet at the undersurface of the lamina, to prevent the sudden downward recoil of the lamina and spinal cord injury.

The lamina is morselized and is used as local bone graft for spinal fusion. Each facet joint and the lateral mass are decorticated using the burr, and the local bone graft is placed within the facet joint before instrumentation. Two 3.5-mm lordotic contoured rods are applied to the screws. The remaining local bone graft is then packed beneath and lateral to the rods, to secure spinal fusion (Fig. 34-7). A cross-link between the two rod systems may be placed to avoid potential dynamic infolding of the posterior cervical muscle or postlaminectomy membrane into the spinal cord, with resulting postlaminectomy spinal cord compression.

A single low-suction drain is used. A four- to five-multilayer posterior cervical muscle closure using interrupted 1.0 polyglactin 910 (Vicryl) suture is recommended. This technique reduces surgical dead space, postoperative bleeding, and wound infection and provides better muscle function preservation. The authors place 1 g of vancomycin powder prophylactically in the muscle and subcutaneous layers of the posterior surgical wound in patients at risk of postoperative wound infections. Patients at risk include those whose surgical procedures last for more than 4 hours, patients undergoing revision surgical procedure, and patients who are immunocompromised.[15]

After the surgical procedure, a soft cervical collar is applied to the patient for comfort. The patient is taught to perform trapezius and rotator cuff stretching exercises to reduce postoperative upper back discomfort. The surgical drain is removed when the drain output is less than 50 mL, to reduce the risk of postoperative epidural hematoma.

Complications

Postoperative complications after laminectomy and fusion may be related to the lamina removal technique or spinal instrumentation. Lateral mass screw insertion may cause less surgical morbidity when compared with cervical pedicle screw insertion. C5 palsy resulting in postoperative deltoid weakness is a specific complication of the posterior cervical surgical approach. The incidence of self-limiting C5 palsy may range from 5% to 12%. Patients at risk for postoperative C5 palsy may include those with preoperative C4-C5 foraminal stenosis, C4-C5 T2-weighted MRI spinal cord signal change, or myelopathic symptoms for more than 12 months preoperatively. Prophylactic bilateral posterior C4-C5 foraminotomies performed together with laminectomy and spinal fusion may reduce the incidence of postoperative C5 palsy.[16]

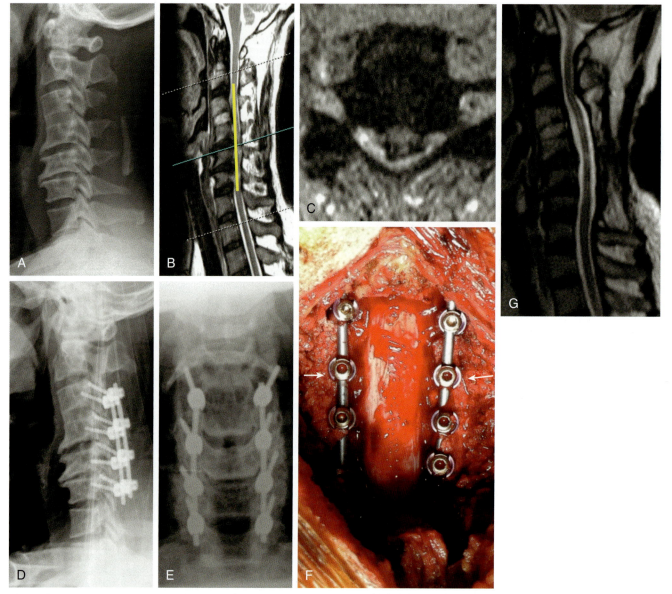

FIGURE 34-7 A 69-year-old man presented with chronic neck pain, K-line–negative, multilevel spinal cord compression with cervical myelopathy. **A,** Preoperatively, the patient has reduced cervical lordosis. **B,** K-line–negative alignment is seen on magnetic resonance imaging (MRI). **C,** Axial view shows spinal cord compression by the disko-osteophytic complex anteriorly. **D** and **E,** Postoperative radiographs of C3 to C6 laminectomies with lateral mass screw fixation. **F,** Intraoperative image of C3 to C6 laminectomies with lateral mass screw fixation. The *arrows* mark the application of local bone graft placed beneath and lateral to the rods, in additional to the facet bone graft, to ensure fusion. **G,** Postoperative MRI showing the decompressed spinal cord.

Results

Cunningham and associates, in a systematic literature review from 1980 to 2008, concluded that neurologic recovery was similar in patients who underwent surgical procedures using either an anterior cervical or a posterior cervical approach.[17] Chen and colleagues reported postoperative results for an average of 4.8 years; the results showed that 71% of the 83 patients studied had good neurologic improvement after laminectomy and fusion for the treatment of cervical myelopathy resulting from OPLL. Postoperative nerve root palsy was the main complication in the study.[18]

In another systematic review using a Cochrane database, Anderson and co-workers concluded that postoperative functional recovery is similar after both laminectomy and laminoplasty for patients with CSM and OPLL. In contrast to laminectomy, postoperative kyphotic spinal deformity does not occur after laminectomy and spinal fusion.[19] Woods and colleagues, in a retrospective matched cohort study of 121 patients, reported that neck pain and gait improvements were similar after either laminoplasty or laminectomy and spinal fusion. Patients who underwent laminectomy and spinal fusion appeared to have more postoperative complications when compared with patients who underwent laminoplasty.[17,20,21]

In a report from a prospective multicenter AOSpine International study of CSM involving 174 patients, the trend was toward better improvement in modified Japanese Orthopaedic Association (mJOA) and Neck Disability Index (NDI) scores in patients who underwent laminoplasty than in those who underwent laminectomy and spinal fusion. However, the study did not include cervical sagittal spinal alignment as a variable factor in influencing the outcome.[22] Further subgroup analysis including sagittal cervical spinal alignment may affect the surgical outcome between laminoplasty and laminectomy and spinal fusion. Fujiyoshi and colleagues reported that, in patients with K-line–negative or kyphotic OPLL, those who underwent laminectomy and spinal fusion had better outcomes than did patients who underwent laminoplasty.[5]

REFERENCES

1. Clark C: *The cervical spine*, ed 4, Philadelphia, 2005, Lippincott Williams & Wilkins.
2. Rhee J M, Riew K D: Evaluation and management of neck pain, radiculopathy, and myelopathy, *Semin Spine Surg* 17:174–185, 2005.
3. Ratliff J K, Cooper P R: Cervical laminoplasty: a critical review, *J Neurosurg* 98(Suppl):S230–S238, 2003.
4. Fujiyoshi T, Yamazaki M, Kawabe J, et al.: A new concept for making decisions regarding the surgical approach for cervical ossification of the posterior longitudinal ligament: the K-line, *Spine (Phila Pa 1976)* 33:E990–E993, 2008.
5. Fujiyoshi T, Yamazaki M, Konishi H, et al.: *The outcome of posterior decompression surgery for patients with cervical myelopathy due to the K-line (–) type OPLL: laminoplasty vs posterior decompression with instrumented fusion. Presented at the 37th annual meeting of the Cervical Spine Research Society (CSRS), Salt Lake City, 2009.*
6. Yonenobu K, Oda T: Posterior approach to the degenerative cervical spine, *Eur Spine J* 12(Suppl):S195–S201, 2003.
7. Rao R D, Gourab K, Kenny S D: Operative treatment of cervical spondylotic myelopathy, *J Bone Joint Surg Am* 88:1619–1640, 2006.
8. Liu G, Buchowski J, Bunmaprasert T, et al.: Revision surgery following cervical laminoplasty: etiology and treatment strategies, *Spine (Phila Pa 1976)* 34:2760–2768, 2009.
9. Taniyama T, Hirai T, Enomoto M, et al: Modified K-line in MRI predicts insufficient decompression of cervical laminoplasty. Presented at the 40th annual meeting of the Cervical Spine Research Society (CSRS), Chicago, 2012.
10. Takeuchi K, Yokoyama T, Aburakawa S, et al.: Axial symptoms after cervical laminoplasty with C3 laminectomy compared with conventional C3-C7 laminoplasty, *Spine (Phila Pa 1976)* 30:2544–2549, 2005.
11. Hosono N, Sakaura H, Mukai Y, et al.: En bloc laminoplasty without dissection of paraspinal muscles, *J Neurosurg* 3:29–33, 2005.
12. Abumi k, Itoh H, Taneichi H, et al.: Transpedicular screw fixation for traumatic lesions of the middle and lower cervical spine: description of the techniques and preliminary report, *J Spinal Disord* 7:19–28, 1994.
13. Rao R D, Marawar S V, Stemper B D, et al.: Computerized tomographic morphometric analysis of subaxial cervical spine pedicles in young asymptomatic volunteers, *J Bone Joint Surg Am* 90: 1914–1921, 2008.
14. Yukawa Y, Kato F, Yoshihara H, et al.: Cervical pedicle screw fixation in 100 cases of unstable cervical injuries: pedicle axis views obtained using fluoroscopy, *J Neurosurg Spine* 5:488–493, 2006.
15. Caroom C, Tullar J, Jones J: Intra-wound vancomycin powder reduces surgical site infections in posterior cervical fusion. Presented at the 40th annual meeting of the Cervical Spine Research Society (CSRS), Chicago, 2012.
16. Liu G, Yeom JS, Shen HX, Riew RD: Is C5 palsy following cervical laminoplasty preventable by bilateral foraminotomy? Presented at the 35th annual meeting of the Cervical Spine Research Society (CSRS), San Francisco, 2007.
17. Cunningham M R, Hershman S, Bendo J: Systematic review of cohort studies comparing surgical treatments for cervical spondylotic myelopathy, *Spine (Phila Pa 1976)* 35:537–543, 2010.
18. Chen Y, Guo Y, Chen D, et al.: Long term outcome of laminectomy and instrumented fusion for cervical ossification of the posterior longitudinal ligament, *Int Orthop* 33:1075–1080, 2009.
19. Anderson P, Mats P, Groff M, et al.: Laminectomy and fusion for the treatment of cervical degenerative myelopathy, *J Neurosurg Spine* 11:150–156, 2009.
20. Heller J G, Edward C C II, Murakami H, et al.: Laminoplasty versus laminectomy and fusion for multilevel cervical myelopathy: an independent matched cohort analysis, *Spine (Phila Pa 1976)* 26:1330–1336, 2001.
21. Woods B, Hohl J, Lee J, et al.: Laminoplasty versus laminectomy and fusion for multilevel cervical spondylotic myelopathy, *Clin Orthop Relat Res*(469)688–695, 2011.
22. Fehlings M, et al: Laminoplasty vs. laminectomy and fusion to treat cervical spondylotic myelopathy: outcomes of the prospective multicenter AOSpine International CSM Study. Presented at the 40th annual meeting of the Cervical Spine Research Society (CSRS), Chicago, 2012.

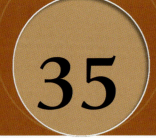

35

Cervical Laminoplasty

Benjamin F. Sandberg, Dino Samartzis, and Francis H. Shen

CHAPTER PREVIEW

Chapter Synopsis

Many techniques have been developed for the surgical management of compressive cervical myelopathy. Laminoplasty is a posterior canal expanding procedure that in selected patients allows for spinal cord decompression, avoids the loss of cervical range of motion, maintains spinal stability without the need for spinal fusion, and potentially avoids the complications associated with scar membrane formation. Various laminoplasty techniques have been developed; however, the two most commonly described and investigated are the open-door and French-door techniques. The purpose of this chapter is to review the indications for surgery, surgical techniques, and complications and outcomes of cervical laminoplasty.

Important Points

Regardless of the specific technique described, the goal of cervical laminoplasty is to expand the spinal canal while maintaining structural stability and alignment by repositioning the lamina.

By preserving the posterior elements and muscular attachments, the risk of postlaminectomy kyphosis, loss of motion, and adjacent segment degeneration is decreased with cervical laminoplasty.

Postoperative C5 palsy is a known complication of posterior cervical laminoplasty.

Surgical and Clinical Pearls

Whenever possible, the facet joints, facet capsule, and extensor attachments to C2 should be preserved to reduce the risk of junctional kyphosis.

If foraminotomies are considered, they should be performed before the laminoplasty on the hinge side and after the laminoplasty on the open side.

Early postoperative range of motion may reduce the risk of postoperative axial neck pain.

Surgical and Clinical Pitfalls

Laminoplasty should not be performed in patients with kyphotic cervical sagittal alignment.

Patients with a large component of preoperative neck pain should be carefully counseled preoperatively and may have a relative contraindication to laminoplasty.

Care should be taken during opening of the laminoplasty to prevent fracture of the hinge side trough.

Many techniques have been developed for the surgical management of compressive cervical myelopathy. They can be divided into anterior, posterior, and circumferential procedures. In the patient with neutral to lordotic cervical sagittal alignment, posterior decompressive procedures remain a good surgical option.[1-4] Available posterior cervical procedures include laminoforaminotomy, laminectomy, laminectomy and fusion, and laminoplasty.

Although laminoforaminotomy procedures are a viable surgical option for the management of cervical radiculopathy, they are not adequate for the management of myelopathy and symptomatic spinal cord compression.

Laminectomy alone, without stabilization, has fallen out of favor because of the risk of postlaminectomy kyphosis and associated neural compression. As a result, laminectomy and fusion and laminoplasty remain the primary posterior surgical options for the management of cervical myelopathy.

Although laminectomy and fusion remain excellent techniques for management of cervical myelopathy, by definition the inclusion of spinal fusion along with instrumentation results in the loss of cervical motion. Furthermore, although controversial, the development of postlaminectomy membrane has been identified as a potential source of late neurologic regression. As a result, laminoplasty has evolved in an attempt to address these concerns.

In selected patients, laminoplasty allows for spinal cord decompression, avoids the loss of cervical range of motion (ROM), maintains spinal stability without the need for spinal fusion, and potentially avoids the complications associated with scar membrane formation.[1-4] Various techniques have been developed; however, the two most commonly described and investigated are the open-door and French-door techniques (Figs. 35-1 and 35-2).[5,6] The purpose of this chapter is to review the indications for surgery, surgical techniques, and complications and outcomes of cervical laminoplasty.

History and Examination Findings

The history and examination of the patient for a cervical laminoplasty are analogous to those in any other patient with cervical myelopathy or myeloradiculopathy and are covered more fully in Chapters 13 and 14, respectively. In the history, patients classically report gradually progressive changes in gait and upper extremity clumsiness. Patients may describe weakness or stiffness in the lower extremities or difficulty with fine motor skills manifested by changes in handwriting or difficulty with buttons or zippers. Bowel dysfunction and bladder dysfunction are late findings and are rarely presenting symptoms. Neck stiffness and axial neck pain are commonly associated nonspecific findings, but it is important to address the proportion of pain resulting from facet arthrosis or disk degeneration because this will not be improved by surgical treatment.[1,3]

The physical examination is directed at determining the pattern of deficits, namely upper motor neuron dysfunction, manifested by weakness and incoordination in the upper and lower extremities. Gait examination is critical and classically demonstrates stiffness or spasticity. Hyperreflexia and pathologic reflexes such as the Babinski sign and patellar clonus are supportive findings. Examination maneuvers such as heel-toe walking, repetitively making a fist, or holding finger adduction and extension can elicit myelopathic signs. Particular attention should be paid to deltoid function preoperatively because postoperative C5 root palsy is a known complication of all cervical spine procedures, and in particular with posterior canal expanding procedures such as laminoplasty and laminectomy and fusion.[7]

Several scoring methods have been developed to standardize the assessment of cervical spondylotic myelopathy. The Japanese Orthopedic Association's (JOA) scoring system is the most frequently used, with higher scores

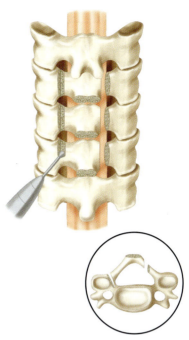

FIGURE 35-1 Schematic drawing of open-door laminoplasty. Note the open complete trough on one side and an incomplete hinge trough on the contralateral side. (From Lee YP, Patel N, Garfin SR: Cervical spondylosis–spinal stenosis: laminoplasty versus laminectomy and fusion. In Jandial R, Garvin SR, editors: *Best evidence for spine surgery: 20 cardinal cases.* Philadelphia, 2012, Saunders.)

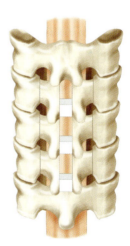

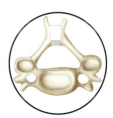

FIGURE 35-2 Schematic drawing of French-door laminoplasty. Note the sagittal split down the midline of the spinous process held open with bone and incomplete hinge troughs on both sides. (From Lee YP, Patel N, Garfin SR: Cervical spondylosis–spinal stenosis: laminoplasty versus laminectomy and fusion. In Jandial R, Garvin SR, editors: *Best evidence for spine surgery: 20 cardinal cases.* Philadelphia, 2012, Saunders.)

relating to greater disability. The modified JOA score was developed and is frequently used in Western societies because the original JOA system includes considerations such as the ability to use chopsticks.[8,9]

Imaging Studies

Initial imaging should begin with anteroposterior and lateral plain upright cervical radiographs. Coronal and sagittal alignment should be noted. Because posterior cervical canal expanding procedures rely on posterior spinal cord drift to achieve decompression, lordotic sagittal alignment is required. Patients with kyphotic alignment will not achieve sufficient decompression because of continued anterior compression even after laminoplasty.[10] Neutral sagittal alignment remains a relative contraindication and should be considered on an individualized basis. Lateral upright flexion and extension cervical radiographs are also valuable and may identify the presence of hypermobility, cervical spondylolisthesis, or other evidence of cervical instability that may preclude proceeding with primary cervical laminoplasty (Figs. 35-3 and 35-4).

Although scoliotic deformity in the coronal plane is not an absolute contraindication to laminoplasty, it should be considered a relative contraindication. Limited information is available to determine whether appropriate posterior spinal cord drift can occur in a patient with substantial cervical scoliosis but with maintained lordosis. These cases should be considered on an individual basis as well.

Magnetic resonance imaging remains the advanced imaging study of choice. In patients with cervical myelopathy, magnetic resonance imaging may reveal evidence of myelomalacia (Fig. 35-5). In addition, careful attention should be paid to sagittal alignment and the location and level of compression. As discussed earlier, kyphotic sagittal alignment is a contraindication to proceeding with cervical laminoplasty. In addition, the number of levels of compression is important to assess. Patients with three levels or more of compression may benefit from a posteriorly based decompressive procedure.[4] The surgeon should also carefully determine whether the compression is anterior, posterior, or circumferential.

In general, the surgical approach should address the site of the compressive disorder. For example, a large one- or two-level anterior cervical disk herniation may be best addressed with an anterior spine surgical procedure, rather than posterior laminoplasty. One exception may be if the anterior compression is secondary to ossification of the posterior longitudinal ligament (OPLL).[8] In these cases, provided the sagittal alignment is lordotic, the preference of some surgeons may still be to perform a posteriorly based canal expanding procedure. The pathophysiology, challenges, and concerns of managing OPLL are covered more completely in Chapter 16.

A computed tomography scan, with or without myelography, may have benefit in selected cases. It can help determine whether the compression is bony or ligamentous. In patients who have undergone previous surgical procedures, or when a question of congenital bony malformations arises, computed tomography scans can better define the bony anatomy and identify conditions

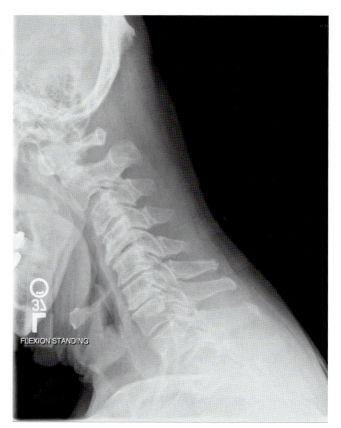

FIGURE 35-3   Preoperative flexion lateral radiograph of the cervical spine.

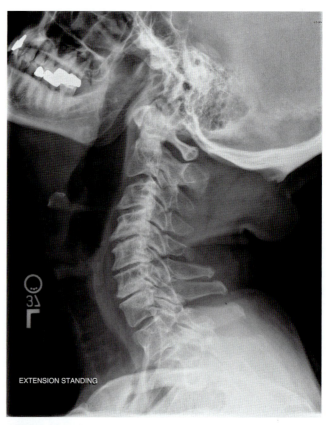

FIGURE 35-4   Preoperative extension lateral radiograph of the cervical spine.

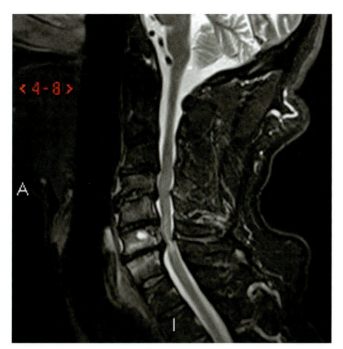

FIGURE 35-5   Preoperative T2-weighted sagittal magnetic resonance imaging of cervical spine. Notice the evidence of spinal cord signal change, particularly at C6 to C7.

that may preclude laminoplasty as a surgical option.[11] However, the use of this imaging modality in routine laminoplasty is not necessary.

Indications and Contraindications

Indications

- Cervical myelopathy or myeloradiculopathy
- Multilevel cervical spondylosis with resultant spinal cord compression
- Symptomatic OPLL
- Cervical canal stenosis narrower than 12 mm in anteroposterior diameter[2]

Contraindications

- Kyphotic deformity
- Predominant neck pain symptoms
- One- or two-level disease[3]
- OPLL with established kyphosis, hypermobility, evidence of cervical spondylolisthesis, or other evidence of cervical instability[4]

Relative Contraindications

- Neutral sagittal spinal alignment
- Coronal plane scoliotic deformity
- Rheumatoid arthritis

Overview of Current Types of Laminoplasty

Although several types of laminoplasty have been described, they can be broadly divided into the two categories of open-door and French-door techniques. In both techniques, hinges are formed at the junction of the lateral mass and the lamina. The lamina is expanded laterally or in the midline in the open-door and French-door techniques, respectively. Regardless of the surgical technique described, the goal of cervical laminoplasty is to perform decompression of the spinal cord by repositioning the lamina while maintaining structural stability and alignment of at the spine.

By preserving the posterior elements and muscular attachments, the risk of postlaminectomy kyphosis, loss of motion, and adjacent segment degeneration is decreased.[3,12] In addition, this technique may allow for earlier mobilization and rehabilitation compared with other surgical options while avoiding graft-related complications such as graft fracture, extrusion, dislodgment, and settling. By preserving the lamina, the risk of postoperative scar that is frequently seen after laminectomy is avoided, as is the potential development of postlaminectomy membrane. As discussed earlier, laminoplasty does not address neck pain, and in fact it may even aggravate those symptoms, particularly in the immediate postoperative period as a result of extensive muscle dissection.

In open-door laminoplasty, the spinal canal is expanded by placing a complete (opening) trough on one side and a partial greenstick trough on the contralateral (hinge) side. In general, the opening side of the lamina is usually placed on the more symptomatic (stenotic) side, or the side with the worse radicular symptoms. The trough is made at the junction of the lamina and lateral mass junction. Care should be taken not to violate the facet joint capsule. Once the troughs have been made, the lamina is gently opened to the desired degree.[5]

The original expansive open-door laminoplasty technique used sutures to hold the hinge open and maintain the decompression (Fig. 35-6). This technique remains in use, but it can be complicated by a "spring back" phenomenon and subsequent neurologic deterioration.[13] In an attempt to address this complication, bone grafts, hydroxyapatite, and other spacers have been developed to maintain patency of the open door. Hydroxyapatite spacers have been shown to have equal bone bonding and fusion rates as autograft, and neurologic recovery rates are similar to those in other reports using traditional laminoplasty.[14,15] Finally, titanium miniplates have been used either alone or in conjunction with the various spacers; however, they can be associated with increased operative time, blood loss, and other potential complications.[16]

Conversely, the French-door technique uses a midline sagittal split of the spinous processes to decompress the spinal cord and an incomplete hinge trough on both sides (Fig. 35-7). The technique was introduced by Kurokawa and uses bone blocks between the halves of the spinous process to maintain decompression.[6] Hydroxyapatite spacers and anchor sutures have also been used as alternatives to autograft.

Surgical Technique

Patient Positioning

The setup for cervical laminoplasty is similar to that for other posterior cervical procedures and should be based

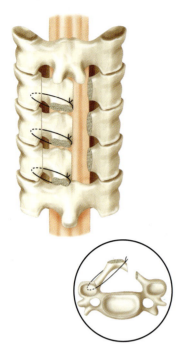

FIGURE 35-6 Schematic of open-door laminoplasty with wiring though the facet joint and lamina to hold the laminoplasty open. (From Lee YP, Patel N, Garfin SR: Cervical spondylosis–spinal stenosis: laminoplasty versus laminectomy and fusion. In Jandial R, Garvin SR, editors: *Best evidence for spine surgery: 20 cardinal cases.* Philadelphia, 2012, Saunders.)

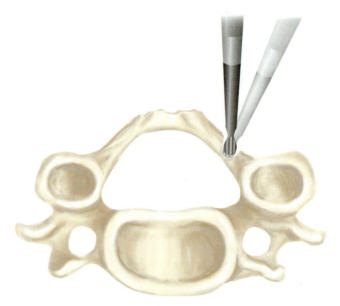

FIGURE 35-8 Perform trough at the lamina-facet junction. Notice that if the burr is positioned too vertically and too laterally, the trough can enter the medial edge of the lateral mass. This can result in excessive bleeding from the cancellous edge of the lateral mass or on the hinge side, with difficulty in opening the lamina. This complication can be prevented by either holding the burr more perpendicular to the lamina or placing the trough slightly more medially. (From Brown C, Lowenstein JE, Yoon TS: Cervical laminoplasty. In Vaccaro AR, Baron EM, editors: *Operative techniques: spine surgery,* Philadelphia, 2008, Saunders.)

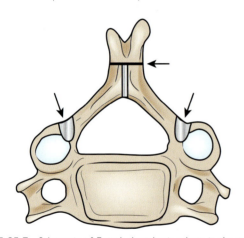

FIGURE 35-7 Schematic of French-door laminoplasty in the axial plane demonstrating the location of the sagittal split and troughs.

Exposure

A longitudinal midline incision is made from the C2 to C7 spinous processes.

The subcutaneous fat and deep cervical fascia are dissected, exposing the nuchal ligament, which is then divided in the midline, with care taken to protect the supraspinous and interspinous ligaments. Staying within the midline in the nuchal ligament helps to decrease bleeding.

The lamina is exposed by dissecting subperiosteally from the spinous process to the lateral mass. Care is taken to protect the facet capsule, the soft tissue attachments to the facet joints, and the extensor muscle attachments of the C2 spinous process. This aspect is important to help reduce the risk of junctional kyphosis and segmental instability. The senior author prefers to preserve the spinous processes whenever possible.

Laminoplasty

Depending on the laminoplasty technique described, either an open (complete) trough or hinge (incomplete) trough is made on each side. This is performed at the lamina-facet junction (Fig. 35-8). The complete trough is typically made with a combination of a burr and a Kerrison rongeur. The lamina is thinned until a 1- or 2-mm Kerrison rongeur can be safely passed. The ligamentum is gently divided at each level.

In the case of the hinge trough, the outer cortex is sequentially thinned with a burr. Once troughs are completed on both sides, the ligamentum flavum is divided at the superior and inferior aspect of the laminoplasty, and the lamina is carefully hinged open. This can be performed using a combination of an angled curet under the

on the surgeon's preference and individualized to the patient. At the authors' institution, the radiolucent table with a Mayfield attachment is used. Consideration for fiberoptic intubation and neurophysiologic monitoring should be performed according to the protocol of the institution and the surgeon. The operating table should be placed in the reverse Trendelenburg position. This allows for improved visualization and decreases bleeding. The patient's shoulders are taped, and imaging is obtained as needed to confirm visualization.

Head positioning varies. However, neutral positioning during the surgical procedure prevents excessive spinal cord compression while allowing for increased space between the lamina and improving the ability to complete the troughs and perform any necessary foraminotomies.

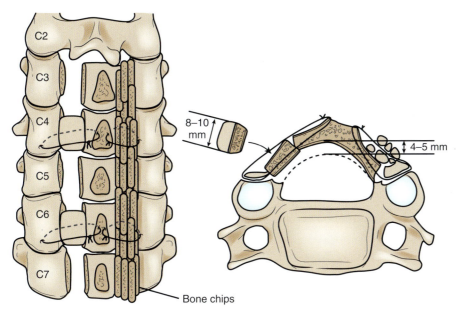

FIGURE 35-9 Example of a structural bone block placed to hold the laminoplasty open.

lamina on the open side, or on the spinous process in the French-door technique. The multiple fine attachments commonly found from the dura to the undersurface of the lamina are carefully dissected free as necessary.

The hinge side trough can be deepened as necessary to help open up the laminoplasty; however, care should be taken to do this sequentially, to avoid inadvertent fracture of the lamina on the hinge side. If this occurs, plating systems exist to achieve fixation of the hinge side back to the lamina-facet junction. If the French-door technique is being used, the base of the spinous processes is split sagittally down to the inner cortex. In this case, bilateral hinge troughs are created to allow for opening of the lamina from the midline.

Foraminotomy

Occasionally, foraminotomy may be required in addition to laminoplasty. This may be indicated for patients with myeloradiculopathy with significant neuroforaminal stenosis. Because of the association of C5 root palsy with posterior canal expanding procedures, some surgeons have advocated performing bilateral C4-C5 foraminotomies. The argument for routine prophylactic decompression, however, remains controversial.

If a foraminotomy is being considered, typically performing it on the open trough side of the laminoplasty is easiest. This procedure is usually performed after the lamina is elevated and the laminoplasty is complete. If the foraminotomy must be performed on the hinge side, then consideration should be given to performing it before the laminoplasty. Performing the foraminotomy after the laminoplasty on the hinge side places the lamina at risk of fracturing. Care should be taken to preserve at least 50% of the facet joint to reduce the risk of instability. A more complete description of posterior cervical keyhole laminoforaminotomy is given in Chapter 36.

Spacers and Fixation Techniques

The use of bone graft or other mechanical spacers varies and has included autologous spinous process, allograft iliac crest bone graft, rib, and biologic spacers such as hydroxyapatite (Fig. 35-9).[14,15,17] The addition of fixation

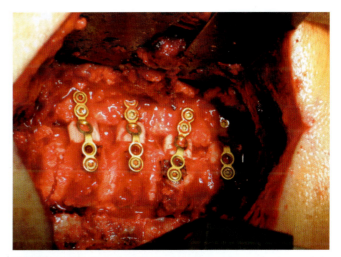

FIGURE 35-10 Example of laminoplasty plate and screw implants to help secure bone in place and maintain the laminoplasty. (From Kim PD, Bae H: Posterior cervical laminoplasty. In Vaccaro AR, Baron EM, editors: *Operative techniques: spine surgery*, ed 2, Philadelphia, 2012, Saunders.)

includes the use of wiring and plate and screw constructs (Fig. 35-10). These techniques were developed to help address the concern for repeat closure of the laminoplasty site. The decision whether to include the use of a spacer and mechanical fixation varies from patient to patient and on the experience and preference of the surgeon. Newer descriptions use plate fixation without any bone on the opening trough side (Fig. 35-11).

Closure

Deep drains are placed. The fascia and subcutaneous tissue are closed in layers, and the subcutaneous tissue and skin are closed in a routine manner.

Postoperative Care

Postoperative care has been debated in the literature, in particular with regard to the duration of immobilization following the surgical procedure. Some research has

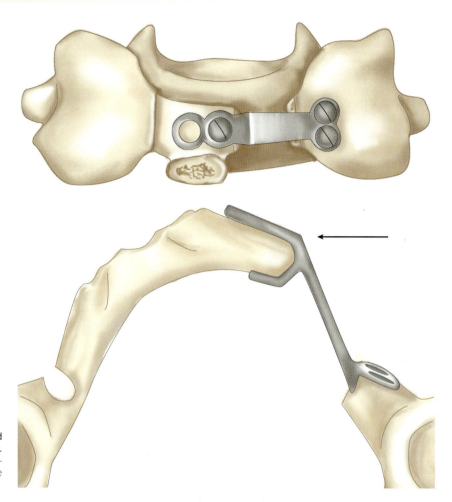

FIGURE 35-11 Example of a laminoplasty plate and screw construct that does not use structural bone. (From Brown C, Lowenstein JE, Yoon TS: Cervical laminoplasty. In Vaccaro AR, Baron EM, editors: *Operative techniques: spine surgery,* Philadelphia, 2008, Saunders.)

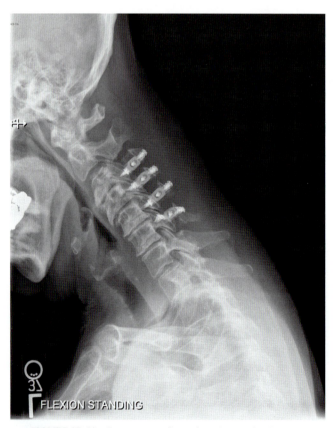

FLEXION STANDING

FIGURE 35-12 Postoperative flexion lateral cervical radiograph.

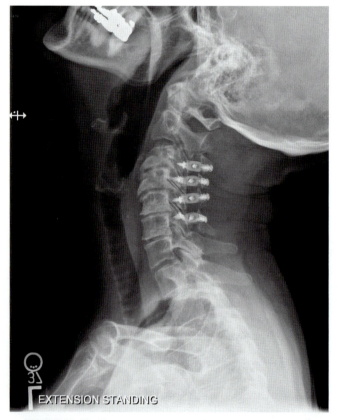

EXTENSION STANDING

FIGURE 35-13 Postoperative extension lateral cervical radiograph.

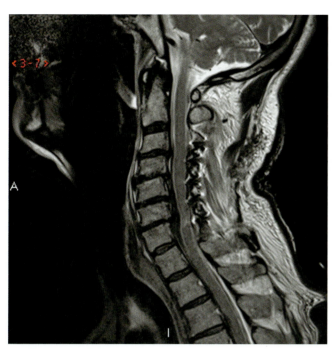

FIGURE 35-14 Sagittal T2-weighted magnetic resonance imaging (MRI) after open-door laminoplasty. The patient was asymptomatic. Notice some residual myelomalacia; however, improvements are evident in spinal cord edema and in space available for the spinal cord compared with preoperative MRI shown in Figure 35-5.

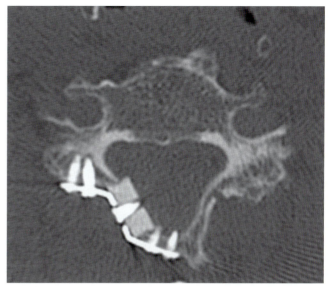

FIGURE 35-15 Axial computed tomography scan after open-door laminoplasty demonstrating good placement of the bone and plate and screw construct with improvement of the sagittal spinal canal diameter.

found a correlation with ROM loss and long-term axial pain symptoms.[18] This finding has led some investigators to encourage early postoperative mobilization, which has been the authors' preference as well (Figs. 35-12 and 35-13). Advanced imaging is not routinely required; however, it can be obtained as needed to assess the decompression, the improvement or persistence of spinal cord signal change, bony osteotomies, and the location of the instrumentation (Figs. 35-14 and 35-15).

Complications

Laminoplasty was developed to avoid the complications of laminectomy that result from loss of the posterior protective elements. However, axial pain, C5 palsy, spinal canal restenosis, and loss of cervical lordosis all complicate laminoplasty and have been the target of many technical improvements.[1]

Axial pain is defined as pain from the nuchal to the periscapular or shoulder region, and its incidence varies widely in the literature from 5.2% to 61.5%.[19] The origin of the increased pain does not appear to be clearly understood. However, early mobilization, reconstruction of the extensor musculature, anatomic reconstruction of semispinalis cervicis, and preservation of the C7 spinous process and its extensor musculature have all been associated with less axial pain, but more research is required to understand the etiology fully.[19]

Postoperative C5 root palsies have been well described after both anterior and posterior spine surgical procedures. In particular, however, these palsies are associated with posterior canal expanding procedures such as laminectomy and fusion and laminoplasty. Clinically, these disorders are defined as loss of deltoid or biceps strength without other neurologic symptoms. The incidence of C5 palsy is also widely variable, with an average of 4.6%.[20] Most patients develop symptoms within 2 weeks of the surgical procedure, but the duration also varies between 15 and 821 days or longer.[20] Prophylactic foraminotomy has been described, but not all investigators agree about its effectiveness.[21]

The incidence of spinal canal restenosis and recurrence of myelopathy has been reported to be as high as 40%, but data are lacking to determine the absolute rate because repeat neuroimaging is infrequently ordered without recurrent symptoms.[1] Radiographic evidence of restenosis does not always correlate with clinical recurrence or progression of symptoms or necessitate additional surgical intervention.

Loss of cervical lordosis and of ROM is noted in virtually all studies of laminoplasty, with a mean decrease in ROM of 50%.[1] Loss of cervical alignment, and in severe cases, more specifically postoperative kyphotic deformity can decrease neurologic recovery by preventing posterior migration of the spinal cord. Patients at high risk for postoperative kyphosis are those with myelopathy associated with cervical spondylosis, preoperative lordosis of less than [10] degrees, and a kyphotic angle during flexion that exceeds the lordotic angle in extension.[10] The combination of all three risk factors was associated with a 66.7% chance of developing postoperative kyphotic deformity.[10]

Results

Laminoplasty is a well-established technique for posterior spinal cord decompression. A significant amount of evidence supports its use in the appropriate clinical situations. Most studies use preoperative and postoperative

JOA scores to calculate neurologic recovery, which quantifies patients' recovery compared with perfect recovery using the following formula:

Recovery rate $(\%)$:

$$\left[\frac{(\text{Postoperative score} - \text{Preoperative score})}{(17 - \text{preoperative score})}\right] \times 100$$

Classic open-door laminoplasty as described by Hirabayashi and colleagues is the most extensively studied procedure and has been shown to have a mean neurologic recovery rate of 60%, with 77% of patients showing improvement.[1] The French-door laminoplasty as described by Kurokawa and associates has also been extensively studied and has a mean neurologic recovery rate of 52%, with 81% of patients showing improvement.[1]

A randomized controlled trial comparing the two techniques failed to demonstrate a difference in neurologic recovery between French-door and open-door techniques. However, axial pain relief and patients' sense of improvement were greater with the French-door rather than with the open-door technique.[1] Neurologic recovery using the open-door technique has been shown to be stable over time, with a recovery rate of 72% at 10 years.[22] However, 44% of patients deteriorated at least one point on the JOA score from maximal neurologic recovery at 10-year follow-up.[22]

Future clinical investigations continue to expand. More specifically, they include correlation of ROM and axial neck pain and optimal postoperative mobilization, role in the preservation of the C7 spinous process, and preservation of the semispinalis cervicis musculature.

REFERENCES

1. Ratliff JK, Cooper PR: Cervical laminoplasty: a critical review, *J Neurosurg* 98:230–238, 2003.
2. Steinmetz MP, Resnick DK: Cervical laminoplasty, *Spine J* 6(Suppl):274S–281S, 2006.
3. Cunningham MR, Hershman S, Bendo J: Systematic review of cohort studies comparing surgical treatments for cervical spondylotic myelopathy, *Spine (Phila Pa 1976)* 35:537–543, 2010.
4. Hale JJ, Gruson KI, Spivak JM: Laminoplasty: a review of its role in compressive cervical myelopathy, *Spine J* 6(Suppl):289S–298S, 2006.
5. Hirabayashi K, Watanabe K, Wakano K, et al.: Expansive open-door laminoplasty for cervical spinal stenotic myelopathy, *Spine (Phila Pa 1976)* 8:693–699, 1983.
6. Yoshida M, Otani K, Shibasaki K, Ueda S: Expansive laminoplasty with reattachment of spinous process and extensor musculature for cervical myelopathy, *Spine (Phila Pa 1976)* 17:491–497, 1992.
7. Takemitsu M, Cheung KM, Wong YW, et al.: C5 nerve root palsy after cervical laminoplasty and posterior fusion with instrumentation, *J Spinal Disord Tech* 21:267–272, 2008.
8. Hirabayashi K, Miyakawa J, Satomi K, et al.: Operative results and postoperative progression of ossification among patients with ossification of cervical posterior longitudinal ligament, *Spine (Phila Pa 1976)* 6:354–364, 1981.
9. Keller A, von Ammon K, Klaiber R, Waespe W: Spondylogenic cervical myelopathy: conservative and surgical therapy, *Schweiz Med Wochenschr* 123:1682–1691, 1993. [in German].
10. Suk KS, Kim KT, Lee JH, et al.: Sagittal alignment of the cervical spine after the laminoplasty, *Spine (Phila Pa 1976)* 32:E656–E660, 2007.
11. Baron EM, Young WF: Cervical spondylotic myelopathy: a brief review of its pathophysiology, clinical course, and diagnosis, *Neurosurgery* 60(Suppl):S35–S41, 2007.
12. Okada M, Minamide A, Endo T, et al.: A prospective randomized study of clinical outcomes in patients with cervical compressive myelopathy treated with open-door or French-door laminoplasty, *Spine (Phila Pa 1976)* 34:1119–1126, 2009.
13. Hirabayashi K, Satomi K: Operative procedure and results of expansive open-door laminoplasty, *Spine (Phila Pa 1976)* 13:870–876, 1988.
14. Tanaka N, Nakanishi K, Fujimoto Y, et al.: Expansive laminoplasty for cervical myelopathy with interconnected porous calcium hydroxyapatite ceramic spacers: comparison with autogenous bone spacers, *J Spinal Disord Tech* 21:547–552, 2008.
15. Kihara S, Umebayashi T, Hoshimaru M: Technical improvements and results of open-door expansive laminoplasty with hydroxyapatite implants for cervical myelopathy, *Neurosurgery* 57:348–356, 2005.
16. O'Brien MF, Peterson D, Casey AT, Crockard HA: A novel technique for laminoplasty augmentation of spinal canal area using titanium miniplate stabilization: a computerized morphometric analysis, *Spine (Phila Pa 1976)* 21:474–483, 1996.
17. Itoh T, Tsuji H: Technical improvements and results of laminoplasty for compressive myelopathy in the cervical spine, *Spine (Phila Pa 1976)* 10:729–736, 1985.
18. Chiba K, Ogawa Y, Ishii K, et al.: Long-term results of expansive open-door laminoplasty for cervical myelopathy: average 14-year follow-up study, *Spine (Phila Pa 1976)* 31:2998–3005, 2006.
19. Wang SJ, Jiang SD, Jiang LS, Dai LY: Axial pain after posterior cervical spine surgery: a systematic review, *Eur Spine J* 20:185–194, 2011.
20. Kaneyama S, Sumi M, Kanatani T, et al.: Prospective study and multivariate analysis of the incidence of C5 palsy after cervical laminoplasty, *Spine (Phila Pa 1976)* 35:E1553–E1558, 2010.
21. Sasai K, Saito T, Akagi S, et al.: Preventing C5 palsy after laminoplasty, *Spine (Phila Pa 1976)* 28:1972–1977, 2003.
22. Sakaura H, Hosono N, Mukai Y, et al.: Long-term outcome of laminoplasty for cervical myelopathy due to disc herniation: a comparative study of laminoplasty and anterior spinal fusion, *Spine (Phila Pa 1976)* 30:756–759, 2005.

36

Posterior Cervical Endoscopic Laminoforaminotomy

Tim E. Adamson

CHAPTER PREVIEW

Chapter Synopsis	The surgical treatment of unilateral cervical radiculopathy with a minimally invasive, microendoscopic technique is reviewed. Important surgical techniques, as well as indications and contraindications, are discussed.
Important Points	Indications:
	Unilateral one- or two-level refractory cervical radiculopathy
	Concordant symptoms and physical examination findings
	Radiographic imaging confirmation of nerve root compression
	Contraindications:
	Bilateral radiculopathy
	Cervical myelopathy
	Alignment abnormalities or instability
Clinical and Surgical Pearls	Sitting position with neck neutral to slightly flexed
	Vertical navigation: "disk level"
	Horizontal navigation: "locating the pedicle"
	Treatment of the symptomatic disorder
Clinical and Surgical Pitfalls	Avoid the interlaminar space when dilating for the cylinder.
	Limit facet resection to 50% or less.
	Limit spinal cord manipulation.
	Be aware of a split rootlet.

The surgical treatment of cervical radiculopathy with posterior cervical laminoforaminotomy has been used for more than 80 years. The original description by Stookey, and the series by Frykholm and Murphey in the 1940s and 1950s, validated the procedure as a safe and effective treatment option.[1] Following the introduction of the anterior approach for anterior cervical decompression and fusion by Cloward, Smith, and Robinson in the 1960s, the anterior approach was rapidly adopted for the treatment of not only radiculopathy but also myelopathy, instability, and alignment abnormalities. Only after time did it become apparent that anterior cervical decompression and fusion had a unique set of complications from the anterior approach and was also associated with a higher rate of developing adjacent-level disease than natural history would suggest.[2] Even though some patients had severe muscle spasm after the posterior approach, the lower incidence of adjacent-level disease and avoidance of the anterior approach risks continued to lead some surgeons to favor its use.[3-5]

In the late 1990s, as spine surgery quickly evolved into minimally invasive techniques, the Microendoscopic Diskectomy (MED) system of Foley and Smith was adapted for cervical use.[6] The author's experience and that of other investigators since that time showed the technique to be very effective for the treatment of cervical radiculopathy, with complication and reoperation rates lower than can be achieved with anterior cervical decompression and fusion.[7-9]

Preoperative Considerations

History

Cervical radiculopathy manifests in patients with a very typical history of neck and arm pain with or without sensory change and weakness affecting a cervical nerve root pattern. The sudden onset of symptoms without a specific inciting event is typical of acute soft disk herniation (Fig. 36-1). A more chronic cyclic pattern with months to years of arm symptoms is typical of spondylotic foraminal stenosis (Fig. 36-2). Because of the common occurrence of recovery without surgical intervention, it is important to carry out a formal period of conservative therapy including antiinflammatory medications, physical therapy, and, frequently, epidural steroid injections. The exception to this approach is the patient who presents with severe weakness or has progression of weakness while undergoing conservative therapy.

Signs and Symptoms

On many occasions, the patient's description of signs and symptoms suggests a specific cervical root pattern. The subjective sensory symptoms are frequently more helpful than the objective changes identified on examination. Symptoms of burning dysesthesias into the thumb are very characteristic of a C6 root disorder, but results of objective light touch and pinprick testing may be unremarkable. Each pattern of pain can usually be matched to a specific root.

Physical Examination

The physical examination frequently confirms an already suspected root disorder, based on the history provided by the patient. The simultaneous finding of a specific motor, sensory, and reflex pattern can be very helpful but is not as common as weakness and reflex change without persistent sensory change. A careful and thorough examination is the most helpful way to identify a specific symptomatic nerve root in a patient with multiple levels of spondylotic foraminal stenosis.

Imaging

Magnetic resonance imaging (MRI) is the most commonly used form of imaging for cervical radiculopathy. The presence of concordant root compression in the lateral canal or medial foramen is an absolute requirement for a patient to be considered a candidate for surgery. As useful as MRI is, it is associated with overestimation of central canal stenosis and frequently does not provide clear axial images of the foramen. In this setting, computed tomography (CT) scanning with intrathecal contrast is very helpful for clear visualization of the foramen. Many foraminal disk herniations missed on MRI are easily seen with CT. Flexion and extension lateral cervical spine radiographs are important whenever concern exists for instability. CT myelography is used in patients with severe spondylosis or a body habitus that limits image quality.

Indications

The presence of refractory unilateral radiculopathy involving one or possibly two adjacent roots is the primary indication for posterior cervical laminoforaminotomy. Imaging studies must confirm concordant nerve root compression in the lateral canal or foramen. Even patients with quite large disk herniations with the apex of the rupture at or lateral to the lateral border of the spinal cord (not the thecal sac) are surgical candidates.

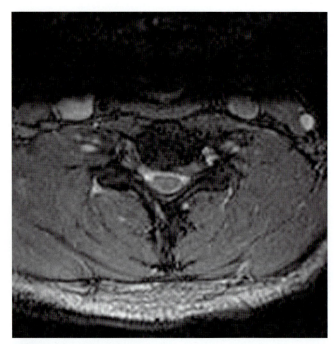

FIGURE 36-1 Axial magnetic resonance imaging demonstrating a left C6-C7 foraminal disk herniation.

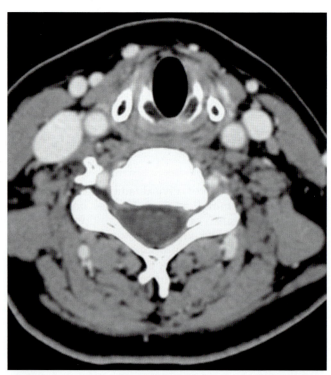

FIGURE 36-2 Axial computed tomography image demonstrating left C5-C6 foraminal spondylotic stenosis.

Contraindications

The presence of bilateral radicular symptoms or myelopathic changes on examination is an absolute contraindication to posterior cervical laminoforaminotomy. Severe alignment abnormalities and instability on flexion and extension are also contraindications. The presence of chronic neck pain or suboccipital headaches is a relative contraindication in that these conditions may not improve without fusion.

Procedure

See Box 36-1.

Anesthesia and Positioning

Balanced general endotracheal anesthesia is used for the procedure. Once induction of anesthesia has occurred, the patient is given a 500-mL normal saline bolus and then is carefully positioned in a semirecumbent sitting position with the head secured in the Mayfield-Kees headholder. The head is placed in neutral rotation and is slightly flexed to straighten the spine but not open the interlaminar space. The table adjustments are then used to orient the neck vertically and to place the operative level at a comfortable position for the surgeon (Fig. 36-3). Sequential compression stockings and end-tidal carbon dioxide monitoring are used, but evoked potential monitoring and ultrasound imaging are not. A C-arm fluoroscopy unit is positioned at the foot of the bed and is placed to provide a lateral projection of the cervical spine from C1 down (Fig. 36-4). The C-arm is incorporated into the sterile draping (Fig. 36-5), to allow for intermittent use throughout the case (averaging 6 to 10 seconds/level).

Operative Technique

One of the primary principles of minimally invasive spine surgery is to orient the procedure in three dimensions without the ability to visualize the anatomy directly. When posterior cervical laminoforaminotomy is performed, this is of utmost importance. The risks of unexpectedly entering the spinal canal and injuring the spinal cord cannot be emphasized enough. In addition, the risk of inadvertently resecting an entire facet joint could predispose the patient to iatrogenic postoperative instability.

The two most important steps in safely and effectively completing the procedure are successful "vertical navigation," to target the symptomatic disk level, followed by "horizontal navigation," which depends on localization of the medial and lateral walls of the pedicle. This procedure ensures confidence that the affected nerve root is adequately decompressed and that no more of the facet is resected than necessary.

Vertical Navigation

At the start of the procedure, a spinal needle is laid against the side of the drapes in line with the C-arm image and is adjusted up and down to coincide with the surgical level.

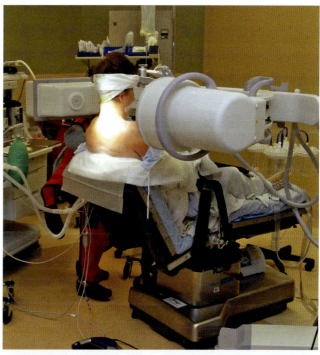

FIGURE 36-3 The sitting position with the head secured in the Mayfield-Kees headholder is used to provide exposure to the posterior cervical spine.

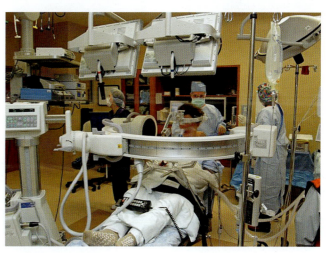

FIGURE 36-4 The fluoroscopy unit is positioned from the foot of the bed to allow lateral imaging counting from C1 caudally.

BOX 36-1 Surgical Steps

Positioning
The sitting position provides the best visualization (fluid drainage).
The patient's neck should be neutral to slightly flexed.

Vertical Navigation: "Disk Level"
Fluoroscopy is used to identify the target disk level.
The trajectory is defined by passing a needle to the cephalad lamina.
The sequential dilators start at the lamina and then shift over the facet.

Horizontal Navigation: "Locating the Pedicle"
Early in the laminoforaminotomy, the pedicle is identified.
This confirms mediolateral orientation and identification of the nerve.

Treating the Pathologic Features
The foraminotomy is enlarged to ensure nerve decompression.
Disk fragments are removed when identified, usually in the axilla.

Closure
Single layer closure of subcutaneous fascia is done with polyglactin 910 (Vicryl).
Skin adhesive is used as a dressing and for closure.

Once the rough alignment is determined, the needle is introduced through the skin approximately one fingerbreadth off the midline to the affected side. The needle is then passed through the muscle, with the target being the cephalad lateral mass (e.g., C5 lateral mass if the operative level is C5-C6). This method provides the safest target and the largest bone surface. Then the author prefers to advance the needle down to the bone with spot fluoroscopy images. Live fluoroscopy can be used but is not really necessary. The ideal trajectory is one the places the tip of the needle slightly cephalad to the entry point. This trajectory facilitates the drainage of blood and irrigation during the procedure. The needle trajectory is then visualized from the outside before it is removed.

Following this, a 16- to 18-mm skin incision is made, centered approximately one fingerbreadth off the midline and placed obliquely or horizontally to correspond to the Langer lines of the level or any existing skin creases. This site aids in a more cosmetic scar after healing. Special attention must be paid to the length of the incision. Too long an incision is not a problem, but when it is less than the diameter of the operative cylinder (15 to 16 mm), the dilators will overstretch the skin and result in a scar that looks somewhat like a smallpox vaccination.

A Kirschner wire (K-wire) is then passed through the incision and along the same path as the spinal needle, again using spot fluoroscopy images. Once the K-wire is docked on the lateral mass, constant mild inward pressure is maintained to keep the tip seated against the bone and to prevent migration. The first dilator is passed carefully over the wire. A combination of inward pressure and rotation is used to seat the dilator against the bone. The K-wire is then removed. The tip of the dilator is then used to carry out subperiosteal stripping of the muscle over the lateral mass and is then shifted caudally to palpate the "step-off" off the facet. Fluoroscopy is used to confirm the level. The superficial and deep facial layers of the neck resist passing the remaining dilators, much more so than in the lumbar spine.

Releasing of the fascia can be accomplished by passing a pair of sharp-tipped scissors along the outside of the dilator and spreading the fascia to release it. The author prefers this method instead of passing a knife along the tract because the knife cuts the fibers rather than displaces them. Once the fascia is released, the remaining dilators are passed, and the operative cylinder is introduced. At this point, using fluoroscopy, the cylinder is shifted caudally over the target disk level (Fig. 36-6). The cylinder is then securely anchored to the table mount.

If the subperiosteal preparation was correctly done, a large pituitary rongeur can be used to remove a small core of muscle at the base of the cylinder that has been freed from the underlying bone and trapped by the tip of the cylinder. Once the core of muscle has been removed, the microendoscope is positioned in the cylinder at the 12-o'clock position to keep it out of the way as much as possible and at the best position to keep it away from pooling blood or irrigation. The endoscope is then

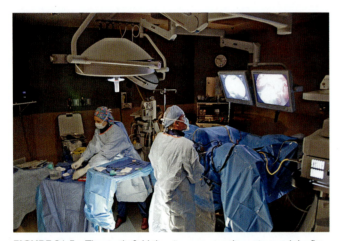

FIGURE 36-5   The sterile field then incorporates the patient and the fluoroscopy unit so that imaging may be performed intermittently throughout the procedure.

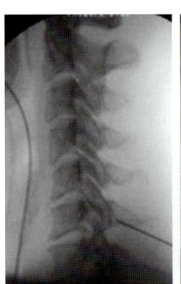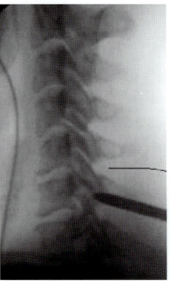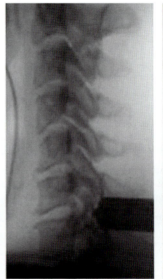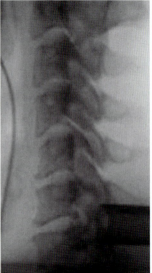

FIGURE 36-6   Lateral fluoroscopy is used to place the Kirschner wire and dilators to the back of the facet complex. The wire and smaller dilators are targeted to the cephalad lateral mass.

oriented so that the screen's up, down, left, and right designations match the position of the patient (Fig. 36-7).

Horizontal Navigation

At this point, the exposed bone of the medial facet at the target level should be identifiable, but the mediolateral orientation may be a challenge. Finding the slope of the cephalad lamina joining with the superior articular process is frequently very helpful, although in patients with extensive spondylosis, it is not always reliable. In those cases, the facet joint may be severely degenerated and not as recognizable, or the patient may have "shingling" in which the cephalad lamina and articular process settle lower over the caudal lamina and articular process. This feature is easily identified on the lateral fluoroscopy image when the "step-off" of the target facet sits caudal to the disk space. If the junction of the lamina and facet is not easily identified, it can be helpful to target more medially and identify the lateral spinal canal first and then work laterally into the foramen, to prevent inadvertently taking too much facet.

A high-speed electric drill with a 2.5-mm round cutting burr is then used to initiate the laminoforaminotomy. The image quality with the endoscope is clear enough to visualize removal of the outer cortex and cancellous bone of the both lateral lamina and into the junction of the facet joint (Fig. 36-8). A thin shell of inner cortex is left in place, except for a small area over the lateral canal in the inferior lamina. Once the epidural space is identified, and a small window is created with the burr, a 2-mm thin-footed Kerrison rongeur is then used to widen the decompression and allow visualization of the underlying margin of the lateral thecal sac and the origin of the nerve root. At this point, the pedicle must be located to complete the horizontal navigation.

A nerve hook is passed lateral from the thecal sac, and the medial wall of the pedicle is palpated. From there, the cephalad margin of the pedicle can be palpated and the foramen located. An additional fluoroscopy image can be used for confirmation. Bony decompression is then finished using the Kerrison rongeur (Fig. 36-9). The nerve root is "unroofed" laterally until a nerve hook placed along the cephalad margin of the pedicle can palpate the caudal curve, thus signifying the lateral margin of the pedicle. At this point, most cases of spondylotic foraminal stenosis have been decompressed, and one third to one half of the medial facet has been removed. In some patients with severe spondylosis and more lateral stenosis, the facet has remodeled so much that it is much wider

or nearly fused. Confirming the anatomic features on the preoperative imaging can frequently allow the decompression to be carried further than the lateral margin of the pedicle, but this should not be done routinely.

Addressing the Pathologic Features

In most cases of spondylosis, completion of the laminoforaminotomy addresses the stenosis. However, in cases of soft disk herniation, the laminoforaminotomy is just the access to the disorder. The safest way to access disk herniation is through the axilla of the nerve root at the lateral edge of the thecal sac. A nerve hook is passed caudally along the medial aspect of the pedicle and is advanced to the floor of the spinal canal. At this point, the nerve hook is rotated medially under the sac and is then rotated cephalad under the origin of the root sleeve and slid laterally along the root. This maneuver is important, especially in the lower levels, which are more likely to have a split rootlet arising from the sac. Failure to identify a split root can result in nerve root damage.

Palpation with the nerve hook is sensitive enough to identify a contained herniation versus a spondylotic spur underlying the root. Extruded fragments can easily be mobilized with the nerve hook and removed with a micropituitary rongeur. Contained herniations sometimes must

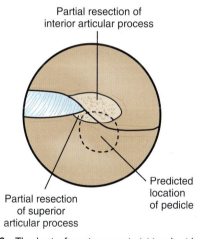

FIGURE 36-8 The laminoforaminotomy is initiated with a high-speed electric drill until a small area over the lateral canal is opened.

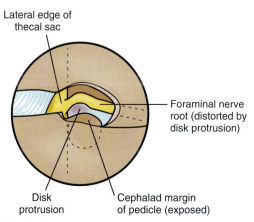

FIGURE 36-9 The laminoforaminotomy is completed with Kerrison rongeurs until the root and axilla are clearly visualized.

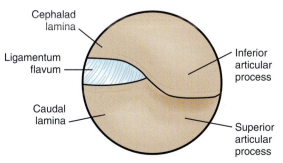

FIGURE 36-7 The endoscopic image is oriented on the screen to match the patient's orientation relative to the surgeon.

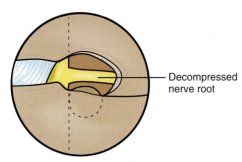

FIGURE 36-10 At the completion of the laminoforaminotomy, the root is fully decompressed to the lateral margin of the pedicle.

be mobilized from the overlying posterior longitudinal ligament, and a small, downward-pushing curet can be very helpful for this maneuver. When a spondylotic spur is identified, the results of simple laminoforaminotomy have been just as good as attempts to mobilize or tamp the spur down.

Once the decompression or diskectomy has been completed (Fig. 36-10), hemostasis is obtained with bipolar electrocautery or hemostatic foam. The wound is copiously irrigated with normal saline, and a pledget of Depo-Medrol soaked Gelfoam is placed over the foraminotomy site. The cylinder is discontinued, and the wound is closed in a single layer using three inverted interrupted absorbable sutures in the subcutaneous fascia. The incisional area is infiltrated with 20 mL of 0.25% bupivacaine (Marcaine) for postoperative analgesia, and the wound sealed with a skin adhesive.

Following the procedure, the patient is allowed to recover and usually is discharged to home after 3 hours.

Postoperative Considerations

Following discharge, the patient is asked to resume a normal routine gradually. No immobilization is used, and the patient is encouraged to start with passive range of motion as quickly as comfortable. The patient may resume driving after 3 to 5 days when neck soreness subsides. A 15-pound lifting limit is kept for the initial 3 weeks. At that point, a follow-up appointment is used to assess healing of the wound, and a formal neck strengthening and mobilization exercise book is provided for the patient to pursue a home program. Some patients with slowly resolving symptoms or physically demanding occupations are placed in formal physical therapy. By 4 to 6 weeks, most patients are back to full, unrestricted activity.

Results

The posterior cervical microendoscopic laminoforaminotomy has been in use since the late 1990s, with personal experience of more than 1400 cases. The author reviewed the experience of the first 10 years (Box 36-2), and almost 1000 patients. Formal follow-up evaluations revealed that more than 90% of patients obtained relief of preoperative weakness, numbness, and pain; 91% of patients stated that they would have the surgical procedure again, and 85%

BOX 36-2   Results

10-year experience with 962 patients

90% relief of preoperative radicular symptoms (pain, weakness, numbness)

91% of patients stating they would have the surgical procedure again

85% of patients had discontinued all prescription pain medications at 3 wk or less

Same Level Reoperation Rates

Soft disk herniation	5.6%	(mean at 2.8 yr)
Spondylotic stenosis	9.5%	(mean at 3.0 yr)
Adjacent-level surgical procedure	3.4%	

---

had discontinued all prescription pain medications at 3 weeks or less. Reoperation at the same level was necessary in 5.6% (mean, 2.8 years) of patients with soft disk herniations and 9.5% (mean, 3 years) of patients with spondylotic cases. Adjacent-level surgical procedures were necessary in only 3.4% of patients, a much more favorable rate than the up to 25% seen with anterior decompression and fusion. Complications consisted of superficial wound infection requiring postoperative antibiotics in 1.6% and dural tears not requiring any additional treatment in 0.8%. Less than 1% of patients had transient worsening of weakness, which resolved within 6 months. The major complications consisted of one case of Brown-Séquard spinal cord injury, one case of reflex sympathetic dystrophy, and one deep infection requiring secondary washout, for a total major complication rate of 0.4%. Posterior cervical microendoscopic laminoforaminotomy has become a standard for the surgical treatment of unilateral radiculopathy that is both safe and effective, with lower risks of immediate and delayed complications and quicker returns to full activity than can be obtained with anterior decompression and fusion.

REFERENCES

1. Murphey F, Simmons JC: Ruptured cervical disc: experience with 250 cases, *Am Surg* 32:83–88, 1966.
2. Hilibrand AS, Carlson GD, Palumbo MA, et al.: Radiculopathy and myelopathy at segments adjacent to the site of a previous anterior cervical arthrodesis, *J Bone Joint Surg Am* 81:519–528, 1999.
3. Clarke MJ, Ecker RD, Krauss WE, et al.: Same-segment and adjacent segment disease following posterior cervical foraminotomy, *J Neurosurg Spine* 6:5–9, 2007.
4. Henderson CM, Hennessy RG, Shuey HN Jr, Shackleford EG: Posterior lateral foraminotomy as an exclusive operative technique for cervical radiculopathy: a review of 846 consecutive cases, *Neurosurgery* 13:504–512, 1983.
5. Williams RW: Microcervical foraminotomy: a surgical alternative for intractable radicular pain, *Spine (Phila Pa 1976)* 8:708–716, 1983.
6. Foley KT, Smith MM: Microendoscopic discectomy, *Tech Neurosurg* 3:301–307, 1997.
7. Adamson TE: Microendoscopic posterior cervical laminoforaminotomy for unilateral radiculopathy: results of a new technique in 100 cases, *J Neurosurg Spine* 95:51–57, 2001.
8. Fessler R, Khoo LT: Minimally invasive cervical microendoscopic foraminotomy: an initial clinical experience, *Neurosurgery* 51(Suppl):S37–S45, 2002.
9. Hilton D Jr: Minimally invasive tubular access for the posterior cervical foraminotomy with three dimensional microscopic visualization and localization with anterior/posterior imaging, *Spine J* 7:154–158, 2006.

Osteotomies of the Cervical Spine 🎥

37

Justin K. Scheer, Yoon Ha, Vedat Deviren, Sang-Hun Lee, William R. Sears, and Christopher P. Ames

CHAPTER PREVIEW

Chapter Synopsis	Cervical deformity correction commonly includes kyphosis correction, regional sagittal balance restoration, and correction of the chin-brow vertical angle to restore horizontal gaze, decrease cantilever forces at the cervical thoracic junction, and decrease spinal cord tension-induced myelopathy. Rigid deformity requires osteotomy and release to achieve adequate correction. This chapter reviews commonly used and advanced techniques to correct semirigid and rigid deformities.
Important Points	Given complexities of the regional anatomy, osteotomy techniques that are common in the thoracic and lumbar spine must be adapted to the cervical region.
	Craniocervical junction osteotomy: C0-C2
	Smith-Petersen osteotomy (SPO): subaxial flexible deformity
	Pedicle subtraction osteotomy (PSO): mid- to low subaxial rigid deformity, osteotomy on C7 or T1
	Circumferential osteotomy: high to mid-subaxial rigid fixed deformity
Clinical and Surgical Pearls	At the craniocervical junction, an anterior approach with initial anterior linear osteotomy, posterior release and reduction of facet joint subluxation, and segmental stabilization may be used.
	Smith-Petersen osteotomy, PSO, or circumferential osteotomy may be used at the midcervical to cervicothoracic junction to achieve the desired correction.
	If significant ventral compressive disease (disk, osteophyte) is present, a ventral decompressive procedure may first be performed before correction of the deformity.
Clinical and Surgical Pitfalls	Intraoperative imaging guidance systems and intraoperative neuromonitoring can help prevent complications related to the osteotomy.
	All posterior approaches may reduce but do not eliminate swallowing dysfunction.
	The 360 and 540 techniques are best for restoring mid-subaxial lordosis.
	C7 PSO is best for correction of cervical sagittal imbalance.
Videos	Video 37-1: Decancellation Procedure in C7 Pedicle Subtraction Osteotomy
	Video 37-2: Lateral Wall of Vertebral Body Dissected with Penfield Number 1
	Video 37-3: Closure of Decancellated C7 Vertebra in C7 Pedicle Subtraction Osteotomy
	Video 37-4: Mobilization of the Vertebral Bodies during the Anterior Portion of the Circumferential 540 Osteotomy Procedure
	Video 37-5: Protecting the Vertebral Artery during the Anterior Portion of the Circumferential 540 Osteotomy Procedure

The causes of cervical deformity are diverse and may include systemic conditions, such as ankylosing spondylitis and rheumatoid arthritis, as well as neuromuscular, degenerative, posttraumatic, neoplastic, and iatrogenic conditions.[1] Surgical intervention should be considered if the patient does not respond to a conservative treatment protocol or shows evidence of deteriorating myelopathy, radiculopathy, or functional impairment, such as inability to achieve horizontal gaze, swallowing dysfunction related to head position, tension- or kyphosis-induced myelopathy, or neck pain resulting from head imbalance.[2-6] The spinal cord may be decompressed effectively by an anterior, posterior, or combined approach, but full decompression may require deformity correction, as in cases of kyphosis. Supplemental posterior fixation minimizes the risk of anterior dislodgment of the graft even in the presence of solid anterior fixation.[7] Treatment of these complex cervical deformities is challenging and requires a clear understanding of the disease and the patient. Surgeons must be comfortable with remobilizing the spinal column anteriorly and posteriorly, with vertebral artery anatomy, and with methods of anterior and posterior correction.

Significant, irreducible deformity of the cervical spine may be sufficient to require corrective osteotomy. At the craniocervical junction, neurologic or functional impairment associated with the deformity may be best managed by osteotomy and fixation. Rigid deformities of the cervical spine below the craniocervical junction are more likely to require some type of osteotomy to correct the deformity and restore horizontal gaze.

This chapter details the preoperative considerations and surgical procedures of four cervical osteotomies: (1) craniocervical junction osteotomy using sequential anteroposterior approaches, (2) Smith-Petersen osteotomy (SPO), (3) cervicothoracic junction pedicle subtraction osteotomy (PSO), and (4) cervical circumferential osteotomy.

Preoperative Considerations in Rigid Cervical Deformity

History

Patients may give a history of past trauma, sometimes associated with an intercurrent illness of ankylosing spondylitis or rheumatoid arthritis, as well as previous cervical spine surgery or degenerative and neoplastic disorders.

Signs and Symptoms

Symptoms may include suboccipital headache and neck stiffness, occipital neuralgia, symptoms of myelopathy, or progressive deformity leading to functional impairment, such as difficulty with looking forward or with eating and drinking. Patients may report low back pain and standing fatigue resulting from use of compensatory muscles to elevate pelvic tilt to alter gaze angle.

Physical Examination

Assessment of the patient with cervical kyphotic deformity should include a comprehensive neurologic examination.

Signs of myelopathy may be evident because of past injury, compression, or spinal cord tension secondary to stretch induced by kyphosis. In addition to a complete neurologic examination, the surgeon should assess the patient's regional and overall global alignment. Assessment of the location of the kyphotic deformity should include evaluation of not only the craniocervical relationship, but also the thoracolumbar spine and lumbopelvic relationships. The angle from the brow to chin relation to the vertical line with the hips and knees extended and the neck in its fixed or neutral position (chin-brow to vertical angle) can be used to measure the degree of flexion deformity.

Clinical and radiographic assessments should be performed with the patient's hips and knees in the extended position to obtain a better understanding of the sagittal alignment and the location of the deformity. This is important because occasionally the focus of the deformity lies within the thoracolumbar spine or lumbar pelvis. In addition, examination of the pelvis may reveal hip flexion contractures. Occasionally, lumbar sagittal deformities must be corrected first. Correction of lumbar imbalance alters head position substantially, especially in rigid deformities such as ankylosing spondylitis. However, all corrective lumbar osteotomies change the T1 slope angle to some extent and therefore change cervical alignment and often cervical C2 sagittal vertical axis.

Imaging

The deformity should be evaluated by anteroposterior and lateral cervical radiographs along with dynamic lateral flexion and extension views. The deformity is then accurately measured (i.e., sagittal angle determination), and any other abnormalities are noted (e.g., subluxation and pseudarthrosis).[2,8,9] The surgeon should obtain full-length posteroanterior and lateral 36-inch scoliosis radiographs to examine overall sagittal and coronal balance in these patients.[2,9,10] The authors assess cervical, thoracic, and lumbar sagittal alignment individually and globally, define the effect of regional imbalance on cervical balance, and determine whether it is a primary, secondary, or compensatory cervical deformity. The degree of required correction depends on the angle of the cervical deformity (the chin-brow to vertical angle), the C2 plumb line, and the desired final lordosis.[3,9,11-13]

The goals of treatment are to obtain balance, horizontal gaze, and spinal cord decompression and to normalize spinal cord tension. Dynamic (i.e., flexion and extension) radiographs permit assessment of the overall flexibility of the cervical spine that is paramount when designing a treatment strategy. Computed tomography (CT) scans of the cervical spine are also useful in determining the presence of fusion or ankylosis of the facet joints and disks and allow assessment of fixation points such as C2 and upper thoracic pedicles.

All patients should be evaluated with preoperative magnetic resonance imaging or CT myelography. These image modalities permit the evaluation of compressive disease. If significant ventral compressive disease (disk, osteophyte) is present, a ventral decompressive procedure may first be performed before correction of the deformity.

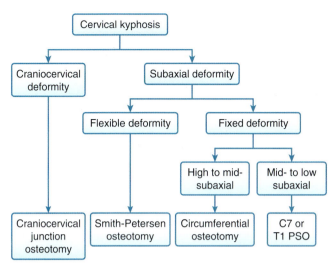

FIGURE 37-1   Flow chart of the surgical decision-making process in cervical kyphosis.

Decision for Planning of Osteotomy

When planning surgical deformity correction for cervical kyphosis, the surgeon should consider whether the deformity is rigid or fixed and whether the patient has neurologic symptoms. Figure 37-1 demonstrates the surgical decision-making process in cervical deformity osteotomy. In the craniocervical junction, osteotomy is indicated when the deformity is irreducible and sufficient to result in severe pain or in functional or neurologic impairment that cannot be relieved with a surgical decompression or stabilization procedure alone. In flexible subaxial deformity, posterior stabilization (usually C2 to T2) is advocated; when deformity is semirigid Smith-Petersen osteotomy should be considered.

However, in the clinical setting of rigid cervical kyphosis (high cervical to midcervical kyphosis) with neurologic symptoms, the spinal cord is usually tethered over the subaxial kyphotic segment, thus leading to neurologic symptoms and myelopathy. Therefore, segmental kyphosis correction (circumferential osteotomy) is mandatory to untether and decompress the spinal cord. In the setting of rigid cervical kyphosis in the mid- to low cervical spine with cervical sagittal imbalance, C7 or T1 PSO may be sufficient.

Craniocervical Junction Osteotomy

At the craniocervical junction, it is unusual for osteotomy to be required, and little has been published on the subject in the surgical literature.[14] However, cases exist, usually in the posttraumatic setting and in association with other conditions such as ankylosing spondylitis or end-stage rheumatoid arthritis with fixed atlantoaxial deformity, in which neurologic or functional impairment associated with the deformity may be best managed by osteotomy and fixation.

Indications and Contraindications

Osteotomy is indicated when the deformity is irreducible (possibly following a trial of traction) and sufficient to result in severe pain and functional or neurologic impairment that cannot be relieved with a surgical decompression or stabilization procedure alone. The procedure is contraindicated in the presence of significant osteoporosis or debilitating comorbidities.

Figure 37-2 is a case example of craniocervical junction osteotomy. Plain radiographs at the atlantoaxial level reveal substantial kyphotic deformity, possibly in the presence of an old odontoid fracture, with subluxation or dislocation of the C1-C2 joints (see Fig. 37-2, A to C). The patient may have bony union across the subluxed joints or involving other elements of the atlantoaxial complex.

Surgical Techniques

1. The ease of surgical access to the ventral aspect of C2 is an important consideration when choosing between an anterior-posterior approach and a posterior-only approach. Grundy and Gill described a posterior-only approach in cases in which the anticipated anterior access may be difficult.[14] Preoperative planning of the intended osteotomy orientation is also important when considering the type of anterior approach. An osteotomy, which is oriented obliquely backward and upward from the base of C2 (Fig. 37-3, A), enables satisfactory exposure through a high anterior retropharyngeal approach. This approach is described later.

2. Anesthesia and positioning: The patient usually requires awake endoscopic intubation and is positioned supine for the first (anterior) stage of the surgical procedure. It is preferable to use an operating table such as the Jackson table (Mizuho OSI, Union City, Calif.), which permits rotation of the patient to the prone position for the second surgical stage, and to secure the patient's head in a Mayfield three-point head holder. Access for adjustment of the head and neck position should be maintained throughout the procedure. Intraoperative image-guided surgical navigation, such as with an O-Arm/Stealth (Medtronic, Dallas, Tex.), Iso-C (Siemens, Erlangen, Germany), or similar system may facilitate the surgeon's orientation and placement of the osteotomy. Intraoperative neuromonitoring may be helpful during deformity reduction.

3. A high anterolateral skin incision is made for a retropharyngeal approach to the C2 vertebral body.
   a. A retropharyngeal approach to the ventral aspect of the C2 vertebral body is used, with fluoroscopic confirmation of position.
   b. The longus colli muscles are mobilized bilaterally.
   c. The old fracture line is identified (when present). The bilateral extents of the fracture line are defined, and the surgeon endeavors to dissect upward to define the lateral aspects of the odontoid process bilaterally (Fig. 37-3, B). This maneuver is important to mobilize the odontoid with the osteotomy completely and to avoid injury to the vertebral arteries.
   d. The osteotomy is made through the old fracture line by using a high-speed drill with a small cutting burr. Frequent position and orientation checks are made with fluoroscopic or image guidance.

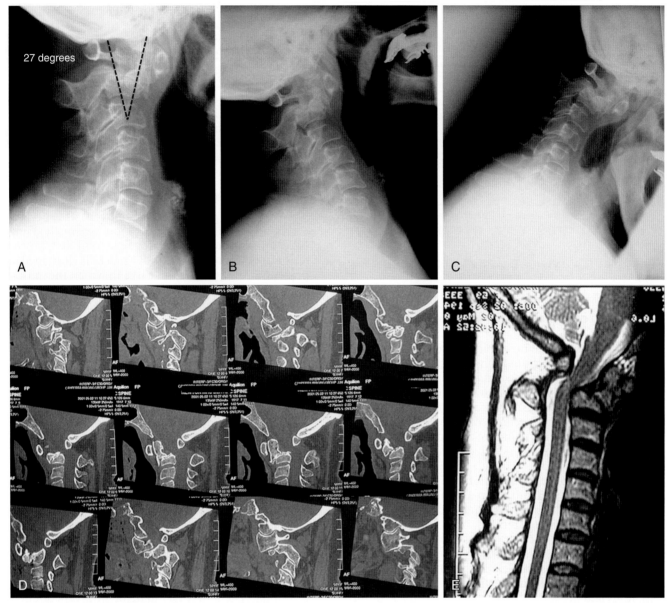

FIGURE 37-2   A 59-year-old woman with a history of rheumatoid arthritis and severe suboccipital neck pain and early signs of myelopathy 6 months after a motor vehicle accident resulting in a type III odontoid fracture that was managed conservatively in a SOMI brace. Plain radiograph, computed tomography, and magnetic resonance imaging show development of fixed 27 degree kyphotic deformity (**A** to **C**), bilateral facet joint dislocations (**D**), and spinal cord compression (**E**).

The osteotomy is extended through to the back of the odontoid and bilaterally. The surgeon should take care not to venture too widely, to avoid injury to the vertebral arteries. If necessary, navigation may be used.

e. Depending on whether bony union of the posterior elements of the C1-C2 complex is present, an attempt may be made at this stage to open up the fracture line and correct the deformity by using intervertebral spreaders.

f. The anterior wound is then closed over a suction drain before the patient is turned to the prone position.

g. Through a midline suboccipital incision, subperiosteal dissection of the posterior elements of C1 to C3 is performed with identification of the C2 nerve roots.

h. While controlling any hemorrhage from the venous plexus around the C2 nerve roots, the superior articular surfaces of C2 are exposed, and the posterior edges of the C1 lateral masses, adjacent to the inferior joint surfaces, are defined on each side. If any bony union has occurred between the C1 and C2 joints, this is divided with the high-speed drill or osteotome (Fig. 37-4). Dissectors are then carefully inserted into the dislocated C1-C2 joints and are used to lever back the C1 lateral masses gently onto C2 while the surgical assistant and anesthesiologist adjust the patient's head position in the Mayfield headholder.

i. It is helpful to remove the articular cartilage from the C2 joint surfaces before reducing the dislocation. Subsequently, the articular cartilage is removed with a small, angled curet from the inferior surface

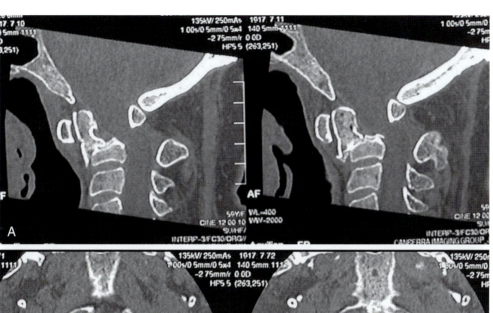

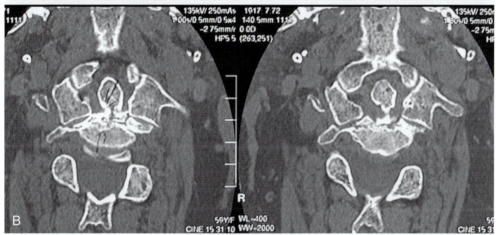

FIGURE 37-3 Computed tomography sagittal and coronal reconstructions showing the orientation of the planned osteotomy (**A**) and the bilateral extent of the base of the osteotomy (**B**).

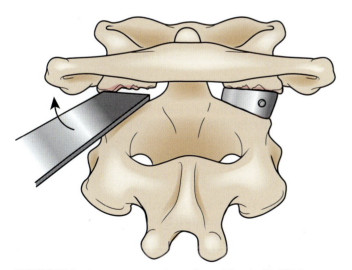

FIGURE 37-4 An osteotome may be used to mobilize the C1-C2 joint space from the anterior or posterior approach in cases of fixed atlantoaxial deformity.

of the C1 lateral masses. Cancellous bone graft is then placed into the C1-C2 joint spaces.
   j. Depending on the surgeon's preference and the vertebral artery anatomy, the C1-C2 segment is then stabilized using either transarticular screws (with additional posterior wiring) or a C1 lateral mass and C2 pars screw construct.[15-17]

   k. Further bone graft is placed over the decorticated posterolateral elements before posterior wound closure, in layers, over a vacuum drain.
4. Depending on how the patient is tolerating the procedure and the time available, the patient may be repositioned supine immediately or later, as a delayed procedure, for placement of bone graft into the anterior osteotomy site. This will have opened up into a wedge-shaped defect following the posterior deformity correction (Fig. 37-5, *A*). Suitably fashioned allograft or iliac crest autograft is inserted into the wedge-shaped osteotomy site and secured with a small locking plate (Fig. 37-5, *B*). Subsequent, standard postoperative care is given following segmental atlantoaxial stabilization and fusion (Fig. 37-6).
5. The patient is then returned, ventilated, to the intensive care unit.

Smith-Petersen Osteotomy

Semirigid Deformity (e.g., Spondylitic Joints and Disks but No Segmental Bridging Bone in a Patient with Good Bone Quality)

The Smith-Petersen extension osteotomy technique, described in 1945, has been used extensively and was previously considered the prototype procedure for reconstruction of sagittal imbalance in patients with deformity

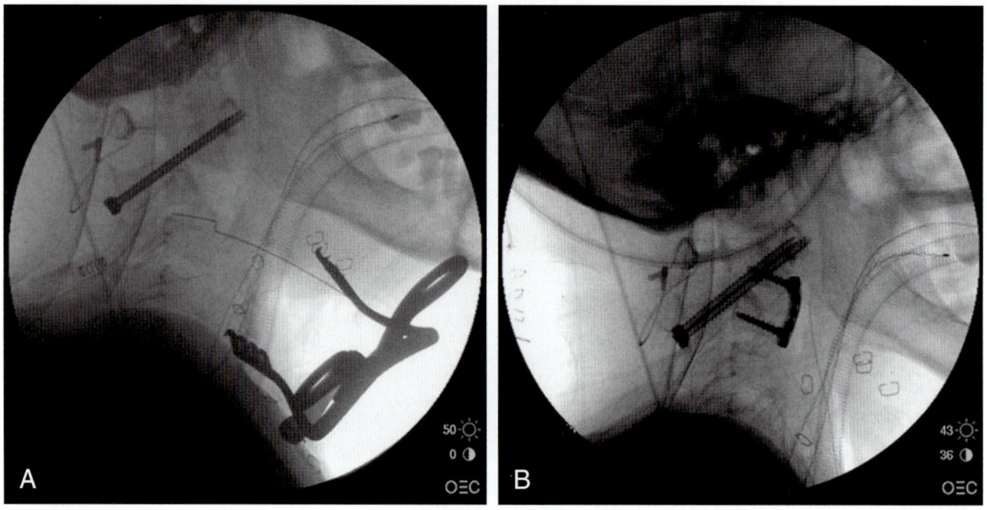

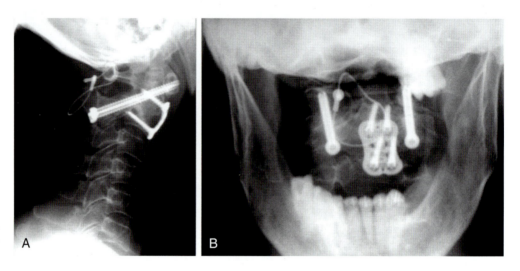

FIGURE 37-5 Intraoperative fluoroscopic images showing an anterior wedge defect resulting from posterior relocation of dislocated facet joints and transarticular screw fixation (**A**) and following anterior bone grafting and plate fixation (**B**).

FIGURE 37-6 Six-month postoperative lateral (**A**) and anteroposterior (**B**) plain radiographs.

above the thoracolumbar junction.[18] Inspired by the lumbar osteotomy performed by Smith-Petersen, Urist in 1958 first reported his experience of cervical osteotomy on one patient with severe flexion deformity of ankylosing spondylitis.[19] It is important to distinguish between opening wedge osteotomy (the classic Smith-Petersen osteotomy used for patients with ankylosing spondylitis at C7) and the procedure involving complete facet removal and posterior closure over a mobile disk space that is more commonly used for semirigid cervical deformity and is sometimes more appropriately called the cervical Ponte osteotomy.

If the deformity is partially correctable with traction or posture (i.e., neck extension), a dorsal-alone Smith-Petersen osteotomy/Ponte strategy may be used.[12,20,21] Traction may be used to reduce the deformity and then may be continued into the operating room. Because this osteotomy uses some cantilever force on the prebent rod to achieve lordosis and segmental osteotomy closure, a stiffer cobalt chromium rod is recommended over a 3.5 titanium rod. Usually, these cases involve fusion from C2 to T2 or T3 (see the case example in Figs. 37-7 and 37-8).

Ankylosing spondylitis may produce an extreme fixed flexion deformity at the cervicothoracic junction. This extreme deformity may place the chin in close proximity to the chest and thus may interfere with eating and respiration. Some investigators have advocated treating this deformity by using Smith-Petersen osteotomy with anterior osteoclasis and gentle extension of neck intraoperatively that results in the classic opening wedge.[11,12,20,21]

Opening Wedge Osteotomy (Ankylosing Spondylitis)

Indications and Contraindications

Severe flexion deformities of the cervical spine, in which patients have loss of horizontal gaze, difficulty with personal hygiene and function, and dysphagia, are corrected by traction or neck extension. Ankylosing spondylitis with fixed deformity is treated with Smith-Petersen osteotomy with anterior osteoclasis. Standing 36-inch radiographs are critical in determining whether lumbar or thoracic kyphosis also exists. If so, and if global imbalance is present, the thoracolumbar deformity usually should be corrected first because this procedure by itself may restore horizontal gaze. If lumbar sagittal deformity is present

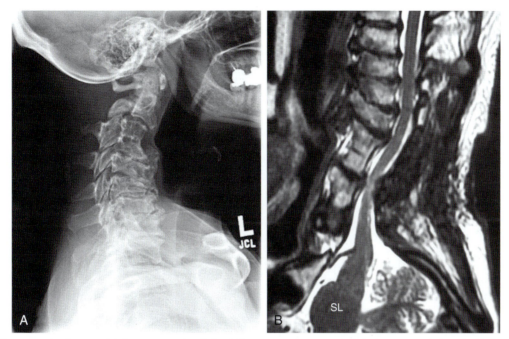

FIGURE 37-7 Case example of semirigid deformity treated with Smith-Petersen osteotomy and cobalt chromium rods (see Fig. 37-8). Preoperative lateral radiograph showing cervical kyphosis (**A**) and preoperative sagittal magnetic resonance imaging showing spinal stenosis (**B**).

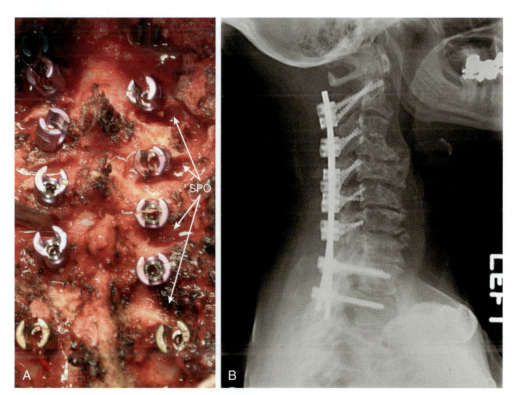

FIGURE 37-8 Case example of semirigid deformity treated with Smith-Petersen osteotomy (SPO). Intraoperative photograph displaying the cervical kyphotic correction using multiple SPOs (**A**) and a postoperative lateral radiograph showing correction of the cervical kyphosis and the use of a cobalt chromium rod (**B**).

and cervical osteotomy is performed first, then secondary lumbar correction may lead to an unacceptably high (gaze on the ceiling) issue, and flexion osteotomy may then be needed.[22]

Surgical Techniques (C7 Smith-Petersen Osteotomy with Anterior Osteoclasis for Fixed Low Cervical Deformity in Ankylosing Spondylitis)

1. Classically, the patient is positioned sitting. However, at the authors' institution, patients are positioned prone in a halo ring. The kyphotic head position is accommodated by additional rolls and pads as needed to elevate the patient's thorax. Transcortical motor-evoked potentials (MEPs), somatosensory-evoked potentials (SSEPs), and electromyography (EMG) are used.

2. An incision is made posteriorly, and the paraspinous muscles are dissected in a subperiosteal fashion, thus exposing the spinous processes, laminar facets, and lateral processes of C4 to T2. If the bone is very soft, fixation is extended to bicortical C2 screws. Preoperative standing films allow determination of the apex of the upper thoracic kyphosis, and the fixation is extended below this apex as needed.

3. After exposure, the osteotomy is performed. A complete C7 laminectomy and partial C6 and T1 laminectomies are performed. The resection is carried laterally to include the removal of the C7 pedicle with rongeurs. All resected bone is saved for reuse later to create the bone graft.

4. The residual portions of the C6 and T1 laminae must be carefully bevelled and undercut to avoid any impingement or kinking of the spinal cord on closure of the osteotomy. Furthermore, the area near the C8 nerve root is curved to provide ample room for the nerve root on closure.

5. The surgeon grasps the halo and extends the patient's neck gradually with closure of the osteotomy posteriorly as the osteoclasis across C7 to T1 occurs anteriorly. An audible snap and sensation of the osteoclasis are usually heard. Also at this time, rotation malalignment and lateral tilt are corrected.

6. A prebent rod is placed and locked down. The C8 foramen is inspected to make sure the nerve is free after complete closure. At the C7-T1 area, the posterior aspects of the spine may then be decorticated. The autologous bone graft from the resection is packed bilaterally onto the decorticated areas.

Cervicothoracic Junction Pedicle Subtraction Osteotomy (Dorsal Approach)

For patients with fixed cervicothoracic kyphosis, a 360-degree release and fusion or an osteotomy typically is used to correct the kyphosis.[3] Such cervical osteotomies were performed at C7 or T1 because of the absence of the vertebral artery at this level. Preoperative CT angiography is performed to rule out an aberrant vertebral artery position at C7.

Several authors have reported successful results with a single-level dorsal decancellation osteotomy, also known as the "eggshell" procedure or PSO.[3,13, 23,24] Once the osteotomy is closed, bone contact occurs in all three columns, and the spinal canal is effectively shortened. Thus, the PSO procedure can provide excellent sagittal correction while simultaneously forming a stable construct and minimizing neural compression.

Indication

Fixed sagittal malalignment of the cervical spine (mid- to low subaxial cervical spine) affecting horizontal gaze, persistent pain related to cervical sagittal imbalance despite conservative treatment, and high pelvic tilt causing low back pain driven by cervical deformity are indications for this procedure.

Surgical Techniques (C7 Pedicle Subtraction Osteotomy)

1. The patient is prone in a halo ring.

2. Transcortical-MEPs and SSEPs, as well as EMG neuromonitoring, are used.

3. A standard posterior surgical approach is made to the cervical spine, thus creating an incision from C2 to T3 to T5, depending on the location of the kyphotic apex.

4. A posterior incision is made from C2 to T3 to T5 and is taken sharply through the skin and down to the fascia. The paraspinous muscles are dissected in a subperiosteal fashion, thereby exposing the spinous processes, laminar facets, and lateral processes of the cervical spine and transverse processes in the thoracic spine.

5. After exposure, the spine is instrumented accordingly (C2 bicortical pedicle screws, cervical lateral mass screws, and thoracic pedicle screws). It is preferable to extend the fixation to C2 to obtain bicortical screw placement for a stronger fixation point than at the lateral masses of the inferior vertebrae. Furthermore, it is preferable to have the caudal extent of the fusion terminate at either T3 or T5, depending on the extent of thoracic kyphosis, to ensure that the apex of the kyphotic deformity is within the fusion. Depending on the surgeon's preference, various types of fusion rods may be used such as stainless steel and titanium; however, cobalt chromium rods are preferred.

6. The osteotomy begins with the Smith-Petersen type by performing facet release and removal of the facets of C6 to C7 as well as C7 to T1 (Fig. 37-9, *I*). The nerve roots at C7 and C8 are then identified and are followed out the foramen, as well as carrying the osteotomy completely laterally, thus isolating the C7 pedicle.

7. After the bilateral facetectomies and isolation of the C7 pedicle, the C7 pedicle is skeletonized and removed with Lempert rongeurs. Sequential lumbar or custom wedge-shaped spinal taps are used to decancellate the C7 vertebral body combined with osteotomes and downward-pushing curets to attempt a 30-degree wedge (Fig. 37-9, *II* and *III*, and Video 37-1).

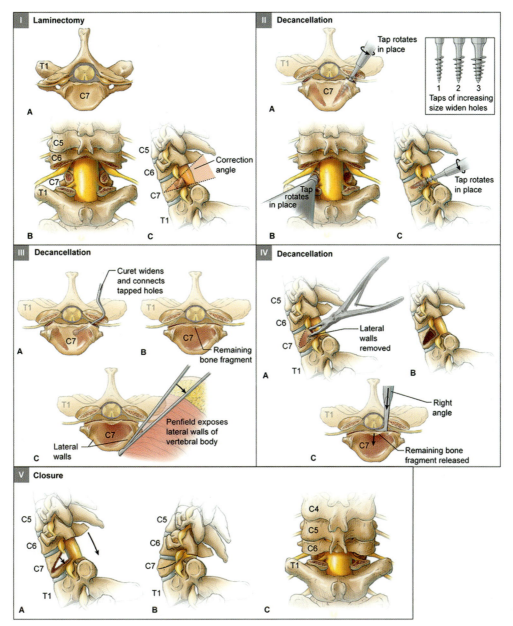

FIGURE 37-9   C7 pedicle subtraction osteotomy technique. (Copyright University of California, San Francisco. Drawn by Kenneth Xavier Probst.)

8. The lateral wall of the C7 vertebral body is then dissected with a Penfield number 1 retractor and is visualized (see Fig. 37-9, *III*, and Video 37-2). The C7 lateral wall is removed with needle-nose rongeurs and osteotomes through the pedicle hole reamed out by the taps, followed by removal of the medial column (Fig. 37-9, *IV*).

9. After completion of the osteotomy, the patient's head is then loosened from the table, and the halo ring is used to extend the head and close the osteotomy (Fig. 37-9, *V*, and Video 37-3).

10. The wound is closed, and the patient is taken to the surgical intensive care unit.

Results

PSO at the cervicothoracic junction has two key benefits compared with the traditional Smith-Petersen osteotomy.

First, PSO results in greater biomechanical stability (producing a mechanically stiffer result) than does Smith-Petersen osteotomy.[25,26] Smith-Petersen osteotomy generally results in disk disruption or, in cases of ankylosing spondylitis, osteoclasis through a fused disk space or the anterior cortex of the vertebral body. The result is a significant anterior gap in which the anterior longitudinal ligament is completely torn or the autofused anterior bridging osteophyte has been fractured.

PSO leaves the anterior longitudinal ligament intact. In addition, PSO has a wedge component that cleaves the vertebral body to create a larger bone-on-bone load-bearing interface even when compared with Smith-Petersen osteotomy that is fully closed posteriorly. This greater bone-on-bone contact significantly increases stiffness, especially in compression, and may provide better fusion rates in patients who do not have ankylosing spondylitis because PSO provides a substantial load-bearing surface area in uniting the anterior, middle, and posterior columns on closure.[25,26] No secondary anterior grafting is required. Second, PSO results in a more controlled closure than does Smith-Petersen osteotomy because no sudden osteoclastic fracture is necessary.

In the authors' surgical series of 11 patients who received cervicothoracic PSO, this procedure resulted in excellent correction of cervical kyphosis and chin-brow to vertical angle (CBVA) with a controlled closure and improvement in health-related quality-of-life measures even at early time points.[3] The mean preoperative and immediate postoperative values (± SD) for cervical sagittal imbalance were 7.9 ± 1.4 cm and 3.4 ± 1.7 cm. The mean overall correction was 4.5 ± 1.5 cm (42.8%), the mean PSO correction was 19.0 degrees, and the mean CBVA correction was 36.7 degrees. A significant decrease was seen in both the Neck Disability Index (51.1 to 38.6; $P = 0.03$) and visual analog scale scores for neck pain (8.1 to 3.9; $P = 0.0021$). The Short Form 36 (SF-36) physical component summary scores increased by 18.4% (30.2 to 35.8) without neurologic complications.

Complications

Because of the advances in surgical technique, anesthesia, and intraoperative neuromonitoring, cervicothoracic junction PSO has been considered a safe, reproducible, and effective procedure for the management of cervicothoracic kyphotic deformities.[3] Cervicothoracic PSO has reported complications that include neurologic deficits, sudden subluxation, and even death.[10,12,20] Daubs and colleagues found that increasing age was a significant factor in predicting a complication for patients who were more than 60 years old. However, in the authors' series, 8 of 11 patients were more than 60 years old, and these patients had no perioperative neurologic deficits, and perioperative medical complications occurred in only 2 of 11 cases.[27] The lower medical complication rate and decreased incidence of dysphagia may reflect the all-posterior nature of this technique. Posterior-only deformity corrections have also been associated with lower complication rates in thoracolumbar surgery compared with staged anterior and posterior procedures (Table 37-1).

Cervical Circumferential Osteotomy

In the clinical setting of rigid cervical kyphosis with neurologic symptoms, the spinal cord is usually tethered over the subaxial kyphotic segment, thus leading to neurologic symptoms and myelopathy. Therefore, segmental kyphosis correction is needed to untether and decompress the spinal cord in the mid-subaxial region. This is a three-stage technique: posterior-anterior-posterior (Figs. 37-10 to 37-12).

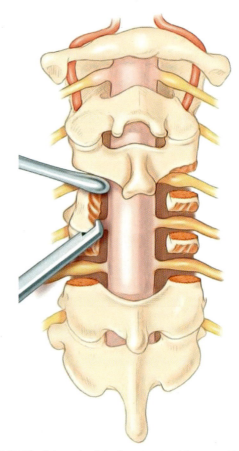

FIGURE 37-10 Schematic of the first stage involving removal of previous instrumentation, central and foraminal decompressions, multiple posterior osteotomies, and posterior reinstrumentation (not depicted here). This is also the so-called "cervical Ponte" osteotomy, which can be performed in a single stage to loosen semirigid deformities with mobile disks.

Table 37-1 Summary of Patient Demographic and Clinical Characteristics

Case No.	Age (yr), Sex	Diagnosis	Operation	Complications
1	70, M	Chin-on-chest deformity	C7 PSO	Pneumonia
2	56, M	Cervical kyphosis and cervical myelopathy	C7 PSO	
3	82, F	Chin-on-chest deformity	C7 PSO	
4	80, M	Chin-on-chest deformity	C7 PSO	Pneumonia
5	73, F	Fixed coronal and sagittal plane cervical deformity	C6 and C7 PSO	
6	69, M	Cervical kyphosis	C7 PSO	Dysphagia/PEG
7	59, F	Chin-on-chest deformity	C7 PSO	
8	75, M	Cervical kyphosis	C7 PSO	
9	94, F	Chin-on-chest deformity	T1 PSO	
10	63, M	Chin-on-chest deformity	C7 PSO	Rod fracture at 4 mo
11	52, M	Chin-on-chest deformity	C7 PSO	

PEG, Percutaneous endoscopic gastrostomy; *PSO*, pedicle subtraction osteotomy.

These stages can be performed during a single anesthetic regimen or in a delayed fashion according to the extension of the planned procedure and the condition of the patient. All stages are performed while the patient is under general anesthesia, and they use neuromonitoring with standard MEPs and SSEPs.

1. First stage (see Fig. 37-10): A standard posterior approach (laminectomy, facetectomy, and insertion of pedicle screw and lateral mass screw) to the cervical spine is performed for the predetermined levels.
2. Second stage (see Fig. 37-11 and Video 37-4): An anterior approach to the anterior cervical vertebrae is used for the decompression and remobilizing the cervical spine.
3. Third stage (see Fig. 37-12): The patient is again positioned prone, and the previous posterior incision is reopened. Final correction of the deformity is gained.

Indications and Contraindications

Fixed mid-subaxial kyphotic deformity results from degenerative or inflammatory conditions or often from previous fixation in a kyphotic position (Fig. 37-13, *A*). Cervical sagittal imbalance secondary to failed anterior procedures as a result of nonunions or graft subsidence is increasingly common. The surgeon should achieve enough correction of sagittal imbalance and regional lordosis to allow dorsal spinal cord migration and decreased cord tension.

Surgical Procedure

First stage

1. After a standard posterior cervical approach, previous instrumentation can be removed, and the fusion mass can be explored to search for any sites of nonunion.
2. Laminectomies can be done as needed, especially around the apex of the deformity to allow for free movement of the spinal cord after the correction of the deformity. Previous laminectomy scar is removed down to the dura.
3. Through the same approach, the necessary foraminotomies are performed, dictated by the patient's preoperative clinical and radiographic picture. Bilateral osteotomies, including the cephalad part of the superior facet and caudad aspect of the inferior facet, are performed at the apical levels of the kyphosis. Care must be taken to carry the resection lateral enough to release all the fusion mass or facets and generously decompress the exiting nerve root (see Fig. 37-10).
4. Segmental instrumentation is placed in the form of lateral mass or pedicle screws, depending on the level and surgeon's preference.
5. The incision is closed in the standard fashion postoperatively; the patient can be mobilized with the use of a hard collar until the next stage.

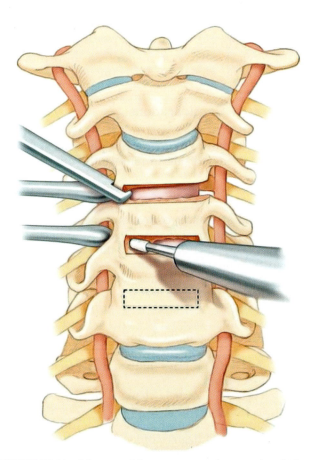

FIGURE 37-11 Schematic of the anterior second stage with multiple osteotomies and diskectomies involving resection of the uncovertebral joins and protection of the vertebral artery. An anterior, overcontoured plate can also be used to produce anterior translation at the apex of the deformity (not depicted here).

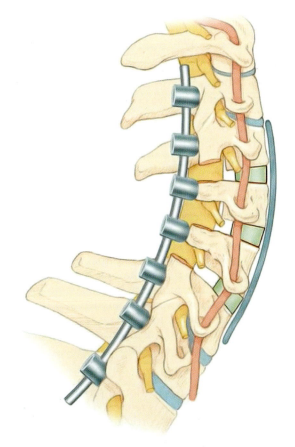

FIGURE 37-12 Schematic of the final correction after the third stage and rod placement.

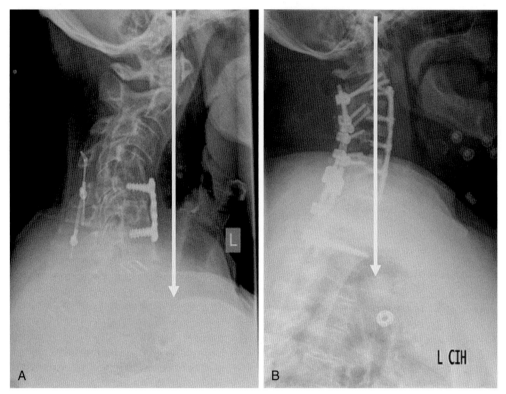

FIGURE 37-13   Preoperative (**A**) and postoperative (**B**) lateral radiographs demonstrating a case example of a 540 circumferential procedure.

Second Stage

1. The patient is turned to the supine position, and an anterior cervical approach is performed through previously operated tissue planes. Any anterior instrumentation used in earlier operations can be removed at this time.
2. Anteriorly based osteotomies are performed as needed, depending on the presence of ankylosed or fused segments, the necessity of anterior decompression, and the overall deformity. For improved correction, the osteotomies must be carried out lateral to the uncovertebral joints, with protection of the vertebral artery from the burr with a Penfield number 4 dissector[28] (see Fig. 37-11 and Video 37-5).
3. After complete release, lordosing distraction is applied at each osteotomy site with Caspar pins and a laminar spreader inserted in the disk space.
4. Interbody lordotic grafting (autograft, allograft, or cages as preferred) is performed.
5. A plate spanning the osteotomies is overcontoured and is fixed initially at the apical level by parallel screws, to conform the apical segment into more lordosis as the screws are tightened and the spine is sequentially reduced to the plate.
6. The rest of the screws are placed and secured, and the incision is closed in standard fashion.

Third Stage

1. The patient is again positioned prone, and the previous posterior incision is reopened.
2. Bony surfaces are decorticated with bone grafting and rod placement (see Figs. 37-12 and 37-13, *B*). Compression at the osteotomies may be performed if deemed necessary.

3. Following closure, the patient is immobilized in a hard cervical collar. Placement of a feeding tube can be done at the end of the procedure if problems with swallowing are anticipated.

Postoperative Considerations

The patient is kept intubated and is nursed in a head-up position to reduce postoperative pharyngeal edema until it is considered safe to remove the endotracheal tube.

Results

A gradual and acceptable correction is achieved through the summation of correct positioning, multiple osteotomy sites, plated anterior segmental translation, and posterior instrumented compression.

Based on the authors' 14 cases of surgical experiences, osteotomies were performed at 3.9 (3 to 6) levels anteriorly and 6.6 (3 to 18) levels posteriorly. The estimated blood loss was on average 1484 mL (range, 400 to 4600 mL). The average stay in the hospital was 19 days (range, 3 to 55 days), and the intensive care unit stay was 6.2 days (range, 0 to 15 days). Days intubated averaged 3.8 days (range, 0 to 15 days).

The average C2-C7 angle changed from 12.4 degrees of kyphosis (range, 58 of kyphosis to 30.9 degrees of lordosis) to an average of 14.9 degrees of lordosis postoperatively (range, 9.4 degrees of kyphosis to 35.1 degrees of lordosis). The average angular correction was 27.7 degrees (range, 1.9 to 74.6 degrees). The average preoperative C2-C7 translation improved from 46.9 mm (range, 2 to 86.2 mm) to 26 mm (range, 57 to 3 mm), for an average 20.8 mm of correction (Table 37-2).

Table 37-2 Demographic Data Including Patient Age, Cause of Deformity, Comorbidities, Radiographic Results, and Complications

Patient	Age (yr)	Cause of Deformity	Levels Fused	Comorbidities	Complications	Preoperative C2-C7 Angle (degrees)	Postoperative C2-C7 Angle (degrees)	Angular Correction (degrees)	Preoperative C2-C7 Translation (mm)	Postoperative C2-C7 Translation (mm)
1	65	Failed fusion after trauma to C6-C7	C3-T2			−30.9	−32.8	1.9	2	45
2	37	Inveterate fracture-dislocation at C6-C7	C3-T2			3.3	9.4	−6.1	51	38
3	60	Postlaminectomy kyphosis and C2-C3 fusion	C3-T1			34.9	−3	37.9	17	17
4	63	Failed ACDF	C3-T1	CAD	Prolonged FT	17.9	−7	24.9	68	29
5	59	Failed C4-C7 AP fusion, OPLL	C3-T1		Crest wound infection, CSF leak needing reoperation, acute SDH, tracheostomy	1.1	−15.7	16.8	50	40
6	60	Postlaminectomy kyphosis, prior ACDF	C3-T3		Wound infection, postoperative halo	6.4	−35.1	41.5	93	57
7	49	Prior C5-C7 ACDF, C3-T1 PSF	C2-T3		Prolonged FT	−13.5	−34	20.5	41	23
8	23	C2 and C7 fractures treated in halo	C5-C7	GERD		3	−15.7	18.7	80.9	36
9	62	Degenerative	C6-T2	HBP, ulnar nerve compression	Mild hoarseness	5.3	−29.4	34.7	15	−3
10	68	Multiple AP fusions and laminectomies	C2-T2	HBP, GERD, DM, CAD, COPD, hypothyroidism, hyperlipidemia	Retained drain, UTI	22.2	−13.2	35.4	58	31
11	65	Degenerative, chin-on-chest deformity	C1-T12	CAD, COPD, HBP, osteoporosis, GERD	PMN, unstable angina	58	−16.6	74.6	86	16.6
12	48	Multiple AP cervical fusions	C4-T4	HC, COPD, soft tissue defect posteriorly	Durotomy repaired, L PTX, C5 right neurapraxia	22.7	−9.3	32	61	26
13	67	Multiple AP cervical fusions	C2-T2	Depression, tobacco use	Prolonged delirium	43.2	0.9	42.3	11	9
14	47	Chronic C6-C7 jumped facets, C6-C7 laminectomy	C4-T2			0	−7.1	7.1	23	0
					Averages	12.4	−14.9	27.7	46.9	26

ACDF, Anterior cervical diskectomy and fusion; *AP,* anteroposterior; *CAD,* coronary artery disease; *COPD,* chronic obstructive pulmonary disease; *CSF,* cerebrospinal fluid; *DM,* diabetes mellitus; *FT,* feeding tube; *GERD,* gastroesophageal reflux; *HBP,* high blood pressure; *HC,* hepatitis C; *OPLL,* ossification of the posterior longitudinal ligament, *PSF,* posterior spinal fusion; *PTX,* pneumothorax; *SDH,* subdural hematoma; *UTI,* urinary tract infection.

Table 37-3 Major Complications of the Various Osteotomies

Technique (Reference)	Number of Patients Reported	Overall Complication Rate	Mortality Rate	Neurologic Complication Rate	Complications
PSO (Deviren et al[3])	11	4/11	0	0	1 dysphagia/PEG 1 rod fracture, 2 pneumonias
360 (Nottmeier et al[29])	41	2/41	0	2/41	1 quadriparesis, 1 C8 radiculopathy
540 (Ames et al[30])	14	5/14	0	1/14	1 incidental durotomy, 1 persistent CSF leak, 1 superficial wound infection, 1 infection at iliac bone harvest site, 1 C5 palsy
Circumferential (Mummaneni et al[31])	30	11/30	2/30	0	2 wound infections, 1 fall with fracture of C6, 1 plate dislodgment, 1 transient dysphonia, 1 intraoperative CSF leak, 3 perioperative tracheostomies and gastrostomies, 2 deaths
OWO (Simmons et al[12])	131	55/131	4/131	21/131	2 intraoperative neurologic complications, 1 hemiparesis, 16 C8 radiculopathies, 2 C8 nerve root irritations, 6 pseudarthroses, 5 pneumonias, 4 deep vein thromboses with pulmonary embolism, 15 halo pin infections, 4 deaths
Anterior-posterior (O'Shaughnessy et al[32])	20	7/20	0	4/20	2 durotomies, 3 transient C5 palsies, 1 head-holder failure with resultant quadriplegia, 1 late progression of deformity at the caudal junctional end

CSF, Cerebrospinal fluid; *PEG,* percutaneous endoscopic gastrostomy; *PSO,* pedicle subtraction osteotomy.

Complications

In the authors' surgical series, one case of incidental durotomy occurred, and it was repaired during the same surgical procedure. One patient had persistent cerebrospinal fluid leak postoperatively and was taken back to the operation room for repair. One superficial wound infection occurred, as well as one infection at the iliac crest bone harvest site. The first infection resolved with irrigation and débridement and oral antibiotics. The second infection was managed with a wound vacuum system and oral antibiotics (Table 37-3). Other complications not directly related to the surgical procedure were one case of acute subdural hematoma that required craniotomy and one case of pneumothorax secondary to line placement.

From the standpoint of neurologic complications, one patient had postoperative right C5 palsy interpreted to be secondary to root stretching after deformity correction.

Conclusions

Cervical spinal deformity is very diverse and has many causes. Surgical intervention should be considered if the patient does not respond to a conservative treatment protocol or shows evidence of deteriorating myelopathy, radiculopathy, or functional impairment. Significant, irreducible deformity of the cervical spine may be sufficient to require corrective osteotomy. At the craniocervical junction, neurologic or functional impairment associated with the deformity may be best managed by osteotomy and fixation. Rigid deformities of the cervical spine below the craniocervical junction are likely to require some type of osteotomy to correct the deformity and restore horizontal gaze. Given the complexities of the regional anatomy, the osteotomy techniques that are common in the thoracic and lumbar spine must be adapted to the cervical region.

The four cervical osteotomies discussed in this chapter are (1) craniocervical junction osteotomy using sequential anterior and posterior approaches (C0-C2), (2) Smith-Petersen osteotomy (subaxial flexible deformity), (3) cervicothoracic junction PSO (mid- to low subaxial rigid deformity with the osteotomy at C7 or T1), and (4) cervical circumferential osteotomy (mid- to low subaxial rigid deformity with the osteotomy at C7 or T1). At the craniocervical junction, an anterior approach with initial anterior linear osteotomy, posterior release and reduction of facet joint subluxation, and segmental stabilization may be used. At the midcervical to cervicothoracic junction, Smith-Petersen osteotomy, pedicle subtraction osteotomy, or circumferential osteotomy may be used to achieve the desired correction. However, if significant ventral compressive disease (disk, osteophyte) is present, a ventral decompression procedure may first be performed before the correction of the deformity. Circumferential (360 and 540) techniques are best for restoring mid-subaxial lordosis. C7 PSO is best for correction of cervical sagittal imbalance. The authors also recommend intraoperative imaging guidance systems and intraoperative neuromonitoring, which can help prevent complications related to the osteotomy.

Treatment of complex cervical deformities is challenging and requires a clear understanding of the disease and the patient. Surgeons must be comfortable with remobilizing the spinal column anteriorly and posteriorly, with vertebral artery anatomy, and with methods of anterior and posterior correction.

REFERENCES

1. Steinmetz MP, Stewart TJ, Kager CD, et al.: Cervical deformity correction, *Neurosurgery* 60:S90–S97, 2007.
2. Chi JH, Tay B, Stahl D, Lee R: Complex deformities of the cervical spine, *Neurosurg Clin N Am* 18:295–304, 2007.
3. Deviren V, Scheer JK, Ames CP: Technique of cervicothoracic junction pedicle subtraction osteotomy for cervical sagittal imbalance: report of 11 cases, *J Neurosurg Spine* 15:174–181, 2011.

4. Epstein NE: Evaluation and treatment of clinical instability associated with pseudoarthrosis after anterior cervical surgery for ossification of the posterior longitudinal ligament, *Surg Neurol* 49:246–252, 1998.

5. Hilibrand AS, Carlson GD, Palumbo MA, et al.: Radiculopathy and myelopathy at segments adjacent to the site of a previous anterior cervical arthrodesis, *J Bone Joint Surg Am* 81:519–528, 1999.

6. Mason C, Cozen L, Adelstein L: Surgical correction of flexion deformity of the cervical spine, *Calif Med* 79:244–246, 1953.

7. Chapman JR, Anderson PA, Pepin C, et al.: Posterior instrumentation of the unstable cervicothoracic spine, *J Neurosurg* 84:552–558, 1996.

8. Edwards CC 2nd, Riew KD, Anderson PA, et al.: Cervical myelopathy: current diagnostic and treatment strategies, *Spine J* 3:68–81, 2003.

9. Mummaneni PV, Deutsch H, Mummaneni VP: Cervicothoracic kyphosis, *Neurosurg Clin N Am* 17:277–287, 2006.

10. Mummaneni PV, Mummaneni VP, Haid RW Jr., et al.: Cervical osteotomy for the correction of chin-on-chest deformity in ankylosing spondylitis: technical note, *Neurosurg Focus* 14:e9, 2003.

11. Belanger TA, Milam RA, Roh JS, Bohlman HH: Cervicothoracic extension osteotomy for chin-on-chest deformity in ankylosing spondylitis, *J Bone Joint Surg Am* 87:1732–1738, 2005.

12. Simmons ED, DiStefano RJ, Zheng Y, Simmons EH: Thirty-six years experience of cervical extension osteotomy in ankylosing spondylitis: techniques and outcomes, *Spine (Phila Pa 1976)* 31:3006–3012, 2006.

13. Suk KS, Kim KT, Lee SH, Kim JM: Significance of chin-brow vertical angle in correction of kyphotic deformity of ankylosing spondylitis patients, *Spine (Phila Pa 1976)* 28:2001–2005, 2003.

14. Grundy PL, Gill SS: Odontoid process and C1-C2 corrective osteotomy through a posterior approach: technical case report, *Neurosurgery* 43:1483–1486, 1998. discussion 1486–1487.

15. Goel A, Laheri V: Plate and screw fixation for atlanto-axial subluxation, *Acta Neurochir (Wien)* 129:47–53, 1994.

16. Harms J, Melcher RP: Posterior C1-C2 fusion with polyaxial screw and rod fixation, *Spine (Phila Pa 1976)* 26:2467–2471, 2001.

17. Jeanneret B, Magerl F: Primary posterior fusion C1/2 in odontoid fractures: indications, technique, and results of transarticular screw fixation, *J Spinal Disord* 5:464–475, 1992.

18. Smith-Petersen MN, Larson CB, Aufranc OE: Osteotomy of the spine for correction of flexion deformity in rheumatoid arthritis, *Clin Orthop Relat Res*(66)6–9, 1969.

19. Urist MR: Osteotomy of the cervical spine: report of a case of ankylosing rheumatoid spondylitis, *J Bone Joint Surg Am* 40:833–843, 1958.

20. McMaster MJ: Osteotomy of the cervical spine in ankylosing spondylitis, *J Bone Joint Surg Br* 79:197–203, 1997.

21. Simmons EH: The surgical correction of flexion deformity of the cervical spine in ankylosing spondylitis, *Clin Orthop Relat Res*(86)132–143, 1972.

22. Smith JS, Shaffrey CI, Lafage V, et al.: Spontaneous improvement of cervical alignment after correction of global sagittal balance following pedicle subtraction osteotomy, *Neurosurg Spine* 17:300–307, 2012.

23. Danisa OA, Turner D, Richardson WJ: Surgical correction of lumbar kyphotic deformity: posterior reduction "eggshell" osteotomy, *J Neurosurg* 92:50–56, 2000.

24. Kim YJ, Bridwell KH, Lenke LG, et al.: Results of lumbar pedicle subtraction osteotomies for fixed sagittal imbalance: a minimum 5-year follow-up study, *Spine (Phila Pa 1976)* 32:2189–2197, 2007.

25. Scheer JK, Tang JA, Buckley JM, et al.: Biomechanical analysis of osteotomy type and rod diameter for treatment of cervicothoracic kyphosis, *Spine (Phila Pa 1976)* 36:E519–E523, 2011.

26. Scheer JK, Tang JA, Deviren V, et al.: Biomechanical analysis of cervicothoracic junction osteotomy in cadaveric model of ankylosing spondylitis: effect of rod material and diameter, *J Neurosurg Spine* 14:330–335, 2011.

27. Daubs MD, Lenke LG, Cheh G, et al.: Adult spinal deformity surgery: complications and outcomes in patients over age 60, *Spine (Phila Pa 1976)* 32:2238–2244, 2007.

28. Wang VY, Aryan H, Ames CP: A novel anterior technique for simultaneous single-stage anterior and posterior cervical release for fixed kyphosis, *J Neurosurg Spine* 8:594–599, 2008.

29. Nottmeier EW, Deen HG, Patel N, Birch B: Cervical kyphotic deformity correction using 360-degree reconstruction, *J Spinal Disord Tech* 22:385–391, 2009.

30. Ames CP, Weber MH, Tay BK, et al: Circumferential osteotomy for fixed cervical sagittal imbalance: a novel surgical technique. *Oper Neurosurg*, 2011.

31. Mummaneni PV, Dhall SS, Rodts GE, Haid RW: Circumferential fusion for cervical kyphotic deformity, *J Neurosurg Spine* 9:515–521, 2008.

32. O'Shaughnessy BA, Liu JC, Hsieh PC, et al.: Surgical treatment of fixed cervical kyphosis with myelopathy, *Spine (Phila Pa 1976)* 33:771–778, 2008.

SECTION 6

Fixation Techniques

Occipitocervical Fixation

38

Giac Consigilieri, Mark P. Garrett, and Volker K.H. Sonntag

CHAPTER PREVIEW

Chapter Synopsis	Occipitocervical fixation techniques have evolved significantly from early occipitocervical wiring techniques to the current rod-screw-occipital plate constructs. Indications for occipitocervical fixation include traumatic injuries, congenital malformations, rheumatoid arthritis, and oncologic processes involving the craniovertebral junction. Judicious clinical decision making and meticulous surgical technique are necessary to manage patients requiring occipitocervical fixation.
Important Points	Surgical indications
	Imaging findings
	Surgical techniques
Clinical and Surgical Pearls	Construct selection should be based on individual anatomic considerations.
	Proper occipitocervical head position should be confirmed before fixation.
	Image guidance should be considered in cases of abnormal anatomy.
	Preoperative vascular imaging should be obtained in cases of abnormal anatomy.
	Proper C1 lateral mass screw length should be ensured to facilitate rod placement.
	The surgeon should consider using rib (versus iliac crest) autograft to reduce donor site morbidity. Proper wiring techniques should be used to secure the allograft construct.
Clinical and Surgical Pitfalls	Fixation in excessive flexion or extension can result in swallowing difficulty or poor visualization of the ground, or both.
	Improper identification of the keel or midline for occipital screw placement can result in cerebellar screw violation.
	Inadequate occipital screw tapping can result in loose occipital screws.
	High-riding or proud occipital instrumentation can result in hardware erosion.
	C1 lateral mass or C2 pedicle screw misplacement can result in vertebral artery injury. Image guidance should be used when the anatomy is mobile.

Occipitocervical fixation (OCF) is a maximally invasive surgical technique that results in significant loss of flexion, extension, and rotation. Therefore, surgical indications for OCF are either conditions that result in cervicomedullary compression, the treatment of which would cause instability, or entities that themselves result in overt instability at the occipitocervical junction. These surgical indications include traumatic injuries, rheumatoid arthritis (RA), congenital malformations, and primary and metastatic neoplastic lesions of the craniocervical junction. The earliest description of occipitocervical fusion was by Foerster in 1927. In subsequent decades, additional reports described similar bone onlay techniques.[1-4] Occipitocervical techniques have evolved extensively since their initial description, and competent spine surgeons should possess a mastery of these techniques in their surgical armamentarium.

Preoperative Considerations

Traumatic Injuries of the Craniovertebral Junction

Traumatic injuries of the craniovertebral junction include occipitoatlantal dislocation (OAD), occipital condyle fractures, atlas fractures, and axis fractures and dislocations.

Occipitoatlantal Dislocation

Considerable force is required to cause OAD, and patients often present with significant head, spinal cord, or multisystemic traumatic injuries. Mechanical ventilation, which can be needed as a result of brainstem compromise, often makes neurologic assessment difficult. Cranial nerve deficits or vertebral artery injury can be present. Despite the significant nature of the injury, some patients may have no neurologic deficits.[5]

Once OAD is suspected based on examination or mechanism of injury, strict cervical spine precautions are mandatory to prevent further complications. Sandbags should be used for initial head immobilization because rigid cervical collars can further distract the occipitoatlantal joint. The authors agree with other investigators who recommend early halo fixation once the diagnosis of OAD is confirmed.[6-8] Even if surgical fixation is planned, a halo vest minimizes motion of the cervical spine during intubation and positioning.

A wide range of sensitivities has been reported for the techniques used to diagnose OAD,[9-12] and none of these criteria is fail proof. Available methods include the Power ratio, the X-line method, the condylar gap method, the basion-dens interval (BDI), and the basion-axial interval (BAI). A universal theme underlying the difficulties of diagnosing OAD using plain lateral cervical radiographs is the ability to visualize the anatomic landmarks required for application of these methods. Dedicated studies using computed tomography (CT) to diagnose OAD have supported the use of the BDI (with 10 mm as the cutoff)[9] and the occipital condyle–C1 interval (CCI) (>4 mm is abnormal) as the diagnostic tests of choice.[13]

The increased use of magnetic resonance imaging (MRI) in trauma patients raises the question of how to interpret equivocal findings in the occipitoatlantal region. The primary dilemma is how to treat patients with equivocal occipitoatlantal joint disruptions noted on MRI whose measurements on CT are normal. Further research may uncover a less severe but still unstable occipitoatlantal joint injury that threatens the neural structures enough to warrant internal fixation of the occiput to the cervical spine.

Once the diagnosis of OAD has been established, OCF is the appropriate treatment. Contraindications to treatment include medical instability in patients.

Occipital Condyle Fractures

The initial neurologic evaluation of patients presenting with occipital condyle fractures is often confounded by a concomitant head injury.[14] Other patients can become symptomatic with neurologic injury or just neck pain.[15-18] CT of the cervical spine is critical in diagnosing these fractures, which are often missed on plain radiographic imaging.[19] Most isolated occipital condyle fractures can be treated with either a hard collar or halo immobilization. Surgical intervention is indicated in cases of concurrent ligamentous injury and instability on dynamic imaging.[20,21]

Atlas and Axis Fractures

Patients with atlas fractures often present with neck pain, although symptoms can include difficulty swallowing related to retropharyngeal edema or neurologic deficit related to vertebral artery injury or lower cranial nerve injury.[22,23] Although plain radiographs can detect an atlas fracture, fine-cut CT with sagittal and coronal reformatted scans can rule out pseudospread of the atlas, and MRI can be used to evaluate the integrity of the transverse ligament.[24,25] Surgical fixation is rarely indicated for isolated C1 fractures.[26] C1 fractures associated with C2 fractures demonstrating dynamic instability, an atlantodens interval (ADI) greater than 5 mm, more than 11 degrees of C2-C3 angulation, or an incompetent transverse ligament may require OCF.[26] Isolated axis fractures rarely require OCF.

Rheumatoid Arthritis

RA is the most common inflammatory disease of the spine. One percent of the world's population is affected by RA, and 50% of these patients have cervical spine involvement.[27] Two of the most common spinal findings in patients with RA are basilar invagination and atlantoaxial instability. The degree of involvement of the cervical vertebral junction is related to the length and severity of the disease.[28] Patients with RA who have involvement of the craniovertebral junction can present with neck pain, cervical deformity, or progressive neurologic decline.[29] However, in more recent years, disease-modifying antirheumatic drugs have made a major impact on the natural history of RA in the cervical spine.[27,29] Dynamic imaging, MRI, and CT are all critical in assessing instability, the degree of cervicomedullary compression, and abnormal bony anatomy.

Preoperative considerations in patients with RA are critical because of the potential multisystemic involvement of the disease. A significant cohort of patients can have cardiovascular involvement, including pericarditis, valvular dysfunction, and conduction abnormalities.[30] Furthermore, patients with RA should be evaluated for pulmonary involvement before surgical intervention,[31] especially patients with pulmonary fibrosis, who tend to have worse outcomes than do other patients with RA.[32]

Pain, myelopathy, spinal cord compression, and symptomatic vertebral artery compression are all indications for OCF in patients with RA and atlantoaxial instability. Patients with basilar invagination undergo surgical procedures to ameliorate neurologic symptoms to prevent progressive neurologic decline. Contraindications to surgical treatment include significant medical comorbidities.

Congenital Malformations

Congenital malformations of the craniovertebral junction include basilar invagination, atlas assimilation, C1 congenital anomalies, atlantoaxial fusion, and odontoid process anomalies. These anomalies occur in isolation or in known syndromes such as Klippel-Feil syndrome, Down syndrome, and Chiari malformations.[33,34] Indications for OCF include instability, spinal cord compression, and progressive neurologic decline.[34]

Neoplasms of the Craniocervical Junction

Neoplasms of the craniocervical junction range from primary tumors, including osteoid osteomas, osteoblastomas, osteochondromas, hemangiomas, aneurysmal bone cysts, plasmacytomas, osteosarcomas, chondrosarcomas, giant cell tumors, Ewing tumors, hemangiopericytomas, and chordomas to metastatic tumors. Patients with tumors in this region often have a late presentation. These patients typically seek treatment for neck pain that can be exacerbated by motion. They also have prominent nocturnal pain and persistent, progressive pain. These patients rarely exhibit neurologic symptoms because of the generous subarachnoid space at the craniocervical junction. Diagnosis is commonly made with MRI. Dynamic imaging can reveal craniocervical instability related to bony destruction associated with the lesion. Indications for OCF in patients with lesions at the craniocervical junction include atlantoaxial instability, pain, and neurologic dysfunction.

Surgical Technique

Positioning

Before patients are positioned for the surgical procedure, appropriate leads are placed if monitoring of somatosensory- or motor-evoked potentials is planned. Depending on the degree of instability, the patient should be transferred to the prone position on the surgical bed in a hard cervical collar or halo brace. The head is positioned in a neutral to slightly flexed position. Excessive flexion could result in discomfort and swallowing difficulty for the patient, and excessive extension results in poor visualization of the ground. The head is rigidly fixed to the surgical bed with a Mayfield skull clamp or the halo ring (Fig. 38-1). If intraoperative navigation is to be used, the stereotactic reference frame should be attached to the Mayfield skull clamp. The occiput, neck, upper thoracic, and infrascapular region should be prepared in sterile fashion for a midline incision and harvest of a rib graft.

Exposure

A routine midline skin incision is made to access the occipital bone and the vertebral levels to be included in the fusion (Fig. 38-2). Dissection proceeds to expose a 5- to 6-cm width of the occipital bone and foramen magnum. The posterior ring of C1 is exposed laterally in a subperiosteal fashion by using the sulcus arteriosus as a landmark to identify and protect the horizontal portion of the vertebral artery on the superior aspect of C1. Dissection is also extended laterally over the remaining cervical levels until the lateral edges of the facet joints are visualized. If necessary, the posterior aspect of the C1 lateral masses can be exposed by using bipolar cautery and sharp dissection ventrally along the medial inferior aspect of the lateral ring of C1. The C1 lateral mass can usually be exposed by identifying and retracting the C2 nerve root, but if necessary it can be sacrificed with minimal consequence.[35]

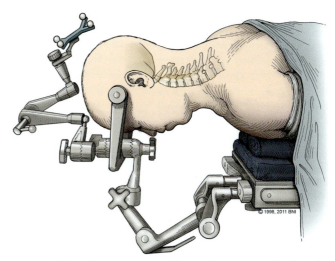

FIGURE 38-1   For occipitocervical fusion the patient is placed in the prone position with the head secured in the Mayfield skull clamp. The head should be placed in the neutral to slightly flexed position. If stereotactic navigation is required, the reference frame can be securely attached to the Mayfield apparatus. (Used with permission from Barrow Neurological Institute, Phoenix, Ariz.)

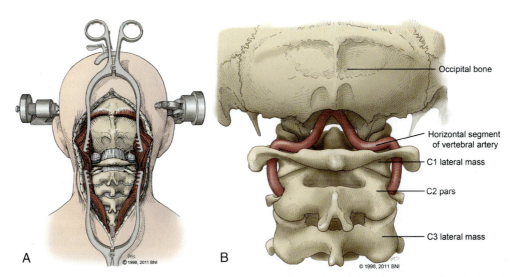

FIGURE 38-2   A, Surgical exposure for occipitocervical fixation. The exposure begins at the nuchal line and widens inferiorly along the occipital bone to accommodate an occipital plate. Care is taken not to injure the vertebral artery when exposing the posterior ring and lateral masses of C1. As needed, the pars of C2 and the lateral masses of the remaining cervical levels can be fully exposed for instrumentation. **B,** Posterior view of the occipitocervical junction illustrating the relationship of the vertebral artery with the bony anatomy. (Used with permission from Barrow Neurological Institute, Phoenix, Ariz.)

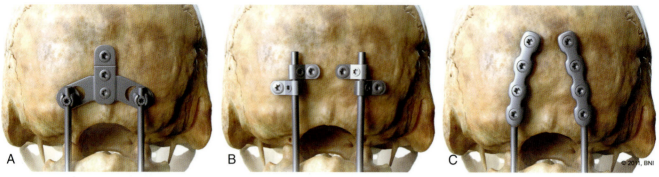

FIGURE 38-3   Multiple options exist for fixation of the construct to the occiput including a midline occipital plate (**A**), occipital clamps (**B**), and a unified plate-rod construct (**C**). (Used with permission from Barrow Neurological Institute, Phoenix, Ariz.)

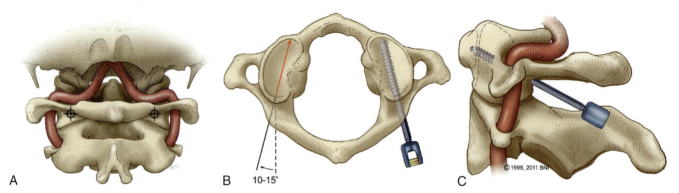

FIGURE 38-4   Landmarks for placement of the C1 lateral mass screw. Exposure of the lateral mass should define the medial and lateral aspect so the entry point can be placed at the midpoint of the lateral mass (**A**). The trajectory of the screw should be 10 to 15 degrees medial (**B**) and directed at the anterior tubercle of C1 in the sagittal plane (**C**). (Used with permission from Barrow Neurological Institute, Phoenix, Ariz.)

Occipital Instrumentation

Many devices, such as midline plates, clamp constructs, or plate and rod constructs, have been developed for occipital fixation (Fig. 38-3). The authors' current practice uses an occipital plate that allows fixation by midline occipital keel screws, typically, a 10-mm screw. The thickness of the keel should be measured preoperatively on the CT scan. Intraoperative navigation can be helpful to identify regions of greatest thickness along the keel.

Occipital keel screws are strongest when placed bicortically, but care must be taken to avoid a penetrating screw injury that can result in cerebrospinal fluid leak, cerebellar injury, or venous sinus injury. Because of the thickness of the occipital keel, drilling with a manual drill requires patience. Care must be taken to avoid applying excessive force with the drill and plunging through the bone. Use of a drill guide set to the appropriate depth and a manual drill allows the surgeon to receive tactile feedback and to confirm bicortical placement. The drill hole is then tapped, and the appropriately sized blunt occipital screw is placed to secure the plate to the occiput.

The size of the midline occipital plate is chosen so that the rod attachment points are aligned with the cervical screws. Modern occipital plates often have rod attachment points that rotate and slide to allow easy connection of the cervical construct to the occipital plate. The occipital plate should be placed 5 to 10 mm superior to the posterior edge of the foramen magnum for placement of the rib or other graft material.

Atlantoaxial Instrumentation

If the patient's anatomy is appropriate, instrumentation should include the C1 level to provide an additional point of fixation to the fusion construct. When a fracture or abnormal anatomy increases the risk of placing a C1 lateral mass screw, that screw should be excluded from the construct. Multiple techniques for upper cervical spine instrumentation exist, including C1-C2 transarticular screws, C1 lateral mass screws, C2 interarticularis pars or pedicle screws, C2 laminar screws, and laminar wiring techniques.

The authors prefer the C1 lateral mass and C2 pedicle or pars screw and rod construct to the transarticular technique, although both offer similar biomechanical stability.[36] The risk for vertebral artery injury is higher with the transarticular technique, and the patient's vascular anatomy often precludes its use. The choice of technique should be based on anatomic and safety considerations.

When a C1 lateral mass screw is used, the entry point is placed at the midline of the posterior aspect of the lateral mass at its junction with the inferior surface of the posterior C1 ring (Fig. 38-4). A small area of the undersurface of the posterior ring can be drilled to improve clearance for the drill and screw. A manual drill and drill guide are used to drill the hole while fluoroscopic guidance can be used to verify the depth and trajectory. The trajectory of the drill should be 10 to 15 degrees medial and aimed directly at the anterior tubercle of C1. The anatomy of the anterior ring on preoperative imaging helps guide the depth of

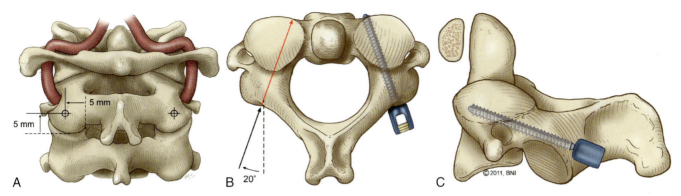

FIGURE 38-5   Landmarks for placement of the C2 pedicle screw. When measured from the medial border of the C2-C3 facet joint, the entry point for the pedicle screw is 5 mm lateral and 5 mm superior (**A**). The trajectory of the screw is 20 degrees medial along the axial plane (**B**) and 10 to 20 degrees cephalad along the sagittal plane (**C**). (Used with permission from Barrow Neurological Institute, Phoenix, Ariz.)

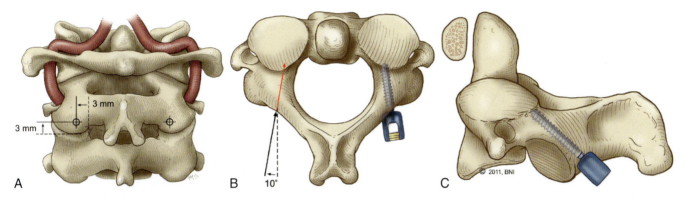

FIGURE 38-6   Landmarks for placement of the C2 pars screw. When measured from the medial border of the C2-C3 facet joint, the entry point for the pars screw is 3 mm lateral and 3 mm superior (**A**). The trajectory of the screw is 10 degrees medial along the axial plane (**B**) and 40 degrees cephalad along the sagittal plane (**C**). On lateral fluoroscopy, the tip of the pars screw should not advance beyond the plane of the posterior aspect of the body of C2, to ensure that the vertebral artery is not put at risk. (Used with permission from Barrow Neurological Institute, Phoenix, Ariz.)

the drill. If the curvature of the anterior arch is minimal or "flat," the tip of the screw on lateral fluoroscopy should be aligned with the anterior tubercle. If the curvature of the anterior arch is significant or "steep," a screw aligned with the anterior tubercle on lateral fluoroscopy will breach the anterior surface of C1 and place the carotid artery at risk.[37] A partially threaded screw is inserted so that its threaded portion is buried in the lateral mass and its smooth portion extends beyond the C2 nerve root to a height that is level with the remaining cervical screws.

Options for screw placement at C2 include a pars interarticularis screw, pedicle screw, or laminar screw. The authors prefer to place pedicle screws or pars screws, depending on the anatomy of the vertebral artery, and to use laminar screws or wires on the rare occasion when placement of neither pedicle screws nor pars screws is possible.

The entry points for the C2 pars and pedicle screws differ slightly. When measured from the medial aspect of the C2-C3 facet joint, the entry point for the pars screw is 3 mm lateral and 3 mm superior, whereas that of the pedicle screw is 5 mm lateral and 5 mm superior. This difference results in a slightly higher and more medial approach for the pedicle screw, which is inserted along a trajectory of 20 degrees medial and 10 to 20 degrees cephalad (Fig. 38-5). The pars screw trajectory is 10 degrees medial and 40 degrees cephalad and does not

extend beyond the region of the pars, to avoid injury to the vertebral artery (Fig 38-6). The transarticular screw uses the same entry point and trajectory as the pars screw, but it extends through the C1-C2 joint into the lateral mass of C1. On lateral fluoroscopy the trajectory of the pars-transarticular screw should be directed at the anterior tubercle of C1 (Fig. 38-7).

When screws are placed in the pars interarticularis or pedicle of C2, it is helpful to use a Penfield number 4 dissector to palpate the medial border of the pars and pedicle in the spinal canal. This maneuver orients the surgeon to the border of the spinal canal and confirms medial placement of the screw within the pars or pedicle, thereby decreasing the risk of vertebral artery injury, as well as avoiding a medial breach into the spinal canal.

Subaxial Instrumentation

Sometimes the fusion construct must be extended below the level of C2 because of injury at these levels or because of the need for additional fixation in the presence of severe instability. For levels C3 to C6, lateral mass screws are placed. The entry point on the lateral mass is slightly medial and inferior to the midpoint. A manual drill with drill guide set to the appropriate depth is used to drill a hole that is oriented 30 degrees cephalad and 30 degrees lateral (Fig. 38-8). This trajectory decreases the risk of vertebral artery injury. Depending on the anatomy, either C7

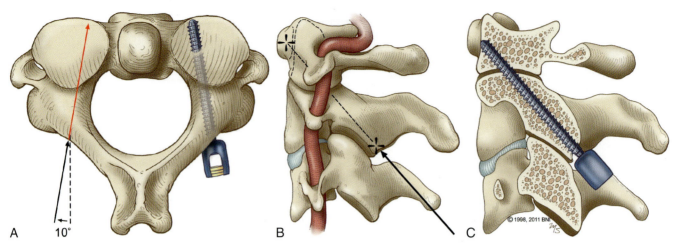

FIGURE 38-7   Landmarks for placement of the C1-C2 transarticular screw. The entry point for the transarticular screw is the same as that of the C2 pars screw (see Fig. 38-6). The trajectory of the screw along the axial plane is 10 degrees (**A**). The trajectory of the screw along the sagittal plane is approximately 40 degrees and should be directed at the anterior tubercle of C1 on lateral fluoroscopy (**B**) to ensure good purchase in the lateral mass of C1 (**C**). (Used with permission from Barrow Neurological Institute, Phoenix, Ariz.)

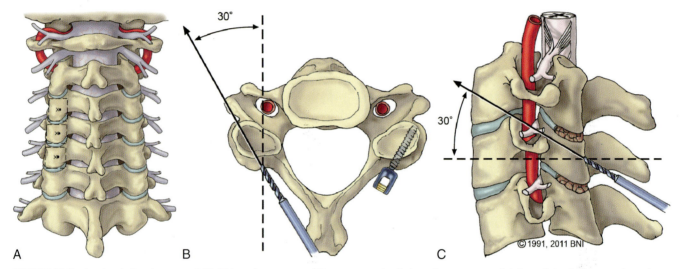

FIGURE 38-8   Landmarks for placement of C3-C6 lateral mass screws. The entry point for the lateral mass screw is slightly medial and inferior to the midpoint of the lateral mass (**A**). The trajectory of the screw is 30 degrees lateral along the axial plane (**B**) and 30 degrees cephalad along the sagittal plane (**C**). (Used with permission from Barrow Neurological Institute, Phoenix, Ariz.)

lateral mass screws or pedicle screws are placed. Often, however, neither type of screw is suitable, so the level is excluded from the construct. Should the construct need to extend into the thoracic spine, pedicle screws are placed.

Rod and Graft Placement

For uncomplicated placement of the rods, appropriately sized cervical screws should be placed so that all the screw heads are well aligned. The shape of the rod should be contoured to match the cervical curvature and to minimize the pull-out force as the rod is secured to the screws. The rod also must accommodate the 90- to 120-degree angle between the occipital plate and the cervical spine. As an alternative to bending a straight cervical rod manually, the surgeon can use prebent and adjustable rods with a joint that can be secured. Once all the screw caps have been secured, they should be tightened to their final position while counter torque is applied to the rod to prevent the construct from dislodging (Fig. 38-9).

Preparation for fusion should include decortication of all exposed facet joints that are to be included in the fusion. A variety of fusion substrates, including autologous bone graft, can then be placed across and in the joint spaces. A bone graft can be placed between the occiput and C1 lamina and secured with braided cables (Fig. 38-10). When the C1 lamina has been removed, an alternative is placement of a long graft from the base of the occiput to C3 (Fig. 38-11). The authors prefer to harvest a rib graft for this purpose, given its lower rate of donor site morbidity when compared with iliac crest bone graft.[38] The inferior aspect of the occiput and the lamina at C2 and C3 are decorticated, and the rib graft is secured down to the cervical spine by using braided cables fastened to the rod construct.

Occipital and Laminar Wiring Techniques

When spinal anatomy precludes the use of screws, occipital and sublaminar wires can be placed to secure the rod to the

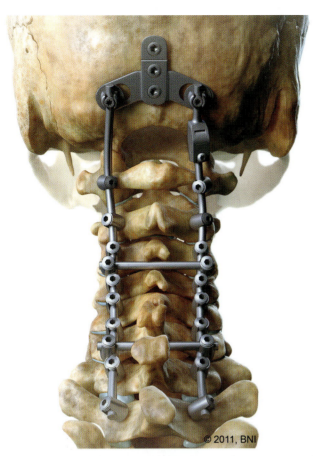

FIGURE 38-9 Illustration depicting a posterior view of a construct extending from the occiput to T1. To accommodate the angle between C1 and the occiput, a standard rod can be manually bent (left) or a hinged rod can be used and secured at the desired angle (right). Two crosslink rods have been placed at C3 to C4 and C6 to C7. (Used with permission from Barrow Neurological Institute, Phoenix, Ariz.)

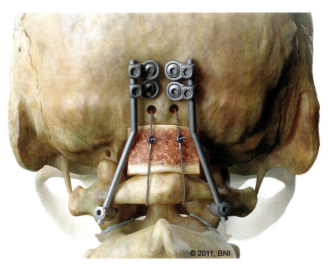

FIGURE 38-10 Illustration depicting a posterior view of an occipital-to-C1 fusion construct. This particular construct uses occipital clamps attached to the rods that extend to C1 lateral mass screws. A bone graft is secured with cables between the occiput and the lamina of C1. (Used with permission from Barrow Neurological Institute, Phoenix, Ariz.)

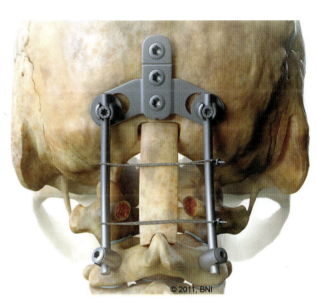

FIGURE 38-11 Illustration depicting a posterior view of an occipital-to-C2 fusion construct with placement of a rib graft. This construct is generally used when laminectomy of C1 is required or if the fusion construct extends beyond C1. A shelf is drilled at the base of the occipital bone where the rib graft can fit securely. A notch is drilled at the distal end of the graft that fits over the spinous process and lamina of C2. Cables are used to secure the rib graft in this position. (Used with permission from Barrow Neurological Institute, Phoenix, Ariz.)

construct. After appropriate exposure, the laminae of the cervical vertebrae are often notched medially as close to the spinous processes as possible with a Kerrison rongeur to facilitate passage of sublaminar wires. Care must be taken not to weaken the posterior elements when placing a notch for wire passage. A Kerrison rongeur is used to remove the posterior rim of the foramen magnum. Two or three burr holes are drilled in the occiput 5 to 10 mm superior to the enlarged rim of the foramen magnum. The burr holes are waxed, and the dura is dissected from the inner table of the skull toward the foramen magnum. If facets are to be wired, drill holes are placed through the inferior facets into the joints. Sublaminar wires or facet wires are then placed.

Wiring is performed with 24-gauge, double-stranded wire (three turns per centimeter) or braided wire cable. Sublaminar wire placement can be facilitated by carefully passing the blunt end of a large needle attached to 2-0 polyglactin 910 (Vicryl) or silk suture under each lamina. The suture is tied to the end of the wire, and both are carefully passed under the lamina using a simultaneous feeding-and-pulling technique. A wide-diameter, stainless steel, threaded Steinmann pin or custom-made titanium grooved rod (5/32-inch diameter) is bent into a U shape, and then secondary curves are fashioned to fit the lordotic contour of the occipitocervical region. Fixation is achieved by securing the pin to the occiput with suboccipital wires and to the cervical spine with sublaminar or facet wires (Fig. 38-12). Sublaminar wires are positioned at the most lateral aspects of the laminae during fixation. The use of such wiring techniques is an excellent option for occipital or cervical fixation when screw placement is not possible.

Postoperative Considerations

Given the amount of muscular detachment that occurs during exposure of the posterior cervical spine, postoperative

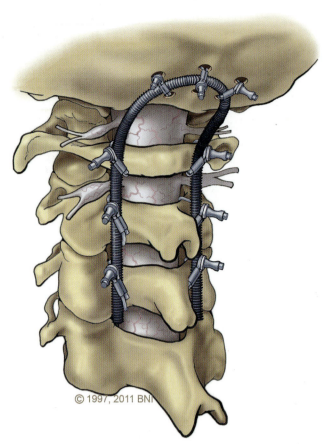

FIGURE 38-12 Illustration showing a threaded Steinmann pin secured to the craniocervical junction with suboccipital and sublaminar wires. (Used with permission from Barrow Neurological Institute, Phoenix, Ariz.)

pain management is critical after OCF. Adequate pain control is necessary so that severe discomfort does not prevent early postoperative mobilization. Physical and occupational therapies are often required. Depending on the medical and neurologic status of the patient, a brief period of inpatient rehabilitation may be necessary to aid in recovery of strength and function.

Complications that are common to other spinal procedures can occur: infection, wound breakdown, graft dislodgment, and pseudarthrosis. Patients should be placed in a rigid cervical collar unless concern exists for significant instability or poor bone quality, in which case halo immobilization may be necessary. The length of immobilization with a cervical collar is determined on a case-by-case basis, but patients typically remain in their collar for 6 weeks. Fusions rates for OCF are very high, approaching 100%,[39] but patients should be followed up radiographically to rule out delayed instability or hardware failure. Dynamic radiographs are obtained 6 weeks and 3 months postoperatively.

Results

The authors' experience with the threaded Steinmann pin fusion technique in the craniocervical junction included 39 patients with occipitocervical instability: RA (n = 12), congenital anomalies (n = 12), trauma (n = 10), tumor

(n = 4), and osteogenesis imperfecta (n = 1). At a mean follow-up of 38.9 months, 37 patients (97%) had a stable postoperative occipitocervical construct: 35 osseous unions, 2 fibrous unions, and 1 nonunion occurred. Postoperatively, 1 patient died of pulmonary complications.[40]

A later look at survivors of occipitoatlantal injuries at the authors' institution included 22 patients (of 28 total initial OAD survivors) who survived until discharge to rehabilitation and for whom follow-up data were available (mean follow-up, 13 months). Fixation techniques involved placement of a Steinmann pin and sublaminar wires in 15 patients, 2 different screw-rod constructs in 6 patients, and autologous rib or split-thickness skull graft wiring in 2 patients. At final follow-up, all patients had intact hardware and radiographic evidence of fusion.[41]

Winegar and colleagues performed a systematic literature review of OCF techniques and outcomes that included 34 articles describing 799 patients.[42] Surgical indications included the treatment of inflammatory diseases in 396 patients (49.6%), congenital anomalies in 84 patients (10.5%), tumor in 67 patients (8.4%), trauma in 63 patients (7.9%), and other causes of occipitocervical instability not further specified in 189 patients (23.7%). Of the 799 patients, 404 (51%) were treated with wiring-rod fixation, 195 (24%) were treated with screw-plate constructs, 150 (19%) underwent treatment with posterior wiring and onlay grafting, and 50 patients (6%) were treated with screw-rod constructs. Fusion status was recorded for 554 (69%) of the total case population. Successful fusion was reported in 517 (93.33%) of 554 patients. Arthrodesis was achieved in 95.9% (187 of 195) of patients with wiring-rod constructs, in 94.7% (162 of 171) of those with screw-plate constructs, in 93.02% (40 of 43) of those with screw-rod constructs, and in 88.3% (128 of 145) of those with wiring–onlay bone grafting constructs.

REFERENCES

1. Foerster O: *Die Leitungsbahnen des Schmerzgefuhls und die chirurgische Behandlung der Schmerzzustande*, Berlin, 1927, Urban & Schwarzenberg.
2. Elia M, Mazzara JT, Fielding JW: Onlay technique for occipitocervical fusion, *Clin Orthop Relat Res* (280):170–174, 1992.
3. Kahn EA, Yglesias L: Progressive atlanto-axial dislocation, *JAMA* 105:348–352, 1935.
4. Rand CW: *The neurosurgical patient: his problems of diagnosis and care*, Springfield, Ill, 1944, Charles C Thomas.
5. Horn EM, Feiz-Erfan I, Lekovic GP, et al.: Survivors of occipitoatlantal dislocation injuries: imaging and clinical correlates, *J Neurosurg Spine* 6:113–120, 2007.
6. Steinmetz MP, Lechner RM, Anderson JS: Atlantooccipital dislocation in children: presentation, diagnosis, and management, *Neurosurg Focus* 14:ecp1, 2003.
7. Farley FA, Graziano GP, Hensinger RN: Traumatic atlanto-occipital dislocation in a child, *Spine (Phila Pa 1976)* 17:1539–1541, 1992.
8. Evarts CM: Traumatic occipito-atlantal dislocation, *J Bone Joint Surg Am* 52:1653–1660, 1970.
9. Dziurzynski K, Anderson PA, Bean DB, et al.: A blinded assessment of radiographic criteria for atlanto-occipital dislocation, *Spine (Phila Pa 1976)* 30:1427–1432, 2005.
10. Harris JH Jr, Carson GC, Wagner LK: Radiologic diagnosis of traumatic occipitovertebral dissociation. 1. Normal occipitovertebral relationships on lateral radiographs of supine subjects, *AJR Am J Roentgenol* 162:881–886, 1994.
11. Harris JH Jr, Carson GC, Wagner LK, Kerr N: Radiologic diagnosis of traumatic occipitovertebral dissociation. 2. Comparison of three methods of detecting occipitovertebral relationships on lateral radiographs of supine subjects, *AJR Am J Roentgenol* 162:887–892, 1994.

12. Lee C, Woodring JH, Goldstein SJ, et al.: Evaluation of traumatic atlantooccipital dislocations, *AJNR Am J Neuroradiol* 8:19–26, 1987.

13. Pang D, Nemzek WR, Zovickian J: Atlanto-occipital dislocation. Part 2. The clinical use of (occipital) condyle-C1 interval, comparison with other diagnostic methods, and the manifestation, management, and outcome of atlanto-occipital dislocation in children, *Neurosurgery* 61:995–1015, 2007.

14. Link TM, Schuierer G, Hufendiek A, et al.: Substantial head trauma: value of routine CT examination of the cervicocranium, *Radiology* 196:741–745, 1995.

15. Chou CW, Huang WC, Shih YH, et al.: Occult occipital condyle fracture with normal neurological function and torticollis, *J Clin Neurosci* 15:920–922, 2008.

16. Cottalorda J, Allard D, Dutour N: Fracture of the occipital condyle, *J Pediatr Orthop B* 5:61–63, 1996.

17. Desai SS, Coumas JM, Danylevich A, et al.: Fracture of the occipital condyle: case report and review of the literature, *J Trauma* 30:240–241, 1990.

18. Stroobants J, Fidlers L, Storms JL, et al.: High cervical pain and impairment of skull mobility as the only symptoms of an occipital condyle fracture: case report, *J Neurosurg* 81:137–138, 1994.

19. Noble ER, Smoker WR: The forgotten condyle: the appearance, morphology, and classification of occipital condyle fractures, *AJNR Am J Neuroradiol* 17:507–513, 1996.

20. Tuli S, Tator CH, Fehlings MG, Mackay M: Occipital condyle fractures, *Neurosurgery* 41:368–376, 1997.

21. Young WF, Rosenwasser RH, Getch C, Jallo J: Diagnosis and management of occipital condyle fractures, *Neurosurgery* 34:257–260, 1994.

22. Sherk HH, Nicholson JT: Fractures of the atlas, *J Bone Joint Surg Am* 52:1017–1024, 1970.

23. Kesterson L, Benzel E, Orrison W, Coleman J: Evaluation and treatment of atlas burst fractures (Jefferson fractures), *J Neurosurg* 75:213–220, 1991.

24. Suss RA, Zimmerman RD, Leeds NE: Pseudospread of the atlas: false sign of Jefferson fracture in young children, *AJR Am J Roentgenol* 140:1079–1082, 1983.

25. Dickman CA, Greene KA, Sonntag VK: Injuries involving the transverse atlantal ligament: classification and treatment guidelines based upon experience with 39 injuries, *Neurosurgery* 38:44–50, 1996.

26. Hadley MN: Isolated fractures of the atlas in adults, *Neurosurgery* 50:S120–S124, 2002.

27. Matteson EL: Cervical spine disease in rheumatoid arthritis: how common a finding? How uncommon a problem? *Arthritis Rheum* 48:1775–1778, 2003.

28. Dreyer SJ, Boden SD: Natural history of rheumatoid arthritis of the cervical spine, *Clin Orthop Relat Res* (366):98–106, 1999.

29. Choi D, Casey AT, Crockard HA: Neck problems in rheumatoid arthritis: changing disease patterns, surgical treatments and patients' expectations, *Rheumatology (Oxford)* 45:1183–1184, 2006.

30. Dedhia HV, DiBartolomeo A: Rheumatoid arthritis, *Crit Care Clin* 18:841–854, 2002. ix.

31. Anaya JM, Diethelm L, Ortiz LA, et al.: Pulmonary involvement in rheumatoid arthritis, *Semin Arthritis Rheum* 24:242–254, 1995.

32. Hakala M: Poor prognosis in patients with rheumatoid arthritis hospitalized for interstitial lung fibrosis, *Chest* 93:114–118, 1988.

33. Semine AA, Ertel AN, Goldberg MJ, Bull MJ: Cervical-spine instability in children with Down syndrome (trisomy 21), *J Bone Joint Surg Am* 60:649–652, 1978.

34. Klimo P Jr, Brockmeyer D: Congenital anomalies of the cervical spine, *Neurosurg Clin N Am* 18:463–478, 2007.

35. Squires J, Molinari RW: C1 lateral mass screw placement with intentional sacrifice of the C2 ganglion: functional outcomes and morbidity in elderly patients, *Eur Spine J* 19:1318–1324, 2010.

36. Melcher RP, Puttlitz CM, Kleinstueck FS, et al.: Biomechanical testing of posterior atlantoaxial fixation techniques, *Spine (Phila Pa 1976)* 27:2435–2440, 2002.

37. Wait SD, Ponce FA, Colle KO, et al.: Importance of the C1 anterior tubercle depth and lateral mass geometry when placing C1 lateral mass screws, *Neurosurgery* 65:952–956, 2009.

38. Sawin PD, Traynelis VC, Menezes AH: A comparative analysis of fusion rates and donor-site morbidity for autogeneic rib and iliac crest bone grafts in posterior cervical fusions, *J Neurosurg* 88:255–265, 1998.

39. Nockels RP, Shaffrey CI, Kanter AS, Azeem S, York JE: Occipitocervical fusion with rigid internal fixation: long-term follow-up data in 69 patients, *Spine (Phila Pa 1976)* 7:117–123, 2007.

40. Apostolides PJ, Dickman CA, Golfinos JG, et al.: Threaded Steinmann pin fusion of the craniovertebral junction, *Spine (Phila Pa 1976)* 21:1630–1637, 1996.

41. Horn EM, Feiz-Erfan I, Lekovic GP, et al.: Survivors of occipitoatlantal dislocation injuries: imaging and clinical correlates, *J Neurosurg Spine* 6:113–120, 2007.

42. Winegar CD, Lawrence JP, Friel BC, et al.: A systematic review of occipital cervical fusion: techniques and outcomes, *J Neurosurg Spine* 13:5–16, 2010.

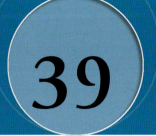

39

C1 Lateral Mass and C2 Pedicle Screw Fixation

Joseph P. Gjolaj and Francis H. Shen

CHAPTER PREVIEW

Chapter Synopsis	Although many different fixation techniques have been developed to manage atlanto-axial instability, C1 lateral mass–C2 pedicle screw fixation has emerged as a preferred treatment, based on its comparative biomechanical strength and modest risk of neurologic or vascular injury, as well as the ability to perform intraoperative reduction.
Important Points	Surgical indications include atlantoaxial instability caused by trauma, tumors, infection or inflammatory disease, or congenital abnormalities.
	Alternative fixation techniques include halo vest immobilization, Brooks or Gallie wiring procedures, and Magerl transarticular screw fixation.
	The C1 lateral mass–C2 pedicle screw technique is typically used for "stand-alone" fixation, but it may be supplemented by rigid cervical collar immobilization in the early postoperative period.
Clinical and Surgical Pearls	Reduction of the C1-C2 joint is not required before screw placement and can be subsequently achieved through repositioning of the patient's head or direct manipulation of the C1 and C2 instrumentation before rod placement.
	C1 lateral mass screws typically have a 10-mm proximal smooth shank, which increases mechanical strength and theoretically decreases the risk of C2 nerve root neuralgia.
	C1 lateral mass and C2 pedicle screws are placed with the use of both direct visualization and fluoroscopic guidance.
	Because of its modularity, C1 lateral mass–C2 pedicle screw fixation can be extended cranially to the occiput or caudally to the subaxial spine, if needed.
Clinical and Surgical Pitfalls	Preoperative evaluation of atlantoaxial bony anatomy with advanced imaging (computed tomography or magnetic resonance imaging, or both) is crucial to ensure that the C1 lateral masses and C2 pedicles can safely accommodate screw placement.
	Bleeding from the epidural venous plexus near the C1-C2 joint is common, but it can be controlled with bipolar cautery, FLOSEAL, and cottonoid patties.
	C2 pedicle screw placement poses the greatest risk of vertebral artery injury, but a superior and medial trajectory decreases this risk.

Atlantoaxial instability can result from multiple disorders, including trauma, tumors, infection and inflammatory conditions, and congenital abnormalities. Regardless of the pathologic process, surgical treatment is often indicated. Surgeons have tended away from halo vest immobilization, which has been associated with significant morbidity and poor patient tolerance,[1] and toward internal fixation techniques performed through a posterior approach. Multiple techniques have been described, including two different posterior

wiring procedures described by Brooks and Gallie and C1-C2 transarticular screw fixation described by Magerl.[2-4]

Although posterior wiring techniques are, in some ways, technically less difficult, they do involve insertion of wires or cables into the spinal canal, a maneuver that poses a risk of spinal cord injury. These techniques also require the use of structural allograft to improve stability and achieve fusion. Even with the addition of halo vest immobilization, however, the rate of pseudarthrosis is up to 30%,[5] as a result of the inferior biomechanical properties of this construct.[4]

The transarticular screw technique provides more stability, based on biomechanical studies, and is also associated with a very high rate of fusion.[2] However, this technique requires reduction of the C1-C2 facet joints bilaterally before screw placement. Additionally, anomalous vertebral artery anatomy, seen in up to 20% of patients, increases the risk of vascular injury and may even preclude the use of this technique.[3]

The most contemporary technique for atlantoaxial fixation was first described by Dr. Jürgen Harms.[6] This technique involves individual screws placed in the lateral masses of C1 and the pedicles of C2 bilaterally connected with rods. The advantages of this technique, also known as the Harms technique, include ability to perform intraoperative reduction and fixation of C1-C2, increased biomechanical strength, and minimized risk of injury to the spinal cord and vertebral artery compared with other fixation techniques. Since its first description in 2001, the Harms technique has been extensively validated in the spinal literature and is now widely used for atlantoaxial fixation.[6-11]

Preoperative Considerations

History

Although atlantoaxial instability is most commonly seen as a result of trauma, it can also be noted inpatients with infection and inflammatory processes, malignant disease, or congenital anomalies. The history of present illness can often help distinguish among these causes. Undoubtedly, all patients who have sustained high-energy injuries require cervical immobilization until atlantoaxial or cervical instability can be excluded. Unfortunately, other causes of atlantoaxial or cervical instability are not as obvious and, without thorough evaluation, can easily be missed.

Signs, Symptoms, and Physical Examination

Signs and symptoms of atlantoaxial instability differ depending on the chronicity of the instability. Patients with acute instability as a result of high-energy trauma may present with only neck pain, but they may also have signs of spinal cord injury. These signs can include upper or lower extremity loss of sensation or motor strength. More importantly, patients may have difficulty breathing because of the high neurologic level of injury. As a consequence, some patients may not survive the injury if medical assistance does not arrive in time or if Advanced Trauma Life Support (ATLS) protocols are not followed.

Patients with chronic atlantoaxial instability typically report neck pain and often describe pain radiating from the upper part of the neck posteriorly into the occipital area, also known as an occipital headache. This pain is caused by irritation or impingement of the C2 or greater occipital nerve root or roots. Because atlantoaxial instability may cause significant stenosis, the patient may also present with symptoms of myelopathy including poor balance, upper or lower extremity weakness, hyperreflexia, or other upper motor neuron findings.

Imaging

As a part of the initial evaluation, imaging studies to define the extent of the injury and amount of instability are required. Plain static radiographs help to define the overall spinal alignment, and dynamic radiographs may help quantify instability in patients with chronic atlantoaxial instability. In patients with instability caused by acute injury, a fine-cut computed tomography (CT) scan may delineate the extent of the bony injury in greater detail. This modality may also be useful in patients with chronic instability in whom plain radiographs are inadequate.

In either acute or chronic instability, a magnetic resonance imaging (MRI) study is very useful for multiple reasons. It can help determine the severity of soft tissue or ligamentous injury in traumatic conditions. It can also help distinguish between spinal infection or inflammatory conditions and malignant disease as a cause of atlantoaxial instability. Additionally, MRI helps establish the severity of nerve or spinal cord compression. Finally, advanced imaging modalities such as fine-cut CT and MRI help to detail the patient's bony and vascular anatomy, to determine whether the C1 lateral mass–C2 pedicle screw technique can be safely used.

Indications and Contraindications

Indications for surgical stabilization of atlantoaxial instability include acute, progressive neurologic compromise from any origin that causes instability at the C1-C2 level. Other indications include an anterior atlantodens interval (AADI) of greater than 3 mm in adults and greater than 4 to 5 mm in children, as defined by flexion radiographs. Persistent neck pain or occipital headache related to C2 nerve root irritation or impingement that is a result of chronic atlantoaxial instability (i.e., odontoid pseudarthrosis) is another indication for surgical stabilization.

Contraindications to use of the C1 lateral mass–C2 pedicle screw technique include bony or vascular anomalies that prohibit safe screw placement. One such example is the presence of a ponticulus posticus, or arcuate foramen at C1, which may be identified by radiographs in approximately 15% of pateints.[12] This bony bridge, through which the vertebral artery courses posteriorly, may not be easily identified intraoperatively and can lead to vertebral artery injury if C1 lateral mass screw placement is attempted.

Surgical Technique

Once adequate general anesthesia is achieved, the patient is positioned prone with the neck held in appropriate alignment with cranial tongs. The atlantoaxial position is confirmed using fluoroscopic imaging. Reduction of any atlantoaxial malalignment may be performed at this time through the use of cranial tongs. Alternatively, reduction may be performed later in the procedure once instrumentation has been placed; this is an advantage of the Harms technique.

Next, the posterior cervical spine is exposed using sharp dissection and electrocautery from the base of the occiput to approximately the C3 level. The inferior portion of the ring of C1 and lamina of C2 are exposed to their lateral borders. The C1-C2 articulation can then be dissected. This step must be performed with caution because significant bleeding may arise from the epidural venous plexus and obscure the C1-C2 joint. This bleeding may be effectively controlled with a combination of bipolar electrocautery, FLOSEAL (or other absorbable gelatin and thrombin mixture), and cottonoid patties.

The C1-C2 joint will now be visible. Identification of this joint is crucial for accurate placement of the C1 lateral mass screw. The C2 nerve must be retracted caudally to expose the entry point for the C1 screw, which is located at the midpoint of the posteroinferior aspect of the C1 lateral mass, where it meets the C1 posterior arch (Fig. 39-1).[10,13] The entry point should be marked with a small, high-speed burr to avoid any slippage of the drill bit. Next, the pilot hole is drilled in a straight-ahead or 10-degree convergent trajectory in the mediolateral direction and parallel to the plane of the C1 posterior arch in the craniocaudal direction.[6,10,13,14] The drill tip should be directed toward the anterior arch of C1 on lateral fluoroscopic imaging, to avoid screw violation of the C1-C2 joint caudally or the occipital-C1 joint cranially (Fig. 39-2).[15] Intraoperative landmarks and preoperative axial CT images are indispensable aids in safe screw placement. A blunt probe is used to check the integrity of the pilot hole. Then the hole is tapped, and a 3.5-mm polyaxial screw of an appropriate length is inserted bicortically into the lateral mass of C1 (Fig. 39-3).

The length of the C1 screw should be determined preoperatively by measurements on a fine-cut CT scan. Typically, a 10-mm smooth shank (unthreaded) portion of the C1 screw stays above the lateral mass itself. This functions to decrease irritation to the C2 nerve root and permits the

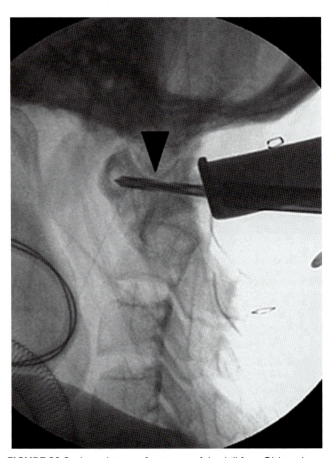

FIGURE 39-2 Lateral image of trajectory of the drill for a C1 lateral mass screw. The tip (*arrowhead*) is directed toward the anterior arch of C1 on the lateral image to avoid violating the C1-C2 joint caudally and the occipital-C1 joint cranially.

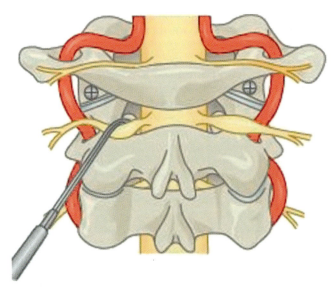

FIGURE 39-1 Schematic drawing of the entry point for a C1 lateral mass screw, which is at the midpoint of the mediolateral lateral mass at the junction where it meets the posterior arch of C1. (From Jarvers JS, Franck A, Glasmacher S, Josten C, et al: Minimally invasive posterior C1/2 screw fixation using C1 lateral mass screws and C2 pedicle screws with 3D C-arm–based navigation. *Oper Tech Orthop* 25:2-8, 2013.)

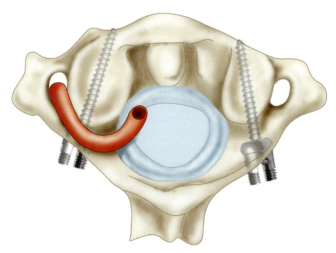

FIGURE 39-3 Axial schematic view demonstrating the position and trajectory of a C1 lateral mass screw. (From Tomycz ND, Okonkwo DO: Occipitocervical fusion. In Jandial R, McCormick P, Black PM, editors: *Core techniques in operative neurosurgery*, Philadelphia, 2011, Saunders.)

polyaxial portion of the screw to rest above the posterior arch of C1.[6] As with placement of all instrumentation, screw position is verified by fluoroscopic imaging.

Next, a small instrument such as a Penfield number 4 or Penfield number 1 dissector can be used to identify

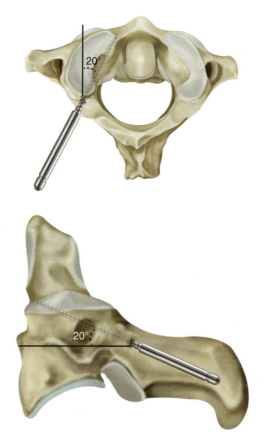

FIGURE 39-4   Axial schematic views demonstrating the position and trajectory of a C2 pedicle screw. (From Kim DH, Vaccaro AR, Dickman CA, et al, editors: *Surgical anatomy and techniques to the spine*, ed 2, Philadelphia, 2013, Saunders.)

the medial border of the C2 pars. This technique helps delineate the entry point for the C2 pedicle screw, which is in the cranial and medial quadrant of the isthmus surface of C2 (Fig. 39-4).[6] After the entry point is marked with a high-speed burr, the pilot hole is drilled bicortically. The trajectory of the drill bit is approximately 20 to 30 degrees convergent and cephalad, typically guided by the superior and medial surface of the C2 isthmus.[14] A blunt probe is used to check the integrity of the pilot hole. After the hole is tapped, a 3.5-mm polyaxial screw of an appropriate length is inserted bicortically.

At this point, reduction of the C1 ring may be performed by either repositioning of the patient's head using cranial tongs or by direct manipulation of the C1 and C2 vertebrae with the screws. Once adequate alignment is achieved, the screws are then fixed to the rods to maintain the alignment (Fig. 39-5). For definitive fusion, the posterior aspects of C1 and C2 are decorticated, and autograft or allograft bone is placed over the decorticated surfaces. Intraarticular fusion has also been described, involving decortication of the joint surfaces between C1 and C2.[6] However, this step poses an additional risk to neurovascular structures and should be performed only under direct vision.

The C1 lateral mass–C2 pedicle screw fixation technique can also be performed for temporary stabilization without definitive fusion, as initially described by Harms for a small number of patients.[6] Implant removal, if performed at an appropriate time interval, may allow the patient to regain atlantoaxial motion. Postoperatively, patients may benefit from cervical collar immobilization for the first 2 to 3 weeks as tolerated.

Results

The C1 lateral mass–C2 pedicle screw fixation technique has yielded satisfactory results in numerous case

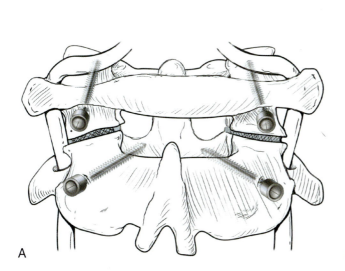

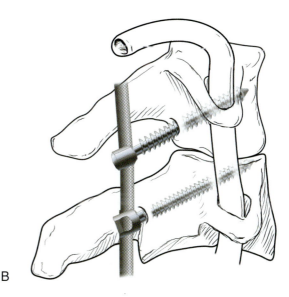

FIGURE 39-5   Posterior (**A**) and lateral (**B**) schematic views of a final C1 lateral mass–C2 pedicle screw construct. (From Moulton AW: Clinically relevant spinal anatomy. In Errico TJ, Lonner BS, Moulton AW, editors: *Surgical management of spinal deformities*, Philadelphia, 2009, Saunders.)

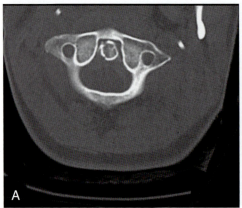

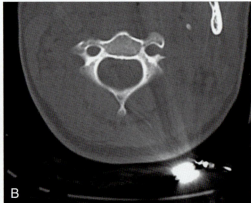

FIGURE 39-6   Sagittal T2-weighted magnetic resonance imaging (**A**) and fine-cut computed tomography sagittal reconstruction (**B**) of a 20-year-old female patient who sustained a type 2 odontoid fracture with associated spinal cord signal change.

FIGURE 39-7   Fine cut axial C1 (**A**) and C2 (**B**) images demonstrating normal anatomy without associated fractures.

series.[6,7,9-11] Harms reported on 37 patients who were the first to undergo this procedure. In this series no vertebral artery injuries, dural lacerations, or neurologic deteriorations occurred as a result of the procedure. One patient had a deep wound infection, which was successfully treated with surgical débridement and intravenous antibiotics. In routine clinical follow-up, the investigators reported no cases of implant failure, and at final follow-up (1 year postoperatively), all patients exhibited radiographic fusion.

Harms' initial case series included two patients who underwent temporary stabilization without fusion using this technique. Both were younger patients in whom preservation of atlantoaxial mobility was desired. Removal of instrumentation was performed in a second-stage procedure at approximately 3 to 4 months, after which time one of the two patients displayed evidence of preserved C1-C2 motion on dynamic MRI evaluation.

CLINICAL CASE

A typical case, which was treated at the author's institution, is herein described. The patient is an athletic 20-year-old woman who sustained an odontoid fracture as a result of a motor vehicle accident. Imaging studies including computed tomography (CT) scan and magnetic resonance imaging show an acute type 2 odontoid fracture with associated spinal cord signal change posterior to the C2 vertebral body (Fig. 39-6). Fine-cut axial CT images show otherwise normal C1 and C2 bony anatomy (Fig. 39-7). Based on these findings, as well as the patient's age, high activity level, and desire for operative fixation in lieu of prolonged rigid cervical collar immobilization, surgical stabilization using the C1 lateral mass–C2 pedicle screw fixation technique was performed (Figs. 39-8 and 39-9).

As described earlier, clinical outcomes verify that the C1 lateral mass–C2 pedicle screw fixation technique remains a viable solution for surgical treatment of atlantoaxial instability caused by trauma, malignant disease, infections, and inflammatory processes or congenital abnormalities. Although the goal of this technique is typically arthrodesis of the C1-C2 joints, temporary stabilization may also be an option.

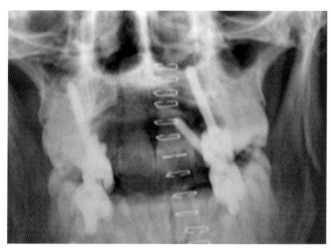

FIGURE 39-8 Anteroposterior postoperative radiograph of a C1 lateral mass–C2 pedicle screw construct.

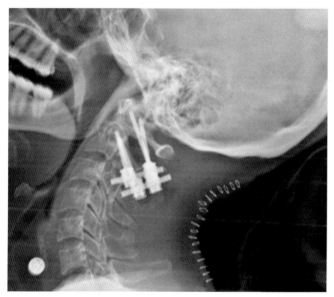

FIGURE 39-9 Lateral postoperative radiograph of a C1 lateral mass–C2 pedicle screw construct.

REFERENCES

1. Bradley J F 3rd, Jones M A, Farmer E A, et al.: Swallowing dysfunction in trauma patients with cervical spine fractures treated with halo-vest fixation, *J Trauma* 70:46–50, 2011.
2. Grob D, Jeanneret B, Aebi M, et al.: Atlanto-axial fusion with transarticular screw fixation, *J Bone Joint Surg Br* 73:972–976, 1991.
3. Jun BY: Anatomic study for ideal and safe posterior C1-C2 transarticular screw fixation, *Spine (Phila Pa 1976)* 23:1703–1707, 1998.
4. Papagelopoulos PJ, Currier B L, Hokari Y, et al.: Biomechanical comparison of C1-C2 posterior arthrodesis techniques, *Spine (Phila Pa 1976)* 32:E363–E370, 2007.
5. Farey I D, Nadkarni S, Smith N: Modified Gallie technique versus transarticular screw fixation in C1-C2 fusion, *Clin Orthop Relat Res* (359):126–135, 1999.
6. Harms J, Melcher R P: Posterior C1-C2 fusion with polyaxial screw and rod fixation, *Spine (Phila Pa 1976)* 26:2467–2471, 2001.
7. Aryan H E, Newman C B, Nottmeier E W, et al.: Stabilization of the atlantoaxial complex via C-1 lateral mass and C-2 pedicle screw fixation in a multicenter clinical experience in 102 patients: modification of the Harms and Goel techniques, *J Neurosurg Spine* 8:222–229, 2008.
8. Claybrooks R, Kayanja M, Milks R, Benzel E: Atlantoaxial fusion: a biomechanical analysis of two C1-C2 fusion techniques, *Spine J* 7:682–688, 2007.
9. Gunnarsson T, Massicotte E M, Govender P V, et al.: The use of C1 lateral mass screws in complex cervical spine surgery: indications, techniques, and outcome in a prospective consecutive series of 25 cases, *J Spinal Disord Tech* 20:308, 2007.
10. Seal C, Zarro C, Gelb D, Ludwig S: C1 lateral mass anatomy: proper placement of lateral mass screws, *J Spinal Disord Tech* 22:516–523, 2009.
11. Xie Y, Li Z, Tang H, et al.: Posterior C1 lateral mass and C2 pedicle screw internal fixation for atlantoaxial instability, *J Clin Neurosci* 16:1592–1594, 2009.
12. Young JP, Young PH, Ackermann MJ, et al.: The ponticulus posticus: implications for screw insertion into the first cervical lateral mass, *J Bone Joint Surg Am* 87:2495–2498, 2005.
13. Puttlitz C M, Goel V K, Traynelis VC, Clark C R: A finite element investigation of upper cervical instrumentation, *Spine (Phila Pa 1976)* 26:2449–2455, 2001.
14. Schulz R, Macchiavello N, Fernández E, et al.: Harms C1-C2 instrumentation technique: anatomo-surgical guide, *Spine (Phila Pa 1976)* 36:945–950, 2011.
15. Yeom J S, Buchowski J M, Park K W, et al.: Lateral fluoroscopic guide to prevent occipitocervical and atlantoaxial joint violation during C1 lateral mass screw placement, *Spine J* 9:574–579, 2009.

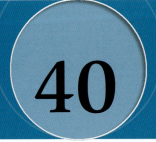

40 C1-C2 Transarticular Screws

Joshua E. Heller and Vincent Arlet

CHAPTER PREVIEW

Chapter Synopsis	Placement of the C1-C2 transarticular screw (Magerl technique) remains a viable alternative for the surgical management of a variety of atlantoaxial disorders. Although the operation is technically demanding, a careful understanding of the procedure and its limitations, as well as a thorough understanding of each patient's individualized bony and vascular anatomy, can help reduce the risk of complications. Proper preoperative radiographic evaluation including x-ray studies, computed tomography (CT), and CT angiography or magnetic resonance angiography is necessary. When used in the appropriate patient, the Magerl technique yields excellent results with high fusion rates and relatively low complication rates. The purpose of this chapter is to review the indications for surgery, the surgical technique, and the relative advantages and disadvantages of C1-C2 transarticular screw fixation.
Important Points	Indications for C1-C2 transarticular screw fixation include acute or chronic atlantoaxial instability in patients in whom conservative treatment has failed.
	Biomechanically, transarticular fixation provides superior biomechanical stabilization compared with other C1-C2 fixation techniques, particularly in axial rotation and lateral bending.
	Advanced imaging, including multiplanar reformatted CT scan, should be reviewed to determine whether screw placement is feasible and safe.
	Attention should be paid to the course and caliber of the vertebral artery, particularly around the C1-C2 joint and the C2 isthmus.
Clinical and Surgical Pearls	Adequate fluoroscopy should be ensured with the technologist after positioning of the patient.
	The Mayfield clamp should be adjusted to ensure proper positioning, including rotation.
	Reduction of C1-C2 before drilling must be obtained.
	A rigid drill guide tube should be used.
	Fluoroscopy should be used through each stage of the procedure, and the surgeon should be mindful of inadvertent Kirschner wire migration when using cannulated screw systems.
Clinical and Surgical Pitfalls	Lack of understanding of the patient's bony and vascular anatomy can lead to complications including bleeding, stroke, or neurologic injury (hypoglossal nerve).
	Improper positioning and inadequate preparing or draping of the upper thoracic area make the tunneling of instruments at the appropriate trajectory difficult.
	Failure to obtain adequate visualization of the C2-C3 facet joint and the mediolateral extent of the C2 isthmus may make placement of the C1-C2 transarticular screw difficult.
	The greater danger in using this technique is vertebral artery injury. The risk of spinal cord injury is extremely low. The drill trajectory should therefore "hug" the medial aspect of the isthmus as much as possible to avoid inadvertently entering the foramen transversarium.

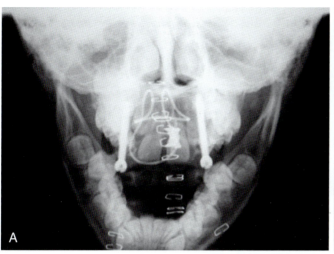
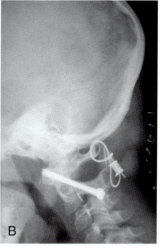

FIGURE 40-1 Anteroposterior (**A**) and lateral radiographs (**B**) of a 7-year-old girl treated for recurrent rotary subluxation with transarticular screw fixation and posterior C1-C2 fusion using graft and wiring technique.

The preferred method for C1-C2 posterior fixation by many spine surgeons has become the C1 lateral mass, C2 pars, or pedicle screw and rod construct (Harms-Goel) discussed in the previous chapter.[1,2] Although several factors have led to that method's increasing popularity, surgeons' familiarity with screw-based instrumentation systems ubiquitously used in the subaxial cervical spine has likely played a significant role. Despite being used less frequently than in years past, the C1-C2 transarticular technique originally described by Magerl offers some unique advantages over other atlantoaxial stabilization methods, and some experts consider it the gold-standard for posterior fixation in the treatment of atlantoaxial instability.[3-5] Regardless, every practicing spine surgeon should gain an understanding of the surgical technique and associated anatomy for placement of the C1-C2 transarticular screw.

The method employs the posterior placement of screws through each pars interarticularis (isthmus) of C2 directly across the C1-C2 facet joint into the C1 lateral mass. This technique provides excellent fixation in all degrees of freedom, particularly axial rotation and lateral bending.[6] When this technique is combined with an interspinous graft and cable construct such as the Sonntag modification of the Gallie fusion, biomechanical strength is further increased, and postoperative halo immobilization is not required[6] (Fig. 40-1). The resulting construct was shown to be superior to other C1-C2 stabilization techniques in published biomechanical studies.[6]

The technique for transarticular screw placement can be technically demanding, and it requires the spine surgeon to have familiarity with the procedure and its limitations, as well as an excellent understanding of the individual patient's bony and vascular anatomy.[7] Proper preoperative radiographic evaluation including x-ray studies, computed tomography (CT), and CT angiography or magnetic resonance angiography (MRA) is necessary. When used in the appropriate patient, the Magerl technique yields excellent results, with high fusion rates (96%) and relatively low complication rates (8%).[3]

BOX 40-1   Indications for Transarticular Screw Fixation

Trauma
Jefferson fractures (C1 burst) with transverse ligament disruption unstable odontoid fractures: type II and shallow type III unstable hangman's fractures

Inflammatory Disease
Rheumatoid arthritis

Infection

Tumor

Congenital Abnormalities
Os odontoideum

Acquired Disorders
Iatrogenic: postsurgical

Indications and Contraindications

Transarticular fixation is indicated for acute or chronic atlantoaxial instability, whether it be caused by trauma, inflammatory disease, infection, congenital disease, or iatrogenic destabilization (Box 40-1). The technique can be combined with occipital or subaxial fixation, or both, if necessary (Fig. 40-2).

Several patient-related factors are used to determine whether the technique is technically feasible. Of utmost importance, the pars interarticularis of C2 must be of adequate size to allow for safe passage of the screw through it without risking injury to adjacent structures (i.e., the vertebral artery and spinal cord). Variations in vertebral artery anatomy (e.g., a large, medially directed vessel or an aberrant vessel that loops into the isthmus of C2) can make the risk of arterial injury associated with screw placement unacceptably high (Fig. 40-3). A thorough review of the preoperative advanced diagnostic imaging is necessary.

The size of the pars interarticularis and the pedicle of C2 may be underappreciated on viewing a standard axial CT image. A standard axial cut, usually across the spinal

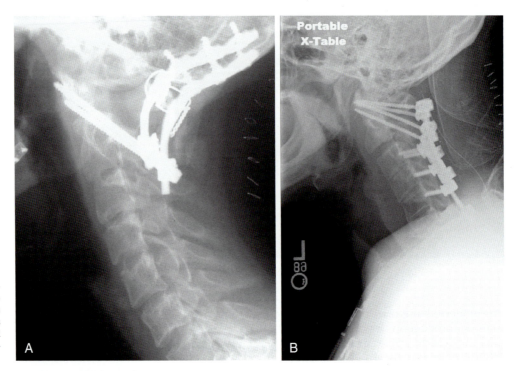

FIGURE 40-2 Transarticular fixation incorporated in occipital cervical fixation (**A**) and subaxial fixation (**B**). Note the use of C1 lateral mass screws in addition to the C1-C2 transarticular screws and subaxial instrumentation in **B**.

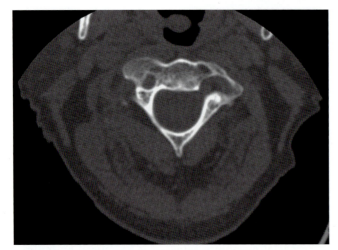

FIGURE 40-3 Axial computed tomography image demonstrating the bony appearance of a large vertebral artery. Transarticular screw fixation may be inappropriate in this patient.

canal, may lead the surgeon to conclude falsely that safe placement of a transarticular screw is not possible. Modern diagnostic imaging software with multiplanar reconstruction and reformatting functions allows the surgeon to determine the width of the pars interarticularis in the plane of trajectory of the C1-C2 screw. When the pars is viewed in this manner, the adequacy of the isthmus can be better demonstrated, and screw length can be measured (Fig. 40-4). Alternatively, image guidance software can be used in a similar manner to demonstrate the adequacy of the pars in screw trajectory planning.[4]

Additional contraindications to transarticular screw placement include the presence of significant thoracic kyphosis, which makes placement of proper screw trajectory impossible to achieve, and the inability to obtain high-quality intraoperative fluoroscopic images. Furthermore, as for all instrumented fusion procedures, soft, osteoporotic bone can be considered a relative contraindication.

Technique

General anesthesia is induced, and the patient is endotracheally intubated with spinal precautions maintained. Additional vascular access is obtained as necessary, and a Foley catheter is inserted if it is not already in place. If intraoperative neuromonitoring (motor-evoked potentials, somatosensory-evoked potentials, and electromyography) is to be used, leads are applied, and baseline values are obtained. Intraoperative neuromonitoring is currently considered an option for C1-C2 fixation because evidence supporting its use is lacking. If the patient has any preoperative neurologic deficit or significant spinal canal compromise, the use of monitoring to ensure that no deleterious changes occur with positioning is reasonable. The authors' preference is to use monitoring in all cases.

Mayfield three-point fixation is applied to the skull, and the patient is positioned prone on the operating room table by using two large gel bolsters or, alternatively, a radiolucent spine frame, which allows the abdomen to hang free. Care is taken to reduce pressure on the knees, and the elbows are padded to protect the ulnar nerves. The patient's body is secured to the operating room table with arms maintained at the side. The bed is placed in a slight "concord" position with reverse Trendelenburg (head above heart).

During body positioning, the surgeon maintains in-line stabilization of the head and neck with slight manual traction on the Mayfield clamp. The Mayfield clamp is then secured to the table with the neck maintained in

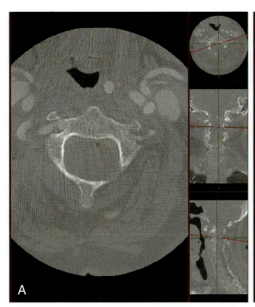
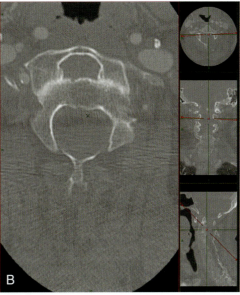

FIGURE 40-4 Multiplanar reconstruction reformatted computed tomography angiography images. On initial inspection of the axial image (**A**), one could think that transarticular fixation is not feasible. However, on review of an image in the plane of the path of a potential transarticular screw (**B**), the adequacy of the pars interarticularis is well demonstrated.

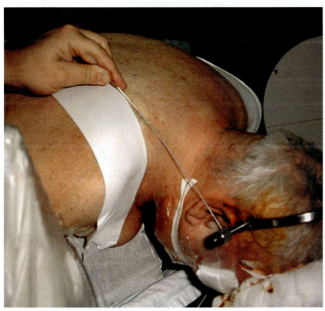

FIGURE 40-5 Positioning for transarticular screw fixation. Note the patient positioned prone on the operating table with Gardner-Wells traction. The surgeon is demonstrating the approximate trajectory of a transarticular screw with a Kirschner wire.

a neutral position and the head translated dorsally and flexed (e.g., "military tuck"). This position ideally allows for both reduction of atlantoaxial dislocation and proper trajectory of instrumentation. Adjustments can be made using the Mayfield as deemed necessary, including correction of rotation, which is best assessed by evaluating the evenness of the external auditory meatuses. Some degree of C1-C2 dislocation can be addressed intraoperatively, and 100% reduction is not necessary with positioning alone. Alternatively, if traction is required to maintain reduction of the fracture or for correction of significant cervical deformity, the patient can be positioned prone with traction applied to a halo ring or Gardner-Wells tongs (Fig. 40-5).

Lateral fluoroscopy is used following positioning to ensure proper alignment of the C1-C2 complex and to mark the incision. An additional image should be obtained with a Kirschner wire (K-wire) held adjacent to the patient's neck in the trajectory of the planned transarticular screw. This image gives three important pieces of information. First, it can be used to mark the approximate location of the entry point for tunneling of instruments. Second, it gives the surgeon an understanding of the proper drill angle for placement of the screw. Third, and most importantly, it determines the intraoperative feasibility of the technique. If the patient's anatomy makes it difficult to obtain the correct angle for screw placement, either positioning will need to be adjusted or an alternative C1-C2 fusion technique will need to be performed.

Surgical preparation and draping include the upper thoracic spine to approximately T5 level, to ensure the ability to achieve proper screw trajectories through percutaneous stab incisions. In addition, if iliac crest bone graft is to be used (gold standard for arthrodesis), the iliac crest site is prepared and draped as well. Antibiotics are given within 1 hour of skin incision, and in accordance with The Joint Commission's Universal Protocol, a time-out is performed.

A midline dorsal incision is made from just below the inion of the occiput to the tip of the C3 spinous process to allow adequate exposure of C1 and C2. Deeper dissection is performed within the avascular median raphe. Self-retaining retractors (Weitlaner and cerebellar) are used to aid dissection. Deep musculature is elevated from the dorsal aspects of the occiput, C1, and C2 by using subperiosteal technique to minimize bleeding. Exposure includes the spinous process, lamina, and isthmus of C2 to the C2-C3 facet, as well as the posterior arch of C1. The entirety of the dorsal elements of C2 should be exposed so proper landmarks can be identified. Caution should be taken when using electrocautery, particularly out laterly (on the lateral aspect of the isthmus of C2 and laterally on the posterior arch of C1) and on the superior aspect of the posterior arch of C1, to prevent inadvertent injury to the vertebral artery. The isthmus and pedicle

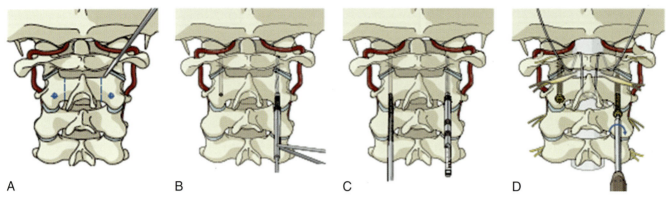

A   B   C   D

FIGURE 40-6 Series of images demonstrating placement of a C1-C2 transarticular screw. Starting position (**A**), proper trajectory for drilling (**B**), tapping and measurement of screw length (**C**), and screw insertion (**D**). (From Aebi M, Arlet V, Webb JK, editors: *AOSpine manual*, vol 1: *Principles and techniques*, New York, 2007, Thieme.)

of C2 are exposed rostrally to the C1-C2 joint using a small dissector such as a number 1 or number 4 Penfield dissector. A number 4 Penfield dissector can be used to elevate the greater occipital nerve (C2 nerve root) during this exposure to gain a better view of the C2 pedicle and the C1-C2 facet joint. This region contains a very robust venous plexus, and bleeding should be anticipated. This bleeding can be controlled with cautious bipolar electrocautery and the use of surgical hemostatic products such as FLOSEAL.

In nearly all cases, given enough time, even robust bleeding ceases with the use of a gelatinous surgical hemostat tamponaded with a small cottonoid patty. This exposure also allows the surgeon to scrape the cartilage and decorticate the bony surfaces within the C1-C2 joint with a small curet or a 2-mm diamond burr to achieve anterior interfacet arthrodesis. This technique is extremely useful, especially when posterior wiring for fusion is not possible (i.e., C1 posterior arch fractures). To help with visualization of the C1-C2 joint, the surgeon can also drill a small K-wire approximately 1 cm deep in the lateral mass of C1 just cephalad to the joint. This maneuver allows the assistant safely to reflect the C2 nerve cephalad while allowing the operating surgeon to work within the joint space. Alternatively, the C2 nerve root can be ligated and sacrificed.

Once adequate exposure of C1 and C2 is completed, fluoroscopy is used to plan the upper thoracic stab incisions, which are necessary in most cases for proper trajectory of screw placement. This can best be done by holding a K-wire adjacent to the patient's neck in the plane of the proposed screw. Where the K-wire crosses the skin of the upper thoracic spine (typically T1 or T2) is marked, and two small incisions approximately 2 cm lateral to the midline are made. Several options are available to the surgeon regarding the percutaneous tunneling of the instruments and screws into the surgical field. K-wires can be passed through two approximately 1-cm incisions, over which cannulated instruments can be used (most common method). Alternatively, tubular systems can allow the use of noncannulated instruments and screws through slightly larger incisions. In either case, the drilling and tapping should be done with the aid of a rigid guide tube.

The entry point for the screw is within the C2 isthmus at a point approximately 3 to 4 mm rostral to the C2-C3 facet joint and approximately 3 mm lateral to the medial portion of the joint (spinal canal) (Fig. 40-6, *A*). Adequate exposure of the C2-C3 joint is thus essential, but care should be taken not to disrupt the joint itself. A high-speed drill or awl is used to create a small entry hole through the cortex. The guide for drill or K-wire is then docked at the starting point, and fluoroscopy is used to help in visualizing the correct angle, approximately 45 degrees cephalad, up the isthmus of C2 as drilling commences. This angle allows the screw to remain dorsal to the vertebral artery throughout its path through the C2 isthmus. The surgical assistant uses a small instrument within the canal (i.e., a small nerve hook) to help in the visualization of the medial portion of the C2 pars and pedicle. The posterolateral extent of the isthmus should also be clearly visualized, but the vertebral artery should not be exposed.

Adequate lateral and medial visualization allows the surgeon to plan the correct trajectory up the isthmus, with essentially a neutral (0 to 5 degrees) lateral to medial trajectory in the sagittal plane (Fig. 40-6, *B*). The proper sagittal angle is essential to prevent inadvertent injury to the vertebral artery and hypoglossal nerve.[8] Before placement of the K-wire or drilling, any residual C1-C2 dislocation must be corrected. This can be done intraoperatively through manipulation of the posterior elements of C1 and C2. To help in the reduction of the C1 vertebral body, a sublaminar wire can be passed under the posterior arch of C1 and gently pulled back before drilling the C1-C2 facet. The drill bit is left in place to maintain reduction while the opposite side is drilled, and a screw is placed (to use this technique, a second drill bit is required). Alternatively, posterior cable placement and grafting can be completed before screw placement to aid in maintenance of correction. The surgeon must recognize any incompetence in the posterior arch of C1 before attempting any maneuvers that involve C1 manipulation.

Fluoroscopy is used to help place the K-wire or drill up the C2 isthmus, across the C1-C2 joint, and into the anterior aspect of the C1 lateral mass to a point approximately 3 to 4 mm posterior to the anterior tubercle of C1. Drilling to this depth and not beyond is done to avoid inadvertent injury to the internal carotid artery or the hypoglossal nerve. The decision whether to use hand drilling or power drilling is based on the individual surgeon's preference. However, some surgeons believe that power drilling allows for easier passage of the drill bit across the cortices of the C2 superior articular facet and the C1 inferior articular facet, thereby reducing bending and the potential for errant screw placement. In addition, the oscillating feature of the power drill can prevent soft tissue from being inadvertently wound into the drill bit, and this reduces the risk of associated neurovascular injury secondary to a malpositioned drill bit. Short pulses with the drill can also give the surgeon increased tactile feel. If a K-wire (cannulated) technique is to be used, care must be taken to ensure that the wire does not migrate anteriorly when passing or using instruments over it. Fluoroscopy should be used at each step of the procedure. Typically, a long, 2.5-mm diameter drill bit is used, as well as a 3.5-mm diameter tap and fully threaded screws. After drilling, the depth for the screw is measured (Fig. 40-6, *C*). The mean optimal screw length has been determined to be 38.1 ± 2.2 mm.[8] Screw lengths outside this range are possible; however, they should alert the surgeon to possible screw malposition. The drill hole is tapped, and the screw is placed (Fig. 40-6, *D*). The procedure can be tailored to patients with soft, osteoporotic bone by using self-drilling screws without tapping.

Following bilateral screw placement, the procedure for C1-C2 posterior interspinous grafting is performed in patients with competent C1 posterior arch. Alternatively, arthrodesis can be achieved across the C1-C2 facet joint through decortication and bone grafting as described earlier.

Advantages and Disadvantages of C1-C2 Fixation Techniques

Although the trend has been toward increased use of the C1 lateral mass–C2 pars or pedicle fixation (Harms-Goel) technique for posterior C1-C2 fixation in more recent years, the Magerl C1-C2 transarticular screw technique should be included in the spine surgeon's armamentarium. Investigators have reported that the Harms technique may be less dangerous with regard to vertebral artery injury, and this may be true in some patients.[2] However, when assessing the safety of the various C1-C2 fixation techniques, most surgeons are likely basing their decision on the axial CT scans. The authors have found that when CT data are reformatted in the plane of the pathway for transarticular screw placement, the pars interarticularis is often of large enough caliber, and the likelihood of vertebral artery injury is low. This observation is in agreement with a report by Bransford and associates that demonstrated a very low rate of transverse foramen encroachment and vertebral artery injury with transarticular screws.[9]

In addition, the authors have recognized several situations in which the Harms-Goel technique (C1 lateral mass and C2 pedicle screws) may put the vertebral artery at higher risk for injury. The surgeon must remember that the vertebral artery passes beneath the posterior arch of C1 in up to 5% of the population, and a C1 lateral mass screw can be potentially very dangerous in these instances. Furthermore, the authors believe that fixation of C1 and C2 must be individualized according to the patient's bony anatomy. In some cases, such as patients with congenital malformations of the upper cervical spine, a combination of approaches may be best (i.e., a transarticular screw on one side and a Harms-Goel technique on the opposite side).[10,11]

A further advantage of transarticular screw fixation is that sacrifice of the C2 nerve is not required. The Harms-Goel technique often requires greater occipital nerve sacrifice, which may be troubling to some patients postoperatively. Finally, the implant cost can be significantly lower with transarticular screw fixation (two fully threaded screws, as opposed to four polyaxial screws and dual rods).

Conclusions

Placement of the C1-C2 transarticular screw remains a viable alternative for the surgical management of a variety of atlantoaxial disorders. Although this operation is technically demanding, a careful understanding of the procedure and its limitations, as well as a thorough understanding of each patient's individualized bony and vascular anatomy, can help reduce the risk of complications. Proper preoperative radiographic evaluation including x-ray studies, CT, and CT or MRA is necessary. When used in the appropriate patient, the Magerl technique yields excellent results with high fusion rates and relatively low complication rates.

REFERENCES

1. Goel A, et al.: Techniques in the treatment of craniovertebral instability, *Neurol India* 53:525–533, 2005.
2. Harms J, Melcher RP: Posterior C1-C2 fusion with polyaxial screw and rod fixation, *Spine (Phila Pa 1976)* 26:2467–2471, 2001.
3. Haid RW Jr, Subach BR, McLaughlin MR, et al.: C1-C2 transarticular screw fixation for atlantoaxial instability: a 6-year experience, *Neurosurgery* 49:65–68, 2001. discussion 69–70.
4. Haid RW, Jr: C1-C2 transarticular screw fixation: technical aspects, *Neurosurgery* 49:71–74, 2001.
5. Jeanneret B, Magerl F: Primary posterior fusion C1/2 in odontoid fractures: indications, technique, and results of transarticular screw fixation, *J Spinal Disord* 5:464–475, 1992.
6. Sim HB, et al.: Biomechanical evaluations of various C1-C2 posterior fixation techniques, *Spine (Phila Pa 1976)* 36:E401–E407, 2011.
7. Bransford RJ, Lee MJ, Reis A: Posterior fixation of the upper cervical spine: contemporary techniques, *J Am Acad Orthop Surg* 19:63–71, 2011.
8. Ebraheim NA, et al.: The optimal transarticular C1-2 screw length and the location of the hypoglossal nerve, *Surg Neurol* 53:208–210, 2000.
9. Bransford RJ, et al.: Posterior C2 instrumentation: accuracy and complications associated with four techniques, *Spine (Phila Pa 1976)* 2011 36:E936–E943, 2011.
10. Elgafy H, et al.: Biomechanical analysis comparing three C1-C2 transarticular screw salvaging fixation techniques, *Spine (Phila Pa 1976)* 35:378–385, 2010.
11. Yanni DS, Perin NI: Fixation of the axis, *Neurosurgery* 66(Suppl):147–152, 2010.

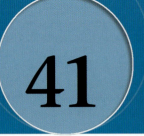

41

C2 Translaminar Screw Fixation

Clinton J. Burkett and Christopher I. Shaffrey

CHAPTER PREVIEW

Chapter Synopsis	C2 translaminar screws are an effective method for fixation of the C2 vertebra. Compared with other techniques, this procedure is technically less demanding and has potentially fewer risks. A thorough history and examination, as well as a careful assessment of the anatomy of the C2 lamina, are still required preoperatively to minimize complications. The goal of this chapter is to review preoperative considerations, surgical technique, and results for C2 translaminar screw fixation.
Important Points	The patient's C2 laminar anatomy must demonstrate the ability to accommodate a screw.
	Unlike other C2 fixation techniques, the translaminar screw does not place the vertebral arteries at risk.
	A history of previous surgical procedures or of congenital cervical spinal abnormalities may be an absolute or relative contraindication to the placement of translaminar screws.
Clinical and Surgical Pearls	The translaminar screw starting point is typically at the junction of the spinous process and the lamina.
	The first screw should be placed as close to the superior margin of the C2 lamina as possible.
	The second screw can be placed at the inferior portion of the lamina to prevent interference with the previously placed contralateral translaminar screw.
	Decortication of the C2 lamina does not affect the stability of the translaminar screw.
Clinical and Surgical Pitfalls	Congenital abnormalities may have other associated disorders, such as occipitalization or absent posterior elements, that may preclude or alter the surgical decision-making process.
	Laminae less than 3.5-mm thick may be at risk for anterior or posterior screw penetration.
	During placement of the screw, the alignment of the drill can be kept slightly posterior to ensure that any potential cortical violation would occur posteriorly through the surface of the lamina rather than anteriorly into the spinal canal.

Bilateral crossing C2 translaminar screws can be an attractive option when contemplating fixation of the C2 vertebra (axis). The procedure is not technically demanding and provides rigid fixation. Traditional posterior wiring methods are also technically simple, but they are associated with suboptimal fusion rates resulting from limited stiffness.[1] Translaminar screws are not as affected by variations in a patient's anatomy and do not risk injury to the vertebral arteries, unlike other technically demanding C2 screw fixation options (C1-C2 transarticular screws, C2 pedicle screws).[2-4]

In an attempt to reduce the risk of injury to the vertebral artery during placement of the C2 pedicle screw, the C2 pars interarticularis fixation, which uses a shorter screw (14 to 16 mm) and a slightly different trajectory, has been suggested to be less risky to the vertebral arteries than longer pedicle screw placement. However, the biomechanical strength of the C2 pars screw has not been proven, and anatomic variations may also prevent placement of this screw.[5] Therefore, developing an understanding of the anatomy and technique for placement of C2 translaminar screw fixation can provide an additional method for rigid fixation of the axis that may be incorporated with occipitoatlantal or subaxial instrumentation. The goal of this chapter is to review preoperative considerations, surgical technique, and results for the placement of C2 translaminar screw fixation.

Preoperative Considerations

The indications for surgery and the use of translaminar screws for stabilization of disorders of the cervical spine remain the same as for other cervical procedures. Although described more completely in other chapters, patients with myelopathy, radiculopathy, myeloradiculopathy, tumors, infection, or trauma with associated cervical instability are potential candidates.

The history and examination should include evaluation for standard signs and symptoms of myelopathy or radiculopathy. Motor weakness, sensory deficits, and reflex changes can help identify the disorder. In addition to the standard history and examination, particular attention should also include evidence of previous posterior cervical spinal surgical procedures or congenital abnormalities that may have resulted in the resection or absence of the C2 lamina, which could preclude the use of translaminar screws. In addition, a search for subtle examination findings such as a low-lying hairline, webbed neck, and decreased range of motion can identify abnormalities such as Klippel-Feil syndrome. This syndrome is associated with congenitally fused cervical segments and frequently with occipitalization, and it may alter the surgical technique selected.

Imaging studies should start with plain radiographs and include cervical spine anteroposterior, lateral, and flexion and extension dynamic imaging studies to assess overall alignment, degenerative disease, osteophytes, range of motion, and stability.

Advanced imaging, in the form of magnetic resonance imaging (MRI), can provide information about the intervertebral disks, cranial and spinal nerve roots, supporting ligaments, presence of a syrinx, Chiari malformation, and information on the spinal cord caliber and quality, among other things. Although MRI is typically the imaging study of choice for identifying disease, the addition of a computed tomography (CT) scan, with or without a myelogram, can be particularly useful when deciding to place translaminar screws.

The CT scan can help provide additional information about the presence and extent of the bony compression, presence of ossification of the posterior longitudinal ligament (OPLL), and in revision cases, presence of a solid fusion or pseudarthrosis. More specifically, with regard to translaminar screws, preoperative CT imaging of the cervical spine is important to ensure that a patient's anatomy can accommodate a screw (length and width) before screw placement is attempted[6] (Fig. 41-1).

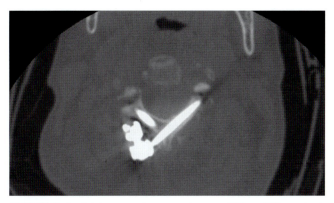

FIGURE 41-1   Axial computed tomography scan of bilateral C2 translaminar screws.

Indications and Contraindications
Indications

Traumatic fracture, traumatic ligamentous laxity, rheumatoid arthritis, congenital disorders, neoplasm, pseudarthrosis, degenerative disease, C1-C2 subluxation, os odontoideum, type II odontoid process fracture, and unfavorable anatomy for C2 transarticular screw or pedicle screw placement are frequent indications for consideration of placement of C2 translaminar screws.

Contraindications

This procedure is contraindicated in patients with earlier C2 laminectomy, C2 posterior element fracture, C2 lamina that is less than 3.5-mm thick, and congenital and anatomic variants with absent or dysplastic C2 lamina. In addition, an anomalous vertebral artery that places its course within the trajectory of the C2 translaminar screw is also a contraindication to placement of a screw, at least on the side of the anomalous anatomy.

Surgical Technique

Anesthesia and Positioning

After induction of general anesthesia and setup of intraoperative neuromonitoring, a Mayfield (Integra, Plainsboro, NJ) three-pin skull clamp is placed, and the patient is placed in the prone position on a Jackson table (Mizuho OSI, Union City, Calif.) with the head and cervical spine in neutral position. The Mayfield clamp is then secured to the C-Flex head positioning system (Allen Medical Systems, Acton, Mass.) and is adjusted as needed for final alignment.

Surgical Steps

A posterior midline incision is made, and subperiosteal dissection of the C1 (axis) posterior arch and the other adjacent areas to be instrumented (subocciput, atlas, or subaxial spine) is carried out in the usual fashion (Box 41-1). If included in the construct, the posterior arch of C1 is dissected to expose the lateral masses bilaterally. The spinous process, laminae, and medial aspect of the lateral masses of C2 are exposed.[7] The spinous process, laminae, and lateral masses are then exposed as needed for the subaxial vertebrae to be included in the construct.

1. Use of a high-speed drill to open a small cortical window at the junction of the C2 spinous process and lamina on the right, close to the superior margin of the C2 lamina (Fig. 41-2).
2. A hand drill is then used, aligned with the downslope of the contralateral lamina, to drill through the cortical window into the contralateral lamina (*left*) to a depth of 30 mm (Fig. 41-3).
3. A ball-tip feeler is then used to palpate the hole to ensure that no cortical violation into the spinal canal has occurred (Fig. 41-4).
4. A 4.0 × 30 mm polyaxial screw (Mountaineer, DePuy, Raynham, Mass.) is then placed along the same trajectory (Fig. 41-5).
5. The small cortical window on the left is made again at the junction of the spinous process and lamina. However, the window is placed at the inferior portion of the lamina to prevent interference with the previously placed contralateral (*right*) translaminar screw (Fig. 41-6).
6. A hand drill is then used, aligned with the downslope of the contralateral lamina, to drill through the cortical window into the contralateral lamina (*right*) to a depth of 30 mm (Fig. 41-7).
7. A ball-tip feeler is then used to palpate the hole to ensure that no cortical violation into the spinal canal has occurred (Fig. 41-8).
8. A 4.0 × 30 mm polyaxial screw (Mountaineer, DePuy, Raynham, Mass.) is then placed along the same trajectory (Fig. 41-9).

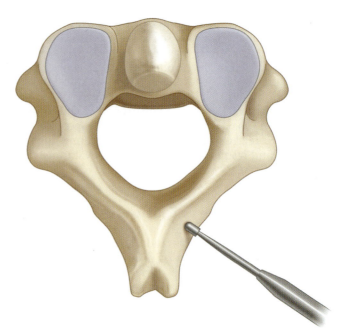

FIGURE 41-2 Surgical step 1. (Modified from Wright NM: C2 translaminar screw fixation. In Vaccaro AR, Baron EM, editors: *Operative techniques: spine surgery*, ed 2, Philadelphia, 2012, Saunders.)

For constructs that include the atlas, C1 lateral mass screws are placed according to the technique described by Harms.[4] If necessary, bilateral C2 neurectomies can be performed before placement of C1 lateral mass screws to enhance surgical exposure of the C1-C2 joint.[8] For constructs that include the subocciput, screws are placed bicortically for rod connection. For constructs that include the subaxial spine (C3 to C6), lateral mass screws are placed using the technique described by Magerl.[9]

C2 fixation begins with use of a high-speed drill to open a small cortical window at the junction of the C2 spinous process and lamina on the right, close to the superior margin of the C2 lamina[7] (Fig. 41-2). A hand drill is then used, aligned with the downslope of the contralateral lamina, to drill through the cortical window into the contralateral lamina to a depth of 30 mm[7] (Fig. 41-3). The alignment of the drill can be kept slightly less than the downslope of the contralateral lamina to make sure that any potential cortical violation would occur posteriorly through the surface of the lamina rather than anteriorly into the spinal canal.[7]

A ball-tip feeler is then used to palpate the hole to ensure that no cortical violation into the spinal canal has occurred (Fig. 41-4). In the authors' experience, typically a 4.0 × 30 mm polyaxial screw (Mountaineer, DePuy, Raynham, Mass.) can be placed along the same trajectory (Fig. 41-5). Depending on the screw system used, the path can be tapped before screw insertion. The head of the screw should sit at the junction of the spinous process and lamina on the right.[7]

The procedure is then repeated starting on the contralateral (left) side. The small cortical window on the left is made again at the junction of the spinous process and lamina (Figs. 41-6 to 41-9). However, the window is placed at the inferior portion of the lamina to prevent interference with the previously placed contralateral (right) translaminar screw.

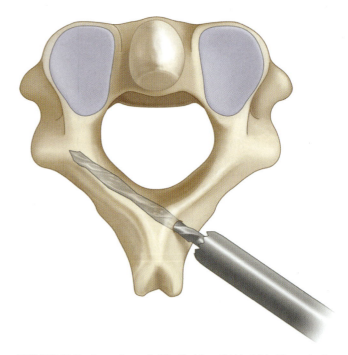

FIGURE 41-3 Surgical step 2. (Modified from Wright NM: C2 translaminar screw fixation. In Vaccaro AR, Baron EM, editors: *Operative techniques: spine surgery*, ed 2, Philadelphia, 2012, Saunders.)

Rods are then measured and cut to fit the construct (which should keep the patient's head and cervical spine in neutral alignment if attained during the original positioning with the head holder). C1 lateral mass screws or subaxial lateral mass screws, or both, are connected to the ipsilateral C2 screw head (which fixates the rod to the contralateral C2 lamina).[7]

The wound is then irrigated copiously. The exposed laminar surfaces and facet joints are decorticated with

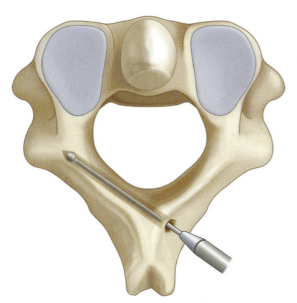

FIGURE 41-4 Surgical step 3. (Based on Wright NM: C2 translaminar screw fixation. In Vaccaro AR, Baron EM, editors: *Operative techniques: spine surgery*, ed 2, Philadelphia, 2012, Saunders.)

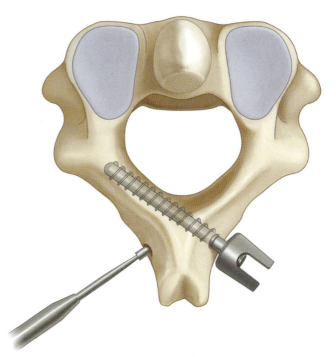

FIGURE 41-6 Surgical step 5. (Based on Wright NM: C2 translaminar screw fixation. In Vaccaro AR, Baron EM, editors: *Operative techniques: spine surgery*, ed 2, Philadelphia, 2012, Saunders.)

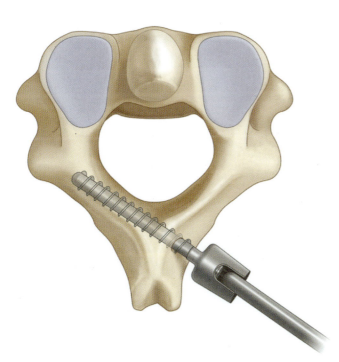

FIGURE 41-5 Surgical step 4. (Modified from Wright NM: C2 translaminar screw fixation. In Vaccaro AR, Baron EM, editors: *Operative techniques: spine surgery*, ed 2, Philadelphia, 2012, Saunders.)

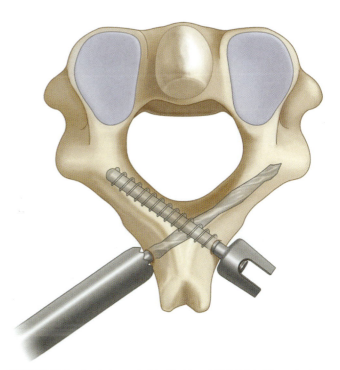

FIGURE 41-7 Surgical step 6. (Modified from Wright NM: C2 translaminar screw fixation. In Vaccaro AR, Baron EM, editors: *Operative techniques: spine surgery*, ed 2, Philadelphia, 2012, Saunders.)

a high-speed drill, which does not affect the stability of the C2 translaminar screw construct.[10] Local autograft and allograft are laid down along the decorticated laminar surfaces and facet joints for fusion. A subfascial drain is placed. The muscle is closed in three layers. The fascia, subcutaneous layer, and skin are closed in the usual fashion.

Postoperatively, patients are typically immobilized in a hard cervical collar, and upright radiographs of the cervical spine in anteroposterior and lateral views are obtained to confirm adequate position of instrumentation (Figs.

41-10 and 41-11). The drain is discontinued on postoperative day 2 or 3, and patients are discharged to home once they have adequate mobility. Cervical collars are discontinued at 6 weeks, and patients return to clinic at 6 weeks, 3 months, 6 months, and 1 year, and flexion and extension lateral radiographs are obtained to assess for fusion.

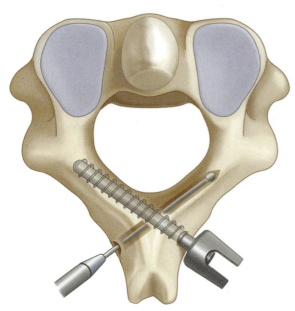

FIGURE 41-8   Surgical step 7. (Based on Wright NM: C2 translaminar screw fixation. In Vaccaro AR, Baron EM, editors: *Operative techniques: spine surgery*, ed 2, Philadelphia, 2012, Saunders.)

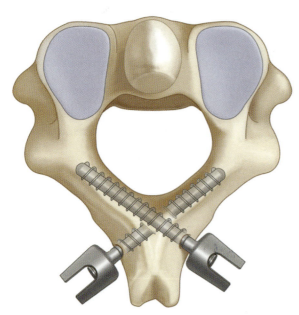

FIGURE 41-9   Surgical step 8. (Based on Wright NM: C2 translaminar screw fixation. In Vaccaro AR, Baron EM, editors: *Operative techniques: spine surgery*, ed 2, Philadelphia, 2012, Saunders.)

Results

In published reports, clinical results of C2 translaminar screws have been promising. In Dorward and Wright's series over the course of 7 years, 52 consecutive patients underwent C2 translaminar screw fixation, and no vascular or neurologic complications were sustained from screw placement.[11] A 97.6% overall fusion rate was achieved.[11] In Wang's series of 30 patients, no vascular or neurologic complications resulted from screw placement.[12] However, 11 patients demonstrated some degree of posterior laminar disruption, and 1 patient

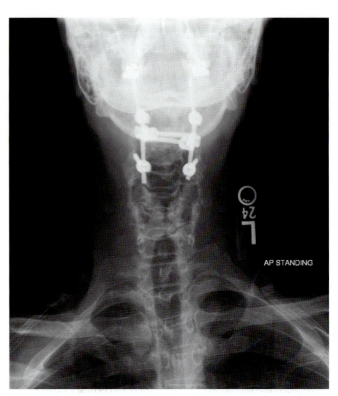

FIGURE 41-10   Anteroposterior radiograph of C1-C3 fusion with bilateral C2 translaminar screws.

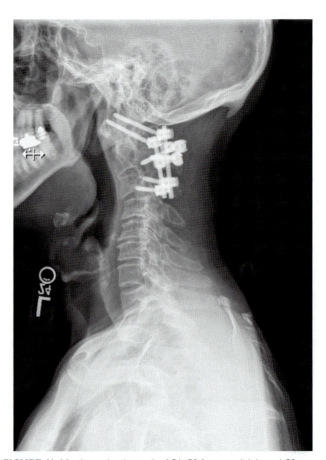

FIGURE 41-11   Lateral radiograph of C1-C3 fusion with bilateral C2 translaminar screws.

Table 41-1 Study Results

Reference	Number of Patients	Vascular Injuries	Neurologic Injuries	Dorsal Breaches	Ventral Breaches
Dorward and Wright[11]	52	0	0	0	3
Wang[12]	30	0	0	11	1
Hong et al[13]	21	0	0	1	0
Sciubba et al[14]	16	0	0	0	0

sustained anterior laminar disruption that was revised.[12] A 6.7% rate of early instrumentation failure may have resulted from using 3.5-mm screws rather than 4.0-mm screws.[12]

Hong and colleagues reported 29 C2 translaminar screws placed in 21 patients, who had no neural or vascular injuries, no anterior breaches, and 1 posterior breach without revision.[13] These investigators reported a 100% fusion rate over 18.9 months.[13] Sciubba and associates reported 16 patients who underwent C2 translaminar screws and found no neurologic or vascular complications from screw placement.[14] Over a minimum 18-month follow-up, 2 patients required revision surgical procedures as a result of pseudarthrosis or fixation failure[14] (Table 41-1).

REFERENCES

1. Menendez JA, Wright NM: Techniques of posterior C1-C2 stabilization, *Neurosurgery* 60(Suppl 1):S103–S111, 2007.
2. Wright NM: Translaminar rigid screw fixation of the axis: technical note, *J Neurosurg Spine* 3:409–414, 2005.
3. Jeanneret B, Magerl F: Primary posterior fusion C1/2 in odontoid fractures: indications, technique, and results of transarticular screw fixation, *J Spinal Disord* 5:464–475, 1992.
4. Harms J, Melcher RP: Posterior C1-C2 fusion with polyaxial screw and rod fixation, *Spine (Phila Pa 1976)* 26:2467–2471, 2001.
5. Sim HB, Lee JW, Park JT, et al.: Biomechanical evaluations of various C1-C2 posterior fixation techniques, *Spine (Phila Pa 1976)* 36:E401–E407, 2011.
6. Wang MY: C2 crossing laminar screws: cadaveric morphometric analysis, *Neurosurgery* 59, 2006. ONS84–8; discussion ONS8.
7. Wright NM: Posterior C2 fixation using bilateral, crossing C2 laminar screws: case series and technical note, *J Spinal Disord Tech* 17:158–162, 2004.
8. Hamilton DK, Smith JS, Sansur CA, et al.: C-2 neurectomy during atlantoaxial instrumented fusion in the elderly: patient satisfaction and surgical outcome, *J Neurosurg Spine* 15:3–8, 2011.
9. Magerl F, Grob D, Seemann D: Stable dorsal fusion of the cervical spine (C2-Th1) using hook plates. In Kehr P, Weidner A, editors: *Cervical spine*, New York, 1987, Springer, pp 217–221.
10. Hong JT, Takigawa T, Udayakunmar R, et al.: Biomechanical effect of the C2 laminar decortication on the stability of C2 intralaminar screw construct and biomechanical comparison of C2 intralaminar screw and C2 pars screw, *Neurosurgery* 69, 2011. ONS1–6, discussion ONS7.
11. Dorward IG, Wright NM: Seven years of experience with C2 translaminar screw fixation: clinical series and review of the literature, *Neurosurgery* 68:1491–1499, 2011. discussion 1499.
12. Wang MY: Cervical crossing laminar screws: early clinical results and complications, *Neurosurgery* 61:311–315, 2007. discussion 315-316.
13. Hong JT, Yi JS, Kim JT, et al.: Clinical and radiologic outcome of laminar screw at C2 and C7 for posterior instrumentation: review of 25 cases and comparison of C2 and C7 intralaminar screw fixation, *World Neurosurgery* 73:112–118, 2010.
14. Sciubba DM, Noggle JC, Vellimana AK, et al.: Laminar screw fixation of the axis, *J Neurosurg Spine* 8:327–334, 2008.

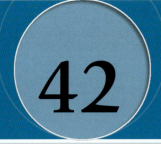

42

Cervical Pedicle Screws

Oliver M. Stokes, Bronek M. Boszczyk, and Kuniyoshi Abumi

CHAPTER PREVIEW

Chapter Synopsis	Cervical pedicle screws offer a biomechanical advantage over other types of posterior cervical instrumentation, but at the expense of increased risk of iatrogenic neurovascular injury. Careful preoperative planning with evaluation of three-dimensional imaging and meticulous surgical technique, however, leads to a low incidence of complications, particularly in experienced hands in high-volume centers. The purpose of this chapter is to review the preoperative considerations, surgical technique, complications, and results for cervical pedicle screw fixation.
Important Points	This procedure is indicated for most cervical disorders requiring stabilization.
	It is contraindicated in patients with narrow or absent pedicles.
	It is contraindicated where the pedicle is destroyed by trauma or tumor.
	Preoperative computed tomography is essential to assess pedicle morphology.
	Three-dimensional imaging of vertebral arteries is indicated if any suspicion exists of involvement in a pathologic process or an aberrant anatomic course.
Clinical and Surgical Pearls	Portals are used percutaneously to probe, sound, and tap the pedicle.
	The entry point is determined by local bony anatomy.
	The trajectory of insertion is guided by direct visualization of the medial cortical pedicle wall, the outer cortex of the ipsilateral lamina, and the direction of the contralateral lamina.
	The entry point and trajectory in the sagittal and transverse planes are confirmed by oblique orthogonal intraoperative fluoroscopy.
Clinical and Surgical Pitfalls	Injury to the vertebral artery is best avoided by careful selection of patients. Cases of aberrant arterial anatomy or disadvantageous pedicle morphology can usually be determined preoperatively.
	The surgeon should avoid injury to the spinal cord by decompressing developmentally narrow spinal canals before kyphosis correction.
	The surgeon should avoid iatrogenic foraminal stenosis secondary to excessive reduction of translational deformity by prior foraminotomy.

Posterior cervical instrumentation is frequently indicated for the treatment of conditions of traumatic, degenerative, cancerous, or inflammatory origin. This instrumentation has evolved from wires to facet and lateral mass screws and laterally based pedicle screws. The evolution in cervical instrumentation has coincided with the increased availability and higher resolution of three-dimensional medical imaging. Cervical pedicle screws, first described in the 1960s as C2 pedicle screw insertion for osteosynthesis of a hangman fracture,[1] and popularized by Abumi and colleagues for reconstructive surgery of the subaxial cervical spine in 1994,[2] offer a biomechanical advantage over other techniques that makes them an attractive option to surgeons,[3] but at the expense of increased risk of iatrogenic damage to the adjacent neurovascular structures. Cervical pedicle screws offer a potential benefit in patients with deficient or dysplastic lateral masses or laminae.

Studies performed since the 1990s in an attempt to reduce the risks of pedicle screw insertion have addressed pedicle morphology, optimal entry point, and trajectory, and preoperative and intraoperative imaging. Nonetheless, the technique is inherently risky. Preoperative radiologic evaluation of the pedicles and adjacent neurovascular structures is mandatory, as is meticulous operative technique. The purpose of this chapter is to review the preoperative considerations, surgical technique, complications, and results for cervical pedicle screw fixation.

Preoperative Considerations

History

When considering the use of pedicle screws to stabilize the cervical spine, the surgeon should take a focused history directed toward the potential for congenital vertebral anomalies and abnormalities of the vertebral arteries. Cervical malignant disease or spondylodiskitis can involve the arteries in the pathologic process. Furthermore, vertebral artery injury is associated with 0.5% of all cases of blunt trauma, and this rate approaches 30% to 40% in patients with cervical fractures because of the tortuous semiosseous course of the artery.

Signs and Symptoms

Damage to the dominant vertebral artery from trauma or involvement of the artery in a pathologic process can lead to symptoms and signs of posterior circulation stroke or transient ischemic attack. The presence of any of these features should direct the clinician to the potential for involvement of the vertebral artery and necessitates imaging of the arteries.

Physical Examination

The focus and the extent of the physical examination should be directed by the nature of the disorder for which the operative intervention is being considered. The patient is observed for the syndromic features of conditions with known cervical spine involvement and for cutaneous manifestations of systemic diseases such as neurofibromatosis. In cases of deformity correction, the cervical alignment is assessed, and consideration is given to the overall spinal balance. Assessment of horizontal gaze is paramount in correction of cervical kyphosis, to help calculate the amount of correction required intraoperatively. A detailed neurologic examination then follows to exclude ischemic posterior circulation stroke secondary to vertebral artery occlusion, spinal cord compression or injury, and radicular pattern nerve root dysfunction.

Imaging

Plain anteroposterior, lateral, and oblique radiographs may provide an indication of when pedicle cannulation would be difficult, for example, by the gross absence of a pedicle as a result of infiltration by tumor or involvement of a pedicle in a fracture. However, plain radiography alone provides insufficient detail of pedicle morphology. Fine-cut (1.0 to 1.5 mm) computed tomography (CT) with bone windows is recommended to aid surgical planning. Morphometric studies have shown that the outer diameter

of most cervical pedicles is greater than 5 mm.[4] Investigators have recommended that pedicle screw placement should not be attempted if the outer pedicle diameter is less than 4 mm,[5] when screw placement may be impossible. The lateral pedicle cortex is typically thinner than the medial, thus increasing the risk of violation of the foramen transversarium. Furthermore, the relative expansion of the dominant vertebral artery may be associated with a narrower pedicle than on the contralateral side of the same vertebra (Fig. 42-1). Evaluation of the axial sections of the CT scan through the pedicles allows for detection of sclerotic pedicles, pedicles infiltrated with tumor (Fig. 42-2), or pedicles involved in fractures (Fig. 42-3). Pedicle screw insertion is not recommended in any of these conditions.

Magnetic resonance imaging (MRI) is performed for diagnosis and in preoperative planning for most cervical disorders. The addition of magnetic resonance angiography (MRA) sequences allows identification of the dominant vertebral artery and provides increased detail of the precise course of the arteries. The vertebral artery occasionally loops into the vertebral body (Fig. 42-4), and ipsilateral

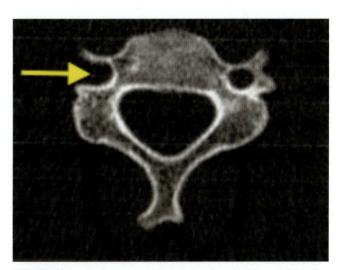

FIGURE 42-1 Axial computed tomography of a subaxial cervical vertebra showing the relative expansion of the right transverse foramen (*arrow*) by the dominant right vertebral artery and consequent narrowing of the ipsilateral pedicle.

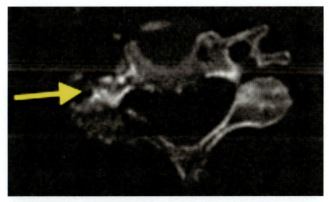

FIGURE 42-2 Axial computed tomography through C5 showing the infiltration of the right pedicle by metastatic lung carcinoma (*arrow*). Note the loss of integrity of the medial and lateral pedicle walls. Attempts to insert a screw through this pedicle would be associated with an increased risk of neurovascular damage resulting from the loss of bony integrity of the pedicle.

pedicle screw insertion is not advised in such patients. MRA should be performed whenever CT or MRI results suggest anomalies in the course of the vertebral arteries or when the arteries may be involved in the disease process.

Furthermore, preoperative CT and MRI can be helpful in patients with preexisting foraminal stenosis when cervical instrumentation is being used to correct deformity. The presence of foraminal stenosis in these cases is a relative indication for prophylactic foraminotomy as a result of the high incidence of iatrogenic neural injury in kyphosis correction.

Indications and Contraindications

Cervical pedicle screws are indicated for potentially all conditions of the cervical spine in which stabilization is required, including subaxial deformity correction

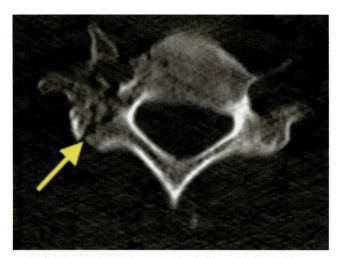

FIGURE 42-3 Axial computed tomography through C6 showing involvement of the right pedicle and lateral mass (*arrow*) in a fracture. Pedicle screw insertion here would be complicated by the loss of normal anatomy and consequent difficulties in identifying the entry point. The risk of neurovascular damage correlates with the degree of involvement of the pedicle walls in the fracture.

(Fig. 42-5), occipitocervical reconstruction, trauma, metastatic or primary malignant disease, rheumatoid or seronegative destructive spondyloarthropathy, and accompanying posterior cervical decompression by laminectomy to address myelopathy secondary to cervical spondylosis, ossification of the yellow ligament, or ossification of the posterior longitudinal ligament.

Cutaneous infection on the posterior aspect of the neck is a relative contraindication. The procedure should be undertaken only in institutions where the appropriate facilities are available, including preoperative and intraoperative imaging and intensive care. When cervical pedicle screws are used to facilitate deformity correction, dual modality spinal cord monitoring is mandatory. Cervical pedicle screws are not recommended when abnormalities are present in the structure or course of the vertebral artery, particularly if they involve the dominant artery. Cervical pedicle screws are also contraindicated in pedicle aplasia or dysplasia, in which the pedicle architecture has been destroyed by tumor, trauma, or infection and when the angle of the pedicle axis from the sagittal plane is extremely oblique.[5] Corticated pedicles are a relative contraindication; an insertion tunnel can be created using a Kirschner wire or high-speed burr, but this requires precision, and caution is recommended.

Surgical Technique

Anesthesia and Positioning

Insertion of cervical pedicle screws mandates prone positioning of the patient on the operating table, general anesthesia, and endotracheal intubation.

The patient's head rests in a horseshoe or is held more firmly with a three-point fixator such as a Mayfield clamp. The use of spinal cord monitoring is dictated according to the indication for surgery, but it is recommended for deformity correction. The patient's arms are positioned

FIGURE 42-4 A, Axial computed tomography through C3 showing a chondrosarcoma (*yellow arrow*) emanating from the right lateral aspect of the vertebra. The left foramen transversarium is enlarged (*red arrow*). This finding suggests an abnormality of the vertebral artery anatomy. **B**, Coronal magnetic resonance angiography of the same patient's neck. The right vertebral artery (*yellow arrow*) has been embolized in preparation for resection of the chondrosarcoma. The left vertebral artery loops abnormally toward the midline (*red arrow*) at the level of the C3 vertebral body.

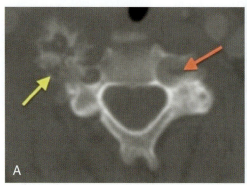

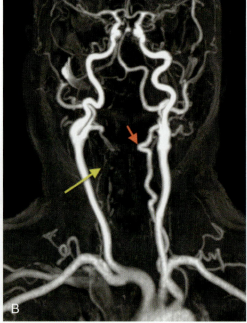

next to the trunk, and tape is applied to the skin on the back if the body habitus necessitates. A bandage or tape is placed over the shoulders, applied to the acromion, to pull the shoulders caudally. This maneuver increases the field of view for lateral intraoperative fluoroscopy. The authors recommend the use of a Montreal mattress and cushioning beneath the pelvis and ankles to prevent pressure sores. The use of thromboembolic deterrent stockings and of continuous pneumatic compression devices applied to the lower limbs is dictated by the incidence of deep vein thrombosis in the ethnicity of the patient.

The surgeon should stand at the head end of the patient to enable the symmetric insertion of pedicle screws. The C-arm fluoroscope is positioned on the right of the patient, with the monitor, the assistant, the operating room nurse, and the instrumentation trays on the left. The authors recommend the use of long tubing to connect the endotracheal tube to the anesthetic machine and the use of long tubes for blood pressure monitoring and for the delivery of intravenous fluids if appropriate. This tubing can all be affixed to or under the operating table, with the anesthesiologist and anesthetic machine positioned at the foot of the table.

Surgical Landmarks, Incisions, and Portals

Cervical pedicles are orientated at approximately 46 degrees from the sagittal plane.[4] Therefore, because of the tension in the soft tissues of the posterior neck, pedicle screw insertion typically requires a long midline posterior cervical incision, longer than would be needed for posterior wiring or lateral mass screws. An alternative method of screw insertion is to make a midline incision of the length required to expose the posterior bony elements, including the cranially adjacent lamina to the most cranial vertebra to be included in the construct and the most caudal lamina included in the construct; the screws are

then inserted percutaneously (Fig. 42-6), aided by portals. If portals are not available, the authors recommend the use of endotracheal tubes, cut to length customized to the patient's neck, to act as portals, thus providing for the smooth passage of instruments. This technique has the potential advantage of giving the surgeon increased tactile feedback from the pedicle probe and pedicle sounder.

Specific Steps

The fluoroscopically assisted freehand technique requires accurate visualization of the bony pedicle entry point. This procedure is aided by meticulous subperiosteal

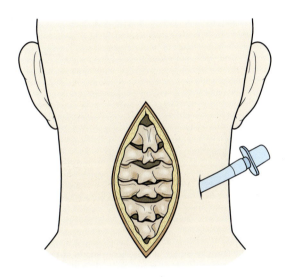

FIGURE 42-6 Schematic diagram of the posterior cervical spine. An endotracheal tube has been cut to length and inserted through a mini-lateral incision to act as a portal to provide for the smooth passage of instruments.

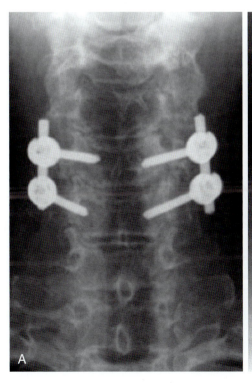
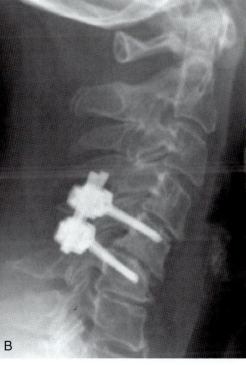

FIGURE 42-5 A, Anteroposterior plain radiograph of the cervical spine showing a pedicle screw and rod construct stabilizing a posttraumatic progressive focal kyphotic deformity. **B**, Lateral plain radiograph of the cervical spine showing a pedicle screw and rod construct stabilizing a posttraumatic progressive focal kyphotic deformity.

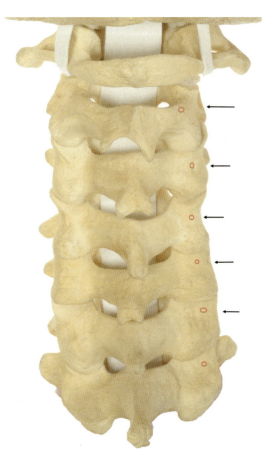

FIGURE 42-7 Posterior aspect of a Sawbones model of the cervical spine, showing the vertebral notches (*black arrows*) and pedicle entry points (*red circles*). (Courtesy Pacific Research Laboratories, Vashon Island, Wash.)

dissection. Because of the variability in the morphology of the lateral masses at each level, the surgeon should study the preoperative CT scan in detail. Furthermore, the location of the entry point for cervical pedicle screws has been shown to be unique at each cervical level (Fig. 42-7), following the enlargement of the spinal cord.[6]

Cannulation of the C2 pedicles can be aided by insertion of a McDonald dissector into the spinal canal above the C2 lamina, medial to the inner surface of the pedicle. This maneuver defines the medial border of the pedicle and projects the trajectory of the pedicle axis. The entry point for C2 cervical pedicle screws is the cranial border of the lamina, which is slightly caudal to the C2 lateral vertebral notch, and the trajectory is at an angle of 15 degrees to the sagittal plane.

The articular masses of the cervical vertebrae have a notch on their lateral aspect that approximates the pedicle. The subaxial C3-C6 pedicles are located at the same level, or just above vertebral notch.[6] The C7 pedicle is, however, located just below the midline of the C7 transverse process. The starting points for the cannulation of the C3-C6 pedicles are lateral to the midpoint of the lateral mass, just beneath the inferior articular process of the vertebra immediately cranially. The authors recommend the use of intraoperative fluoroscopy to confirm the accuracy of the starting point for each pedicle screw. The C-arm is rotated to approximately 45 degrees to the sagittal plane, and it is adjusted to the appropriate degree of lordosis until the pedicle is seen en face, whereby an entry point close to the midpedicle axis can be confirmed (Fig. 42-8). Rotating the C-arm to an orthogonal angle shows a true lateral view of the pedicle (an image perpendicular to the anatomic axis of the pedicle) and provides the craniocaudal trajectory (see Fig. 42-8).

The medial pedicle wall is typically thicker than the lateral. It provides an important tactile reference, and

FIGURE 42-8 Schematic representation of the position of the C-arm relative to the cervical vertebra. First, an intraoperative fluoroscopic image is obtained by rotating the C-arm to approximately 45 degrees to the sagittal plane, and adjusted to the appropriate degree of lordosis, until the pedicle is seen en face (*yellow arrow, top*). Then an image is obtained by rotating the C-arm to an orthogonal angle showing a true lateral view (*yellow arrow, bottom*) of the pedicle (an image perpendicular to the anatomic axis of the pedicle), thus confirming the craniocaudal trajectory for screw insertion.

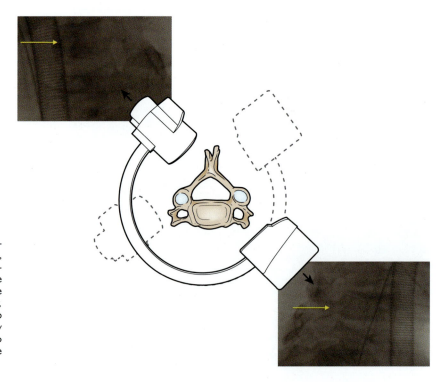

many surgeons choosing to slide the pedicle probe along the medial cortical wall. The local bony anatomy provides a trajectory reference to the sagittal plane. The angle formed between the outer cortex of the lamina and ipsilateral pedicle ranges from 97 degrees at C3 to 87 degrees at C7.[7] The angle of the contralateral lamina has been shown to be within 1 degree of the angle required from the sagittal plane for placement of pedicle screws at C3 to C6 and within 11 degrees at C7.[8]

The use of a high-speed burr and curet allows the creation of a funnel down to the start of the pedicle posteriorly. This tunnel can allow the opening of the pedicle to be seen,[2] with direct visualization of the cortical medial wall and the cancellous flush of blood from the anatomic axis. Furthermore, moving the starting point of the pedicle cannulation closer to the posterior opening of the pedicle, rather than starting cannulation from the level of the lateral mass, increases the degree of freedom of angulation of screw trajectory and allows screws to be inserted at an angle of approximately 25 degrees to the sagittal plane.[5]

Because of the small caliber of cervical pedicles, specially designed pedicle probes, sounders, taps, and screws are used. Screws larger than 4.5 mm are contraindicated. Given the risk of pedicle breach, the hole in the pedicle should be rechecked with the pedicle sounder following tapping and before insertion of the pedicle screw. The authors recommend the insertion of all pedicle screws before any decompression of the neural elements because of the risk of iatrogenic injury secondary to slippage. If the pedicle screws are to be used to correct deformity, consideration should be given to a posterior canal widening laminectomy before connection of the screws to precontoured rods or plates, particularly in the presence of developmental spinal canal stenosis. Care must be taken, when connecting the screws to the longitudinal rods or plates, to observe for potential screw pull out or malposition due to the proximity of neurovascular structures.

Since 2000, the move has been toward the use of technology intraoperatively in spinal surgery to increase the accuracy of implant placement. Early navigation systems were beset with issues such as long setup times and did not enhance the safety or accuracy of screw placement.[9] However, subsequent technologic advances in three-dimensional navigation have been shown not only to improve accuracy and safety of screw placement, but also to enhance identification of optimal bone stock for fixation.[10] Full-rotation, three-dimensional image (O-arm) navigation-assisted screw placement has been shown to facilitate accurate and safe screw placement, but even with these technologic advances, the grade 1 pedicle breach rate is 8.3%, and the grade 2 pedicle breach rate is 2.8%.[11] More recently, advances in robotics have led to a reported 98.9% accuracy of thoracolumbar pedicle screw implantation.[12] However, no reports of accurate or successful use of robots for insertion of cervical pedicle screws have been published.

Postoperative Considerations

Rehabilitation

Cervical pedicle screws offer a biomechanical advantage over other posterior cervical instrumentation constructs

and potentially offer an advantage to patients in enabling earlier mobilization and thereby facilitating faster rehabilitation. The indications for cervical pedicle screw insertion are broad, however, and the specific rehabilitation regimen should therefore be individualized to the patient. Factors to be considered when deciding on the type and duration of external immobilization include patients' comorbidities, number of instrumented levels, indication for surgery, postoperative spinal stability, and quality of bone stock and hence fixation, in addition to consideration of the impact of potential complications of external immobilization on the patient. Ideally, a stable construct with good fixation to bone will have been achieved intraoperatively, and external immobilization can be avoided. Some surgeons prescribe a soft collar for 2 weeks for the patient's comfort, and in patients with severe osteoporosis, the authors recommend the use of a rigid cervical collar for up to 3 months.

Time to return to work also depends on multiple factors. Most patients can return to sedentary employment after 6 weeks, but heavy lifting and physically demanding occupations should be avoided for up to 6 months.

Complications

The insertion of cervical pedicle screws is unfortunately associated with potentially significant complications because of the close proximity of the neural structures and vertebral arteries. The frequency of complication is minimized by thorough preoperative imaging evaluation and meticulous fluoroscopically guided intraoperative technique.

In a reported series of 180 patients, in whom 712 pedicle screws were implanted, the vertebral artery was injured in only 1 patient, in whom the bleeding was stopped with bone wax. A 6.7% pedicle breach rate on CT was reported, but only 2 of the 45 breaches resulted in radiculopathy. In addition to these 3 neurovascular complications, 1 patient had iatrogenic foraminal stenosis resulting from excessive reduction of translational deformity; these findings led to the conclusion that the incidence of clinically significant complications is low.[13]

A retrospective review of 20 patients whose cervical kyphosis was corrected with pedicle screws found that 6 patients had postoperative neurologic defects, developing at a mean of 2.8 days postoperatively and resulting in unilateral muscle weakness of the deltoid and biceps. No cases of misplaced screws were reported. The 6 patients with postoperative deficits had significantly more preoperative kyphosis and the correction angles at C4 and C5 than did the 14 patients without postoperative deficits. Furthermore, the foramen on the side of deficits was significantly smaller than that on the opposite side.[14] Investigators have postulated that severe kyphosis may have a tethering effect on the nerves and have recommended that excessive kyphosis correction should not be performed by posterior surgery, to avoid posterior shift of the spinal cord, and that prophylactic foraminotomies should be considered.[14]

A systematic review compared the complication rates of cervical pedicle screws and lateral mass screws and concluded that the perioperative neurologic and late biomechanical complication rates are low for both methods.

Table 42-1 Summary of Results of Published Studies of 50 or More Patients in Whom a Quoted Number of Pedicle Screws from C3 to C7 Were Implanted by Either Freehand or Navigated Techniques

Author and Year	No. of Patients	No. of Screws	NRI	SCI	VAI	Malposition Requiring Revision	Loss of Screw Fixation to Bone	Metalwork Breakage	Loss of Reduction	Pseudarthrosis
Abumi et al, 2000[13]	180	595	2	0	1	1	0	NR	0	1
Yoshimoto et al, 2009[16]	52	264	0	0	0	NR	NR	NR	NR	NR
Yukawa et al, 2009[17]	144	559	1	0	1	0	1	1	5	NR
Lee et al, 2012[18]	50	277	0	NR	0	NR	NR	NR	NR	NR
Nakashima et al, 2012[19]	84	365	3	0	2	3	5	3	2	2

NR, Not reported; *NRI*, nerve root injury; *SCI*, spinal cord injury; *VAI*, vertebral artery injury.

Vertebral artery injury was found to be significantly more frequently associated with cervical pedicle screws, but it was extremely rare with both techniques.[15]

Results

Cervical pedicle screws offer a biomechanical advantage over other posterior cervical fixation options,[3] but at the expense of increased risk of iatrogenic injury to the adjacent structures, particularly the vertebral artery,[15] albeit at extremely low rates.

The literature contains reports of 5 series of 50 or more patients in whom a quoted number of pedicle screws from C3 to C7 were implanted by either freehand or navigated techniques (Table 42-1).[13,16-19] In all these studies, the reported rates of biomechanical failure of fixation, failure of instrumentation, pseudarthrosis, neurologic injury, or vascular injury are extremely low. The low reported rates of complications, however, are an indication of the frequency of complications in experienced hands in high-volume specialist centers.

REFERENCES

1. Leconte P: Fracture et luxation des deux premieres vertebres cervicales. In Judet R, editor: Luxation congénitale de la hanche: fractures du cou-de-pied rachis cervical. Actualités de chirurgie orthopedique de l'Hôpital Raymond-Poincaré, vol. 3, Paris, 1964, Masson, pp 147–166.
2. Abumi K, Itoh H, Taneichi H, Kaneda K: Transpedicular screw fixation for traumatic lesions of the middle and lower cervical spine: description of the techniques and preliminary report, *J Spinal Disord* 7:19–28, 1994.
3. Johnston TL, Karaikovic EE, Lautenschlager EP, Marcu D: Cervical pedicle screws vs. lateral mass screws: uniplanar fatigue analysis and residual pullout strengths, *Spine J* 6:667–672, 2006.
4. Reinhold M, Magerl F, Rieger M, Blauth M: Cervical pedicle screw placement: feasibility and accuracy of two new insertion techniques based on morphometric data, *Eur Spine J* 16:47–56, 2007.
5. Abumi K, Ito M, Sudo H: Reconstruction of the subaxial cervical spine using pedicle screw instrumentation, *Spine (Phila Pa 1976)* 37:E349–E356, 2012.
6. Karaikovic EE, Kunakornsawat S, Daubs MD, et al.: Surgical anatomy of the cervical pedicles: landmarks for posterior cervical pedicle entrance localization, *J Spinal Disord* 13:63–72, 2000.
7. Bayley E, Zia Z, Kerslake R, Boszczyk BM: The ipsilateral lamina-pedicle angle: can it be used to guide pedicle screw placement in the sub-axial cervical spine? *Eur Spine J* 19:458–463, 2010.
8. Hacker AG, Molloy S, Bernard J: The contralateral lamina: a reliable guide in subaxial, cervical pedicle screw placement, *Eur Spine J* 17:1457–1461, 2008.
9. Ludwig SC, Kowalski JM, Edwards CC 2nd, Heller JG: Cervical pedicle screws: comparative accuracy of two insertion techniques, *Spine (Phila Pa 1976)* 25:2675–2681, 2000.
10. Rajasekaran S, Kanna PR, Shetty TA: Intra-operative computer navigation guided cervical pedicle screw insertion in thirty-three complex cervical spine deformities, *J Craniovertebr Junction Spine* 1:38–43, 2010.
11. Ishikawa Y, Kanemura T, Yoshida G, et al.: Intraoperative, full-rotation, three-dimensional image (O-arm)-based navigation system for cervical pedicle screw insertion, *J Neurosurg Spine* 15:472–478, 2011.
12. Hu X, Ohnmeiss DD, Lieberman IH: Robotic-assisted pedicle screw placement: lessons learned from the first 102 patients, *Eur Spine J* 22:661–666, 2013.
13. Abumi K, Shono Y, Ito M, et al.: Complications of pedicle screw fixation in reconstructive surgery of the cervical spine, *Spine (Phila Pa 1976)* 25:962–969, 2000.
14. Hojo Y, Ito M, Abumi K, et al.: A late neurological complication following posterior correction surgery of severe cervical kyphosis, *Eur Spine J* 20:890–898, 2011.
15. Yoshihara H, Passias PG, Errico TJ: Screw-related complications in the subaxial cervical spine with the use of lateral mass versus cervical pedicle screws, *J Neurosurg Spine* 19:614–623, 2013.
16. Yoshimoto H, Sato S, Hyakumachi T, et al.: Clinical accuracy of cervical pedicle screw insertion using lateral fluoroscopy: a radiographic analysis of the learning curve, *Eur Spine J* 18:1326–1334, 2009.
17. Yukawa Y, Kato F, Ito K, et al.: Placement and complications of cervical pedicle screws in 144 cervical trauma patients using pedicle axis view techniques by fluoroscope, *Eur Spine J* 18:1293–1299, 2009.
18. Lee SH, Kim KT, Abumi K, et al.: Cervical pedicle screw placement using the "key slot technique": the feasibility and learning curve, *J Spinal Disord Tech* 25:415–421, 2012.
19. Nakashima H, Yukawa Y, Imagama S, et al.: Complications of cervical pedicle screw fixation for nontraumatic lesions: a multicenter study of 84 patients, *J Neurosurg Spine* 16:238–247, 2012.

Lateral Mass Screws 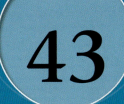 43

Dachuan Wang and Wun-Jer Shen

CHAPTER PREVIEW

Chapter Synopsis	Lateral mass screw–based instrumentation is a well-established technique for cervical spine fusion. Screw placement is constrained by the course of the vertebral artery, the nerve roots, and the anatomy of the facet joints. Many screw trajectories have been described, each with advantages and disadvantages. This chapter provides an overview of pertinent factors and describes the technique of placing cervical lateral mass screws.
Important Points	Lateral mass screws are more robust and versatile than wires. They can be used when the posterior elements are absent or deficient. They are safer and more forgiving than pedicle screws.
	This procedure is contraindicated when the lateral mass is malformed or fractured and in severe osteopenia.
	Different screw trajectories place different neurovascular structures at risk.
Clinical and Surgical Pearls	The lateral margins of the lateral masses should be fully exposed.
	The surgeon should aim from the inferomedial quadrant (close to the center of the lateral mass) in the direction of the superolateral quadrant.
	Burring a pilot hole before drilling can help prevent the drill from slipping.
	Placement of a pin into the facet joint can help demonstrate the cephalad angulation needed to place a Magerl trajectory screw.
	Bicortical purchase provides greater pull-out resistance; however, unicortical screws may be acceptable in degenerative disorders without obvious instability.
Clinical and Surgical Pitfalls	Lateral mass morphology can vary from patient to patient and even within the same patient.
	Facets may be obscured by osteophyte overgrowth.
	The surgeon should expect bleeding from the venous plexus at the lateral border of the lateral masses.
	Roy-Camille screw trajectory at C6 and C7 has a marked risk of entering the caudad facet joint. The margin of safety for this trajectory is smaller than for the Magerl screw trajectory.
	Screws directed too laterally (outward) risk fracturing the lateral mass.
	Common screw lengths are 14 and 16 mm. Suspect screw length measurements over 18 mm as being too long.
Video	Video 43-1: Modified Kurokawa French Door Laminoplasty and Lateral Mass Fusion of C4 to C5 or C6

Indications for cervical surgical fixation include instability secondary to trauma, infection, degenerative spondylosis, osseous metastasis, pseudarthrosis, rheumatoid disease, destruction of bony elements, and extensive laminectomies and other iatrogenic causes. Goals of treatment include preservation of neurologic function, stabilization, maintenance of anatomic alignment, fusion, and early rehabilitation.

Wiring techniques were the first to be developed. Patterns grew complicated, wires evolved into multifilament cables, and rectangular frames were added. However, wires cannot be used when the posterior elements are deficient or after laminoplasty. The degree of stability is poor, and additional external support (e.g., collar, sternal occipital mandibular immobilizer [SOMI brace], halo vest) is often required. Although cervical pedicle screws are biomechanically stronger and provide more rigid fixation than lateral mass screws, the risk of vascular and neurologic injury is higher, the learning curve is steeper, and quite often the pedicle is too small for the screw or does not have a cancellous center.

Since its description in 1972 by Roy-Camille,[1] lateral mass screw–based techniques have become common procedures for posterior stabilization of the subaxial cervical spine. Early designs were simple screw and plate constructs. Because the interfacet distance in the cervical vertebrae is variable, the fixed hole spacing of the plate markedly limits screw positioning. Furthermore, plates are difficult to contour in three dimensions, are not easily extended to the skull or the thorax, and have been known to cause iatrogenic foraminal stenosis through a lag screw effect. Modern system designs are almost all based on polyaxial screws and connected by rods. They allow the surgeon to place screws in the optimal position in the lateral mass while contouring the longitudinal rods to the lateral mass screws. This chapter provides an overview of pertinent factors and describes the technique of placing cervical lateral mass screws.

Lateral Mass Anatomy

A thorough understanding of cervical anatomy is essential. Unlike in the lumbar spine, the cervical nerve root is normally positioned at the lower part of the intervertebral foramen, which corresponds to the middle to lower portion of the lateral mass. On a lateral cervical view, the lateral mass projects as a rhomboid; however, lateral mass morphology can vary from patient to patient and even within the same patient. In particular, compared with C3 to C6, the lateral mass of C7 is more elongated from superior to inferior and is thinner from anterior to posterior (increased height-to-thickness ratio).[2] Pait and colleagues noted in 1995 that the variance in measurements from spine to spine and within the same spine was great enough to render averages clinically unreliable.[3] These investigators proposed that the superolateral quadrant, anterior to which no neurovascular structures are present, be considered the "safe quadrant" and suggested aiming posterior screws in that direction.

Lateral Mass Techniques

Several different techniques have been described for placement of lateral mass screws.[1,4-7] Five trajectories are shown in detail in Figure 43-1, and this list is by no means complete. All the techniques are compromises that attempt to balance anatomic safety and mechanical competence with ease of placement. Nerve roots, the vertebral artery, facet joints, and, to a lesser extent, the spinal cord are at risk during placement of lateral mass screws.[8] Direct anterior trajectories such as the Roy-Camille are technically straightforward, but the screw length (bite) is shorter and at C6 and C7 has a higher chance of violating the inferior facet joint. Screws that angle cranially (Magerl) have a longer, biomechanically stronger screw tract, but they also have a higher chance of damaging the exiting nerve root and of entering the superior facet joint. A more outward (lateral) trajectory, such as used by the An technique,[4] avoids the vertebral artery but has less bone stock available for the screw to traverse (resulting in

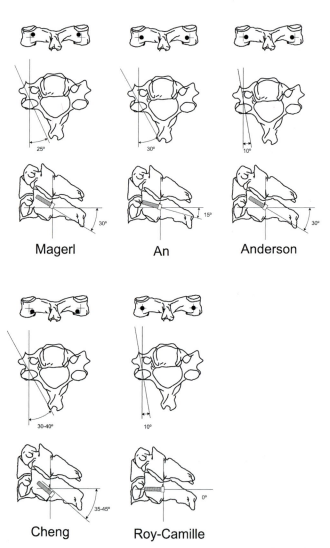

FIGURE 43-1 Comparison of the entry points and screw trajectories described by various authors. The *black dots* indicate the entry points for the lateral mass screws. (From Wu JC, Huang WC, Chen YC, et al: Stabilization of subaxial cervical spines by lateral mass screw fixation with modified Magerl's technique. *Surg Neurol* 70(Suppl I):S25-S33, 2008.)

shorter screw length) and a higher probability of lateral mass fracture.

Trajectory-based methods rely on the surgeon's feel of the angle of screw placement, either freehand or by using a mechanical angle guide or C-arm fluoroscopy. Bayley and colleagues proposed aligning the screw trajectory with a constant anatomic reference plane (i.e., parallel to the ipsilateral cervical lamina).[9] The large degree of lateral angulation (up to 50 degrees) provides a reliable safety margin for neurovascular structures, but many patients do not have sufficient lateral mass width for this technique to be performed. Stevens and associates described a technique that is based on the presence of an intact spinous process.[10] The trajectory is aligned parallel to the tip of the spinous process of the vertebra being instrumented and without any lateral angulation. The authors agree with the concept of using anatomic structures for guidance, and their method is by referencing a guidewire placed in the facet joint for the cranial angle, as described in detail later.

Additional Considerations

Heller and co-workers showed that bicortical purchase provides greater pull-out resistance for lateral mass screws, with a gain of approximately 30%.[11] Stemper and colleagues stated because of superior mechanical stability under single-cycle loading and stiffer response under repeated loading, the use of bicortical lateral mass screws is a superior option for posterior spinal stabilization.[12] The preference at the authors' institution is for bicortical insertion, although for patients with degenerative disorders without obvious instability, unilateral cortical fixation is usually sufficient.

Using fresh frozen spine segments and in-line pull-out testing, Hostin and associates showed that conversion of a stripped lateral mass screw to an alternate trajectory appears to offer no biomechanical advantage over placement of an increased diameter salvage screw using the same trajectory.[13] Conversion to pedicle screw fixation does provide superior biomechanical fixation, but it is technically challenging, associated with a significant breach rate, and is perhaps best used when lateral mass screw salvage is not feasible (e.g., in cases of fracture). The authors' protocol is to attempt salvage of a stripped 3.5-mm lateral mass screw by converting it to a 4.0-mm screw in the same path. If the screw is still loose, an attempt is made to convert to pedicle screw fixation if the authors believe that the screw heads connectors can be made to align. As a last resort, that level can be skipped, and the instrumentation can be extended cranially or caudally as necessary.

Several computer-assisted surgical navigation systems are currently available. Although they are theoretically useful, the authors have not found them to make much difference during lateral mass screw placement and do not use them on a routine basis. Malpositioned screws can be identified by stimulation with an electromyography probe and a search for a sustained burst of neurotonic discharge, but again, the authors do not find this necessary on a routine basis.

All the major orthopedic implant manufacturers have their own screw and rod systems. The surgeon should be aware that rods of the same diameter are not necessarily equally rigid, and special connectors, or a transitional rod with varying rod diameters, may be needed to attach a cervical system to a thoracic system (transition rods).

Surgical Technique

The following case example (**Video 43-1**) describes the procedure for lateral mass screw placement.

CASE EXAMPLE

A 42-year-old male patient presents with central cord syndrome after sustaining a hyperextension injury. Plain films and computed tomography scans do not show any fractures or dislocations, but magnetic resonance imaging reveals stenosis at C4 to C5 or C6 with hyperintense signal in the spinal cord. The lateral masses are anatomically normal. The plan is to perform laminoplasty and fusion of C4 to C5 or C6.

Positioning: After endotracheal intubation, the patient is carefully placed prone on a four-poster or Wilson frame. The neck is held neutral with slight head flexion on a horseshoe support. Adequate padding for the face and eyes is provided. The authors do not routinely use three-point fixation to secure the cranium in patients with degenerative disorders, but the Mayfield head holder can be useful in the setting of trauma or instability. The shoulders are pulled down and held in place with adhesive tape. This maneuver flattens out the skin fold at the base of the neck to facilitate the surgical approach, and it also allows for easier intraoperative imaging. The neck (and iliac crest if needed) is prepared and draped in a sterile fashion (Fig. 43-2).

Incision and Approach: Preincision skin injection with epinephrine for hemostasis is optional. A midline posterior approach to the cervical spine is used. It is important to stay in the midline when reflecting the paraspinal muscles, to maintain a bloodless field. The spinous processes are exposed, and a lateral roentgenogram or intraoperative fluoroscopy is used for level identification. The dissection is carried out subperiosteally, fully exposing the facet joints and the lateral borders of the lateral masses (Fig. 43-3). The soft tissue and the capsular ligaments around the facets must be meticulously removed. However, the facets that are not intended to be fused should be carefully kept intact. Bleeding may be encountered from the venous plexus lateral to the lateral masses. This bleeding can be safely stopped with bipolar cautery.

Decompression: If a laminectomy or laminoplasty is to be performed, it may be done either before or after lateral mass screw site preparation. Those surgeons in favor of placing screws first cite protection of the spinal cord and dura during drilling and use of the intact spinous process and lamina bony landmarks as guides to screw placement. Other surgeons are concerned that the process of placing the instrumentation inevitably shakes an already compressed spinal cord and prefer to decompress first. In this case, a Kurokawa (French door) style laminoplasty is performed first. Gutters are made with a burr at the junction of the lamina and the lateral mass (Fig. 43-4) on both sides, and then the spinous process is split using a 2-mm burr (Fig. 43-5). Decompression is achieved by separation of the lamina halves (Fig. 43-6).

Instrumentation: For screw placement, the center of the lateral mass is marked by a cross that divides it in cephalocaudal and medial to lateral directions (Fig. 43-7). The authors prefer to place the screws parallel to the facets (Magerl-type trajectory). A 1.2-mm Kirschner wire is bent into a 90-degree angle and is inserted into the facet joint (Fig. 43-8). This technique provides a reference for the cephalic angulation needed. The entry point is 1 mm inferior and 1 mm medial to the center of the lateral mass.

With a high-speed burr, a small pilot hole is made (Fig. 43-9), followed by a 2-mm drill that is aimed parallel to the interfacet Kirschner wire in the sagittal plane and 20 to 25 degrees laterally (outward) toward the superolateral ventral corner (Hostin's safe quadrant)[13] (Fig. 43-10). With experience, the surgeon can usually feel the drill penetrating the ventral cortex. A depth gauge is then used to measure the screw tract length and also as a probe to palpate the bony surroundings to ascertain that the whole tract is within the lateral mass (Fig. 43-11). The procedure is repeated for all the lateral masses.

The facet joint cartilage is removed, and the joint is decorticated using a small burr (Fig. 43-12). Autologous bone, taken locally or from the iliac crest, is packed into the facet joints. The dorsal cortex is tapped, and 3.5-mm top-loading polyaxial titanium screws are placed sequentially (in this case, Vertex System, Medtronic Sofamor Danek, Warsaw, Ind.) (Fig. 43-13). Screw length is determined individually for each lateral mass. The most commonly used screw length is 16 mm. The surgeon should suspect that screw length measurements of more than 18 mm are too long.

If the screw is inadvertently stripped, the authors fill the tract with small fragments of bone and then insert a 4.0-mm diameter rescue screw along the same path. The lamina is then decorticated. The connecting rod is contoured into lordosis and applied, screw caps are placed and torqued, and the construct is completed (Fig. 43-14). Crosslinks are applied if needed.

Intraoperative fluoroscopy is not used routinely, but only when patients have severe lateral mass deformity or whenever the surgeon needs confirmation.

As previously discussed, the lateral mass at C7 is shaped differently, being thinner and more elongated. The screws at this level are angled more cranially compared with those at more rostral levels. Most modern polyaxial screw-rod systems can accommodate this steeper trajectory without difficulty. In certain cases, it may be easier to place a pedicle screw at C7 than a lateral mass screw.

Closure: The wound is thoroughly irrigated. Morselized autograft or allograft chips are placed in the lateral gutters as needed. Hemostasis is obtained with cautery. Suction drainage is always used at the authors' institution, with the drain placed deep to the fascia. The muscles and fascia are closed in anatomic layers. The skin is closed, and an occlusive dressing is applied. The drain is usually removed 24 hours postoperatively.

Postoperative Care: A radiograph of the cervical spine is taken immediately after the surgical procedure. Intravenous antibiotics are continued for 24 hours postoperatively. A rigid orthosis is routinely prescribed to be worn for 2 to 3 months. Follow-up radiographic films are taken at intervals (Fig. 43-15).

Conclusions

Several surgical techniques for achieving fixation in the posterior cervical spine exist. Traditional wiring techniques require the presence of the posterior elements, whereas cervical pedicle screws remain technically challenging and place the vertebral artery and spinal cord at risk. Currently, cervical lateral mass screws in the subaxial spine remain the most common fixation technique. Multiple trajectories have been described; however, they are all designed to reduce the risk of injury to neurovascular structures while attempting to avoid lateral mass fracture and facet joint violation. Whenever possible, placement of bicortical fixation provides the greatest biomechanical pull-out strength. However, the surgeon should remember that, ultimately, meticulous attention to decorticating the posterior aspect of the lateral mass and removing the cartilage of the facet joint is necessary to help achieve bony fusion, or else any fixation will eventually fail.

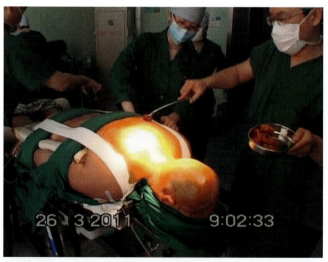

FIGURE 43-2 Patient positioning. The head is supported on a well-padded horseshoe frame, and the shoulders are taped down.

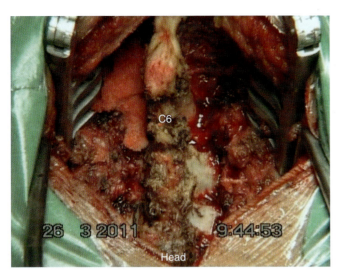

FIGURE 43-3   Approach. The exposure extends to lateral border of the lateral masses. Bleeding may be encountered from the venous plexus lateral to the lateral masses. In this and all subsequent intraoperative figures, the patient's head is toward the bottom of the figure.

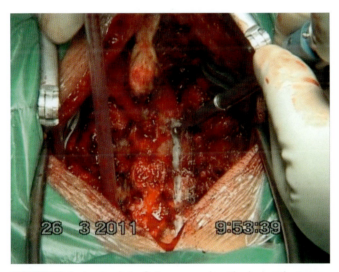

FIGURE 43-4   Laminoplasty. Gutters are made with a burr at the junction of the lamina and the lateral mass.

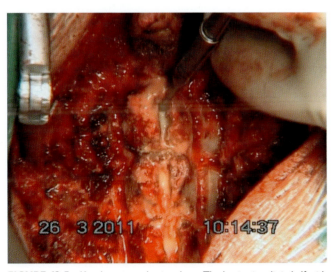

FIGURE 43-5   Kurokawa-type laminoplasty. The lamina is split in half with a 2-mm burr.

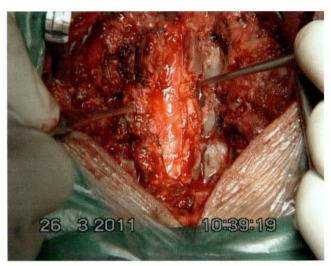

FIGURE 43-6   Decompression. The split lamina halves are separated. The dura is exposed.

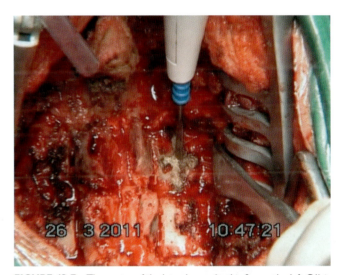

FIGURE 43-7   The center of the lateral mass (in this figure, the left C6) is marked with a cross.

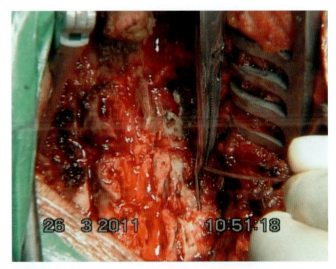

FIGURE 43-8   Determination of sagittal cephalad angulation of the screw. A Kirschner wire is bent and placed in the facet joint (in this figure, the left C4-C5 facet). It serves as a guide for the Magerl trajectory, which is parallel to the facet joint.

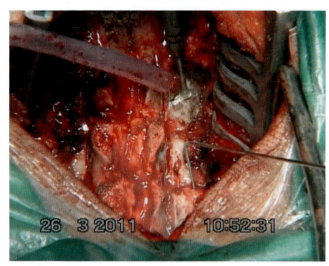

FIGURE 43-9 Pilot hole in the left C6 lateral mass. With a burr, a pilot hole is made 1 mm medial and 1 mm caudad to the center of the lateral mass. This prevents the drill from inadvertently slipping across the hard posterior cortex of the lateral mass in the next step.

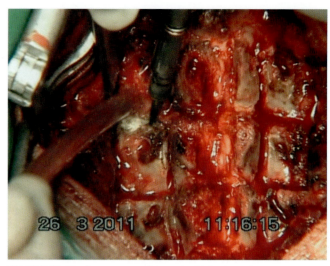

FIGURE 43-12 Facetectomy of the right C5-C6 facet. The facet joint cartilage is removed, and the joint is decorticated using a small burr. Bone graft is then packed into the facet joints.

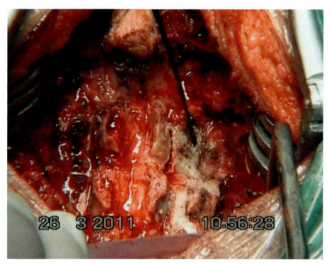

FIGURE 43-10 A 2-mm drill is aimed parallel to the interfacet Kirschner wire in the sagittal plane and 20 to 25 degrees laterally (outward) toward the superior lateral ventral corner of the lateral mass.

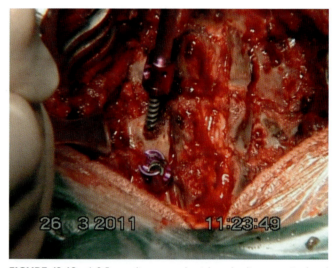

FIGURE 43-13 A 3.5-mm diameter polyaxial top loading screw is placed into the right C5 lateral mass.

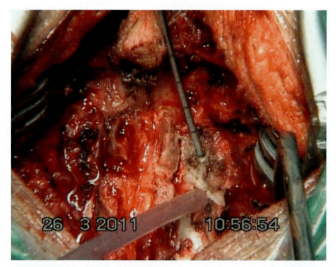

FIGURE 43-11 A depth gauge is used to measure the screw length and also as a probe to palpate the bony surroundings to confirm that the whole tract is within the lateral mass.

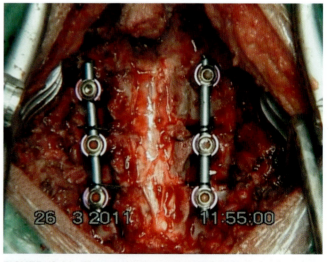

FIGURE 43-14 The completed construct. The lamina halves have been tied to the rod to prevent closure and restenosis.

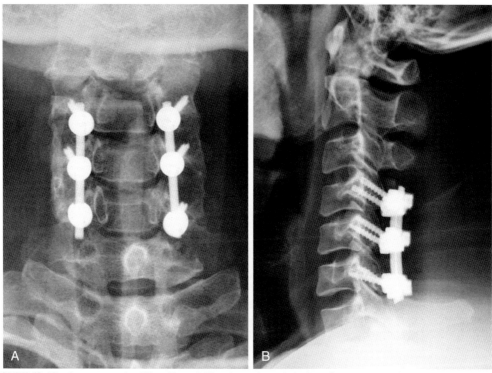

FIGURE 43-15 Anteroposterior (**A**) and lateral (**B**) radiographs with the lateral mass screw rod instrumentation in place.

REFERENCES

1. Roy-Camille R, Gaillant G, Bertreaux D: Early management of spinal injuries. In McKibben B, editor: *Recent advances in orthopedics*, Edinburgh, 1979, Churchill-Livingstone, pp 57–87.
2. Abdullah KG, Steinmetz MP, Mroz TE: Morphometric and volumetric analysis of the lateral masses of the lower cervical spine, *Spine (Phila Pa 1976)* 34:1476–1479, 2009.
3. Pait TG, McAllister PV, Kaufman HH: Quadrant anatomy of the articular pillars (lateral cervical mass) of the cervical spine, *J Neurosurg* 82:1011–1014, 1995.
4. An HS, Gordin R, Renner K: Anatomic considerations for plate-screw fixation of the cervical spine, *Spine (Phila Pa 1976)* 16(Suppl):S548–S551, 1991.
5. Anderson PA, Henley MB, Grady MS, et al.: Posterior cervical arthrodesis with AO reconstruction plates and bone graft, *Spine (Phila Pa 1976)* 16(Suppl):S72–S79, 1991.
6. Jeanneret B, Magerl F, Ward EH, et al.: Posterior stabilization of the cervical spine with hook plates, *Spine (Phila Pa 1976)* 16(Suppl):S56–S63, 1991.
7. Wu JC, Huang WC, Chen YC, et al.: Stabilization of subaxial cervical spines by lateral mass screw fixation with modified Magerl's technique, *Surg Neurol* 70(Suppl 1):S25–S33, 2008.
8. Merola AA, Castro BA, Alongi PR, et al.: Anatomic consideration for standard and modified techniques of cervical lateral mass screw placement, *Spine J* 2:430–435, 2002.
9. Bayley E, Zia Z, Kerslake R, et al.: Lamina-guided lateral mass screw placement in the sub-axial cervical spine, *Eur Spine J* 19:660–664, 2010.
10. Stevens QE, Majd ME, Kattner KA, et al.: Use of spinous processes to determine the optimal trajectory for placement of lateral mass screws: technical note, *J Spinal Disord Tech* 22:347–352, 2009.
11. Heller JG, Estes BT, Zaouali M, et al.: Biomechanical study of screws in the lateral masses: variables affecting pull-out resistance, *J Bone Joint Surg Am* 78:1315–1321, 1996.
12. Stemper BD, Marawar SV, Yoganandan N, et al.: Quantitative anatomy of subaxial cervical lateral mass: an analysis of safe screw lengths for Roy-Camille and Magerl techniques, *Spine (Phila Pa 1976)* 33:893–897, 2008.
13. Hostin RA, Wu C, Perra JH, et al.: A biomechanical evaluation of three revision screw strategies for failed lateral mass fixation, *Spine (Phila Pa 1976)* 33:2415–2421, 2008.

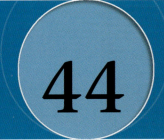

44 Interspinous Wiring

Raghav Badrinath and Jonathan N. Grauer

CHAPTER PREVIEW

Chapter Synopsis	Interspinous wiring techniques were developed as a means of stabilizing traumatic cervical injuries. Although increasingly replaced by newer technologies, such as lateral mass screws and pedicle screws, interspinous wiring remains a useful supplemental or alternative means of posterior cervical fixation. The purpose of this chapter is to review the indications, surgical technique, and postoperative management for cervical interspinous wiring.
Important Points	Wiring offers better stabilization in flexion than in extension or rotation.
	If used by themselves, wiring techniques are generally supplemented with an external orthosis or halo.
	Several techniques have been described, but each involves wiring together of adjacent vertebrae.
	Contraindications include spinous process fracture and lamina fracture or extensive laminectomy.
Clinical and Surgical Pearls	Rogers wiring involves passing a wire through the cephalad spinous process and under the caudal spinous process.
	Bohlman triple wiring involves passing a wire through the spinous processes of both levels being addressed. Two additional wires are passed through the spinous process holes and structural graft on either side of the posterior elements.
	Facet wiring involves passing a wire through a drill hole in the inferior facet of the cephalad level and then around the spinous process of the caudad level.
Clinical and Surgical Pitfalls	Interspinous wiring alone may not provide sufficient fixation. It may be used as an adjunct to other instrumentation or for supplemental external immobilization.
	The most common complications of spinous process wiring are lack of fusion and loss of alignment.

Posterior cervical stabilization using wires was first described by Hadra in 1891 as a means to address instability secondary to fracture and Pott disease.[1] Subsequently, Rogers described the treatment of traumatic cervical instability by using interspinous wiring in 1942.[2] Relatively minor modifications to wiring techniques have been made over the decades, but the general concept remains similar.

Although these techniques are generally referred to as wiring techniques, wires or cables may be considered. Braided cables offer the potential merit of flexibility, strength, and improved fatigue properties.[3] However, these cables may not be readily available, they require specific tools, and they have a tendency to return to a circular shape if loosening occurs. Interspinous wiring provides good support in flexion, but it offers much less in extension and rotation because only the midline spinous processes are stabilized.[4]

Indications and Contraindications

Posterior cervical stabilization has many indications, including, but not limited to, traumatic cervical spine injuries, sagittal deformity, and instability resulting from congenital anomalies or inflammatory arthritis, infection, neoplasms, or anterior nonunion.[4,5] The goals of internal fixation are stabilization, maintenance of alignment, enhancement of fusion, and alleviation of pain.[6]

Interspinous wiring is contraindicated when the spinous processes are fractured or when the laminae are fractured or removed by laminectomy resulting from decompression. In these cases, facet wiring, briefly described later, can be performed. Alternatively, the vertebrae can be stabilized with wires extending from the segment above the level of spinous process fracture to the level below it.

For many applications, newer methods such as lateral mass screws and pedicle screws have replaced wiring techniques in current clinical practice because of their flexibility and ability to be placed despite removal of posterior vertebral elements. Nonetheless, interspinous wiring remains a useful technique as a result of its "low cost, decreased risk of neurologic or vascular injury and relative technical ease of instrumentation placement."[7] This is a good tool to maintain in the armamentarium of cervical stabilization techniques.

Of the applications for which interspinous wiring is considered, the one that is currently most common is for provisional reduction and stabilization of traumatic injuries. By facilitating reduction with the interspinous wire, the alignment of the spine can be improved before placement of lateral mass fixation. The wire is then often left or can even be considered for removal before completing the stabilization construct.

Surgical Technique

Anesthesia, Positioning, and Approach

The indications dictating surgical intervention generally lead the anesthetic and positioning considerations. In the setting of cervical instability, limited extension intubations are typically warranted. The head is generally held in a Mayfield head holder. Positioning reduction is usually achieved as possible. Neuromonitoring is generally considered. A standard midline posterior cervical approach is then performed.

Interspinous Wiring

The two most popular methods of interspinous wiring are the Rogers technique and the Bohlman triple-wiring technique. The oblique facet wiring technique is also described for cases in which laminectomy has been performed or when the spinous process is fractured.

Rogers Wiring

In the Rogers technique, a burr is used to create holes at the base of both sides of the cephalad spinous process near the laminae. A towel clip is passed through these holes to create a path for the wire. A wire (usually 18 or 20 gauge) or cable is passed through the hole (Fig. 44-1, *A*). The wire is looped around the caudad border of the inferior spinous process (Fig. 44-1, *B*).

The wire can then be tightened, thus affording reduction, if required. Spinal alignment is evaluated radiographically. Alternatively, two twists can be used (one on either side of the spinous processes) to ensure symmetric compression with tightening.

If multiple levels need to be fused, the wire can be passed in a figure-of-eight pattern to include the middle level.[8] The lateral masses can then be decorticated and packed with bone graft.[7]

Bohlman Triple Wiring

The Bohlman triple-wire technique builds from the Rogers wiring technique. The first wire is a modified Rogers-type wire. This is passed through holes at the base of both

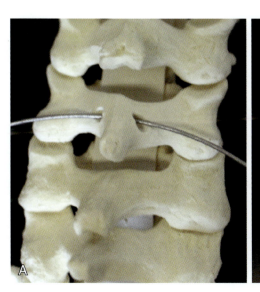 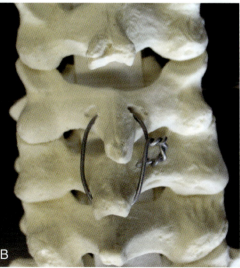

FIGURE 44-1 The Rogers wiring technique. **A,** Burr holes are made through the cephalad spinous process and wire is passed through them. **B,** The wire is wrapped around the inferior edge of the caudad process and tightened.

spinous processes being addressed and is then tightened (Fig. 44-2, *A*). The wire may additionally be looped around the cephalad border of the superior spinous process and the caudad border of the inferior spinous process to provide greater stability and decrease the incidence of wire pull out.

At this point, the technique diverges from the Rogers method. Two subsequent wires are then used to secure structure bone grafts (traditionally corticocancellous iliac crest bone graft) to either side of the spinous processes (Fig. 44-2, *B*). The bone grafts should be long enough to extend across the required fusion length. A burr is used to make two holes in each of the bone grafts. Decortication of the two spinous processes and lamina can be performed. The wires are passed through the holes in the spinous processes used for the primary wire and then through the structural bone graft on either side. These two secondary wires are simultaneously tightened, thereby securing the grafts in close approximation to the lamina (Fig. 44-2, *C*). Cancellous chips are also placed on the exposed lamina or wherever possible.

Facet Wiring

Oblique wiring from one facet to the subadjacent spinous process is an alternative that can be considered if the superior spinous process is not adequate (e.g., as a result of fracture or decompression). The facet joint of the level being addressed is opened with a Penfield instrument. A drill is then used to create a hole through the inferior facet of the superior vertebra. A wire is passed through this hole (Fig. 44-3, *A*) and is obliquely looped around the caudad border of the inferior spinous process and tightened (Fig. 44-3, *B*). This procedure is repeated from the other side as well, to ensure symmetry. Posterior elements are then decorticated, and bone graft is applied.

Postoperative Considerations

Posterior wiring techniques offer only a semirigid means of stabilization. For this reason, these techniques may be supplemented with additional screw fixation. However, if these techniques are used alone, as was their initial intent, patients often have additional stabilization with external collar, cervicothoracic, or halo orthoses.

Complications associated with this procedure are lack of fusion, hyperextension, or construct failure. Failure occurs either through wire failure or spinous process fracture because of excessive loading or excessive tightening, usually in the immediate postoperative period.[9]

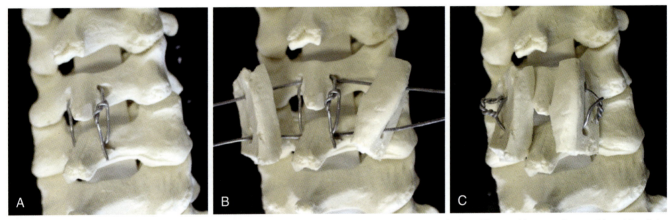

FIGURE 44-2 **A** to **C,** The Bohlman triple-wiring technique is similar to the Rogers technique, with the addition of bone grafts on either side of the spinous process.

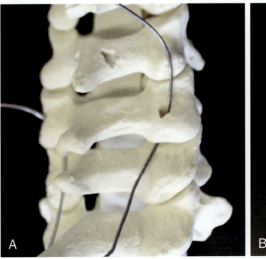
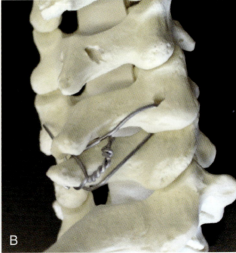

FIGURE 44-3 The oblique facet wiring technique can be used in case of spinous process fracture or extensive laminectomy. This procedure involves wrapping the wire through burr holes on the facet joints (**A**) and around the caudad spinous process (**B**).

Conclusions

Interspinous wiring provides a suitable way of stabilizing the cervical spine and reconstituting the posterior tension band.[9] Wiring can be used by itself in addition to other constructs, especially lateral mass screws, which allow for additional stability in rotation, lateral bending, and extension.[10] The surgeon must decide on the appropriate approach, depending on the particular pathoanatomy, mechanism of injury, and his or her own abilities with fixation devices.[8]

REFERENCES

1. Hadra B: Wiring the spinous processes in Pott's disease, *J Bone Joint Surg* 1:206, 1891.
2. Rogers WA: Treatment of fracture-dislocation of the cervical spine, *J Bone Joint Surg* 24:245, 1942.
3. Weis JC, Cunningham BW, Kanayama M, et al.: In vitro biomechanical comparison of multistrand cables with conventional cervical stabilization, *Spine (Phila Pa 1976)* 21:2108, 1996.
4. Fuji T, Yonenobu K, Fujiwara K, et al.: Interspinous wiring without bone grafting for nonunion or delayed union following anterior spinal fusion of the cervical spine, *Spine (Phila Pa 1976)* 11:982, 1986.
5. Vender JR, Rekito AJ, Harrison SJ, McDonnell DE: Evolution of posterior cervical and occipitocervical fusion and instrumentation, *Neurosurg Focus* 16:1–15, 2004.
6. White AA III: Biomechanical analysis of clinical stability in the cervical spine, *Clin Orthop Relat Res* 109:85, 1975.
7. Arnold PM, Bryniarski M, McMahon JK: Posterior stabilization of subaxial cervical spine trauma: indications and techniques, *Injury* 36:S36–S43, 2005.
8. An HS: Internal fixation of the cervical spine: current indications and techniques, *J Am Acad Orthop Surg* 3:194, 1995.
9. Capen DA, Nelson RW, Zigler J, et al.: Surgical stabilisation of the cervical spine: a comparative analysis of anterior and posterior spine fusions, *Spinal Cord* 25:111–119, 1987.
10. Liu JK, Das K: Posterior fusion of the subaxial cervical spine: indications and techniques, *Neurosurg Focus* 10:1–8, 2001.

SECTION 7

Emerging Technologies

Minimally Invasive Techniques in the Cervical Spine

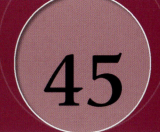

45

Albert P. Wong, Zachary A. Smith, and Richard G. Fessler

CHAPTER PREVIEW

Chapter Synopsis	The goals of individual minimally invasive surgery (MIS) approaches in the cervical spine are to minimize disruption of the normal anatomic structures, to diminish soft tissue disruption, and to prevent both short-term and long-term morbidity while achieving the aims of the surgical procedures. MIS approaches have been shown to be safe for cervical foraminotomies, diskectomies, decompression for stenosis, resection of spinal tumors, and posterior spinal fusion. Patients undergoing MIS procedures typically have decreases in length of hospital stay, surgical blood loss, and postoperative narcotic requirement, as well as improved clinical outcome scores. The purpose of this chapter is to discuss the preoperative considerations, surgical techniques, and complications associated with the most recent MIS approaches available in the cervical spine.
Important Points	A detailed understanding of surgical anatomy is critical to avoid disorientation in MIS approaches.
Clinical and Surgical Pearls	Confirmation of the surgical level of interest with fluoroscopy is essential to avoid becoming disoriented when working in a narrow surgical field.
	Migration or misplacement of the dilators can lead to significant disorientation. Thus, the surgeon must be extremely careful during the initial steps in localization and dilation.
	If endoscope visualization is poor, the surgeon should attempt to irrigate the field and the lens first. If this does not improve visualization, the surgeon should remove the endoscope, clean it directly, and reapply the defogger solution.
Clinical and Surgical Pitfalls	Caution must be used in the region of the medial interlaminar space to avoid inadvertent intrusion into the spinal canal or creation of a cerebrospinal fluid leak.
	A Kirschner wire should not be used for localization or dilation in the cervical spine. The trapezius fascia is incised under direct vision for maximum ease and safety of dilation. The muscle fibers are bluntly split using Metzenbaum scissors before dilation.
	The surgeon should not angle the dilator medially until the working channel is placed.

Cervical spondylosis is a chronic and degenerative consequence of aging that traditionally has been treated with open surgical decompression. Spondylosis can result from degenerative arthritis of the disk space and joints, disk herniation, facet or ligamentous hypertrophy, and spinal instability (Fig. 45-1).[1] Any of these conditions can result in central spinal canal or foraminal stenosis leading to symptoms of cervical myelopathy, radiculopathy, or myeloradiculopathy.[2] Advances in technology have promoted an evolution from open surgery to microsurgical

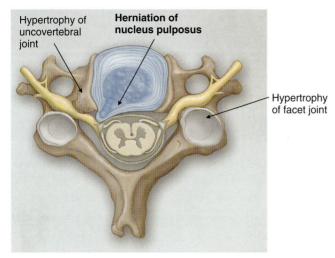

FIGURE 45-1 Hypertrophy of the facets and ligaments or a herniated disk can lead to central stenosis and cervical myelopathy or foraminal stenosis and cervical radiculopathy.

and minimally invasive surgery (MIS) techniques to treat these conditions.[3-12]

Cervical spondylosis can be treated with an anterior approach, a posterior approach, or combined anterior and posterior surgical approach. Historically, the anterior approach to the cervical spine provides a direct solution to ventral disease. This approach is commonly well tolerated and allows the surgeon to approach the ventral cervical spine with minimal muscle dissection. However, soft tissue exposure in the neck is required. Thus, potential complications include anatomic injury to the adjacent carotid artery or jugular vein, esophagus, trachea, thoracic duct, sympathetic plexus, and superior laryngeal, recurrent laryngeal, or hypoglossal nerves, as well as postoperative dysphagia and accelerated adjacent segment level disease.[13,14]

Consequently, posterior approaches to the cervical spine remain popular in the treatment of symptomatic cervical spondylosis. Particularly in the treatment of cervical radiculopathy from foraminal stenosis or lateral disk herniation, posterior cervical laminoforaminotomy remains a standard surgical technique that leads to resolution of clinical symptoms in 92% to 97% of patients.[15,16] For patients with cervical stenosis and myelopathy, cervical laminectomy or laminoplasty results in stable or improved clinical symptoms in 62% to 83% of cases.[27-32] Unfortunately, the traditional open posterior cervical approach requires significant muscle dissection and retraction, resulting in predictable postoperative pain and prolonged recovery time in 20% to 60% of patients.[5,21,33] Therefore, the MIS approach provides an attractive alternative surgical approach to the posterior cervical spine. Specifically in patients with focal disease confined to one to two levels, MIS approaches have excellent outcomes when compared with open cervical procedures.[21]

The fundamental philosophy of MIS in the posterior cervical spine consists of maintaining the normal anatomic structures, preserving the posterior tension band, and minimizing iatrogenic defects.[5,6,34] Sequentially muscle-dilating tubes were developed to access the surgical site through a minimal skin and fascia incision, thereby preserving the normal anatomy and structural integrity of the spine. The incorporation of the microscope or endoscope has enhanced the surgical field of view and facilitates excellent surgical outcomes through these minimally invasive access tubes.

The goal of this chapter is to discuss the most recent MIS approaches available for the cervical spine. The main surgical approach described is the minimally invasive posterior paramedian cervical method (transtubular or transmuscular). A microscope, endoscope, or loupes may be used, depending on the surgeon's preference. This approach is used to perform cervical laminectomy, laminotomy, laminoplasty, foraminotomy, diskectomy, lateral mass screws, tumor resection, or even deformity correction.

Preoperative Considerations

Patients with cervical spondylosis usually present with myelopathy, radiculopathy, or myeloradiculopathy. Myelopathic patients typically describe a chronic and progressive *stepwise decline* in their fine motor function and gait ataxia over a period of months to years. Classic descriptions of fine motor dysfunction include difficulties with buttoning shirts or putting on earrings and trouble with dexterity such as handwriting or typing on a keyboard. Gait ataxia, usually described as a "loss of balance" or "inability to locate the feet" while walking, leads to increased falls. Less common complaints include weakness of hand intrinsic muscles, low back pain, burning paresthesias in the extremities, and bladder or bowel changes. Less than 10% of patients describe having axial or radicular pain as the main symptom.

On physical examination, patients may exhibit signs of extremity weakness, gait imbalance, a positive Romberg sign, hyperreflexia caudal to the site of spinal cord compression, clonus, the Hoffmann sign, or the Babinski sign. Occasionally patients may describe a shooting electrical pain down the spine with neck flexion known as the Lhermitte sign.

In contrast, patients with cervical radiculopathy usually report radiating pain in a dermatomal distribution specific to the compressed nerve root or roots.[35] The pain may radiate from the neck in the midline and extend down to the fingers as burning or electric shooting pain with associated paresthesias. Symptoms are usually acute if they result from trauma, but they may be chronic if they are caused by cervical spondylosis.

On physical examination, patients may have decreased sensation to light touch, pinprick, and vibration in a dermatomal distribution with associated muscular weakness from the compressed nerve root. Patients with chronic compression may have evidence of muscular atrophy or diminished to absent reflexes in the affected nerve root distribution. The radicular pain may be exacerbated and confirmed with the Spurling test (ipsilateral lateral neck flexion and rotation, neck extension with axial loading).

Cervical spondylosis may be seen on radiographs (static or dynamic), but it is more clearly seen on computed tomography (CT) or magnetic resonance imaging (MRI) (or CT myelogram). Evidence of disk degeneration, loss of disk space height, disk herniation, or calcification is usually present. Underlying vertebral body osteophyte formation and hypertrophy of the facets or ligaments also contribute to cervical stenosis. Central canal stenosis may result in myelopathy from spinal cord compression, whereas lateral or foraminal stenosis usually results in radiculopathy from nerve root compression. Additional diagnostic tools include electromyography (EMG) or nerve conduction studies to help localize the level of nerve root compression. For patients with ambiguous myelopathy, EMG and somatosensory-evoked potentials (SSEPs) can help determine whether spinal cord compression with dysfunction is present. Irrespective of the imaging findings, the clinical examination must always match the radiographic findings to ensure an appropriate diagnosis.

Minimally invasive cervical decompression is indicated for patients with myelopathy from cervical stenosis or patients with radiculopathy from nerve root compression. A posterior cervical approach is indicated in cervical nerve root compression from lateral disk herniation, foraminal stenosis, hypertrophy of ligaments or facets, synovial cyst compression, failed indirect anterior cervical decompression, medical contraindication to anterior approach, or patient habitus (short neck). Contraindications to posterior cervical decompression include patients with a straight or kyphotic cervical spine, spinal instability, or inaccessible ventral midline disease.[36,37]

Before any surgical intervention, extensive discussion with the patient and family should be held to ensure appropriate expectations of surgical outcomes. Patients with radiculopathy should have completed a trial of physical therapy, pain management, steroids, or epidural injections before conceding a failure of medical management. Decompression of the nerve root typically results in immediate relief of pain symptoms, but weakness and paresthesias may take longer to improve, and recovery can be incomplete. Similarly, patients with myelopathy should be counseled that the surgical procedure is intended to prevent further neurologic decline and although some patients may experience some improvement, the operation is not designed to return patients to their previously healthy baseline. Orienting patients to realistic expectations is imperative to a successful surgical outcome. All potential risks of the surgical procedure, including intraoperative complications of surgery or anesthesia and postoperative complications (e.g., urinary tract infections, wound infections, venous thrombosis), should be clearly discussed with the patient preoperatively.

This chapter discusses the available MIS approaches to the cervical spine: microendoscopic decompression for stenosis (MEDS), foraminotomy (MEF), diskectomy (MED), and laminoplasty, as well as MIS approaches for spinal tumors.

Operative Setup

The anesthesia and positioning setup is similar for the following posterior MIS cervical approaches unless otherwise stated. General endotracheal anesthesia is performed in a routine manner, except in patients requiring fiberoptic intubation (cervical stenosis with spinal cord

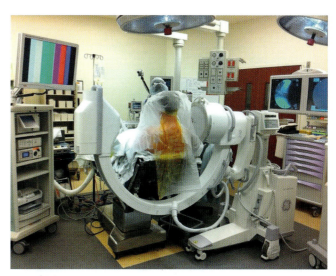

FIGURE 45-2 Patient prepared, draped, and positioned in a sitting position with the C-arm in place.

compression). Neuromonitoring with motor-evoked potentials (MEPs), SSEPs, and free-run EMG is implemented. An arterial line may be added for patients with spinal cord compression to ensure adequate spinal cord perfusion by maintenance of elevated mean arterial pressure. A Foley urinary catheter is generally not needed in patients with one- or two-level disorders. Sequential compression devices are used in conjunction with knee-high compression stockings to minimize the risk of deep venous thrombus formation. Perioperative antibiotics with skin flora (gram-positive bacteria) coverage are given before incision. Muscle relaxants are usually unnecessary after anesthesia induction because MIS approaches require minimal muscle dissection or retraction.

Positioning of the patient in MIS cervical approaches is influenced by the size and length of the neck, shoulder height, and surgical level. The head is secured with the Mayfield head holder in either the prone or upright sitting position. The senior author prefers the sitting position because it reduces epidural bleeding and fluid accumulation in the operative field, decreased airway or facial edema and anesthesia time, and improved visualization of lateral cervical radiographs secondary to gravity traction on the shoulders.

The surgical site is cleaned with alcohol solution, and the midline is approximated by palpation of the spinous processes between two fingers and outlined by a marking pen. The surgical site is then hand scrubbed in sterile fashion with a povidone-iodine (Betadine) solution, painted with alcohol, and reprepared with DuraPrep. The patient is draped in the usual sterile fashion, and the fluoroscopy machine is brought into the field to localize the level of disease (Fig. 45-2).

Minimally Invasive Microendoscopic Foraminotomy or Diskectomy for Foraminal Stenosis or Lateral Disk Herniation

The following steps are similar for microendoscopic foraminotomy, diskectomy, and decompression. Anatomic

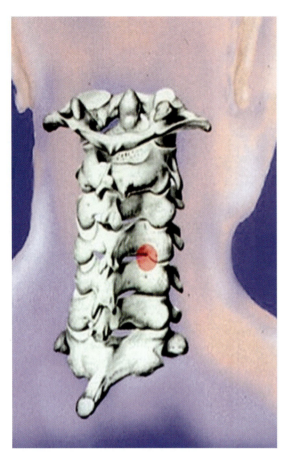

FIGURE 45-3 Cervical spine with a target for a final dilator tube on the ipsilateral facet junction.

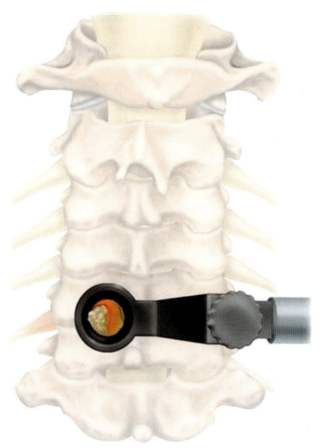

FIGURE 45-4 Minimally invasive tube with the root and disk exposed. (From Hilton DL: Minimally invasive tubular access for posterior cervical foraminotomy with three-dimensional microscopic visualization and localization with anterior/posterior imaging. *Spine J* 7:154-158, 2007.)

landmarks helpful in surgical planning include the angle of the mandible (C2 vertebral body), the first bifid spinous process (C2), and the prominent spinous process (C7). An ipsilateral paramedian line is drawn approximately 1.5 cm from the midline. The fluoroscopy machine is positioned for lateral radiographs, and the surgical level is approximated with a small dilator tube placed over the paramedian line (Fig. 45-3). The point of entry is marked before injecting the skin and underlying fascia with local anesthesia. The skin and fascia are incised (2.0 cm) with a scalpel, and Metzenbaum scissors are used to dissect the paraspinal muscles bluntly down to the facet joint. Placement of sequential tube dilators is then performed (Fig. 45-4). The final tubular retractor (~18 mm) is secured in place with the flexible table-mounted retractor arm, and the final position is confirmed by lateral fluoroscopy (Fig. 45-5). Use of a Kirschner wire (K-wire) before dilator placement is not recommended in the cervical spine. At this point, the microscope, loupe, or endoscope (preference of the senior author) is used to facilitate soft tissue dissection over the lamina-facet junction.

Before using the endoscope, it should be optimally focused, with contrast and brightness adjusted, orientation confirmed with a stationary object (an upright thumb is sufficient), white balanced, and "defogger" applied (Fig. 45-6). The tip of the endoscope should be placed as close as possible to the surgical field (~1 cm away) to improve visualization. Long-handle monopolar electrocautery and suction are used in all minimally invasive tubular systems. Caution should be used with the endoscope because monopolar electrocautery activity adjacent to the endoscope tip may create an "electrical arc" and burn the endoscope lens.

Under improved visual guidance, monopolar electrocautery is used to dissect the soft tissue away from the lamina-facet junction, by working from the rim of the dilation tube toward the center in a 360-degree fashion and staying on bone at all times to prevent inadvertent "plunging" into the spinal canal. A pituitary rongeur is used to remove cauterized soft tissue, and an up-angle curet is used to create a plane between the lamina or facet and the underlying ligamentum flavum. A hemilaminotomy is begun using 1- and 2-mm Kerrison rongeurs. This initial exposure is similar for MED, MEF, and microendoscopic diskectomy.

After the initial exposure, foraminal stenosis can be treated by MEF. The medial one third to one half of the facet is dissected free, and a pneumatic drill is used to thin out the inferior facet of the rostral vertebral body and the superior facet of the caudal vertebral body. A laminotomy "keyhole" is completed in conjunction with the medial facetectomy and exposure of the underlying ligamentum flavum (Fig. 45-7).[38] The

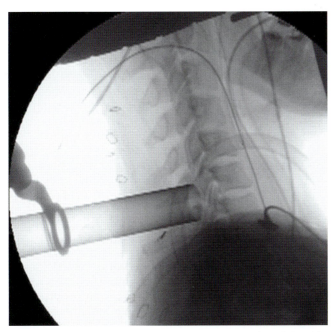

FIGURE 45-5 Fluoroscopic verification of correct placement of the table-mounted retractor after removal of the dilators.

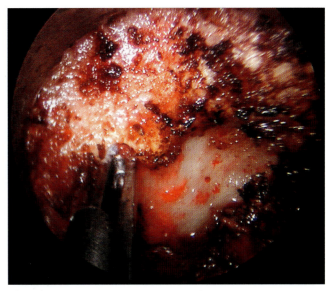

FIGURE 45-7 Intraoperative endoscopic photograph of bony decompression of the lamina-facet junction with a Kerrison-3 punch.

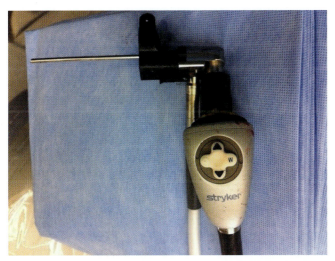

FIGURE 45-6 The microendoscopic system used for microendoscopic decompression for stenosis and foraminotomy (Stryker, Kalamazoo, Michigan).

residual bony fragments are removed with a Kerrison rongeur. The up-angle curet is placed in the cephalad and caudad portions of the foramen and is confirmed with lateral fluoroscopy to ensure that adequate bony decompression of the foramen is complete. The up-angle curet is then used to create a plane between the ligamentum flavum and the underlying thecal sac. A Kerrison rongeur is used to resect the ligament and any residual bone overlying the disk space until the dura and exiting nerve root (both cephalad and caudal surfaces) are visualized. A nerve hook is used to confirm appropriate foraminal decompression before obtaining hemostasis and irrigating the field with antibiotic solution.

Removal of one third to one half of the medial facet at a single level is rarely associated with future spinal instability. If a lateral disk herniation is present, it will be located ventral to the exiting nerve root. To improve access to the disk space, drilling 2 to 3 mm of the superomedial portion of the caudal pedicle improves visualization and mobility for decompression. A small micropituitary rongeur is used to extract the herniated disk fragment, with care taken to avoid traction injury to the nerve root or the thecal sac. A micronerve hook is placed inferior and ventral to the nerve root to gently free away any residual disk fragments for removal. Any disk fragments should be removed if easily accessible but "should not be chased" behind the thecal sac.

Minimally Invasive Microendoscopic Decompression for Cervical Stenosis

The MIS approach to MEDS uses the same initial approach as described previously. After final positioning of the tubular retractor on the lamina-facet junction, the soft tissue over the entire hemilamina is dissected free with monopolar electrocautery until the lateral limit of the lamina-facet junction is reached. Extra care is taken to *avoid violation of the facet capsule* because facetectomy is usually not necessary in MEDS for central canal stenosis. The entire hemilamina is drilled off from the spinous process to the facet, to leave a thin sheet of bone above the ligament. Drilling the superior half of the lamina should be performed with caution because no ligamentum flavum is present to protect the drill from the dura underneath.

An up-angle curet is used to dissect the inferior half of the residual lamina from the underlying ligamentum flavum, and the bony shelf is removed with a Kerrison number two rongeur. The ipsilateral ligamentum flavum is left intact as a protective layer over the thecal sac until final bony decompression is completed. Once the ipsilateral hemilaminectomy is complete, attention is turned

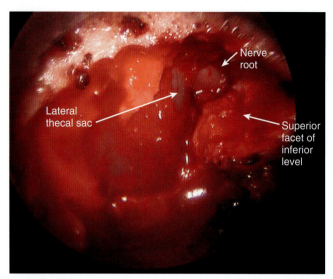

FIGURE 45-8 Intraoperative endoscopic photograph demonstrating decompression of central and foraminal stenosis, with visualization of the thecal sac and exiting nerve root.

toward the contralateral stenosis. The tubular retractor is repositioned toward the contralateral side with 45 degrees of medial angulation. A microcuret or Woodson instrument is used to create a safe plane of dissection on the contralateral side between the overlying spinous process and ligamentum flavum. The drill with a one-sided protective sleeve is used to "undercut" the bony spinous process and contralateral lamina over to the contralateral facet or foramen to ensure adequate central and foraminal decompression. Once the bilateral bony decompression is complete, the contralateral ligamentum flavum is dissected and removed with curets and Kerrison rongeurs.

The Kerrison number 3 rongeur is tilted at an upright angle to "undercut" the ligament underneath the spinous process and contralateral lamina until adequate decompression is confirmed by tactile use of a nerve hook or Woodson instrument. The tubular retractor is now repositioned toward the ipsilateral ligamentum flavum and is removed accordingly with curets and Kerrison rongeurs. With further decompression, the compressed thecal sac may "balloon" into the decompression site and potentially be injured by the Kerrison rongeur during resection, leading to a cerebrospinal fluid (CSF) leak. Continuous plane separation is ensured with intermittent use of the nerve hook or 0.5 by 0.5 inch cottonoid to protect the dura from the Kerrison rongeur. After bilateral decompression has been achieved, the thecal sac should reexpand and be pulsatile (Fig. 45-8). This process decompresses the cervical stenosis with minimal disruption of the "posterior tension band" or contralateral facet or paraspinal muscles. Closure proceeds in typical fashion.

Minimally Invasive Laminoplasty for Cervical Stenosis

The MIS approach to cervical laminoplasty does not incorporate the use of a tubular retractor system as in traditional MIS systems. However, the goal of laminoplasty

is to preserve the posterior tension band during spinal canal decompression, which is the ultimate goal of all MIS approaches.

The traditional approach to cervical laminoplasty starts with a midline incision over the surgical levels of interest. Subperiosteal dissection is completed medial to the lamina-facet junction bilaterally, and the interspinous ligaments are cut above and below the surgical levels. A high-speed drill is used to create a "trough" medial to the lamina-facet junction approximately 10 mm wide, through the outer cortical lamina, cancellous bone, and inner cortical lamina until the ligamentum flavum is exposed on the side ipsilateral to the patient's clinical symptoms.

Attention is now turned toward creating a similar trough on the contralateral side, medial to the lamina-facet junction. However, the trough is not completely drilled through the inner bony cortical lamina, and a residual thin shelf of bone is left untouched. The resulting bony complex should have intact spinous processes and a single side of bony residual lamina. A nerve hook is used to create a safe plane in the trough between the ligament and the underlying dura. A Kerrison number one rongeur is used to deepen the trough through the ligament until the surgical levels are "released" from their ipsilateral lamina-facet junction.

Two caulkers are attached to the spinous processes of the bony complex and are levered toward the side of residual bony laminar shelf while using a Penfield number 1 or Woodson instrument to resect adhesions and ligamentum flavum between the undersurface of the lamina and the thecal sac. Eventually a "greenstick fracture" of the bony residual lamina shelf occurs, completing the opening and decompression of the underlying thecal sac. After adequate decompression and hemostasis are achieved, the bony complex is returned to its original anatomic position with a bony spacer placed within the trough that increases the spinal canal diameter and treats the cervical stenosis.

Each laminar level is reattached to its corresponding lateral mass with a 2-mm cervical miniplate and screw. An assistant is necessary to hold the cervical plate in place with a bayonet while the surgeon carefully secures the screw without accidentally plunging the screwdriver into the interlaminar space or the surgically created trough. After successful completion of the surgical procedure, most of the bony and ligamentous support structures are left intact, and the spinal canal is appropriately decompressed. Closure proceeds in typical fashion.

Minimally Invasive Surgical Approach for Lateral Mass Screws

To date, evidence is insufficient to support or discourage the use of MIS lateral screw placement for cervical spine fusion. This technique has not yet been popularized because of the technical difficulties of the surgical procedure, but it has been performed with success. In some procedures for decompression or spinal tumors, the authors have employed the MIS approach for cervical lateral mass screws for posterior spinal fusion.

The initial approach and setup are similar to those for MEDS except the patient is placed prone on a Jackson table or chest rolls. A paramedian incision is made 1.5 cm off the midline as before, with sequential dilation down to the facet joint of the surgical level of interest. Monopolar cautery is used to clean the soft tissue away from the facet joint and lateral masses of the cephalad and caudad vertebral bodies to be fused.

The start point for the lateral mass is 1 mm inferomedial to the center of the lateral mass (as defined by the mediolateral borders of the lateral mass and superoinferior facets above and below). A hand drill is directed 30 degrees lateral and 30 degrees superior in the direction of the superior facet joint, and drilling is performed down to the measured anteroposterior length of the lateral mass (~12 to 14 mm). The hole is probed to evaluate for a consistent bony floor and all four walls before "tapping" the hole, followed by reprobing. This is performed at the adjacent level for instrumentation, and the screws are placed in an angulation similar to that described for the drill.

A rod is measured and cut to fit the screws and is secured into place with set screw caps. The drill is then used for arthrodesis of the available lateral mass, lamina, and facet joint to enhance bony fusion. Irrigation and hemostasis are completed, followed by fascia and skin closure. Attention is then directed to the contralateral side, and the procedure is performed in similar fashion as described earlier. The end result comprises two paramedian incisions 1.5 cm from the midline, approximately 2 cm in length, with placement of cervical lateral mass screws and arthrodesis while maintaining normal anatomic structures.

Minimally Invasive Surgical Approach for Cervical Tumors

The initial setup and positioning for MIS approach for cervical tumors are similar to those for MED and MEF except the patient is placed prone on chest rolls or on an open Jackson table. The midline and paramedian lines are marked with fluoroscopy as described earlier. The skin and fascia are incised, followed by blunt muscle dissection and placement of sequential tube dilators until the MAST Quadrant (Medtronic, Minneapolis, Minn.) retractor system is secured in place. The remainder of the decompression approach is performed similar to MEDS for cervical stenosis.

Once hemostasis is achieved, the tumor is localized and confirmed with preoperative imaging, intraoperative fluoroscopy anatomic landmarks, ultrasound, nerve stimulation, or intraoperative MRI. If the tumor is extradural, the surgical approach should reveal the mass with ease for resection. If the mass is intradural and extramedullary, a number 15 blade scalpel is used to make a midline incision over the dura, and the dura is tacked laterally with 4-0 Nurolon (Ethicon, Somerville, N.J.) sutures, thus revealing the underlying mass for resection.

If manipulation of the spinal cord is necessary for tumor exposure, resection of the dentate ligaments will provide some additional mobility for retraction. If the tumor is intradural and intramedullary, the dura should be opened as described earlier, and the margins of the tumor should be identified clearly with the microscope or endoscope, ultrasound, nerve stimulation, or intraoperative MRI. Bipolar cautery is used to separate a plane gently between the tumor and normal spinal cord parenchyma, and the tumor is incised with microscissors. The tumor is eventually resected in circumferential fashion, and hemostasis is achieved with bipolar cautery and Gelfoam (Pfizer, New York, N.Y.). Irrigation is performed after tumor resection, the dura is reapproximated with a running 4-0 Nurolon stitch, and the dural incision is covered with fibrin glue (DuraSeal [Covidien, Mansfield, Mass.]) or TISSEEL (Baxter Healthcare, Westlake Village, Calif.). The remainder of the fascia and skin is closed in typical fashion.

Wound Closure and Postoperative Care

After completion of the cervical decompression, meticulous hemostasis is achieved with bipolar cautery, Gelfoam soaked in thrombin, or Surgifoam (Ethicon). The muscles and fascia are injected with local anesthesia for postoperative pain control, and the surgical field is then irrigated with copious amounts of antibiotic solution. Fascial closure is completed with 1-0 or 2-0 polyglactin 910 (Vicryl, Ethicon) sutures, and the subcutaneous layer closed with inverted Vicryl 3-0 sutures. The superficial dermal layer is closed with a running subcutaneous nonabsorbable suture and a skin adhesive (Dermabond, Ethicon) to complete the surgical procedure. An external cervical orthosis is not necessary, and the patient may be discharged from the postanesthesia care unit later the same day, with follow-up in clinic in 10 to 14 days.

Complications

Regardless of the surgical approach (MIS versus traditional open), the surgeon must be comfortable with the surgical anatomy and potential complications. Working through a narrow access tube may decrease the disruption of normal anatomic structures, but it also limits the surgeon's viewpoint and surrounding anatomy.[39] The literature has shown minimally invasive posterior cervical foraminotomy to be a safe procedure associated with minimal complications (1% to 15%), most commonly wound infection and dural tear.[17,21,22,39,40,41] Since incorporating microendoscopic techniques, the senior author has no postoperative infections to date. This result has been attributed to decreased surgical time and hospital stay, decreased blood loss, smaller incisions, and minimal postoperative "surgical dead space" for bacteria to flourish.[21] The durotomy rate has dropped from 8% in the initial series of patients to currently approximately 1% per surgical procedure.

Unintentional durotomies are difficult to repair primarily through an MIS surgical tube and are best treated with indirect techniques. The authors advocate placing a water-insoluble layer on top of the dural defect (muscle, fat, fascia, or a dural substitute) and coating with a dural sealant (fibrin glue or TISSEEL). The patient is placed on flat bed rest for 24 hours for small durotomies, but larger defects may require CSF diversion with a lumbar drain for a few days. The combination of a small incision and lack of surgical dead space has reduced clinically significant pseudomeningoceles or CSF leaks to negligible after a minimally invasive approach.

Neurologic complications that may occur include direct injury to the nerve within the foramen or the spinal cord during decompression procedures in both MIS and open approaches. Unique to MIS approaches is the potential injury with the use of a K-wire during localization. Initial placement should be localized with fluoroscopy, but inattention can easily lead to misplacement of the K-wire medial to the facet into the interlaminar space (spinal cord injury) or lateral to the facet (vertebral artery injury). The K-wire must be controlled at all times and removed immediately after placement of the initial tubular dilator to minimize the potential migration of the K-wire into a "danger zone."

For these reasons, the senior author now advocates blunt muscle dissection with Metzenbaum scissors until the facet joint is visualized and the dilator tube is placed directly over the surgical facet level without ambiguity. This technique eliminates any potential injury caused by the K-wire. With proper knowledge of surgical anatomy and attention to detail, the MIS approach to the cervical spine can be completed safely and quickly, with minimal complications.

Results

MIS techniques have gained popularity since 2000 with similar to improved outcomes when compared with traditional open surgical approaches.[21,42] The minimally invasive, muscle-dilating, and tissue-sparing approach has been successfully applied not only to cervical approaches but also to thoracic and lumbar disorders. Review of outcomes of the authors' patients after MED/MEF for central or foraminal stenosis demonstrates that patients who underwent MIS procedures had significant decreases in operative time, estimated blood loss, hospital stay, and postoperative narcotic requirement.[21]

When comparing the conventional open decompression group with the sitting MEF group, the authors noted a decrease in overall operative time (171 to 115 minutes), a decrease in estimated blood loss (246 to 138 mL), a shorter hospital stay (68 to 8.1 hours), and lower postoperative narcotic morphine equivalent requirements (40 to 9 Eq).[17] When comparing postoperative clinical outcomes, MIS cervical spine surgery has similar to improved scores on the visual analog pain scale (VAS), Short Form-36, and Prolo Scale scores. The authors' results have since been reproduced by other investigators, with similar results.

Conclusions

MIS approaches are not only increasing in popularity but also undergoing rapid evolution in techniques and application for myriad disorders. Benefits of these approaches include a decrease in surgical trauma, preservation of anatomic structures, early functional recovery, excellent cosmesis, and improved clinical outcomes. The future of MIS techniques is bright as new ideas are implemented to incorporate spinal fusion, deformity correction, and tumor resection. Understanding the fundamentals of surgical anatomy and MIS techniques is essential for every practicing and future spine surgeon.

REFERENCES

1. Aldrich F: Posterolateral microdisectomy for cervical monoradiculopathy caused by posterolateral soft cervical disc sequestration, *J Neurosurg* 72:370–377, 1990.
2. Crandall PH, Batzdorf U: Cervical spondylotic myelopathy, *J Neurosurg* 25:57–66, 1966.
3. Fessler RG, O'Toole JE, Eichholz KM, Perez-Cruet MJ: The development of minimally invasive spine surgery, *Neurosurg Clin North Am* 17:401–409, 2006.
4. Fong S, Duplessis S: Minimally invasive lateral mass plating in the treatment of posterior cervical trauma: surgical technique, *J Spinal Disord Tech* 18:224–228, 2005.
5. Gala VC, O'Toole JE, Voyadzis JM, Fessler RG: Posterior minimally invasive approaches for the cervical spine, *Orthop Clin North Am* 38:339–349, 2007. abstract v.
6. Henderson CM, Hennessy RG, Shuey HM Jr, Shackelford EG: Posterior-lateral foraminotomy as an exclusive operative technique for cervical radiculopathy: a review of 846 consecutively operated cases, *Neurosurgery* 13:504–512, 1983.
7. Lawton CD, Smith ZA, Barnawi A, Fessler RG: The surgical technique of minimally invasive transforaminal lumbar interbody fusion, *J Neurosurg Sci* 55:259–264, 2011.
8. Mannion RJ, Nowitzke AM, Efendy J, Wood MJ: Safety and efficacy of intradural extramedullary spinal tumor removal using a minimally invasive approach, *Neurosurgery* 68:208–216, 2011. discussion 216.
9. O'Toole JE, Eichholz KM, Fessler RG: Minimally invasive approaches to vertebral column and spinal cord tumors, *Neurosurg Clin North Am* 17:491–506, 2006.
10. Ogden AT, Fessler RG: Minimally invasive resection of intramedullary ependymoma: case report, *Neurosurgery* 65:E1203–E1204, 2009. discussion E1204.
11. Santiago P, Fessler RG: Minimally invasive surgery for the management of cervical spondylosis, *Neurosurgery* 60:S160–S165, 2007.
12. Tredway TL, Santiago P, Hrubes MR, et al.: Minimally invasive resection of intradural-extramedullary spinal neoplasms, *Neurosurgery* 58:ONS52–ONS58, 2006. discussion ONS52–58.
13. Hilibrand AS, Robbins M: Adjacent segment degeneration and adjacent segment disease: the consequences of spinal fusion? *Spine J* 4:190S–194S, 2004.
14. Ishihara H, Kanamori M, Kawaguchi Y, et al.: Adjacent segment disease after anterior cervical interbody fusion, *Spine J* 4:624–628, 2004.
15. Burke TG, Caputy A: Microendoscopic posterior cervical foraminotomy: a cadaveric model and clinical application for cervical radiculopathy, *J Neurosurg* 93:126–129, 2000.
16. Coric D, Adamson T: Minimally invasive cervical microendoscopic laminoforaminotomy, *Neurosurg Focus* 25:E2, 2008.
17. Fessler RG, Khoo LT: Minimally invasive cervical microendoscopic foraminotomy: an initial clinical experience, *Neurosurgery* 51:S37–S45, 2002.
18. DELETED IN PROOFS.
19. DELETED IN PROOFS.
20. DELETED IN PROOFS.
21. Lawton CD, Smith ZA, Lam SK, et al.: Clinical outcomes of microendoscopic foraminotomy and decompression in the cervical spine, *World Neurosurg* 81:422–427, 2014.
22. O'Toole JE, Sheikh H, Eichholz KM, et al.: Endoscopic posterior cervical foraminotomy and discectomy, *Neurosurg Clin North Am* 17:411–422, 2006.

23. DELETED IN PROOFS.
24. DELETED IN PROOFS.
25. DELETED IN PROOFS.
26. DELETED IN PROOFS.
27. Benglis DM, Guest JD, Wang MY: Clinical feasibility of minimally invasive cervical laminoplasty, *Neurosurg Focus* 25:E3, 2008.
28. Boehm H, Greiner-Perth R, El-Saghir H, Allam Y: A new minimally invasive posterior approach for the treatment of cervical radiculopathy and myelopathy: surgical technique and preliminary results, *Eur Spine J* 12:268–273, 2003.
29. Kumar VG, Rea GL, Mervis LJ, McGregor JM: Cervical spondylotic myelopathy: functional and radiographic long-term outcome after laminectomy and posterior fusion, *Neurosurgery* 44:771–777, 1999. discussion 777–778.
30. Ratliff JK, Cooper PR: Cervical laminoplasty: a critical review, *J Neurosurg* 98:230–238, 2003.
31. Wang MY, Shah S, Green BA: Clinical outcomes following cervical laminoplasty for 204 patients with cervical spondylotic myelopathy, *Surg Neurol* 62:487–492, 2004. discussion 492–493.
32. Yabuki S, Kikuchi S: Endoscopic surgery for cervical myelopathy due to calcification of the ligamentum flavum, *J Spinal Disord Tech* 21:518–523, 2008.
33. Hosono N, Yonenobu K, Ono K: Neck and shoulder pain after laminoplasty: a noticeable complication, *Spine (Phila Pa 1976)* 21:1969–1973, 1996.
34. Hilton DL Jr: Minimally invasive tubular access for posterior cervical foraminotomy with three-dimensional microscopic visualization and localization with anterior/posterior imaging, *Spine J* 7:154–158, 2007.
35. Frykholm R: Deformities of dural pouches and strictures of dural sheaths in the cervical region producing nerve-root compression; a contribution to the etiology and operative treatment of brachial neuralgia, *J Neurosurg* 4:403–413, 1947.
36. Albert TJ, Vacarro A: Postlaminectomy kyphosis, *Spine (Phila Pa 1976)* 23:2738–2745, 1998.
37. Kaptain GJ, Simmons NE, Replogle RE, Pobereskin L: Incidence and outcome of kyphotic deformity following laminectomy for cervical spondylotic myelopathy, *J Neurosurg* 93:199–204, 2000.
38. Caglar YS, Bozkurt M, Kahilogullari G, et al.: Keyhole approach for posterior cervical discectomy: experience on 84 patients, *Minim Invasive Neurosurg* 50:7–11, 2007.
39. Perez-Cruet MJ, Fessler RG, Perin NI: Review: complications of minimally invasive spinal surgery, *Neurosurgery* 51:S26–S36, 2002.
40. Holly LT, Moftakhar P, Khoo LT, et al.: Minimally invasive 2-level posterior cervical foraminotomy: preliminary clinical results, *J Spinal Disord Tech* 20:20–24, 2007.
41. O'Toole JE, Eichholz KM, Fessler RG: Surgical site infection rates after minimally invasive spinal surgery, *J Neurosurg Spine* 11:471–476, 2009.
42. Thongtrangan I, Le H, Park J, Kim DH: Minimally invasive spinal surgery: a historical perspective, *Neurosurg Focus* 16:E13, 2004.

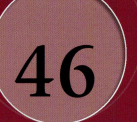

46 Image-Guided Navigation for Cervical Spine Surgery

Iain H. Kalfas

CHAPTER PREVIEW

Chapter Synopsis	Image-guided spinal navigation is a computer-based surgical technology designed to improve intraoperative orientation to the nonvisualized anatomy during both conventional and minimally invasive spinal procedures. This chapter covers the principles of image-guided spinal navigation, current types of navigation systems, and the concept and process of registration. Its clinical application, specifically to C1-C2 transarticular screw fixation, C1-C2 segmental screw fixation, and transoral surgery, is briefly discussed as well.
Important Points	The rate of disruption of the pedicle cortex with traditional techniques ranges from 15% to 31% in the reported literature.
	Image-guided spinal navigation facilitates surgical accuracy by matching spinal image data with its corresponding intraoperative anatomy and is based on the principle that both the image data and the surgical anatomy represent three-dimensional coordinate systems.
	Several classes of navigation systems currently exist, including (1) computed tomography (CT)–based navigation, (2) fluoroscopic navigation, (3) intraoperative isocentric fluoroscopic navigation, and (4) intraoperative CT navigation.
	Registration is the process through which a spatial relationship between the image data and the surgical anatomy is achieved.
Clinical and Surgical Pearls	Image-guided spinal navigation provides the ability to manipulate multiplanar CT or fluoroscopic images to gain a greater degree of orientation of the surgical anatomy.
	Compared with conventional intraoperative imaging, it may eliminate or significantly reduce radiation exposure to the surgical team.
	Passive reflectors attached to surgical instrumentation allow for intraoperative tracking by the workstation and provide real-time feedback.
Clinical and Surgical Pitfalls	Image-guided spinal navigation does not replace the need for thorough preoperative planning.
	Image-guided spinal navigation does not replace the need for a thorough understanding of the spinal anatomy.
	Image-guided spinal navigation does not replace the need for a thorough understanding of correct surgical technique.

The management of spinal disorders has been greatly influenced by the development and use of screw-based fixation devices. Accurate placement of these screws requires the spinal surgeon to have a precise orientation to that part of the spinal anatomy that is not exposed in the surgical field. Although conventional intraoperative imaging techniques, such as fluoroscopy, have proven useful, they are limited in that they provide only two-dimensional imaging of a complex three-dimensional structure. Consequently, the surgeon is required to extrapolate the third dimension based on an interpretation of the images and knowledge of the pertinent anatomy. This situation can result in varying degrees of error when placing screws into that part of the spinal column that is not visualized in the surgical field.

Several studies have shown the unreliability of routine radiography in guiding the appropriate trajectory for placement of pedicle screws in the lumbosacral spine. The rate of disruption of the pedicle cortex by an inserted screw ranges from 15% to 31% in these studies.[1-4] The disadvantage of these conventional radiographic techniques for orienting the spinal surgeon to unexposed spinal anatomy is that they display, at most, only two planar images. Although the lateral view can be relatively easy to assess, the anteroposterior (AP) or oblique view can be difficult to interpret. For most screw fixation procedures, the position of the screw in the axial plane is most important. This plane best demonstrates the position of the screw relative to the neural canal. Conventional intraoperative imaging cannot provide this view.

An additional concern of conventional intraoperative imaging is the radiation exposure experienced by the surgical team and the patient. Rampersaud and colleagues demonstrated that, compared with other orthopedic procedures using intraoperative fluoroscopy, spinal procedures potentially result in a 10- to 12-fold increase in radiation exposure to the surgical team because of such factors as backscatter radiation and the increased energy levels needed to image the lumbar spine. These conditions create a potentially significant hazard to those individuals who perform a high volume of complex spinal surgery.[5]

Computer-assisted spinal surgery, or image-guided spinal navigation, is a computer-based surgical technology designed to improve intraoperative orientation to the nonvisualized anatomy during complex spinal procedures.[6,7] It provides the spinal surgeon with the ability to manipulate multiplanar computed tomography (CT) or fluoroscopy images during the procedure to gain a greater degree of orientation to the surgical anatomy and thereby optimize the precision and accuracy of the surgery. Compared with conventional intraoperative imaging, image-guided spinal navigation eliminates or significantly reduces radiation exposure to the surgical team.

Principles of Image-Guided Spinal Navigation

Image-guided spinal navigation facilitates surgical accuracy by matching spinal image data with its corresponding intraoperative anatomy. It is based on the principle that both the image data and the surgical anatomy represent three-dimensional coordinate systems. Each point in the image data set and in the surgical field has a location in space defined by a specific x, y, and z cartesian coordinate. Using defined mathematical algorithms, a specific point in the image data set can be "matched" with its corresponding point in the surgical field. After matching a limited number of these points together, any point in the surgical field can then be selected and its corresponding point in the images displayed in several planes, to give the surgeon greater orientation to the pertinent surgical anatomy.

Types of Navigational Systems

Currently, four general options are available for the application of image-guided spinal navigation. *CT-based navigation* uses CT images of the patient acquired preoperatively. Conventional intraoperative imaging is not necessary. During navigation the surgeon is presented with reformatted CT images in multiple planes with the selected screw entry point and trajectory superimposed on the images (Fig. 46-1). This information updates in real time as adjustments are made to the selected trajectory in the surgical field.

Fluoroscopic navigation uses a standard AP and lateral image of the spinal anatomy acquired in the immediate pre-operative period. No additional intraoperative imaging is needed. The selected trajectory information is superimposed on the AP and lateral images on the workstation screen (Fig. 46-2). Unlike with CT-based navigation, no axial image is available. The advantage of fluoroscopic navigation is that it uses less radiation than conventional fluoroscopy and does not require a preoperative CT scan, as does CT-based navigation. The disadvantage compared with CT-based navigation is that it does not provide an image in the axial plane.

Intraoperative isocentric fluoroscopic navigation is a variation of standard fluoroscopic navigation. Images are acquired in the immediate preoperative period by rotating the specialized C-arm in a 180-degree arc around the patient. These images can then be reformatted to provide images in the axial and sagittal planes similar to CT-based navigation but without the need to acquire a preoperative CT scan. Although the images are not of the same quality as a standard CT image set, they are adequate for navigation in most cases.

Intraoperative CT navigation is the most recent advance in computer-assisted surgery. It consists of a portable CT scanner that uses flat panel detector technology to improve intraoperative image acquisition and quality. The scanner has a configuration similar to that of a standard C-arm fluoroscope. In addition to being able to acquire standard AP and lateral images, its C-arm configuration can be "closed" to encircle the patient completely. This allows the flat panel detector to be swept in a 360-degree arc around the patient and significantly improves the acquired image quality. Images can be acquired preoperatively or intraoperatively and are reformatted into multiplanar views. The advantage over CT-based navigation is the option of intraoperative reimaging after decompression or instrumentation. The reformatted images are similar in quality to conventional CT imaging and are superior to isocentric C-arm imaging. The use of automated registration makes this form of computer-assisted spinal surgery readily applicable to minimally invasive surgery.

The common components of most navigation systems include an image-processing computer workstation interfaced with a two-camera optical localizer (Fig. 46-3). When positioned during surgery, the optical localizer emits infrared light toward the operative field. A

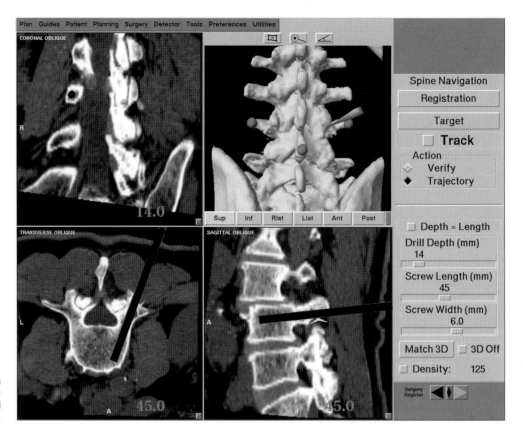

FIGURE 46-1 Workstation screen demonstrating navigation for an L3 pedicle screw using a computed tomography–based navigation system.

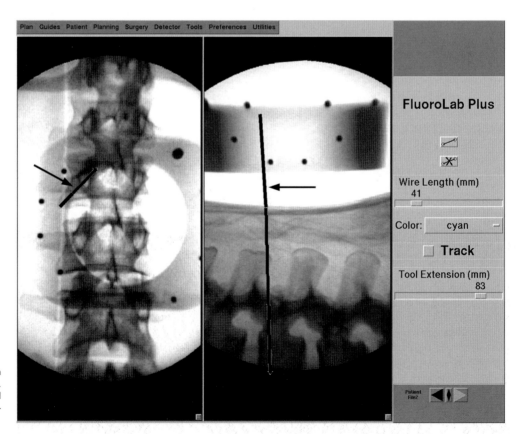

FIGURE 46-2 Workstation screen of a fluoroscopic navigational system. Standard anteroposterior and lateral views are provided with superimposed trajectory lines (*arrows*).

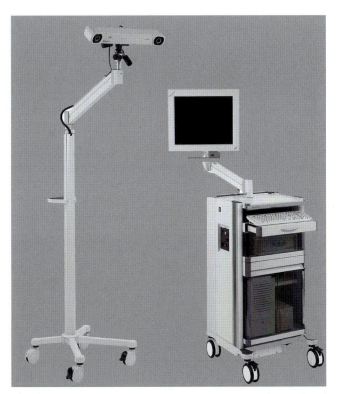

FIGURE 46-3   Image-guided navigational workstation with an infrared camera localizer system.

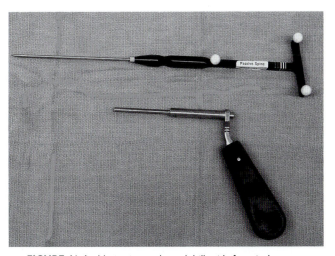

FIGURE 46-4   Navigation probe and drill guide for spinal surgery.

handheld navigational probe mounted with a fixed array of passive reflective spheres serves as the link between the surgeon and the computer workstation (Fig. 46-4). Passive reflectors can also be attached to standard surgical instruments. The spacing and positioning of the passive reflectors on each navigational probe or customized trackable surgical instrument are known by the computer workstation. The infrared light that is transmitted toward the operative field is reflected back to the optical localizer by the passive reflectors. This information is relayed to the computer workstation, which can then calculate the precise location of the instrument tip in the surgical field,

as well as the location of the anatomic point on which the instrument tip is resting.

Registration

Establishing a spatial relationship between the image data and the surgical anatomy is achieved through a process termed *registration*. Three different registration techniques can be used for spinal navigation: paired point registration, surface matching, and automated registration. Each registration technique creates a virtual link between the image data and the surgical anatomy.

Paired point registration involves preoperatively selecting a series of discrete anatomic points in a CT data set that will be easily identified in the surgical field after exposure. These points typically are the tip of a spinous or transverse process or the apex of a facet joint. When the surgical field is adequately exposed, one of the points in the CT image set is selected. The tip of the navigation probe is then placed on the corresponding point in the surgical field, and the reflective spheres on the probe handle are aimed toward the camera. Infrared light from the camera is reflected from the spheres toward the camera. This information is transferred to the computer workstation, which does the calculations to determine the spatial position of the probe's tip and the anatomic structure it is touching. This process effectively links the point selected in the image data with the point selected in the surgical field. When a minimum of three such points are registered, the probe can be placed on any other point in the surgical field and the corresponding point in the image data set will be identified on the computer workstation.[8]

Surface matching registration involves selecting multiple, random (nondiscrete) points on the exposed surface of the spine in the surgical field. This technique does not require prior selection of points in the image set, although several discrete points in both the image data set and the surgical field are typically required to improve the accuracy of surface mapping. The positional information of these points is transferred to the workstation, and a topographic map of the selected anatomy is created and "matched" with the patient's image set.[9]

Automated registration is performed when fluoroscopic navigation, isocentric fluoroscopic navigation, or intraoperative CT imaging systems are used. This technique involves attachment of a reference frame on the exposed spinal anatomy or, with lumbar surgery, the iliac crest. A second reference frame is attached to the CT imaging scanner or fluoroscope. As the images are acquired, the two reference frames allow for registration of the spinal anatomy to be performed automatically without the need for a surgeon's input. When the images are acquired, the CT scanner or fluoroscope can then be removed, and real-time navigation of up to five separate spinal levels can be performed.[10]

Following accurate registration, the navigation probe can be positioned on any surface point in the surgical field. As the probe is tracked by the camera, the computer workstation relates the corresponding image data through the selected anatomic point. When CT-based navigation is used, three separate reformatted CT images centered on the corresponding point in the image data set are displayed. These images allow the surgeon to select the appropriate screw trajectory and entry point in the sagittal, coronal, and axial planes. The appropriate screw length and diameter can also be selected. As the surgeon moves the probe into different positions and angles, the image data updates in real-time to demonstrate the newly selected entry point and trajectory. If fluoroscopic navigation is used, the trajectory line will be superimposed on the preoperatively acquired AP and lateral fluoroscopic images on the workstation monitor.

Clinical Applications

Image-guided spinal navigation was initially evaluated by assessing its accuracy when used to place pedicle screws placed into the thoracic and lumbosacral spines of cadaver specimens.[7] The first study evaluating navigational accuracy in the clinical setting was performed in a series of 30 patients undergoing lumbar pedicle screw fixation. Accuracy of screw insertion was documented by plain film radiography and thin-section CT imaging of the instrumented levels. Satisfactory screw placement was noted for 149 of 150 inserted screws.[6]

Several additional studies also demonstrated the improved accuracy of pedicle screw insertion with the assistance of image-guided navigation.[1,11-13] These studies all demonstrated a statistically significant improvement in the accuracy of pedicle screw placement in the navigation-assisted cohort.

Other applications of image-guided spinal navigation soon developed, directed by the complexity of the procedure and, specifically, by the need to "visualize" the unexposed spinal anatomy. In addition to pedicle screw insertion, other applications in the thoracic and lumbosacral regions evolved including the insertion of iliac wing screws, decompression of spinal metastasis, and anterior thoracolumbar decompression and fixation.[14-16]

The application of this technology to the cervical spine is driven by several surgical challenges. Specifically, these challenges include optimizing the accuracy of C1-C2 transarticular and segmental screw fixation, transoral decompression, corpectomy, and anterior odontoid screw fixation.[17-20] For each of these procedures, image-guided navigation can be used with or without standard intraoperative imaging techniques (i.e., fluoroscopy). With CT-based navigation, it can also be used for preoperative planning because of the capability of multiplanar image manipulation on the navigational workstation.

C1-C2 Transarticular Screw Fixation

This procedure involves the insertion of a screw through the pars interarticularis of C2, across the facet joint, and into the lateral mass of C1. The risks of screw insertion include injury to the vertebral artery if the screw is placed too laterally or ventrally, injury to the spinal cord if the screw is placed too medially, and failure to engage the lateral mass of C1 if the screw trajectory is too ventral. The insertion of a screw on either side may be contraindicated if the pars interarticularis of C2 is too narrow. The procedure is typically performed bilaterally, using fluoroscopic guidance.

The selection of the appropriate screw entry site and trajectory requires a thorough understanding of the atlantoaxial anatomy. Although fluoroscopy provides real-time imaging of the relevant spinal anatomy, the views generated represent only two-dimensional images of a complex three-dimensional anatomic region. Manipulation of the fluoroscopic unit can reduce this problem, but these maneuvers can be cumbersome and time-consuming.

Although CT-based navigation is the most common type of navigational technology applied to this procedure, fluoroscopic, isocentric fluoroscopic, and intraoperative CT navigation can also be used. The CT-based navigation technique involves acquiring a preoperative CT scan that extends from the lower occipital region to C3. The image data are transferred to the computer workstation and can be used to create a preoperative screw trajectory plan. A proposed entry point and target can be selected at the C2 and C1 levels, respectively. The image data set can then be manipulated in multiple planes between these two points to demonstrate the position of a screw placed along the selected trajectory. In addition to a sagittal image that demonstrates the same information provided by lateral fluoroscopy, two other images are presented. One of the images lies perpendicular to the sagittal image along the selected trajectory. It represents an orthogonal view that lies approximately midway between the coronal and axial planes through the spine. This view provides a second image of the selected trajectory.

A third view demonstrates an image oriented perpendicular to the long axis of the probe and therefore the selected trajectory. A cursor superimposed on this image can show the position of the screw tip along the selected trajectory at millimetric increments. By scrolling through this image, the proposed position of the screw along the selected trajectory can be assessed along its entire path. Although this planning technique does not ensure safe screw placement intraoperatively, it can preoperatively alert the surgeon to avoid screw placement in patients with insufficient anatomy and to select an alternate approach.

Intraoperatively, the patient is positioned, and the posterior C1-C2 complex is exposed. A cable and bone graft stabilization procedure at the C1-C2 level is performed before navigation and screw insertion. Performing this step first minimizes any independent motion between C1 and C2 during navigation and makes tap and screw insertion easier. If a reference frame is used, it is typically attached to the spinous process of C2.

Following placement of the graft and cable, three to five registration points are selected at the C2 level. It is not necessary to include registration points at C1. Although the spatial relationship of C1 and C2 may change between the preoperative scanned position and the intraoperative position, the ability of image-guided navigation to facilitate accurate screw placement is not significantly affected. The lateral mass of C1 is a relatively large target. It can be easily accessed by an inserted screw provided atlantoaxial alignment is satisfactory. The technical difficulty of this procedure is the accurate passage of the screw through the narrow pars interarticularis of C2. Although the relative position of C1 and C2 in both the preoperative image set and in the surgical field is important, it is not critical enough to affect navigational accuracy.

Two separate stab incisions are made on either side of the midline at the C7-T1 level. A drill guide is placed through one of the stab incisions and is passed through the paravertebral musculature and into the operative field. A small divot is drilled at the proposed entry site to provide for secure placement of the drill guide. The registration process is performed at the C2 level, and its accuracy is confirmed using the verification step. The probe is passed through the drill guide. As its position is adjusted in the surgical field, the images on the workstation screen adjust accordingly to show the corresponding trajectory in two separate planes and the projected location of the screw tip in the third plane. Orientation to the correct screw position can be assessed rapidly and accurately (Fig. 46-5). Any errors in trajectory or entry point selection can be determined and corrected by adjusting the position of the probe and the drill guide through which it passes. When the correct screw insertion parameters have been selected, the probe is removed from the drill guide, and a drill is inserted. A hole is drilled along the selected trajectory, it is tapped, and the appropriate length screw is inserted. The process is repeated on the opposite side.

Even though image-guided navigation does not guarantee accurate screw placement, it does provide the surgeon with a greater degree of anatomic information than fluoroscopy alone. Conventional fluoroscopy can also be used to provide an additional check on the accuracy of a selected screw trajectory, but the radiation exposure time is far less with navigation compared with using fluoroscopy alone.

C1-C2 Segmental Screw Fixation

As an alternative to transarticular screw fixation, segmental fixation of C1 and C2 can be used for managing atlantoaxial instability.[21] The procedure involves placing a screw into each of the two lateral masses of C1 and two screws through each of the pedicles of C2. The polyaxial screw heads on each side are then connected with rods. Although this approach potentially reduces the risk of injury to the vertebral artery during screw insertion, it does not completely eliminate the risk of injury. As with the transarticular technique, precise anatomic orientation is required to avoid arterial or neural injury. Image-guided navigation can supplement intraoperative fluoroscopy and provide an added degree of orientation for accurate screw insertion.

As with the transarticular screw fixation technique, a preoperative CT scan is obtained. The posterior C1-C2 spine is exposed, and a wire and cable fixation procedure is performed. Registration is performed at C1 for placement of the C1 lateral mass screws. The three registration points typically used at are the midline posterior tubercle and the bilateral landmarks located at the junction of the pedicle of C1 with its lateral mass. Once registered, the correct trajectory into the lateral masses can be displayed on the workstation screen, and the screws can be inserted (Fig. 46-6).

To navigate the placement of screws into the pars and pedicle of C2, the registration points used are the C2 spinous process and the two lateral margins of the C2-C3 facet. The entry point for the screw is located more laterally and the trajectory is aimed more medially than for a transarticular screw. The navigation probe is placed through a drill guide onto this entry point, and the selected trajectory is displayed on the workstation screen. When the correct entry point and trajectory have been selected, the probe is removed, a drill is inserted, and the pilot hole is drilled (Fig. 46-7). The process

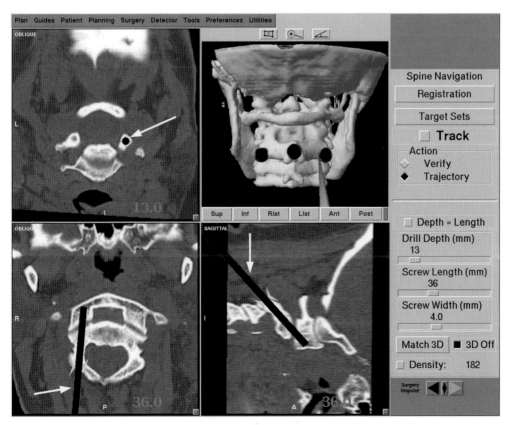

FIGURE 46-5 Workstation screen demonstrating a trajectory for insertion of a C1-C2 transarticular screw. The *lower right screen* shows the trajectory in the sagittal plane. The *lower left screen* represents an orthogonal plane lying between the axial and coronal planes. It conveys the mediolateral trajectory. The *upper left screen* represents a plane that is perpendicular to the two other images. It demonstrates the location of the screw tip inserted along the selected trajectory at the indicated depth. (Screw trajectory and tip location are highlighted by *arrows*.)

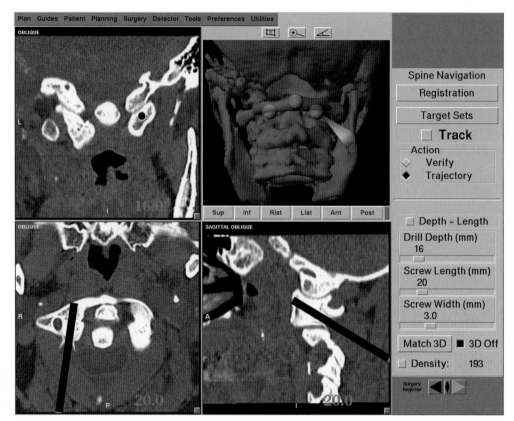

FIGURE 46-6   Workstation screen demonstrating navigational information for placement of a screw into the lateral mass of C1.

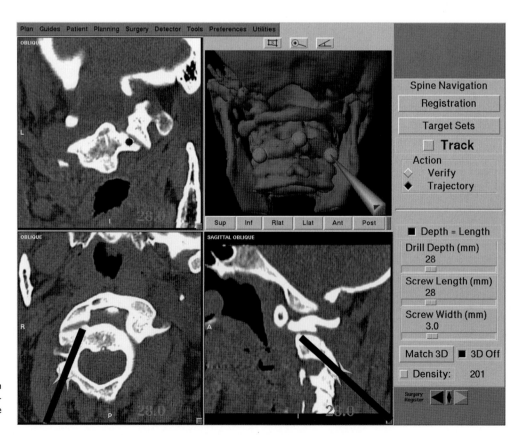

FIGURE 46-7   Workstation screen demonstrating navigational information for placement of a screw into the pedicle of C2.

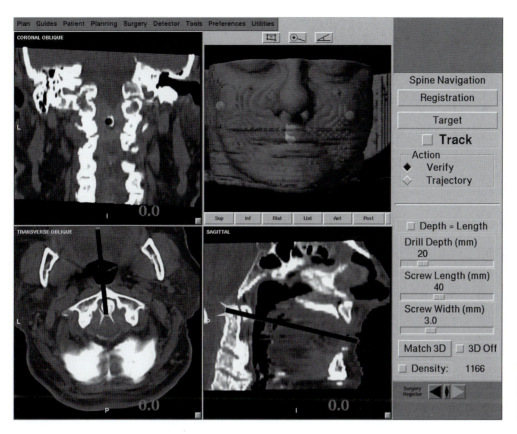

FIGURE 46-8 Workstation screen demonstrating navigational information during transoral decompression. (Probe tip location and trajectory are highlighted by *arrows*.)

is then repeated for the other side. The heads of the screws are then connected with two rods.

Transoral Surgery

Transoral decompression of the upper cervical spine typically requires intraoperative fluoroscopy to help maintain proper anatomic orientation during the decompressive procedure. Although orientation in the sagittal plane is easy to obtain with fluoroscopy, depth and mediolateral orientation are more difficult to assess. Image-guided technology can be used to orient the surgeon in multiple planes during transoral surgical procedures.[16]

Unlike in other spinal applications of image-guidance, discrete registration points are not readily available during transoral surgery. In this setting, surface-mounted markers (fiducials) are applied to the patient before obtaining the preoperative CT scan. Typically, two fiducials are applied to the mastoid processes and two are applied to the lateral orbital margins or to both malar eminences. The nasal septum can also be used as a registration point. Following surgical exposure, registration points in the surgical field such as the anterior arch of C1 or the base of the odontoid can be used.

The patient is positioned in a three-point head holder. Before the patient is draped, the registration process is performed using the surface-mounted fiducials. Because the registration points are not accessible during the procedure, a reference frame is used for transoral navigation. This device allows for changes in intraoperative patient positioning without the need to register again. The reference frame can be attached to the three-point head holder.

During the decompressive procedure, the probe can be intermittently placed into the surgical field. Reformatted sagittal, axial, and coronal CT images are immediately generated and provide the surgeon with precise orientation to the pertinent surgical anatomy. In particular, orientation in the axial plane minimizes the risk of lateral deviation toward the vertebral artery during the decompression (Fig. 46-8). If posterior fixation is performed following transoral decompression, the same CT image data set can be used for C1-C2 screw placement.

Other Cervical Applications

Image-guided navigation has several other applications in the cervical spine. In particular, these procedures include any operation in which intraoperative imaging is required to improve a surgeon's orientation to nonexposed spinal anatomy. Image-guided navigation has been applied to the removal of cervical neoplasms, anterior odontoid screw fixation for the management of nondisplaced odontoid fractures, lateral mass screw fixation in the subaxial spine, cervical corpectomy, and placement of pedicle screws into C7.[17-20]

Conclusions

Image-guided spinal navigation has been successfully applied to spinal surgery. It can be used for both conventional and minimally invasive spinal procedures. By linking digitized image data to spinal surface anatomy, navigational technology facilitates the surgeon's orientation to unexposed spinal structures, thereby improving the precision and accuracy of the surgery and reducing or eliminating the need for conventional intraoperative imaging.

Although image-guided spinal navigation is a versatile and effective technology, it is not a replacement for a surgeon's thorough knowledge of the pertinent spinal anatomy, as well as correct surgical techniques. It merely serves as an additional source of information used by the surgeon to make selected intraoperative decisions.

REFERENCES

1. Amiot L, Lang K, Putzier M, et al.: Comparative results between conventional and computer-assisted pedicle screw installation the thoracic, lumbar and sacral spine, *Spine (Phila Pa 1976)* 25:606–614, 2005.
2. George DC, Krag MH, Johnson CC, et al.: Hole preparation technique for transpedicle screws: effect on pull-out strength from human cadaveric vertebrae, *Spine (Phila Pa 1976)* 16:181–184, 1991.
3. Gertzbein SD, Robbins SE: Accuracy of pedicle screw placement in vivo, *Spine (Phila Pa 1976)* 15:11–14, 1990.
4. Weinstein JN, Spratt KF, Spengler D, et al.: Spinal pedicle fixation: reliability and validity of roentgenogram-based assessment and surgical factors on successful screw placement, *Spine (Phila Pa 1976)* 13:1012–1018, 1988.
5. Rampersaud YR, Foley KT, Shen AC, et al.: Radiation exposure to the spine surgeon during fluoroscopically assisted pedicle screw insertion, *Spine (Phila Pa 1976)* 25:2637–2645, 2000.
6. Kalfas IH, Kormos DW, Murphy MA, et al.: Application of frameless stereotaxy to pedicle screw fixation of the spine, *J Neurosurg* 83:641–647, 1995.
7. Murphy MA, McKenzie RL, Kormos DW, Kalfas IH: Frameless stereotaxis for the insertion of lumbar pedicle screws: a technical note, *J Clin Neurosci* 1:257–260, 1994.
8. Kalfas IH: Spinal registration accuracy and error. In Germano IM, editor: *Advanced techniques in image-guided brain and spine surgery*, New York, 2002, Thieme, pp 37–44.
9. Tamura Y, Sugano N, Sasama T, et al.: Surface based registration accuracy of CT-based image-guided spine surgery, *Eur Spine J* 14:291–297, 2005.
10. Wood MJ, Mannion RJ: Improving accuracy and reducing radiation exposure in minimally invasive lumbar interbody fusion surgery, *J Neurosurg Spine* 12:533–539, 2010.
11. Laine T, Schlenzka D, Makitalo K, et al.: Improved accuracy of pedicle screw insertion with computer-assisted surgery, *Spine (Phila Pa 1976)* 11:1254–1258, 1997.
12. Shin BJ, James AR, Njoku IU, Hartl R: Pedicle screw navigation: a systematic review and meta-analysis of perforation risk for computer-navigated versus freehand insertion, *J Neurosurg Spine* 17:113–122, 2012.
13. Verma R, Krishan S, Haendlmayer K, Mohsen A: Functional outcome of computer-assisted spinal pedicle screw placement: a systematic review and meta-analysis of 23 studies including 5,992 pedicle screws. *Eur Spine J* 19:370–375, 2010.
14. Kalfas IH: Image-guided spinal navigation, *Clin Neurosurg* 46:70–88, 1999.
15. Assaker R, Reyns N, Vinchon M, et al.: Transpedicular screw placement. Image-guided versus lateral-view fluoroscopy: in vitro simulation, *Spine (Phila Pa 1976)* 26:2160–2164, 2001.
16. Kalfas IH: Image-guided spinal navigation: application to spinal metastasis. In Maciunas RJ, editor: *Advanced techniques in central nervous system metastasis*, Lebanon, NH, 1998, AANS Publications, pp 245–254.
17. Welch WC, Subach BR, Pollack IF, Jacobs GB: Frameless stereotactic guidance for surgery of the upper cervical spine, *Neurosurgery* 40:958–964, 1997.
18. Lee G, Massicotte EM, Rampersaud YR: Clinical accuracy of cervicothoracic pedicle screw placement: a comparison of the "open" lamino-foraminotomy and computer-assisted techniques. *J Spinal Disord Tech* 20:25–32, 2007.
19. Bolger C, Wigfield C: Image-guided surgery: application to the cervical and thoracic spine and a review of the first 120 procedures, *J Neurosurg Spine* 92:175–180, 2000.
20. Weidner A, Wahler M, Chiu ST, Ulrich GC: Modification of C1-C2 transarticular screw fixation by image-guided surgery, *Spine (Phila Pa 1976)* 25:2668–2673, 2000.
21. Harms J, Melcher R: Posterior C1-C2 fusion with polyaxial screw and rod fixation, *Spine (Phila Pa 1976)* 26:2467–2471, 2001.

Biologics for Intervertebral Disk Regeneration and Repair

47

Adam L. Shimer and Xudong Joshua Li

CHAPTER PREVIEW

Chapter Synopsis Neck and low back pain is common, and intervertebral disk degeneration is thought to be one of the primary sources for pain generation. Although therapeutic techniques including surgical and non-surgical modalities have been applied, current therapies for disk degeneration may address symptoms but do not restore structure and function. In this chapter, we will review the advancement of biologic therapeutic options for disk degeneration.

Important Points Animal models used for disk degeneration can be placed into three major groups: mechanical compression model, annular injury model, and environmental model.

Treatment strategies differ in different stages of degeneration.

Growth factors, cells, and scaffolds are the major elements in disk tissue engineering and regeneration.

Whole disk replacement is a promising approach for biologic disk replacement.

Despite the advancement in preclinical settings, there is still a long way to clinical application.

Low back and neck pain is ubiquitous and is a prevalent disabler of persons of working age. In fact, more than 100 million work days are lost for this reason every year in the United States, second only behind the common cold. Current treatment for axial pain and intervertebral disk (IVD) degeneration is dominated by symptomatic care such as activity modification, physical therapy, and oral medications. When symptoms are recalcitrant to conservative measures, surgery may be considered. At this time nearly all surgical treatment for predominantly diskogenic axial pain involves removal of the diseased disk, followed by either fusion or metallic disk replacement. No clinically available medical, biologic, or cellular-based treatment is available to slow, halt, or reverse disk degeneration.

IVD degeneration is characterized by a progressive alteration in the mechanical properties, cellular numbers and composition, nutrition, and metabolic profile. Currently, most biologic strategies for treatment of IVD degeneration are centered on one or more of these aspects of the degenerative cascade. Techniques studied have included augmenting trophic factors either by introduction of growth factors or gene-based therapy to transfect native cells to upregulate growth factor production. This chapter reviews the animal models and advances made in the biologic therapeutic options for disk degeneration.

Animal Models

The study of any intervention for a human disease often requires the development and validation of an animal model equivalent. Several models currently exist, although most can be placed into three major groups: mechanical compression model, annular injury model, and environmental model.

Mechanical Compression Model

Repetitive supraphysiologic mechanical stress has been suggested as a promoter of IVD degeneration. Studies of truck drivers suggested an increased rate of IVD degeneration. Lotz and colleagues devised an animal model of IVD degeneration by placing a static compressive load across a mobile tail segment in a mouse and demonstrated "number of harmful responses in a dose-dependent way: disorganization of the an[n]ulus fibrosus; an increase in apoptosis and associated loss of cellularity; and down regulation of collagen II and aggrecan gene expression."[1] Another group used a custom-made external loading device to compress rabbit IVD to yield histologic and radiographic evidence of degeneration. This degeneration was not reversible when the compression was removed for 28 days.

Annular Injury Model

Annular injury that initiates the degenerative cascade is a well-known clinical entity. Research has even suggested that a misplaced needle for anterior cervical level confirmation can lead to iatrogenic degeneration.[2] One of the most widely used animal models for disk degeneration is an annular stab model. Sobajima and associates characterized a rabbit model using a 16-gauge needle puncture of the annulus fibrosus (AF) by magnetic resonance imaging (MRI), plain radiographs, histology, and molecular composition.[3] This technique has been adapted to use a percutaneous, minimally invasive stab model with computed tomography (CT) guidance, thus eliminating a formal surgical approach. A more recent study used a similar approach but with the annular injury provided by diode laser. A similar rate of degeneration was seen compared with needle puncture. Despite their widespread use in basic science and translational research, the annular injury model has been criticized as perhaps not truly reflecting age-related IVD degeneration, and it may more accurately represent posttraumatic disk degeneration.

Environmental Model

Many studies have linked smoking to accelerated rates of IVD degeneration. One study demonstrated that mice exposed to long-term cigarette smoke demonstrate IVD degeneration. This may be a useful model to better understand the pathways linking smoking to IVD degeneration.

Different Treatment Strategies for Different Stages of Disk Degeneration

Different stages of disk degeneration will likely require different treatment strategies. In the early stages of disk degeneration, cells in the nucleus pulposus (NP) area are still abundant. Therefore, a non–cell-based treatment option, such as in vivo gene transfer or growth factor injection targeted at NP regeneration using minimally invasive techniques, may be the most suitable strategy for targeting early disk degeneration.

However, for moderate disk degeneration, most functional NP cells, the target of gene therapy, have already disappeared, so only gene delivery or growth factor injection is insufficient. Thus, ex vivo gene approach or NP tissue engineering will be better for the intermediate stages of disk degeneration.

In the end stages of degeneration, the disk may be virtually nonexistent and replaced with a thin mass of fibrous tissue. Therefore, a tissue-engineered AF, or whole disk, or artificial disk will be needed (Fig. 47-1).

Interventions

The IVD regeneration and repair technology has been developed in three major areas: appliance of growth factors, characterization and use of stem cells, and the development of novel, degradable biomaterials.

Growth Factors

One of the hallmarks of disk generation is the imbalance of the catabolic and anabolic metabolism of extracellular

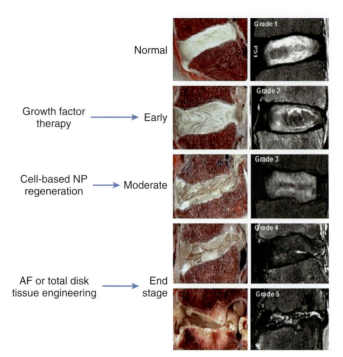

FIGURE 47-1 Three major areas for possible therapeutic intervention in intervertebral disk tissue regeneration and repair. *AF,* Annulus fibrosus; *NP,* nucleus pulposus.

matrix. Thus, scientists are targeting the production of extracellular matrix of disk cells and decreasing the degradation of matrix with growth factors and inhibitors of matrix degrading enzymes. Numerous studies have demonstrated that various growth factors promote disk cell proliferation and glycosaminoglycan synthesis, such as growth differentiation factor-5 (GDF5, also named BMP-14), bone morphogenetic proteins (BMPs), insulin-like growth factor-1 (IGF-1), fibroblast growth factor (FGF), transforming growth factor-β (TGF-β), epidermal growth factor (EGF), platelet-derived growth factor (PDGF), and platelet-rich plasma (PRP)[4] (Table 47-1).

These growth factors can be given by intradiskal injection or delivered with cells or scaffolds. For example, in the cultured disk cells, GDF5 has been shown to promote NP cell proliferation and increase GAG production. Similarly, in a rabbit disk degeneration model, injection of recombinant GDF5 alleviated degenerative progression and restored disk height. Adenovirus GDF5 injection to mice disks increased extracellular protein production and restored disk height and T2-weighted signal in an MRI study (Fig. 47-2).[5]

BMP-7 has also been shown to have a similar function. Indeed, GDF5 and BMP-7 have been approved for a phase I clinical trial of intra-disk injection.[4] The combination of several growth factors can synergistically stimulate matrix synthesis in the disk. In a pilot clinical study, a "cocktail solution" comprising a mixture of agents known to induce the synthesis of proteoglycan was injected into the lumbar disks of 30 patients with chronic low back pain.[6] The evidence clearly showed that growth factors alter the degenerative process in the disk. The response of NP and AF cells may differ in response to growth factors; therefore, optimized combinations of growth factors may

Table 47-1 Growth Factors Used for Disk Repair

Molecular	Method	Outcome
BMP-2	Gene and protein therapy	Increase proteoglycan and collagen production, delay degeneration process
BMP-7	Gene and protein therapy	Increase cell proliferation and proteoglycan synthesis; Restore disk structure and biomechanical function
GDF5	Gene and protein therapy	Increase proteoglycan and collagen synthesis, restore disk height and delay degeneration process
IGF-1	Protein and gene therapy	Enhance proteoglycan synthesis, increase cell proliferation and anti-apoptotic effects; preserve degenerated disk
PDGF	Protein therapy	Increase cell proliferation
TGF-β1	Gene and protein therapy	Increase cell proliferation and proteoglycan production in vitro and in vivo
bFGF	Protein therapy	Increase cell proliferation
Proteinase inhibitor TIMP-1	Gene therapy	Increase proteoglycan synthesis of human degenerated disk cells; delay degeneration changes in rabbits
Sox 9	Gene therapy	Increase collagen in human degenerated disk cells; main rabbit disk cell chondrocyte phenotype and architecture of the NP
Lim mineralization protein-1	Gene therapy	Increases proteoglycan, BMP2, and BMP7 in cultured cells and disk of rabbit with intradiskal injection
Platelet-rich plasma (PRP)	Protein	Increase cell proliferation and matrix production; increase disk height and maintain disk structure
TNF inhibitor	Protein	Decrease MMPs level
Interleukin-1α receptor	Gene and protein therapy	Decrease MMP3 and ADAMTS-4 expression

bFGF, Basic fibroblast growth factor; *BMP,* bone morphogenetic protein; *GDF,* growth differentiation factor; *IGF,* insulin-like growth factor; *MMP,* matrix metalloproteinase; *PDGF,* platelet-derived growth factor; *TGF,* transforming growth factor; *TIMP,* tissue inhibitor of metalloproteinase; *TNF,* tumor necrosis factor.

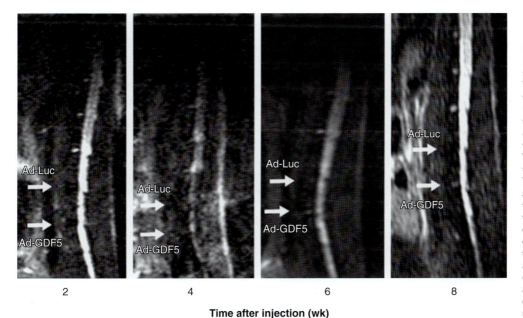

Time after injection (wk)

FIGURE 47-2 Magnetic resonance imaging T2-weighted signal images of the same animal at different time points. The *upper arrow* points to the location where the disk was injected with Ad-Luc (adenovirus–Luciferase vector), whereas the *lower arrow* points to the disk injected with Ad-GDF5 (adenovirus–growth differentiation factor-5). When compared with the adjacent intact disks, both the disks lost the bright T2-weighted signal at the second week after injection. However, the signal of the disk injected with Ad-GDF5 began to reappear at 6 weeks and had become clearer at 8 weeks. In contrast, no signs of recovery of the signal were seen in the disk injected with Ad-Luc. (From Liang H, Ma SY, Feng G, et al.: Therapeutic effects of adenovirus-mediated growth and differentiation factor-5 in a mice disc degeneration model induced by annulus needle puncture, *Spine J* 10:32-41, 2010.)

be needed for individual patients, depending on cells or metabolic pathways. However, some of these growth factors not only stimulate chondrogenic response but also induce osteogenesis. For example, BMP-2, BMP-7, GDF5, and TGF-β have been shown to have osteogenic properties.

Other proteins such as inhibitors of matrix degrading enzyme or inflammatory cytokines have also been investigated for the disk degeneration. The injection of recombinant interleukin-1 (IL-1) receptor antagonist reversed disk degeneration and restored disk height by inhibiting matrix metalloproteinases (MMPs). Tumor necrosis factor (TNF) inhibitors and antibody have shown promising results as well. The N terminal peptide of Link protein was shown to

halt and reverse some of the degeneration in a rabbit disk injury model. Gene therapy methods have also been used to deliver growth factors or inhibitors to the disk space for constant endogenous production and release of the molecules.

Cells

The use of proteins or gene transfer approaches is based on the assumption that enough viable disk cells are available; thus, the protein treatments are not suitable for the moderate stage of disk degeneration, in which the numbers of disk cells that can respond to growth factor and produce matrix are greatly diminished. Three major cell sources have been investigated: autologous disk cells, articular chondrocytes, and mesenchymal stem cells

Table 47-2 Cells Used for Disk Repair

Cell Type	Method	Outcome
Autologous disk cells from sand rat	Cells expanded in vitro and loaded on Gelfoam for transplantation	Cells integrated into the disk and exhibited a spindle-shaped morphology in the AF or a rounded chondrocyte phenotype in NP
Disk chondrocytes from canine	Chondrocytes expanded in vitro and transplanted to the same animal via percutaneous delivery	Disk chondrocytes remained viable and proliferated; normal disk matrix, disk height restored and degeneration retarded
Human disk cells	Disk cells cultured in vitro and returned to patients	Matrix restored and mechanical balance maintained
Rabbit bone marrow MSCs	Cells cultured and labeled with GFP and then transplanted to mature rabbit	Cells proliferated and secreted matrix; NP phenotype markers maintained
Rabbit bone marrow MSCs	Cells cultured in vitro, transfected with LacZ, and then transplanted into rabbit degenerated disk	Matrix produced; disk height restored and degeneration process delayed
Human bone marrow MSCs	Cells expanded in vitro and seed on collagen sponge and then transplanted to human IVD	Symptoms alleviated and disk height restored
Human bone marrow MSC	MSCs expanded in vitro and transplanted to NP area	Pain relieved
Human hematopoietic precursor stem cells	Autologous stem cells intradiskally injected in patient	No improvement for low back pain
Human adipose-derived stem cells	Cells intradiskally injected into rabbit disk space	Cells proliferated and matrixes produced
Mouse embryonic stem cells	Cells differentiated to chondrocyte in vitro; chondrocytes expressing GFP injected into degenerated disk	New notochordal cell population seen in degenerated disks. no inflammation response

AF, Annulus fibrosus *GFP,* green fluorescent protein; *IVD,* intervertebral disk; *MSC,* mesenchymal stem cell; *NP,* nucleus pulposus.

(MSCs) (Table 47-2). Autologous disk cell transplantation demonstrated promising results in rabbit, sand rat, and canine models. In a randomized, multicenter clinical trial, the EuroDisc study, interim 2-year analysis showed safe application and a decreased sum score and disability index in 14 patients who received disk chondrocyte transplantation.[7] However, obtaining the "healthy" disk cells is a challenge, and the survivability of disk cells in the disk tissue is questionable.

Another attractive cell source is the pluripotent stem cell. Adult stem cells are derived from a variety of tissues such as bone marrow, adipose tissue, articular cartilage, muscle, and synovium. Studies have shown that disk cells themselves contain a population of progenitor cells, which would be the ideal cell source. Among the stem cells, bone marrow–derived mesenchymal stem cells (MSCs) have received the most extensive attention. For the MSCs, two approaches are being used: one is expanding the progenitor cells in vitro and then directly injecting into disk; another is differentiating the cells to a chondrocyte-like phenotype, followed by injection. Autologous bone marrow MSCs have not only proliferated and undergone NP cell phenotypic switch months after transplantation in canine, porcine, and rabbit models, but have also preserved disk height and water content.[8-10] Two older Japanese women received a collagen sponge seeded with autologous bone marrow MSCs. Two years after the surgical procedure, symptoms were alleviated, and T2-weighted MRI signal intensity was restored in both patients.[11] Similarly, Orozco and colleagues transplanted autologous expanded bone marrow MSCs into the NP area of 10 patients.[12] Eighty-five percent of patients had rapid improvement of pain and disability in 3 months, comparable to the outcome of spinal fusion. Moreover, co-culture of MSCs with NP cells stimulates both NP cell proliferation and MSC differentiation toward the chondrogenic lineage. Conversely, in another pilot study of 10 patients who received intradiskal injection of autologous

hematopoietic precursor stem cells, little improvement of low back pain was reported at 1-year follow-up.[4]

Autologous human adipose-derived stem cells (ASCs) have generated great interest. ASCs are abundant and easy to manipulate; they also have high plasticity—differentiation along a multitude of lineages, such as chondrocyte, myocyte, and adipocyte lineages. ASC transplant has been demonstrated to be effective in canine, rat, and rabbit animal models. Other stem cell sources are also under investigation, such as neonatal human fibroblast combined with growth factors and umbilical cord stem cells.[4,8]

Despite the encouraging results from animal and human pilot studies, serious concerns about these stem cells remain. For example, it is still not clear whether the differentiated chondrocyte-like cells are close to NP cells. How to control the differentiation direction and how many cells to use are other concerns because these stem cells have osteogenic potential under certain conditions. Finally, the biomechanical properties of these cells are uncertain.

Cell-based gene delivery is also an alternative therapeutic strategy for advanced stages of disk degeneration (Fig 47-3). To overcome the osteogenesis of stem cells, the inducible promoters that are sensitive to the disk environment could be genetically integrated into cells to upregulate chondrogenic genes but suppress the osteogenic genes. For example, one study isolated canine NP cells and infected then with adeno-associated virus (AAV)-htert (human telomerase reverse transcriptase). The NP cells were then injected into disk tissue and transplanted into dogs. Results showed that the composite effectively resisted disk degeneration in a beagle model.

Scaffold

Nucleus Pulposus Tissue Engineering Scaffolds

The loss of NP integrity is one of the earliest events in disk degeneration; thus, NP tissue engineering is crucial for

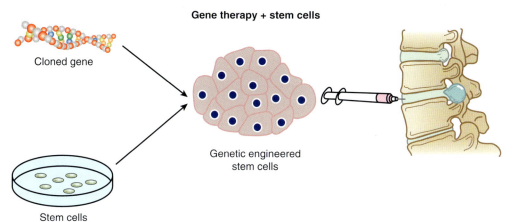

Gene therapy + stem cells

Cloned gene

Genetic engineered
stem cells

Stem cells

FIGURE 47-3 Schematic demonstrating cell-based gene delivery for the treatment of disk degeneration.

functional disk restoration. Scaffolds in tissue engineering are aimed at retaining cells in the desired location and supporting appropriate mechanical properties and/or biochemical signals. Hydrogels have been proposed as ideal candidates for NP replacement because of their mechanical similarity to native tissues.[8] Successful hydrogels for NP tissue engineering require load resistance, easy and minimally invasive implantation, tissue biocompatibility, low viscosity during injection and the ability to solidify at body temperature, and cell growth and matrix production stimulation. Many different native and synthetic biomaterials have been used for NP tissue engineering. Native materials include alginate, agarose, chitosan, chondroitin sulphate, collagen, fibrin, gelatin, hyaluronan, small intestine submucosa, gellan gum, and demineralized bone matrix (DBM); synthetic material include calcium polyphosphate, polyethylene glycol, poly(l-lactic acid), poly(d,l-lactic acid), poly(glycolic acid), and poly(lactic-co-glycolic acid). Synthesis of in situ crosslinkable polymers may provide an alternative method for producing hydrogels. The crosslinking is achieved by redox reactions (thiols), condensations (polyacrylates), or complex formation (alginate, peptides). Natural polymer photo-crosslinking with functional groups (e.g., methacrylates or N-vinyl pyrrolidone) provide a solution to gel transition properties, good biocompatibility, and increased matrix production.[13] Cell survival has been reported to be good to excellent, with most of the reports initially relying on in vitro observations. From those in vitro observations, some of the materials have already been transitioned to in vivo animal experiments, either in ectopic or intradiskal administration.

A cell-free, resorbable nonwoven polyglycolic acid–hyaluronan scaffold was implanted into rabbit and ovine models and showed NP tissue formation and water content improvement. Chitosan/glycerophosphate hydrogel kept viability and functionality of encapsulated bovine NP cells or induced differentiation of human MSCs into NP-like cells even in the absence of a differentiating medium. Hyaluronic acid is the most abundant water absorption molecule in the NP. The bovine NP cells seeded in a thermoreversible hyaluronan-based hydrogel (HA-pNIPAM) exhibited NP phenotype and matrix production in a whole organ culture disk mode. Two hyaluronan-derived materials (HYAFF 120, an ester, and HYADD 3, an amide) seeded with MSCs exhibited a close to normal disk NP structure in a pig lumbar nucleotomy model. The rapid degradation problem of native polymer (e.g., hyaluronan and collagen) may be overcome by crosslinking with a protein crosslink to enhance stability and mechanical properties.

Mechanical properties of the hydrogels can be controlled by varying concentrations and crosslinking processes. This characteristic is one of the crucial criteria for NP tissue engineering. For instance, modified alginate hydrogels were photo-crosslinked and encapsulated with bovine NP cells. Under in vitro culture for 4 weeks, the photo-crosslinked alginate hydrogels showed increased matrix production and Young modulus, and they remained intact up to 8 weeks.[8] A thiol-modified hyaluronan and elastin-like polypeptide (ELP) composite hydrogel with human disk cells exhibited biocompatibility and appropriate biomechanical properties in a rabbit disk degeneration model. One study investigated the time-dependent mechanical properties of gelatin and agar hydrogels with viscoelastic and poroelastic frameworks. The group found that several gel formulations had equilibrium elastic properties comparable to those of the NP tissue under unconfined compression, but permeability values were much greater than those of the native tissue.

Annulus Fibrosus Tissue Engineering Scaffolds

In the bench and preclinical studies, a number of scaffolds have been used for AF tissue engineering.[8,13] They are categorized into two categories: single unit (oriented or non-oriented to simulate the organized lamellae) and biphasic to simulate inner and outer layers of AF.

Native materials such as collagen, glycosaminoglycan, chitosan, and alginate have been used for AF scaffolds in a singular or combination formula. In in vitro observations, these materials were able to support AF cell growth and maintain phenotype. In animal models, these scaffolds loaded with AF cells also demonstrated promising results in disk repair.[8,14] Silk is also a candidate scaffold. Chang and colleagues assessed AF cells spreading and proliferation on different porosity of silk scaffolds.[15] Park and associates seeded porcine AF cells on a lamellar ring silk structure and showed support of AF tissue repair.[16] Silk fibers crosslinked with chondroitin sulfate have also been shown to support human chondrocyte redifferentiation.

The biodegradable synthetic materials have also been investigated for AF scaffolds. Using a direct one-step polycondensation method, the authors were able to create a malic acid–based polyester poly(1,8-octanediol malate) (POM) film and support the proliferation of rat AF cells (Fig. 47-4).[17] In a mouse subcutaneous model, this scaffold showed biocompatibility. Similarly, studies showed that poly-d-l-lactide (PDLLA) foams incorporated with different percentages (0, 5, and 30 wt %) of bioglass particles supported bovine AF cell growth and matrix production.[4]

The electrospinning technique is gaining attention to produce oriented AF microfibers that are ideal for cell function. For example, the polycarbonate polyurethane (PU) and poly-σ-caprolactone (PCL) were electrospun to nanofibers, and both the tensile strength and initial modulus of aligned scaffolds were higher than in the random-fiber scaffold. The tensile strength of silk-elastin link protein was also enhanced with electrospinning. Bioactive nanoparticles dispersed in electrospun microfibers have demonstrated a capacity to modulate the differentiation of human MSCs. Vadala and colleagues created a construct consisting of randomly oriented electrospun poly(l-lactide) (PLLA) fibers incorporated with TGF-β_1.[18] The study showed that bovine AF cells produced a significant amount of collagen and GAG content with the continuous release of growth factor.

To simulate the outer and inner structure of AF tissue closely, the authors' laboratory constructed a biphasic scaffold with a ring-shaped DBM as an outer AF and poly(polycaprolactone triol malate) (PPCLM)–oriented concentric sheets seeded with chondrocytes as an inner AF (Fig. 47-5).[19] The DBM was extracted from

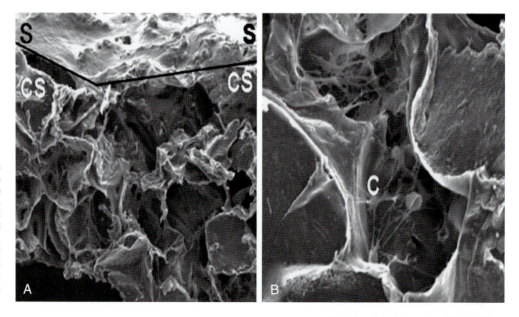

FIGURE 47-4 Scanning electron microscopic images of rat annulus fibrosus cells (C) cultured on the polyester poly (1,8-octanediol malate) (POM) scaffold at 70× (**A**) and 200× (**B**) for 3 weeks. *CS,* Scaffold cross-section; *S,* scaffold surface. (Wan Y, Feng G. Shen FH, et al.: Novel biodegradable poly(1,8-octanediol malate) for annulus fibrosis regeneration, *Macromol Biosci* 7:1217-1224, 2007.)

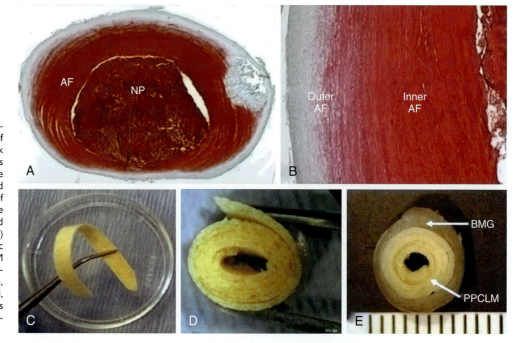

FIGURE 47-5 Horizontal section (**A**) and vertical section (**B**) of normal rabbit intervertebral disk stained with Safranin-O. *AF,* Annulus fibrosus; *NP,* nucleus pulposus. The outer layer (reduced red staining) and inner layer (abundant red staining) of the annulus fibrosus can clearly be seen. **C,** The elastic biomaterial and poly(polycaprolactone triol malate) (PPCLM) is oriented in concentric sheets (**D**) and inserted into a DBM ring to mimic the structure of inner and outer annulus fibrosus (**E**), respectively. (Wan Y, Feng G, Shen FH, et al.: Biphasic scaffold for annulus fibrosus tissue regeneration. *Biomaterials* 29:643-652, 2008.)

cortical bone that mimicked the type I collagen structure and fibril property of the outer AF. PPCLM matrix was oriented in concentric sheets and seeded with chondrocytes to recapitulate the inner layer of the AF, which is rich in type II collagen and proteoglycan. The resulting PPCLM/DBM biphasic scaffold had excellent elasticity, with no permanent deformation after at least 100 press-loading and release cycles. The compressive stress of the DBM/PPCLM scaffold was significantly higher than that of pure PPCLM, with the incorporation of DBM enhancing the compressive strength of the PPCLM scaffold from 0.21 to 1.26 MPa. The gelatinous pulposus of the IVD absorbs and transmits compressive loads into the tensile stretch at the periphery of the AF. In the strain-stress curve, the stress increased linearly with the strain. The tensile stress of the DBM/PPCLM scaffold was 3.37 MPa, which was much higher than that of the pure PPCLM scaffold at 0.06 MPa for three sheets, and it approached that of rabbit AF at 6.95 MPa.

Whole Disk Tissue Engineering

A whole disk tissue can be simulated by combining the different properties of the NP and AF. Different combinations of biomaterials and cells have been used for total disk tissue engineering (Table 47-3).[20] In 2004, Mizuno and associates designed a composite disk in a cylinder shape with polyglycolic acid (PGA) and solvent-cast polylactic acid (PLA) as an outer "AF" ring seeded with AF cells and an alginate hydrogel to serve as the "NP" core.[21] Later, Nesti and colleagues reported the use of hyaluronic acid hydrogel as NP and PLLA electrospun nanofibrous as the AF component loaded with human MSCs.[22] Park and colleagues constructed a whole disk with silk protein for the AF and fibrin/hyaluronic acid gel for the NP seeded with porcine AF cells

and chondrocytes, respectively.[16] By electrospinning, Lazebnik and co-workers fabricated a biphasic IVD by using PCL as the AF and agarose as the NP; both parts were seeded with porcine chondrocytes.[23] See and associates created a silicone NP with BMSC cell sheets surrounded by silk scaffolds to mimic the IVD structure.[24] Rat studies provided some encouraging results for the whole disk tissue engineering. Bowles and associates constructed a biphasic whole IVD using collagen I with ovine AF cells for AF and alginate with NP cells for the NP.[25] The constructs were implanted into athymic rat caudal spine IVD after diskectomy. No significant loss of height was noted from 4.5 to 8 months between reimplanted disks and the engineering construct groups. Proteoglycans and collagen were present throughout the disk construct, and no bridging bone or bony fusion was demonstrated with micro-CT.

Conclusions

Disk degeneration is a common problem, and its clinical manifestation—back pain—is the second most common reason for clinic visits. Current therapies for disk degeneration may address symptoms but do not restore structure and function. With the advance in molecular and cellular biology as well as biomaterials, it is possible to repair disk degeneration with different strategies according to the stages of disease. Despite the promising results achieved in animal and preclinical studies, there is still a long distance to the clinical application of tissue engineering. Four major obstacles remain: first, the biology of disk cells is still not clear; second, the nutrition penetration for the engineered whole disk is a problem; third, the mechanical properties of different scaffolds still need to be optimized; finally, the dose, temporal and special of growth factors, cells, and scaffolds still have a long way to be well characterized.

Table 47-3 Total Disk Tissue Engineering

Total Disk Tissue Engineering References	Material	Results
Mizuno et al, 2004[21]	Polyglycolic acid and polylactic acid as outer AF; an alginate hydrogel as NP	AF and NP cells maintained their phenotypes; the implants formed distinct AF and NP tissue in an athymic mice subcutaneous implant model; mechanical properties similar to native tissue by 16 wk
Nesti et al, 2008[22]	Human MSCs with a hyaluronic acid hydrogel as NP; a poly (L-lactic acid) as AF	MSCs differentiated to chondrocytes
See et al, 2011[24]	Rabbit bone marrow MSCs sheet with silk as AF; a silicon as NP	MSCs produced matrices in in vitro culture; type I collagen predominant in the beginning; collagen II more pronounced in a 4-wk culture
Lazebnik et al, 2011[23]	PCL fiber as AF; agarose as NP seeded with chondrocytes	Cells viable, well distributed around the interface; higher mechanical moduli than agarose hydrogel alone
Bowles et al, 2011[25]	Collagen I with ovine AF cells as AF; polyethylene or alginate with NP cells as NP	In an athymic rat tail model, composite maintained disk height and matrix; integrated with the host body; similar axial load capacity to the native disk
Park et al, 2012[16]	Silk with porcine AF cells as AF, a fibrin-hyaluronic acid gel with porcine chondrocytes as NP	Lamellar scaffolds supported AF-like tissue over 2 wk in culture; porcine chondrocytes formed the NP phenotype after 4 wk of culture with the AF tissue

AF, Annulus fibrosus; *MSC,* mesenchymal stem cell; *NP,* nucleus pulposus; *PCL,* poly-σ-caprolactone.

REFERENCES

1. Lotz JC, Colliou OK, Chin JR, et al.: Compression-induced degeneration of the intervertebral disc: an in vivo mouse model and finite-element study, *Spine (Phila Pa 1976)* 23:2493–2506, 1998.
2. Nassr A, Lee JY, Bashir RS, et al.: Does incorrect level needle localization during anterior cervical discectomy and fusion lead to accelerated disc degeneration? *Spine (Phila Pa 1976)* 34: 189–192, 2009.
3. Sobajima S, Vadala G, Shimer A, et al.: Feasibility of a stem cell therapy for intervertebral disc degeneration, *Spine J* 8:888–896, 2008.
4. Zhang Y, Chee A, Thonar EJ, An HS: Intervertebral disc repair by protein, gene, or cell injection: a framework for rehabilitation-focused biologics in the spine, *PM R* 3:S88–S94, 2011.
5. Liang H, Ma SY, Feng G, et al.: Therapeutic effects of adenovirus-mediated growth and differentiation factor-5 in a mice disc degeneration model induced by annulus needle puncture, *Spine J* 10:32–41, 2010.
6. Klein RG, Eek BC, O'Neill CW, et al.: Biochemical injection treatment for discogenic low back pain: a pilot study, *Spine J* 3:220–226, 2003.
7. Meisel HJ, Siodla V, Ganey T, et al.: Clinical experience in cell-based therapeutics: disc chondrocyte transplantation. A treatment for degenerated or damaged intervertebral disc, *Biomol Eng* 24:5–21, 2007.
8. Chan SC, Gantenbein-Ritter B: Intervertebral disc regeneration or repair with biomaterials and stem cell therapy: feasible or fiction? *Swiss Med Wkly* 142:(w13598), 2012.
9. An HS, Masuda K, Cs-Szabo G, et al.: Biologic repair and regeneration of the intervertebral disc, *J Am Acad Orthop Surg* 19: 450–452, 2011.
10. Hughes SP, Freemont AJ, Hukins DW, et al.: The pathogenesis of degeneration of the intervertebral disc and emerging therapies in the management of back pain, *J Bone Joint Surg Br* 94:1298–1304, 2012.
11. Yoshikawa T, Ueda Y, Miyazaki K, et al.: Disc regeneration therapy using marrow mesenchymal cell transplantation: a report of two case studies, *Spine (Phila Pa 1976)* 35:E475–E480, 2010.
12. Orozco L, Soler R, Morera C, et al.: Intervertebral disc repair by autologous mesenchymal bone marrow cells: a pilot study, *Transplantation* 92:822–828, 2011.
13. Bae WC, Masuda K: Emerging technologies for molecular therapy for intervertebral disc degeneration, *Orthop Clin North Am* 42:585–601, 2011. ix.
14. Mehrkens A, Muller AM, Valderrabano V, et al.: Tissue engineering approaches to degenerative disc disease: a meta-analysis of controlled animal trials, *Osteoarthritis Cartilage* 20:1316–1325, 2012.
15. Chang G, Kim HJ, Kaplan D, Vunjak-Novakovic G, Kandel RA: Porous silk scaffolds can be used for tissue engineering annulus fibrosus, *Eur Spine J* 16(11):1848–1857, 2007 Nov.
16. Park SH, Gil ES, Cho H, Mandal BB, Tien LW, Min BH, Kaplan DL: Intervertebral disk tissue engineering using biphasic silk composite scaffolds, *Tissue Eng Part A* 18(5-6):447–458, 2012 Mar.
17. Wan Y, Feng G, Shen FH, et al.: Novel biodegradable poly(1,8-octanediol malate) for annulus fibrosus regeneration, *Macromol Biosci* 7:1217–1224, 2007.
18. Vadalà G, Mozetic P, Rainer A, Centola M, Loppini M, Trombetta M, Denaro V: Bioactive electrospun scaffold for annulus fibrosus repair and regeneration, *Eur Spine J* 21(Suppl 1), 2012 May.
19. Wan Y, Feng G, Shen FH, et al.: Biphasic scaffold for annulus fibrosus tissue regeneration, *Biomaterials* 29:643–652, 2008.
20. Jin L, Shimer AL, Li X: The challenge and advancement of annulus fibrosus tissue engineering, *Eur Spine J* 22:1090–1100, 2013.
21. Mizuno H, Roy AK, Vacanti CA, Kojima K, Ueda M, Bonassar LJ: Tissue-engineered composites of anulus fibrosus and nucleus pulposus for intervertebral disc replacement, *Spine (Phila Pa 1976)* 29(12):1290–1297, 2004 Jun 15. discussion 1297–1298.
22. Nesti LJ, Li WJ, Shanti RM, Jiang YJ, Jackson W, Freedman BA, Kuklo TR, Giuliani JR, Tuan RS: Intervertebral disc tissue engineering using a novel hyaluronic acid-nanofibrous scaffold (HANFS) amalgam, *Tissue Eng Part A* 14(9):1527–1537, 2008 Sep.
23. Lazebnik M, Singh M, Glatt P, Friis LA, Berkland CJ, Detamore MS: Biomimetic method for combining the nucleus pulposus and annulus fibrosus for intervertebral disc tissue engineering, *J Tissue Eng Regen Med* 5(8):e179–e187, 2011 Aug.
24. See EY, Toh SL, Goh JC: Effects of radial compression on a novel simulated intervertebral disc-like assembly using bone marrow-derived mesenchymal stem cell cell-sheets for annulus fibrosus regeneration, *Spine (Phila Pa 1976)* 36(21):1744–1751, 2011 Oct 1.
25. Bowles RD, Gebhard HH, Härtl R, Bonassar LJ: Tissue-engineered intervertebral discs produce new matrix, maintain disc height, and restore biomechanical function to the rodent spine, *Proc Natl Acad Sci U S A* 108(32):13106–13111, 2011 Aug 9.

48

Biologics for Spinal Fusion

Daniel K. Park, Mihir J. Desai, and S. Tim Yoon

CHAPTER PREVIEW

Chapter Synopsis
Biologics in cervical spine surgery include demineralized bone matrix (DBM), ceramics, allografts containing mesenchymal stem cells, and growth factors. Each of these biologics has different characteristics and different degrees of osteoconductivity, osteoinductivity, and ostegenicity. This chapter reviews the key basic science principles, preclinical studies, and clinical studies that guide the surgeon in the appropriate use of biologics in the cervical spine.

Important Points
A successful spinal fusion requires sufficient bone graft, adequate vascularity to the fusion bed, and mechanical stability at the fusion level.

Unlike posterior cervical spine surgery, bone graft requirements for anterior cervical surgery include the ability for the graft structurally to resist axial compression.

Each graft material differs in properties providing a supply of osteogenic cells, an osteoconductive matrix, and an osteoinductive signal.

Graft materials can also be classified based on their ability to serve as graft extenders, enhancers, or bone graft substitutes.

The most common traditional bone graft is autograft, typically harvested from the iliac crest.

Clinical and Surgical Pearls
In single-level anterior cervical diskectomy and fusion, allograft bone is highly effective with similar fusion rates as compared to autograft bone

DBM allows for natural bone morphogenetic proteins (BMPs) to become available to induce bone formation.

Ceramics are synthetic bone grafts consisting of calcium phosphate biomaterials fused into an osteoconductive structure.

BMPs are multifunctional growth factors that belong to the transforming growth factor-β superfamily and have variable osteoinductive properties.

Clinical and Surgical Pitfalls
DBM has no structural support and must be used with a cage or as a graft enhancer.

Ceramics are brittle and have low impact and fracture resistance.

The quantity and quality of mesenchymal cells available in allograft containing mesenchymal stem cells are unknown.

Knowledge and understanding of the use of BMP in the cervical continue to evolve; BMPs should be used carefully because potential complications remain unknown.

Specifically, the use of recombinant human BMP-2 (rhBMP-2) in the cervical spine remains debated; the optimal concentration, carrier system, and associated complications continue to be investigated.

Surgical fusion of the cervical spine is a common procedure with a myriad of indications. Historically, allograft and autograft bone have been the mainstays of cervical fusion; however, in more recent years, surgeons have begun using a class of bone graft substitutes known as biologics. The biologics include demineralized bone matrix (DBM), ceramics, allografts containing mesenchymal stem cells, and growth factors. Each of these biologics has different characteristics and different degrees of osteoconductivity, osteoinductivity, and ostegenicity. This chapter reviews the key basic science principles, preclinical studies, and clinical studies that guide the surgeon in the appropriate use of biologics in the cervical spine.

Spinal Fusion

For successful spinal fusion to occur, sufficient bone graft, adequate vascularity to the fusion bed, and mechanical stability of the fusion levels are required. Without these components, the rate of nonunion is markedly increased. A key component of the fusion cascade begins at the cellular level. Progenitor cells, which respond to the local environment to produce bone, are the ultimate throughput allowing fusion to occur. These cells can be provided by cellular grafting to the fusion site, as well as through vascularity to the fusion bed.

A sufficient vascular supply to the fusion bed is required to complete the various phases of fusion biology. Adequate vascularity allows a hematoma, rich with various activated growth factors, to accumulate at the fusion bed. The factors ultimately attract progenitor cell migration into the fusion bed. These cells can then differentiate into osteoblasts.

The oxygen tension in the fusion bed also depends on blood supply. Investigators have hypothesized that an abundant blood supply leads to a higher oxygen tension level, which favors osteoblastic differentiation rather than chondrogenic differentiation. Following differentiation, the osteoblasts produce osteoid matrix, which calcifies into bone. The newly formed bone ultimately undergoes remodeling according to Wolff's law, such that reorganization is based on the imposed load.

Mechanical stability is the final requirement for fusion. In bony fracture healing, Perren proposed the interfragmentary strain theory, which states that the amount of strain in the fracture gap determines the type of tissue formed during healing. Strain greater than 100% would lead to nonunion, 10% to 100% would lead to initial fibrous union, and 2% to 10% would lead to cartilage formation and endochondral ossification. Strains less than 2% would lead to direct bone healing.

Furthermore, once tissue forms, the fracture gap could stiffen, which would lower strain and possibly change the tissue characteristics in the gap. Similarly, in fusion healing, a rigid structure is needed to promote the formation of bony tissue rather than a fibrous union. Instrumentation in the spine helps promote bone formation by reducing the "fracture" gap strain between the functional spinal units.[1-3] These findings suggest that a certain amount of rigidity in fixation may facilitate spinal fusion.

Historical Fusion Rates

Anterior Procedures

One of the most common cervical procedures performed is anterior cervical diskectomy and fusion (ACDF). ACDF has been highly successful in the treatment of radiculopathy, myelopathy, and myeloradiculopathy secondary to disk herniation and cervical spondylosis; however, the risk of nonunion following ACDF remains a real concern in certain patient populations.[4] Fusion rates in the literature vary because no standard radiographic criteria exist for determining osseous fusion.[5] Furthermore, successful fusion depends on the number of levels, graft type, and use of instrumentation. The fusion rates for single-level ACDF are much higher than for multilevel fusion. More specifically, for one-, two-, and three-level fusions, the fusion rates are 82% to 100%, 73% to 80%, and 70%, respectively.[6,7] The use of allograft or autograft bone may also play a factor in the fusion rates, but in single-level fusions, this difference appears to be minimal.[8] Instrumentation plays a critical role in fusion, particularly in multilevel constructs, to stabilize the motion segment and prevent graft compression and graft expulsion (Fig. 48-1).

Posterior Procedures

Historically, posterior procedures have yielded high fusion rates. Rates of fusion using iliac crest autograft range from 20% to 100%, depending largely on the segments incorporated, the techniques used, and how fusion was assessed. In contrast to anterior surgery, location with regard to the cervical level being addressed plays a pivotal role in fusion rates in the posterior cervical spine. Occipitocervical constructs using iliac crest bone graft fuse 62% to 100% of the time, whereas atlantoaxial fusion has demonstrated pseudarthrosis rates with iliac crest–based constructs that exceed 40% in some series. Overall, a rate of 80% is quoted for successful atlantoaxial fusion.[9-11] In contrast, for noninstrumented subaxial fusion procedures, fusion is reported in 92% to 100%, with a composite fusion rate of 97%.

As in anterior surgical procedures, the type of graft also plays a role in posterior procedures. Sawin and colleagues reported a fusion rate of 98.7% with autogeneic rib graft compared with 94.2% with iliac crest. The investigators speculated that the rib's morphology contoured well to the cervical lordosis and may have allowed a higher fusion rate. In addition, investigators have hypothesized that a higher concentration of bone morphogenetic protein (BMP) may be found in the rib.[12] Again, instrumentation plays a key role posteriorly because rigid internal fixation has been more successful than wiring constructs.

Summary

With these concepts in mind, a key difference in anterior and posterior cervical surgery exists when considering which type of bone graft is required. Whereas anterior cervical surgical procedures require the bone graft to resist axial compression, structural support is not a required function of bone graft typically used for posterior fusion. Axial compression support is usually needed in anterior surgical procedures because disk material is removed between

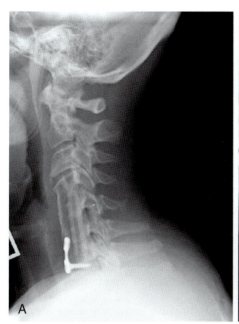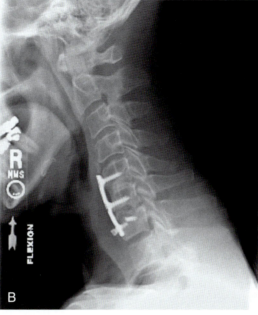

FIGURE 48-1 **A,** This patient underwent C5-C7 corpectomy with fibular allograft and plate. Flowing bone and remodeling can be seen. **B,** This patient underwent a two-level anterior cervical diskectomy and fusion at C5 to C7. The C5-C6 level demonstrates solid fusion with bridging bone; however, the lower level demonstrates clear nonunion. Radiolucencies around the graft and broken screws are visible.

Table 48-1 Properties of Various Bone Graft Substitutes

Material	Osteogenic	Osteoinductive	Osteoconductive	Structural Support
Autogenous cancellous bone	+	−	+	−
Autogenous cortical bone	+	−	±	+
Allograft cortical	−	−	±	+
Allograft cancellous	−	−	+	−
Demineralized bone matrix	−	+	+	−
Ceramic	−	−	+	±
BMP	−	+	−	−

BMP, Bone morphogenetic protein; +, present; −, absent.

the functional spine units, thereby destabilizing the spinal anterior column. The gap formed must be structurally supported to prevent the disk space from collapsing.

Furthermore, anterior cervical graft must have sufficient structural integrity to handle the axial loads without fragmenting, to prevent nonunion or malunion between the functional spinal units. This structural support is typically provided by the cortical component of the bone graft. If purely noncortical bone is used, then a structurally sound device (e.g., a cage) should be used. In contrast, with posterior cervical fusion, the structural integrity of the spine is typically intact (the anterior column remains untouched, and the lateral masses remain intact); therefore, axial loading of the graft is usually not a problem.

Definitions

Each graft material differs in its properties of providing a supply of osteogenic cells, an osteoconductive matrix, and an osteoinductive signal (Table 48-1). The *osteogenic* property of bone graft refers to the cellular component of the graft that participates in bone formation. As such, this property typically refers to osteoblasts or osteoblast precursors such as stem cells or preosteoblasts.

Osteoconductive properties refer to the structural properties of the graft matrix that enhance the attachment, migration, proliferation, and differentiation of stem cells and other cells that contribute to bone healing. Porosity is an important aspect of osteoconductivity. Appropriate pore sizes ranging from 200 to 500 μm are thought to be ideal. The composition of the graft matrix can also affect the osteoconductivity. For instance, with biodegradable grafts, the degradation properties can alter osteoconductive properties.

Osteoinductivity refers to the ability of some substance, usually a growth factor, to stimulate cellular events that transform a potential cell into a differentiated cell that becomes activated and committed to contributing to new bone formation. Marshal Urist defined osteoinductivity by the ability of a substance to form bone at an ectopic location such as fat or muscle tissue. Known naturally occurring osteogenic factors include a subset of the transforming growth factor-β (TGF-β) gene superfamily and some BMPs. The most osteogenic BMP molecules are thought to be BMP-2, BMP-6, and BMP-9. Less osteogenic molecules can form bone at sufficiently high doses, and other BMP molecules do not form bone reliably even at very high doses. Many other growth factors that cannot form bone by themselves but may participate in bone formation TGF-β, insulin-like growth factors, and basic fibroblast growth factor.

In addition to classifying bone graft substances by their osteoconductivity, osteogenicity, and osteoinductivity, another very useful method of describing graft materials is based on their use as bone graft extenders, enhancers, or bone graft substitutes. *Graft extenders* are substances that, when added to autogenous bone, allow for fusion of more levels or the use of smaller amounts of autogenous bone to produce fusion equal to that of autogenous bone graft alone. Therefore, graft materials that are extenders must be used with a certain amount of autograft to be effective. In contrast, *graft enhancers* allow for a higher rate of fusion when they are added to autogenous bone as compared with autogenous bone graft alone. Therefore, graft enhancers must also be used with autograft. *Bone graft substitutes* completely replace autogenous bone and produce equivalent fusion rates. Therefore, by definition, substitutes do not require any autograft bone at all. These terms are valid for only the indication and situation in which the graft material was tested. For instance, rhBMP-2 can serve as a bone graft substitute for anterior lumbar interbody fusion in certain situations; however, the same concentration of rhBMP-2 in the same carrier sponge is ineffective as a bone graft substitute in posterolateral lumbar spinal fusion.

Traditional Bone Grafts

The most common traditional bone graft is an autograft, typically harvested from the iliac crest. These grafts combine osteogenic, osteoinductive, and osteoconductive properties. Autografts can be either cancellous or cortical. Cortical grafts provide mechanical stability, but with less osteoconductivity and fewer osteogenic cells than cancellous graft. Cancellous grafts provide an excellent osteoconductive matrix and more osteogenic cells that can enhance fusion biology, but they have poor structural integrity. Tricortical iliac crest bone, the most popular autograft, has a combination of the useful properties of cortical and cancellous bone and therefore is an excellent choice for anterior cervical fusion. However, autografts have certain disadvantages. These include a limited supply, donor site morbidity, increased operative time, pain, blood loss, increased risk of infection, risk of cutaneous nerve damage, and even a small risk of local fracture.

The use of allograft was popularized to avoid some of the potential pitfalls associated with the morbidity of autologous bone graft harvest. Furthermore, allograft can be pre-processed into various physical shapes and forms, thus optimizing the architectural properties and making it easier for the surgeon to use intraoperatively. Currently, cortical allograft is used for ACDF. In this situation, the allograft has neither osteoinductivity nor osteogenicity and has very poor osteoconductivity. Nevertheless, for a single-level ACDF, allograft bone has been shown to be highly effective, with fusion rates similar to those with autograft bone.

Some disadvantages of allograft include limited supply as a result of limited donor availability, religious and cultural inhibitions, and the theoretical risk of disease transmission. Furthermore, allograft bone is probably not as effective as autograft for multilevel fusion. The reason may be due the absence of osteogenicity of the allograft or possibly decreased host biologic acceptance compared with autograft. However, immunogenicity is typically not considered an important factor for cortical processed allograft bone.

Biologics

Demineralized Bone Matrix

Marshall Urist discovered that demineralizing cortical bone produced a substance that could form bone when it was implanted into an ectopic location. Osteoinductivity was defined by this ability to form ectopic bone, and the discovery of osteoinductive materials led to the identification of BMPs. DBM is essentially acid-treated cortical bone. Careful demineralization of the cortical bone allows the natural BMPs that exist in bone to become biologically available and act to induce bone formation. This is the major advantage of DBM over untreated allograft. DBM, however, does not confer any structural support and must be used with cages or as a graft enhancer with allograft or autograft. Furthermore, all DBM preparations are not created equally because each company's product may differ in the concentration of osteoinductive factors based on the decalcification and preparation process.

Clinically, the evidence for DBMs is limited. An and associates first compared patients undergoing uninstrumented one- to two-level ACDF procedures who had allograft cortical bone combined with DBM versus autograft bone.[13] These investigators found that the allograft-DBM combination resulted in a slightly higher rate of graft collapse and pseudarthrosis. This study, however, had a relatively high nonunion rate for even autograft ACDF, which the investigators attributed to a high percentage of smokers and radiographic methodology.

In contrast, in a prospective study of patients treated with polyetheretherketone (PEEK) cages and Grafton DBM (Osteotech, Inc., Shrewsbury, N.J.), Park and colleagues found single-level and multilevel ACDF fusion rates comparable to those with traditional tricortical iliac crest bone graft. The investigators did not have any complications associated with the use of Grafton and concluded that this substance could be used as a safe alternative to autograft for anterior cervical fusions.[14] Topuz and co-workers followed patients treated with two-level ACDF with PEEK cages and DBM and found a 91% fusion rate and no DBM-specific complications at 3-year follow-up.[15]

Ceramics

Ceramics are a group of synthetic bone grafts consisting of calcium phosphate biomaterials fused into a polycrystalline structure by high temperatures (Fig. 48-2). Most calcium phosphate ceramics have a high degree of biocompatibility, but each ceramic differs slightly in its bioresorbability characteristics. The two most commonly studied ceramics are composed of either hydroxyapatite (HA) or tricalcium phosphate (TCP). The major role of ceramics is osteoconduction. In the late stages of bone formation, ceramics may exert some osteoinductive properties through an affinity to bind osteoinductive proteins onto a stable surface. The minimal macropore size needed for effective bone ingrowth is approximately 100 μm. The primary disadvantage of these implants is that they are brittle, with low impact and fracture resistance.

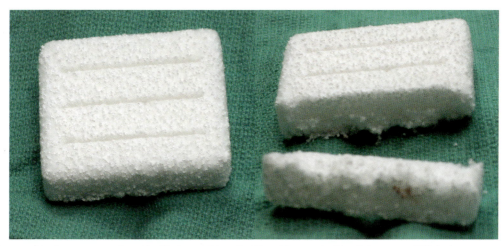

FIGURE 48-2   An example of a ceramic marketed by Medtronic (Memphis, Tenn. Minneapolis, Minn.). It contains 15% hydroxyapatite and 85% tricalcium phosphate admixed with collagen for easier handling characteristics.

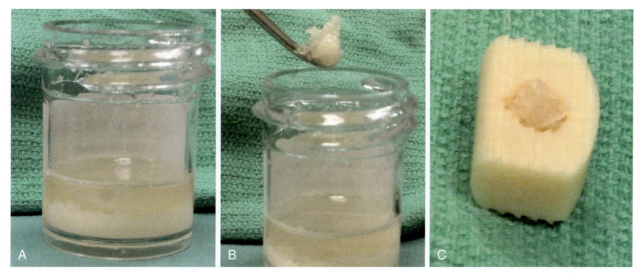

FIGURE 48-3   A, This allograft contains mesenchymal stem cells (Osteocel Plus, NuVasive, La Jolla, Calif.). The allograft is suspended in solution. **B,** The graft material can be collected and then, as an example, packed into a cortical allograft (**C**) for an anterior cervical diskectomy and fusion procedure.

Studies examining the clinical use of ceramics in the cervical spine are limited. Ceramic blocks were evaluated in the goat anterior cervical fusion model, with fusion rates ranging from 50% to 70%.[16,17] Various ceramics, however, have been studied in lumbar spinal fusions with good results.[18,19] One ceramic derived from coral has been tested as a graft in ACDF. Although the initial studies by Thalgott and associates showed 100% incorporation of the graft in the disk spaces, this finding has not been consistently replicated.[20] In fact, because of reports of graft fragmentation, this is not a popular stand-alone graft. Ceramics may play a better role as adjuvant grafts when used in conjunction with autografts or allografts. Ceramics may be useful to fill in voids or gaps left after anterior cervical grafting or as extenders in posterior cervical grafting.

Allograft Containing Mesenchymal Stem Cells

Another bone graft material marketed for fusion is allograft containing mesenchymal stem cells (Fig. 48-3).

The so-called minimally manipulated allograft is processed in a way that depletes nonmesenchymal cells and leaves the mesenchymal cells. These mesenchymal cells are purported to contain stem cells capable of providing the necessary osteoprogenitor cells for bone fusion. These stems cell are also theoretically self-renewing and can differentiate into various cell types depending on the surrounding milieu. Finally, because these cells express low levels of major histocompatibility complex and human leukocyte antigen class II antigens and co-stimulatory molecules, the ability of the host to mount an inflammatory response is diminished.[21,22]

However, the actual quantity and concentration of these stem cells in the allograft are unknown. Furthermore, the importance of this cellular component in contributing to bony fusion is the subject of debate because when these stem cells are combined with various carriers, they provide osteogenic, osteoconductive, and osteoinductive properties.[22,23] Whether the cells actually stay viable in the graft material for prolonged periods post-operatively is also unknown. Investigators have hypothesized that osteogenic cells may produce osteoinductive molecules that promote fusion.

Currently, two products are available for use. Trinity Evolution (Orthofix, Lewisville, Tex.) is an allogenic cancellous bone matrix containing cryopreserved adult stem and osteoprogenitor cells and a demineralized bone component. This product has been used successfully in other orthopedic situations, particularly in the foot and ankle. With respect to use in the cervical spine, the manufacturer is enrolling patients in a prospective trial using allograft mesenchymal stem cells with a structural graft or cage. Definitive studies proving efficacy and safety have not been published.

The other product being marketed is Osteocel Plus (NuVasive, La Jolla, Calif.). Like Trinity Evolution, Osteocel Plus is an allograft cellular bone matrix containing viable allograft mesenchymal stem cells. These cells are retained after proprietary processing within the allogeneic cancellous bone chips. DBM is then added to formulate the mixture and is cryopreserved at temperatures between −60 and −80° C. According to the manufacturer, more than 20,000 patients have been treated with Osteocel in various applications, with no adverse events reported. As with Trinity Evolution, the clinical data in the cervical spine are sparse. Reports noted successful use of Osteocel and PEEK cages in 46 patients undergoing ACDF. The fusion rate was reportedly 100% for 1-level, 97.1% for 2-level, and 83.3% for 3-level procedures. Fusion was determined by flexion and extension radiographs and occurred between 8 and 12 weeks.[24] Currently, the manufacturer of this product is actively recruiting patients to examine its use in lumbar interbody fusions, as well as cervical fusions. Definitive studies proving efficacy and safety have not been published.

Growth Factors: Bone Morphogenetic Protein Family

BMPs are multifunctional growth factors that belong to the TGF-β superfamily. Multiple members of the BMP subfamily have been discovered. The osteoinductive property of BMPs was first identified in the 1960s, and the proteins were purified and discovered to be responsible for bone induction in the late 1980s. Since that time, BMPs have been shown to mediate mesenchymal differentiation, cell proliferation, and chemotaxis, resulting in the transient formation of cartilage and the production of living bone. Not all members of the BMP family of genes possess osteoinductive properties. In the United States, two of the osteoinductive BMPs (BMP-2 and BMP-7) have undergone U.S. Food and Drug Administration (FDA) trials for spine fusion indications.

Leach and Bittar reported on the *off-label* use of rhBMP-7 (OP-1, Stryker, Kalamazoo, Mich.) in anterior cervical fusion surgery.[25] One hundred-twenty three patients were treated with ACDF using interbody cages and BMP-7. No autograft or allografts were used. The primary outcome was the presence of clinical adverse events during the first 30 days, and the secondary outcome was the extent of radiographic evidence of soft tissue swelling. One patient had transient brachialgia and 2 had dysphagia, a complication rate of 2.4%. The investigators concluded that rhBMP-7 could be safely used in anterior spinal fusion in an off-label fashion. The rate of fusion was not reported, however. Initially, OP-1 was approved for use in posterior revision lumbar surgery and received a Humanitarian Device Exemption; however, it did not receive FDA approval for routine use in that clinical situation. Use of rhBMP-7 in the cervical spine remains off-label and controversial today.

Currently, only rhBMP-2 has been approved for use in the spine (Medtronic, Minneapolis, Minn.). Use of rhBMP-2 in the spine is approved only in anterior lumbar surgery with a particular threaded structural cage. Use of rhBMP-2 outside of that clinical indication remains highly controversial and off-label. Furthermore, use of rhBMP-2 in the anterior cervical spine may have significant adverse effects attributable to this agent. The main complications associated with its use in the cervical spine are soft tissue swelling with subsequent dysphagia, dysphonia, and airway compromise, as well as neurologic deficits. These complications resulted in a black box warning by the FDA in 2008 for significant dangers when rhBMP-2 is used in anterior cervical surgical procedures.

Nevertheless, many clinicians have supported the use of rhBMP-2 in the cervical spine as an effective bone graft enhancer. The rationale for its use in the cervical spine stems from success in the off-label use in posterior lumbar fusion situations. rhBMP-2 has been shown to decrease operative time, blood loss, and hospital stay, as well as increase fusion rate, after lumbar spinal fusion. In anterior cervical surgical procedures, use of rhBMP-2 may also help avoid the risks of autograft harvest, increase fusion rate, and eliminate possible disease transmission from allograft.

As stated previously, use of rhBMP-2 in anterior cervical spine surgical procedures has potentially dangerous complications. To date, at least 38 reports of soft tissue swelling in the neck have been reported. The complications generally occurred between day 2 and day 14. The exact cause of the adverse swelling reported is unknown, but it is thought to be secondary to local inflammation triggered by the BMP.

Shields and colleagues reviewed 151 patients (138 with ACDF and 13 with corpectomy) who underwent anterior spinal fusion with rhBMP-2 (2.1 mg/level).[26] rhBMP-2 was placed in the cage and in some cases lateral and anterior to the cage or graft. The investigators reported a complication rate of 23.2% (10% hematoma and 9% prolonged hospital stay for dysphagia or dyspnea). Postoperative hematoma was seen in 15 patients; 8 of these patients required surgical evacuation, and 13 patients needed readmission specific to dysphagia, respiratory compromise, and incisional swelling. Smucker and coworkers also reported a complication rate of 27.5% with adverse swelling affecting 5 patients who required reexploration.[27] The concentration used was 1.5 mg/mL. Theories to explain these complications include dosing and containment within the cage.

With dosing and containment issues considered, studies have demonstrated safer use with rhBMP. Baskin and associates compared InFuse (0.4 mL of a 1.5 mg/mL rhBMP-2 solution, Medtronic Sofamor Danek, Memphis, Tenn.) with fibular allograft to iliac crest bone graft when used within a structural cortical allograft in a randomized, prospective, controlled study.[28] Thirty-three patients were enrolled. No implant-related or device-related adverse events occurred in either group with complete fusion by 6 months postoperatively. Two instances of anterior bone formation at adjacent segments in the rhBMP-2 group and one in the control group were reported. Boakye and colleagues also used InFuse with PEEK cages and reported that 2 of 24 patients had transient dysphagia, which was not attributed to rhBMP. All patients received 10 mg dexamethasone at the start of the procedure.[29]

Tumialan and co-workers also demonstrated safer use of a low dose of rhBMP-2 (as low as 0.7 mg per level); 7% of patients (14 patients) had complications.[30] Four of these patients required repeated operation for evacuation of either a postoperative hematoma or a seroma. Three other patients required readmission within 1 week of the initial surgical procedure for difficulty swallowing or breathing. These patients were treated with a brief course of steroids and then discharged. Fourteen patients (7%) had clinically significant dysphagia that either delayed discharge, altered diet, or required supplemental nutrition. Six patients had mild dysphagia, 3 had moderate, and 5 had severe. Of the 5 with severe dysphagia, 4 required a gastric tube for feeding. This study also had a tiered group because the investigators decreased the amount of rhBMP-2 from an initial 2.1 mg per level to 1.05 mg and then to 0.7 mg per level. In patients with the lowest dose, 5 patients had complications. Three had severe dysphagia, and 2 needed reexplorations. All nondiabetic patients also received 10 mg of dexamethasone (Decadron) at the time of the surgical procedure as protocol.

Another issue with use of rhBMP-2 in the anterior spine is osteolysis. Klimo and Peelle presented 22 patients (38 cervical levels) who underwent spinal fusion using PEEK spacers and varying doses of BMP.[31] Moderate or severe osteolysis in 57% of the levels led to subsidence and loss of alignment. In contrast, Tumialan and associates reported no end plate resorption and subsidence with use of BMP and PEEK cages in the cervical spine.[30] Vaidya and colleagues reported 100% incidence of end plate resorption but only subsidence in 40.5% of cervical levels.[32]

With these complications, the question remains whether BMP should be used in the anterior cervical spine because the historical success rate for fusion in ACDF without BMP is very high. However, some patients have a high risk of nonunion, and the use of rhBMP-2 may be considered. These high-risk patients may have a combination of various risk factors such as smoking or tobacco use, with multilevel disease, osteoporosis, long-term steroid use, revision surgery, or metabolic bone disease. In addition, the use of rhBMP-2 may decrease the need for a combined anterior and posterior fusion surgical procedure in some cases by increasing the anterior fusion rate. Nevertheless, the use of rhBMP-2 in the anterior cervical spine is highly controversial and warrants further research.

rhBMP-2 has also been used in off-label fashion in the posterior cervical spine in both adults and pediatric patients.[33-36] Its use posteriorly also has complications. For example, Shahlaie and Kim reported neurologic decline

associated with significant tissue swelling and seroma formation after the posterior cervical use of rhBMP-2.[34] In addition, Crawford and associates found a higher, but not statistically significant, incidence of posterior wound complications in a study comparing rhBMP-2 with iliac crest bone graft in a retrospective study.[35] The reported complications were increased wound drainage, culture-positive infections, and possibly sterile fluid collections. The average rhBMP-2 per level was 3.6 mg. The rhBMP-2 dose for patients with a wound infection was 2.9 mg per level compared with 3.7 mg for patients without a wound infection. In another large retrospective study, rhBMP-2 was found to be safe. In the group of patients who received rhBMP-2, a new neurologic deficit was found in 6% compared with 4%, wound infection requiring further surgery occurred in 12% versus 0%, and no postoperative hematomas and 6% significant neck swelling were noted compared with 0%; 1.3 mL of a 1.5 mg/mL rhBMP-2 solution was used per level.[33] Nevertheless, the routine use of rhBMP-2 in the posterior cervical spine continues to be controversial, off-label, and experimental and requires further research before widespread use can be supported.

In summary, the use of rhBMP-2 in the cervical spine is not straightforward. The optimal concentration and carrier system must be clarified, and the associated complications need to be investigated. Until the risk and advantages of its use are studied further, any use of rhBMP-2 in the cervical spine remains controversial and off-label.

Conclusions

With further advances and expanding knowledge of the biologic processes of bone fusion, newer technologies in the realm of biologics have the potential to increase fusion rates and minimize the complications of pseudarthrosis. The use of engineered products may eliminate the need for autograft and the morbidity associated with bone graft harvesting. Ultimately, a plethora of options will be at the disposal of the surgeon. However, caution should be advised in using the new technology without understanding how the product works and clinically extrapolating how this technology may benefit the patient. Ultimately, one cannot forget to pursue meticulous fusion bed preparation and to educate patients about controllable factors, such as smoking, to optimize the possibility of fusion. In the near future, advances will likely occur in the more efficient and effective delivery of current biologics.

REFERENCES

1. Perren SM: Biological internal fixation: its background, methods, requirements, potential and limits, *Acta Chir Orthop Traumatol Cech* 67:6–12, 2000.
2. Perren SM: Evolution of the internal fixation of long bone fractures: the scientific basis of biological internal fixation: choosing a new balance between stability and biology, *J Bone JointS urg Br* 84:1093–1110, 2002.
3. Perren SM: Fracture healing: the evolution of our understanding, *Acta Chir Orthop Traumatol Cech* 75:241–246, 2008.
4. Zeidman SM, Ducker TB, Raycroft J: Trends and complications in cervical spine surgery: 1989-1993, *J Spinal Disord* 10:523–526, 1997.

5. Cannada L K, Scherping S C, Yoo J U, et al.: Pseudoarthrosis of the cervical spine: a comparison of radiographic diagnostic measures, *Spine (Phila Pa 1976)* 28:46–51, 2003.

6. Wang J C, McDonough P W, Endow K K, Delamarter R B: Increased fusion rates with cervical plating for two-level anterior cervical discectomy and fusion, *Spine (Phila Pa 1976)* 25:41–45, 2000.

7. Wang J C, McDonough P W, Kanim L E, et al.: Increased fusion rates with cervical plating for three-level anterior cervical discectomy and fusion, *Spine (Phila Pa 1976)* 26:643–646, 2001. discussion 646–647.

8. Samartzis D, Shen F H, Matthews D K, et al.: Comparison of allograft to autograft in multilevel anterior cervical discectomy and fusion with rigid plate fixation, *Spine J* 3:451–459, 2003.

9. Brooks A L, Jenkins E B: Atlanto-axial arthrodesis by the wedge compression method, *J Bone Joint Surg Am* 60:279–284, 1978.

10. Chan D P, Ngian K S, Cohen L: Posterior upper cervical fusion in rheumatoid arthritis, *Spine (Phila Pa 1976)* 17:268–272, 1992.

11. Clark C R, Goetz D D, Menezes A H: Arthrodesis of the cervical spine in rheumatoid arthritis, *J Bone Joint Surg Am* 71:3813–3892, 1989.

12. Sawin P D, Traynelis V C, Menezes A H: A comparative analysis of fusion rates and donor-site morbidity for autogeneic rib and iliac crest bone grafts in posterior cervical fusions, *J Neurosurg* 88:255–265, 1998.

13. An H S, Simpson J M, Glover J M, Stephany J: Comparison between allograft plus demineralized bone matrix versus autograft in anterior cervical fusion: a prospective multicenter study, *Spine (Phila Pa 1976)* 20:2211–2216, 1995.

14. Park H W, Lee J K, Moon S J, et al.: The efficacy of the synthetic interbody cage and Grafton for anterior cervical fusion, *Spine (Phila Pa 1976)* 34:E591–E595, 2009.

15. Topuz K, Colak A, Kaya S, et al.: Two-level contiguous cervical disc disease treated with peek cages packed with demineralized bone matrix: results of 3-year follow-up, *Eur Spine J* 18:238–243, 2009.

16. Zdeblick T A, Cooke M E, Kunz D N, et al.: Anterior cervical discectomy and fusion using a porous hydroxyapatite bone graft substitute, *Spine (Phila Pa 1976)* 19:2348–2357, 1994.

17. Pintar F A, Maiman D J, Hollowell J P, et al.: Fusion rate and biomechanical stiffness of hydroxylapatite versus autogenous bone grafts for anterior discectomy: an in vivo animal study, *Spine (Phila Pa 1976)* 19:2524–2528, 1994.

18. Epstein N E: A preliminary study of the efficacy of beta tricalcium phosphate as a bone expander for instrumented posterolateral lumbar fusions, *J Spinal Disord Tech* 19:424–429, 2006.

19. Lerner T, Bullmann V, Schulte T L, et al.: A level-1 pilot study to evaluate of ultraporous beta-tricalcium phosphate as a graft extender in the posterior correction of adolescent idiopathic scoliosis, *Eur Spine J* 18:170–179, 2009.

20. Thalgott J S, Fritts K, Giuffre J M, Timlin M: Anterior interbody fusion of the cervical spine with coralline hydroxyapatite, *Spine (Phila Pa 1976)* 24:1295–1299, 1999.

21. Schu S, Nosov M, O'Flynn L, et al.: Immunogenicity of allogenic mesencymal stem cells, *J Cell Mol Med* 16:2094–2103, 2012.

22. Grabowski G, Robertson R N: Bone allograft with mesenchymal stem cells: a critical review of the literature, *Hard Tissue* 2:20, 2013.

23. Grabowski G, Cornett C A: Bone graft and bone graft substitutes in spine surgery: current concepts and controversies, *J Am Acad Orthop Surg* 21:51–60, 2013.

24. Mohan V, Templin C, Lorenz M A, Zindrick M R: *Allograft mesechymal stem cells for anterior cervical discectomy and fusion*, Toronto, 2010, International Meeting on Advanced Spine Techniques.

25. Leach J, Bittar R G: BMP-7 (OP-1) safety in anterior cervical fusion surgery, *J Clin Neurosci* 16:1417–1420, 2009.

26. Shields L B, Raque G H, Glassman S D, et al.: Adverse effects associated with high-dose recombinant human bone morphogenetic protein-2 use in anterior cervical spine fusion, *Spine (Phila Pa 1976)* 31:542–547, 2006.

27. Smucker J D, Rhee J M, Singh K, et al.: Increased swelling complications associated with off-label usage of rhBMP-2 in the anterior cervical spine, *Spine (Phila Pa 1976)* 31:2813–2819, 2006.

28. Baskin D S, Ryan P, Sonntag V, et al.: A prospective, randomized, controlled cervical fusion study using recombinant human bone morphogenetic protein-2 with the CORNERSTONE-SR allograft ring and the ATLANTIS anterior cervical plate, *Spine (Phila Pa 1976)* 28:1219–1224, 2003. discussion 1225.

29. Boakye M, Mummaneni P V, Garrett M, et al.: Anterior cervical discectomy and fusion involving a polyetheretherketone spacer and bone morphogenetic protein, *J Neurosurg Spine* 2:521–525, 2005.

30. Tumialan L M, Pan J, Rodts G E, Mummaneni P V: The safety and efficacy of anterior cervical discectomy and fusion with polyetheretherketone spacer and recombinant human bone morphogenetic protein-2: a review of 200 patients, *J Neurosurg Spine* 8:529–535, 2008.

31. Klimo P Jr, Peelle M W: Use of polyetheretherketone spacer and recombinant human bone morphogenetic protein-2 in the cervical spine: a radiographic analysis, *Spine J* 9:959–966, 2009.

32. Vaidya R, Carp J, Sethi A, et al.: Complications of anterior cervical discectomy and fusion using recombinant human bone morphogenetic protein-2, *Eur Spine J* 16:1257–1265, 2007.

33. Hiremath G K, Steinmetz M P, Krishnaney A A: Is it safe to use recombinant human bone morphogenetic protein in posterior cervical fusion? *Spine (Phila Pa 1976)* 34:885–889, 2009.

34. Shahlaie K, Kim K D: Occipitocervical fusion using recombinant human bone morphogenetic protein-2: adverse effects due to tissue swelling and seroma, *Spine (Phila Pa 1976)* 33:2361–2366, 2008.

35. Crawford C H 3rd, Carreon L Y, McGinnis M D, et al.: Perioperative complications of recombinant human bone morphogenetic protein-2 on an absorbable collagen sponge versus iliac crest bone graft for posterior cervical arthrodesis, *Spine (Phila Pa 1976)* 34:1390–1394, 2009.

36. Oluigbo C O, Solanki G A: Use of recombinant human bone morphogenetic protein-2 to enhance posterior cervical spine fusion at 2 years of age: technical note, *Pediatr Neurosurg* 44:393–396, 2008.

Intervertebral Disk Transplantation

49

Jason Pui Yin Cheung, Dino Samartzis, Dike Ruan, and Keith DK Luk

CHAPTER PREVIEW

Chapter Synopsis

The current gold standard for treatment of disk degeneration is spinal fusion. Although effective in controlling pain, spinal fusion leads to restricted spinal motion and potentially to adjacent level degeneration. The goal of management should be to restore the functional spinal unit. This can be done with artificial or biologic disk replacements. Artificial total disk replacements are gaining popularity, and early results are encouraging; however, they are not without their challenges and complications. As an alternative, the concept of allograft disk transplantation began in 1991, and multiple studies were performed to verify this technique in animal models. Experiments on disk autografts, allografts, and fresh frozen allografts have been performed. Viability has been proven with these experiments, and active regeneration of the disk has been noted morphologically. A small-scale clinical trial has also been conducted. Further research is required to expand on issues regarding graft harvesting, preservation techniques, surgical implantation techniques, and immunoreaction, to validate disk transplantation as an option for the treatment of degenerative disk disease.

Important Points

Artificial and biologic disk replacements can help restore the functional spine unit by preserving anatomy, motion, and stability.

Disk transplantation has been studied as an autograft, allograft, and fresh frozen allograft and was successful in retaining cell viability and maintaining mechanical properties.

Disk cells can retain the best overall metabolic activity, elastic modulus, and viscous modulus of a normal disk by a slow cooling rate, in combination of cryoprotective agents with limited incubation time.

Further research is required on graft harvesting, preservation, and surgical implantation techniques and on the immune reaction.

With aging, the nucleus pulposus of the intervertebral disk begins to desiccate, characterized by a loss of aggrecan core proteins, glycosaminoglycan, matrix turnover, and cell numbers that eventually leads to losing the ability to imbibe water. As the nucleus pulposus loses its water content, the disk can no longer distribute forces effectively. The annulus fibrosus buckles under compressive loading, and this leads to disk collapse. Further load on the annulus fibrosus leads to fissuring and cracks. Loss of disk height also leads to overriding facet joints. Uneven loading causes osteophyte formation and joint instability. Pain associated with intervertebral disk degeneration can be caused by bulging or rupturing of the annulus with herniation of disk material irritating the pain fibers in the peripheral part of the annulus. Neural tissues are also implicated in herniated disks as a result of mechanical or chemical irritation. Finally, degenerated facet joints,

together with instability, subluxation, or deformity of the functional spinal unit (FSU), can also produce pain.

If conservative modalities fail, surgical intervention is indicated, especially in those patients with significant neurologic compromise. Classically, the most common surgical treatment for lumbar disk degeneration is spinal fusion.[1,2] Although effective in controlling pain, fusion leads to restriction of the spinal motion and may cause adjacent level degeneration secondary to increased stress and motion at adjacent levels.[3-5] The goals of surgical treatment of lumbar spine degeneration are to relieve any neural compression and to maintain a stable FSU that is free of deformity. Thus, many different types of intervertebral disk implants have been advocated to avoid the effects of spinal fusion and to preserve motion. Artificial disks made of metals, polymers, or combinations of materials have been attempted and are gaining popularity. The early results of total disk replacement (TDR) are encouraging and are at least comparable to the results of spinal fusion.[6-9] However, questions have been raised regarding the implant material, design kinematics, recipient factors, surgical precision, and long-term outcome and salvage options.[10-14] An interesting long-term study of artificial disk replacement showed that the best results occurred in patients who had spontaneous fusion in the replaced disk.[15,16]

Disk replacements can also be biologic, with the goals of preserving anatomy, motion, and stability. Theoretically, one could manufacture a disk scaffold using tissue engineering technology. Appropriate cells with necessary promoter growth factors can be used to populate this scaffold. Regeneration or repair of the disk by using growth factors, gene therapy, and cell therapy is being actively researched.[17] Most experiments are focused on the rejuvenation of the nucleus pulposus by restoring the matrix production through increasing cell numbers. However, this approach has a major flaw because the annulus fibrosus is also structurally and mechanically incompetent when the disk is degenerated to the point of causing symptoms. In addition, the delivery channel in which nutrients reach the disk is also jeopardized. This limits sustained cell viability and the ability for cells to restore the matrix or to repair the damaged annulus fibrosus. Current evidence suggests that cellular therapy is unable to restore the matrix content in advanced disk degeneration but can only maintain it in mild degeneration.[18,19]

The concept of disk transplantation began in 1991 when Olson and associates reconstructed a spinal column defect by using a quadruped model transplantation of a vertebral body together with the two adjacent disks to act as a spacer.[20] Relatively normal mobility and stability of the spinal column were found because of partial revascularization of the intervening vertebral body and the intervertebral disks. The same research group followed up with a fresh autograft disk transfer in a canine model.[21] In this experiment, the morphology and the metabolic functions of the transplanted disks were abnormal, but the structure and function were maintained. The likely cause of these findings was attributed to the rigidly fixed transplanted disks, which jeopardized disk nutrition. Further studies by Katsuura and Hukuda,[22] as well as by Matsuzaki and colleagues,[23] used cryopreserved allografts in quadruped models, but these investigators experienced the same limitation of rigid fixation of the grafts with plates and screws.

Around the same time as the study by Olson and colleagues, Professor Keith DK Luk and investigators at the Department of Orthopaedics and Traumatology at the University of Hong Kong had a similar idea of disk transplantation that avoided constraining the transplanted graft. Experiments were conducted in upright primates, the model closest to human biomechanics. A series of experiments was performed to verify this animal model, disk autograft, disk allograft, and fresh frozen allograft. Further studies were carried out to validate the storage processing technique and implantation technique. A small-scale clinical trial was conducted in 2000 to prove the applicability of this technique in clinical practice. The following discussion provides an account of the evolution of allograft disk transplantation from animal models to the latest clinical trial outcomes, as based on the experience of investigators at the University of Hong Kong and their collaborators.

Animal Models and Graft Experimentation

Autograft Experiment

In 1992, the first autograft experiment was initiated at the Tangdu Hospital, Affiliated Hospital of the Fourth Military Medical University, Xian, China in collaboration with Dr. Dike Ruan. The animal model used was the rhesus monkey. Fourteen male monkeys were followed up for 2, 4, and 6 months, and 2 monkeys were followed up for 12 months. The L3-L4 intervertebral disk was isolated without damaging the surrounding structures, and the composite graft was repositioned into the disk space and anchored to the outer annulus. No rigid internal fixation or external immobilizer was used, and the animal was allowed to move freely. Serial radiographs were used to measure the disk height and observe for any degeneration. A gradual reduction in the disk height was noted postoperatively but was stabilized at 2 to 4 months, and some disk height was regained at the 12-month final follow-up. Autografts were retrieved from the animals and underwent biochemical, histologic, and biomechanical testing. Analysis showed no statistical significant changes of water, proteoglycan, and hydroxyproline contents with time. A continuing drop in water content was reported; an initial drop was followed by an increase in proteoglycan and persistently raised hydroxyproline in the nucleus fibrosus. Viable cells were seen at the annulus fibrosus and nucleus pulposus on histologic examination. The morphology of the annulus was found to be well preserved. The grafted disk had an initial period of hypermobility in all ranges of motion at 2 to 4 months postoperatively but returned to normal by 6 months. Cells in the composite autograft were able to withstand a transient period of ischemia and were able to recover their biochemical and biomechanical function.[24] As a result, a bipedal animal model was found to be a successful model in studies of intervertebral disk transplantation.

Allograft Experiment

Fresh allograft transplants must be examined to see how they behave when sourced from a live or freshly dead donor. The problem of immunogenicity must also be addressed. Similar to the cornea for the eye and the meniscus for the knee, the intervertebral disk is immunologically privileged because of its avascularity. This experiment was confirmed by switching the L3-L4 disks in two monkeys. No rhesus factor or blood grouping was performed for the monkeys, and no immunosuppressants were given, based on the knowledge that allografts have already been used in joint replacement revisions or tumor reconstructions without immunosuppressant agents. The two monkeys in the experiment were of similar age and size and were operated on simultaneously by two teams of surgeons and anesthesiologists to minimize the operating time and the blood loss. In this experiment, problems of repeated subluxation and dislocation secondary to graft size mismatch were reported. From this failure, appropriate graft size matching and press-fit fixation were vital to obtaining stability of the transplant without rigid internal fixation.

Fresh Frozen Allograft

Fresh frozen allografts were used for disk transplantation to confirm the feasibility of the procedure further. Specifically, this experiment was necessary to help resolve issues of organ donation, preservation, physical size, and immunocompatibility of the grafts. Seventeen monkeys were used. Two monkeys were donors of the disks, and 3 others were used as controls. The other 12 monkeys were followed up for 2 to 8 weeks, 6 months, and 24 months. Sections from T10 to L7 were harvested and split into 1- to 2-mm segments along with adjacent end plates. The grafts were measured and were immersed in a dimethylsulfoxide (DMSO) solution and cooled stepwise to −196° C in liquid nitrogen for storage.

After the disk was removed from the recipient, an appropriately sized graft was thawed and placed to fit snugly into the defect. No immunosuppressant was used. Bony union of the end plates was obtained successfully in all cases without any complication of graft subluxation or dislocation. Up to the 24-month final follow-up, the disk height was found to have a slow and progressive reduction with secondary degenerative changes of traction osteophytes. In contrast to the autograft, the water and proteoglycan content had a steady decrease from 6 to 24 months. As compared with the controls, the grafted FSU maintained similar mechanical stability and mobility. Histologic examination was also performed to look for immunoreactivity and showed inflammatory cells infiltration with lymphocytic and fibroblastic proliferation limited only at the osteotomy site. Yet this reaction was significantly reduced at 8 weeks of follow-up. The numbers of cells in both the annulus fibrosus and the nucleus pulposus were similar at early follow-up and at 24-month follow-up, the cells of the nucleus pulposus underwent degeneration with features of irregular nuclear shape, mitochondrial swelling, and karyopyknosis.

This study confirmed that, similar to autografts, a cryopreserved allograft could retain cell viability and maintain mechanical properties.[25] The cryopreservation process could also cause minimal or no immunoreaction during disk transplantation. The minimal immunoreaction seen in this experiment was found only at the bone interface; thus, mechanical washout of the cancellous end plates should be performed before preservation. This experiment found that degeneration of the transplanted allograft still occurred. Further research should refine the preservation protocol to increase cell viability and reduce early graft degeneration.[26] This is important because long-term storage of allografts in a bank is a vital part of allograft transplantation procedures. The use of cryopreservation is necessary for safe preservation of the intervertebral disk allograft.

Cryopreservation Experiments

Two further studies were published to improve knowledge of the cryopreservation process further.

Cryopreservation must retain both mechanical properties and cellular activity, and so this method was refined with different cooling rates, solutions for immersion, and incubation times. The first study, published in 2010, was able to optimize survival of disk cells by modulating cooling rates, cryoprotective agents (CPAs) concentration, and incubation time in porcine lumbar disks.[27] In this study, 52 porcine lumbar disks (L2-L3 to L4-L5) were obtained from 22 pigs. Three different rates of cooling were tested by immersing disk samples in cryopreservation solution in either a precooled glass container filled with 80° C isopropanol, a precooled glass container filled with 4° C isopropanol, or a 16 × 11.5 × 21 cm polystyrene box that was 1.6 cm thick. Three different cryopreservation formulas were also tested, including the traditional formula of 10% DMSO, 10% DMSO with 10% propylene glycol, and 10% DMSO with 0.1% Supercool X-1000. Different precooling intubation time periods between 2 and 4 hours in the cryopreservation solution were also tested. Metabolic activity, mechanical property, and histologic features of the allografts were evaluated by comparing them with fresh specimens. The authors found that a slow cooling rate (−0.3° C/minute), a combination of cryoprotective agents (10% DMSO and 10% propylene glycol), and a limited cryoprotective agent incubation time of 2 hours favored the overall metabolic activity of disk cells up to 60% of the fresh control. The mechanical property and matrix organization were maintained with this method.

The second study, published in 2011, further analyzed the variable cryoprotective agents and their effects on the biomechanical properties of the allografts.[28] Forty disks (from L1 to L6) were harvested from 9 pigs. Corneal Potassium TES 2 solution (CPTES2) was used as the cryoprotective agent carrier solution. Different cryoprotective agent concentrations were used in combination with CPTES2 for cryopreservation. These included CPTES2 only, 10% DMSO in CPTES2 solution, and 10% DMSO with 10% propylene glycol in CPTES2 solution. Disks were incubated at 4° C for 2 hours and were stored after freezing to −80° C and in liquid nitrogen for 4 weeks. All disks were thawed to 37° C in a saline bath before analysis. Uniaxial compression testing and viscoelastic properties were investigated. The results showed that allografts that were cryopreserved with cryoprotective agents were able to preserve the normal elastic modulus and viscous modulus of an intervertebral disk, whereas allografts without cryopreservatives were stiffer. Although this study further confirms that cryopreservation can preserve the mechanical properties of an intervertebral disk allograft, only human studies can truly validate this finding.

Biomechanical Studies on Graft Positioning

Besides the issues surrounding storage, the technical aspects of allograft disk placement and the determination whether malpositioning of the allograft would affect the kinematics of the FSU and lead to early failure were equally important. A biomechanical study addressed the effect of remodeling on the kinematics of the malpositioned disk allograft transplantation.[29]

Eighteen male goats were used in this study. Three goats were selected as donors of their intervertebral disks, whereas the other goats were assigned randomly to control, allograft, and malpositioned allograft groups. All goats were followed up for 6 months. The 3 donor goats were sacrificed, and the entire spinal column of T13 to S1 was harvested en bloc. Preparation included osteotomy at the end plates 1 to 2 mm above and below the disks and washing of the grafts with saline and immersion in 10% DMSO and 10% calf serum for 2 hours at 4° C to preserve cellular viability. The disks were then placed at −15° C for 1 hour, −40° C for 1 hour, and −80° C for 1 hour, after which the disk grafts were preserved in liquid nitrogen at −196° C until implantation.

L4-L5 diskectomy and complete removal of the posterior annulus with preservation of the posterior longitudinal ligament were performed in the recipient goats. The preserved frozen disk allograft of the most compatible size was selected and was positioned into the disk space. For the well-aligned groups, the disk allograft was positioned and aligned to the anterior vertebral margin of the excised disk. For the malaligned group, the allograft implant was placed proud anteriorly by 25% of the allograft's anteroposterior length. Sutures were used to fix the allografts in place by attaching them to the outer annulus.

In vitro three-dimensional kinematics was performed by placing a pure moment of 5 Nm to the top vertebra. This continuous moment was applied at 0.5 degrees per second in the axis of flexion and extension, bilateral and lateral bending, and axial rotation. Five complete loading cycles were applied, with the first four used for preconditioning and the fifth for analysis. Analysis found no significant differences in flexion, axial rotation, and lateral bending. A significant increase in extension motion was observed in both the aligned allograft group and the malpositioned allograft group as compared with the control group. This difference was likely caused by early degeneration in the transplanted allograft in response to its more fibrotic nucleus pulposus resulting from decreased water content. No significant differences in range of motion were noted between the aligned and malpositioned groups. In summary, intervertebral disk allograft transplantation did not compromise the stability of the lumbar spine or motion parameters. In this study, precise positioning of the allograft did not affect the overall survival of the FSU. Despite these promising findings, human studies are ultimately required to validate findings.

Clinical Trial

With the experimental studies showing promising results, a small-scale clinical trial was initiated in 2000 after obtaining approval from the appropriate institutional-national authority and informed consent of the patients. Between March 2000 and January 2001, disk transplantation was performed in the first five subjects with cervical disk herniation and spinal cord compression at the Navy General Hospital in Beijing. Results at 5-year follow-up were published in *The Lancet* in 2007.[30]

The grafts were obtained from three previously healthy young female trauma victims within 2 hours of their death. These hosts were screened to exclude any bone abnormality or degenerative disk disease from radiographs and also any transmissible diseases (hepatitis B and C, tuberculosis, and human immunodeficiency virus infection).

All allografts were immersed in 10% DMSO and 10% calf serum (GibcoBRL/Invitrogen, Carlsbad, Calif.) in a special container and were stored at −196° C in liquid nitrogen. For the recipient, diskectomy, including removal of the posterior longitudinal ligament, was performed for complete decompression of the spinal cord and when the dura was exposed. The defect was measured, and an appropriately sized allograft was thawed in a water bath of 37° C and snugly fitted into the defect. No internal fixation was required, and the postoperative regimen included full-time use of a neck collar for 2 weeks and part-time use for 4 weeks. A single dose of cephalosporin was given as prophylaxis preoperatively and was continued for 3 days postoperatively. No immunosuppressive agents were used. Regular dynamic flexion and extension radiographs and preoperative, postoperative, and final follow-up magnetic resonance imaging (MRI) scans were performed for assessment. Grading of the nucleus pulposus in T2-weighted MRI was performed using the modified Schneiderman scale.[31] The Japanese Orthopedic Association (JOA) scoring system was used for assessing the improvement in neurologic status.

The first five patients (one female and four male) all presented with classic symptoms of pyramidal tract compression. One patient had traumatic cervical disk herniation with acute paraparesis, whereas the other four patients had chronic cervical spondylotic myelopathy. No complications of the procedure, including subluxation or dislocation of the graft or immunoreaction, occurred, but one graft was too anteriorly positioned. However, this malpositioned graft had complete remodeling by the fifth year of follow-up, with creeping substitution as evidenced by relocation of the annulus fibrosus and preservation of the nucleus pulposus (Fig. 49-1). This outcome proved that the allograft was viable and was able to regenerate. All patients improved with surgical treatment. The patient with incomplete paraplegia improved neurologically from Frankel B grade to D grade postoperatively. The JOA score of the other four patients with myelopathy improved from a mean score of 11/17 to 14.8/17. At 5-year follow-up, no patients had significant neck pain, and only one patient had loss of disk height on radiographs. All except one patient had between 7 and 11.3 degrees of motion at the grafted disk site (Fig. 49-2). The remaining patient had spontaneous fusion of the disk after a revision posterior foraminotomy procedure for residual radiculopathy. Using Schneiderman scoring, early degeneration was noted postoperatively. Yet in the final follow-up, the score improved; at least two of the allografts showed a higher T2-weighted signal on MRI than did the original preoperative disk (Fig. 49-3).

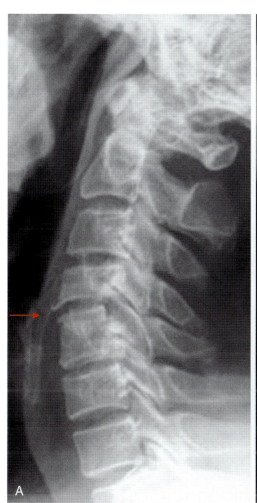
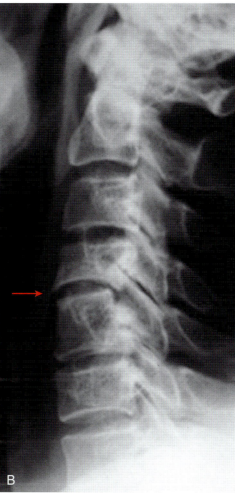

FIGURE 49-1   A, Lateral view of the cervical spine showing a malpositioned C4-C5 allograft 3 months postoperatively. **B,** Lateral view of the same disk showing complete remodeling 6 years postoperatively. (Modified from Ruan D, He Q, Ding Y, et al: Intervertebral disc transplantation in the treatment of degenerative spine disease: a preliminary study. *Lancet* 369:993-999, 2007.)

Surgical Procedure

The patient is placed in the supine position, endotracheal anesthesia is administered, and a Halter traction harness is applied. The spine is exposed with a right-sided Smith-Robinson approach through a transverse or longitudinal incision. After the surgeon verifies the index level with intraoperative fluoroscopy, the anterior longitudinal ligament and any anterior osteophytes are removed. A near-total diskectomy is performed, with removal of the posterior longitudinal ligament and the Luschka joints to ensure complete spinal cord and root decompression. After fashioning the intervertebral gap into a roughly cuboid shape with a high-speed burr, the surgeon measures the dimension of the recipient space either with the patient's neck under 2 to 5 kg of traction or with placement of a temporary internal Caspar distractor. A preserved frozen disk allograft of the most compatible size is then selected and thawed for 30 minutes by immersion into a water bath at 37° C. All the redundant soft tissue on the allograft is then removed while the Luschka joints and annulus fibrosus are kept intact. Before insertion into the slot, the allograft is trimmed with a rongeur, and a high-speed burr is used to fashion the bony end plate as thin as 1 mm. The graft is then carefully knocked into the slot. A free space of 1 to 3 mm is left posterior to the

graft to prevent iatrogenic spinal cord compression. The stability of the graft is checked by rocking it with a Kocher clamp with the distraction released. The position of the graft is confirmed by fluoroscopy. No internal fixation is applied. The wound is then closed in layers over a soft suction drain.

Future Directions

Disk regeneration is applicable in cases of disk degeneration only when patients experience spells of diskogenic pain, neurologic disabilities resulting from mechanical impingement, or spinal instability that requires treatment. This method of treatment should not be expected for all cases of disk degeneration noted on MRI. Currently, artificial disk replacement is a reasonable option for motion preservation operations in patients with degenerative disk disease. Further understanding of the etiology and pathogenesis of degenerative disk disease is required before biologic disk rejuvenation or regeneration surgery can become a standard of care. To date, evidence is inadequate to support that artificial disk surgery has sustainable long-term results superior to those of spinal fusion or to ascertain whether motion preservation can prevent adjacent segment degeneration. Risks of revision

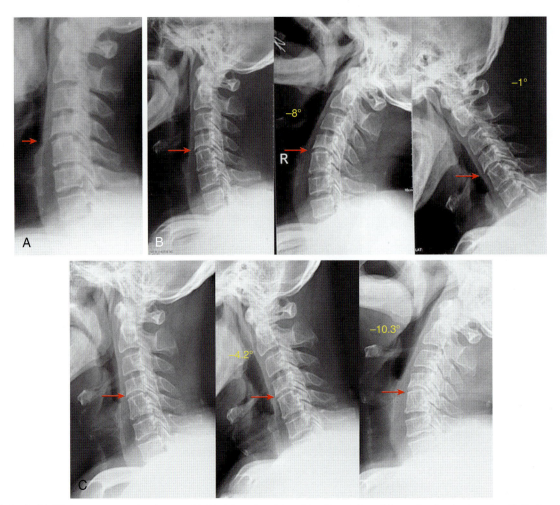

FIGURE 49-2 **A,** C4-C5 degeneration with reduction of disk height and position of the allograft (*arrow*) 6 months after implantation. **B,** Flexion and extension lateral radiographs showing excellent range of motion (*arrows*) 15 months postoperatively. **C,** Flexion and extension lateral radiographs showing that the excellent range of motion (*arrows*) was maintained 10 years postoperatively. (Modified from Ruan DK, Ding Y, He Q, Luk KD: Intervertebral disc transplantation: preserving segment motion and rebuilding stability of the cervical spine. *InSpine* 4:20-24, 2008.)

surgery and salvage procedures are not well established. Thus, clinical application may be limited to older adults. Disk rejuvenation is a more promising idea for young and middle-aged patients.

The intervertebral disk is composed of cranial and caudal bony and cartilaginous end plates, a peripheral annulus fibrosus, and a central nucleus pulposus. Regenerative strategies must include all these structures, the cellular biology as well as the local environment. In degenerative disk disease, the passageways for nutrition to travel through the end plates are jeopardized. Deformation also occurs at the annulus fibrosus. Rejuvenation of only the nucleus pulposus cannot reverse degenerative disk disease because the other two components have had irreversible changes. Disk transplantation, if completely integrated by the recipient and incorporated, would restore the best mechanical and biologic environment for the host. Even if the transplant fails, the disk can provide stability and mobility as an alternative to spinal fusion, as confirmed in a clinical trial.[30] Many questions have yet to be answered about the graft in the long term, such as the change in the host's pain generator and its degenerative process. As compared with the artificial disk implant, the transplanted

disk can encourage remodeling in the recipient that can overcome any technical imperfection arising from a malpositioned disk replacement. With no adverse immune response or osteolysis, revision surgery should not be as challenging because options remain to perform another disk transplantation, disk replacement, or spinal fusion.

The allograft disk can take on the role of a biologic scaffold on which cells can seed after transplantation. Nutritional channels through the bony end plate must be reestablished for the host cells or allogenic stem cells to repopulate. Because degenerative disk disease has a genetic predisposition, host cells are also at risk, and allogenic stem cells may be preferred. Preservation of the allografts maintains cell viability and reduces immunogenicity. Further development of this protocol can help increase the allograft shelf life and help preserve more nucleus pulposus cells. Kinematics of the FSU after transplantation also requires further research, including the mechanical effect of the adjacent segment caused by a malpositioned disk. With remodeling, the kinematics of the allograft should improve and provide protection against degeneration of the adjacent segment. The load endured by the graft at different levels of the spine

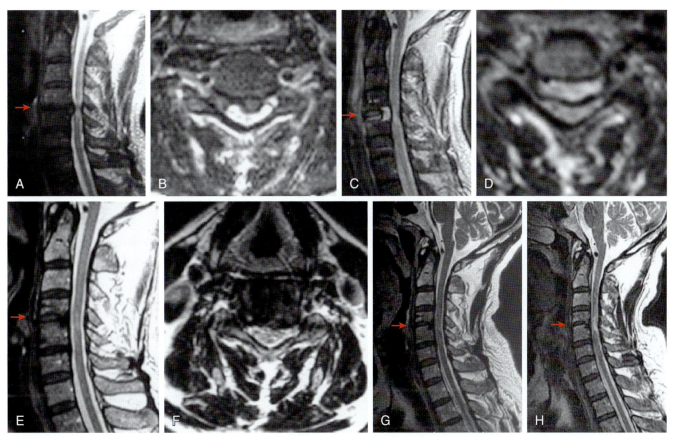

FIGURE 49-3 T2-weighted magnetic resonance imaging scans preoperatively (**A** and **B**), immediately postoperatively (**C** and **D**), 15 months later (**E** and **F**), 6 years later (**G**), and 10 years later (**H**), showing satisfactory spinal cord decompression and status of hydration of the allograft at C4 to C5 (*arrows*). (Modified from Ruan DK, Ding Y, He Q, Luk KD: Intervertebral disc transplantation: preserving segment motion and rebuilding stability of the cervical spine. *InSpine* 4:20-24, 2008.)

(e.g., the lumbar spine) is likely different. Thus, other applications of disk transplantation remain a mystery.

To take on wider clinical applications, remaining concerns and controversies must be further addressed. First, concern about transmissible diseases in any live tissue transplantation must be addressed preoperatively by adequate screening. Possible solutions include sterilizing the allograft with radiation, but its effect on the biology of the organ must be understood. Second, disk degeneration is not life-threatening, as is terminal heart, lung, or kidney failure. Nevertheless, the benefits of disk transplantation could outweigh the risks. Finally, the issue of the availability of suitable donors depends largely on the ethical, cultural, and legal backgrounds of the different countries. With the increasing acceptance of major organ donation in developed countries, no reason exists to assume that donation of musculoskeletal tissues should be any more problematic in the future. The duty of the clinician-scientist is to find the best solution for a disease based on scientific principles, and the responsibility of the community is to debate whether that solution is acceptable.

Conclusions

Intervertebral disk transplantation has developed from animal experiments to clinical applications since the 1990s. Graft harvesting, preservation techniques, surgical implantation technique, and immunoreaction issues have been investigated in these experiments. Further laboratory and clinical research should be expanded on these issues to validate this option of surgery for degenerative disk disease. Despite findings of mild disk degeneration on radiographs in a preliminary clinical trial, the motion and stability of the FSU were preserved. Disk transplantation is an attractive and possible alternative for preserving motion in the management of degenerative disk disease. Further larger-scale clinical trials are needed to verify the benefits and risks.

REFERENCES

1. Brox JI, Sorensen R, Friis A, et al.: Randomized clinical trial of lumbar instrumented fusion and cognitive intervention and exercises in patients with chronic low back pain and disc degeneration, *Spine (Phila Pa 1976)* 28:1913–1921, 2003.
2. Fritzell P, Hagg O, Wessberg P, Nordwall A: 2001 Volvo award winner in clinical studies. Lumbar fusion versus nonsurgical treatment for chronic low back pain: a multicenter randomized controlled trial from the Swedish Lumbar Spine Study Group, *Spine (Phila Pa 1976)* 26:2521–2532, 2001. discussion 2532–2534.
3. Radcliff KE, Kepler CK, Jakoi A, Sidhu GS, Rihn J, Vaccaro AR, Albert TJ, Hilibrand AS: Adjacent segment disease in the lumbar spine following different treatment interventions. *Spine J* 13(10):1339–1349, 2004 Oct.
4. Hilibrand AS, Robbins M: Adjacent segment degeneration and adjacent segment disease: the consequences of spinal fusion? *Spine J* 4:190S–1904S, 2004.
5. Ekman P, Moller H, Shalabi A, Yu YX, Hedlund R: A prospective randomised study on the long-term effect of lumbar fusion on adjacent disc degeneration. *Eur Spine J* 18(8):1175–1186, 2009 Aug.

6. Heller JG, Sasso RC, Papadopoulos SM, et al.: Comparison of BRYAN cervical disc arthroplasty with anterior cervical decompression and fusion: clinical and radiographic results of a randomized, controlled, clinical trial, *Spine (Phila Pa 1976)* 34:101–107, 2009.

7. Huppert J, Beaurain J, Steib JP, et al.: Comparison between single- and multi-level patients: clinical and radiological outcomes 2 years after cervical disc replacement, *Eur Spine J* 20:1417–1426, 2011.

8. Mummaneni PV, Burkus JK, Haid RW, et al.: Clinical and radiographic analysis of cervical disc arthroplasty compared with allograft fusion: a randomized controlled clinical trial, *J Neurosurg Spine* 6:198–209, 2007.

9. Robertson JT, Papadopoulos SM, Traynelis VC: Assessment of adjacent-segment disease in patients treated with cervical fusion or arthroplasty: a prospective 2-year study, *J Neurosurg Spine* 3:417–423, 2005.

10. Dooris AP, Goel VK, Grosland NM, et al.: Load-sharing between anterior and posterior elements in a lumbar motion segment implanted with an artificial disc, *Spine (Phila Pa 1976)* 26:E122–E129, 2001.

11. Lee CK, Goel VK: Artificial disc prosthesis: design concepts and criteria, *Spine J* 4:209S–218S, 2004.

12. Lee CK, Langrana NA: A review of spinal fusion for degenerative disc disease: need for alternative treatment approach of disc arthroplasty? *Spine J* 4:173S–176S, 2004.

13. Rohlmann A, Mann A, Zander T, Bergmann G: Effect of an artificial disc on lumbar spine biomechanics: a probabilistic finite element study, *Eur Spine J* 18:89–97, 2009.

14. Tournier C, Aunoble S, Le Huec JC, et al.: Total disc arthroplasty: consequences for sagittal balance and lumbar spine movement, *Eur Spine J* 16:411–421, 2007.

15. Lemaire JP, Carrier H, Sariali el H, et al.: Clinical and radiological outcomes with the Charite artificial disc: a 10-year minimum follow-up, *J Spinal Disord Tech* 18:353–359, 2005.

16. Putzier M, Funk JF, Schneider SV, et al.: Charite total disc replacement: clinical and radiographical results after an average follow-up of 17 years, *Eur Spine J* 15:183–195, 2006.

17. Alini M, Roughley PJ, Antoniou J, et al.: A biological approach to treating disc degeneration: not for today, but maybe for tomorrow, *Eur Spine J* 11(Suppl 2):S215–S220, 2002.

18. Ho G, Leung VY, Cheung KM, Chan D: Effect of severity of intervertebral disc injury on mesenchymal stem cell-based regeneration, *Connect Tissue Res* 49:15–21, 2008.

19. Leung VY, Chan D, Cheung KM: Regeneration of intervertebral disc by mesenchymal stem cells: potentials, limitations, and future direction, *Eur Spine J* 15(Suppl 3):S406–S413, 2006.

20. Olson EJ, Hanley EN Jr, Rudert MJ, Baratz ME: Vertebral column allografts for the treatment of segmental spine defects: an experimental investigation in dogs, *Spine (Phila Pa 1976)* 16:1081–1088, 1991.

21. Frick SL, Hanley EN Jr, Meyer RA Jr, et al.: Lumbar intervertebral disc transfer: a canine study, *Spine (Phila Pa 1976)* 19:1826–1834, 1994. discussion 1834–1835.

22. Katsuura A, Hukuda S: Experimental study of intervertebral disc allografting in the dog, *Spine (Phila Pa 1976)* 19:2426–2432, 1994.

23. Matsuzaki H, Wakabayashi K, Ishihara K, et al.: Allografting intervertebral discs in dogs: a possible clinical application, *Spine (Phila Pa 1976)* 21:178–183, 1996.

24. Luk KD, Ruan DK, Chow DH, Leong JC: Intervertebral disc autografting in a bipedal animal model, *Clin Orthop Relat Res* (337)13–26, 1997.

25. Flynn J, Rudert MJ, Olson E, et al.: The effects of freezing or freeze-drying on the biomechanical properties of the canine intervertebral disc, *Spine (Phila Pa 1976)* 15:567–570, 1990.

26. Luk KD, Ruan DK, Lu DS, Fei ZQ: Fresh frozen intervertebral disc allografting in a bipedal animal model, *Spine (Phila Pa 1976)* 28:864–869, 2003. discussion 870.

27. Chan SC, Lam S, Leung VY, et al.: Minimizing cryopreservation-induced loss of disc cell activity for storage of whole intervertebral discs, *Eur Cell Mater* 19:273–283, 2010.

28. Lam SK, Chan SC, Leung VY, et al.: The role of cryopreservation in the biomechanical properties of the intervertebral disc, *Eur Cell Mater* 22:393–402, 2011.

29. Lam SK, Xiao J, Ruan D, et al.: The effect of remodeling on the kinematics of the malpositioned disc allograft transplantation, *Spine (Phila Pa 1976)* 37:E357–E366, 2012.

30. Ruan D, He Q, Ding Y, et al.: Intervertebral disc transplantation in the treatment of degenerative spine disease: a preliminary study, *Lancet* 369:993–999, 2007.

31. Schneiderman G, Flannigan B, Kingston S, et al.: Magnetic resonance imaging in the diagnosis of disc degeneration: correlation with discography, *Spine (Phila Pa 1976)* 12:276–281, 1987.

32. Ruan DK, Ding Y, He Q, Luk KD: Intervertebral disc transplantation: preserving segment motion and rebuilding stability of the cervical spine, *InSpine* 4:20–24, 2008.

SECTION 8

Complications

Vascular Injuries

50

Gregory Grabowski, Chris A. Cornett, and James D. Kang

CHAPTER PREVIEW

Chapter Synopsis

Vertebral artery injury during cervical spine surgery is a rare but devastating complication. The vertebral artery is most susceptible to injury anteriorly at C7, laterally from C3 to C7, and posteriorly at C1 and C2. A thorough understanding of normal arterial and osseous anatomy, as well as common aberrancies, can reduce the risk of injury. Despite taking all possible precautions, inadvertent injury to this vessel can still occur, thus making an understanding of treatment options following an injury a necessity for all surgeons performing these procedures. The purpose of this chapter is to review the vertebral normal and anomalous vertebral anatomy, identify points of risk during specific cervical spine procedures, and provide a general treatment algorithm for management of intraoperative vertebral artery injuries.

Important Points

Normal vertebral artery anatomy includes passage anterior to the transverse foramen of C7 and through the foramina of C3 to C6.

The transverse foramen of C2 is an oblique channel through the axis, and the artery courses medially in the vertebral groove on the superior aspect of the atlas.

At a distance ranging from 8 to 18 mm from the midline, the artery abruptly changes course, traveling anteriorly and superiorly toward the foramen magnum.

In the event of injury, repair should be attempted when possible, with tamponade and angiographic coiling as other potential treatment options.

Clinical and Surgical Pearls

During anterior spine surgery, the vertebral artery is most susceptible to injury anterior to C7 and laterally from C3 to C7.

Posterior C1-C2 transarticular screw fixation (Magerl) has a relatively high reported rate of vertebral artery injury and has largely been replaced by C1-C2 fusion with a screw-rod construct (Harms).

Posterior subaxial spine instrumentation has exceedingly low rates of vertebral artery injury, although injury during pedicle screw placement has been reported.

Clinical and Surgical Pitfalls

Numerous vertebral anomalies can place the vertebral artery at risk if they are not recognized preoperatively.

From C3 to C6, the artery is typically protected by the transverse foramen at the level of the uncovertebral joint. However, care should be taken while exposing the C7 uncovertebral joint, given the anterior position of the vertebral artery at this level.

The presence of an aberrant entry level of the vertebral artery places it at risk anteriorly at potentially any level if this aberrant anatomy is not recognized preoperatively.

During anterior cervical corpectomy, the recommended width of decompression is approximately 16 mm.

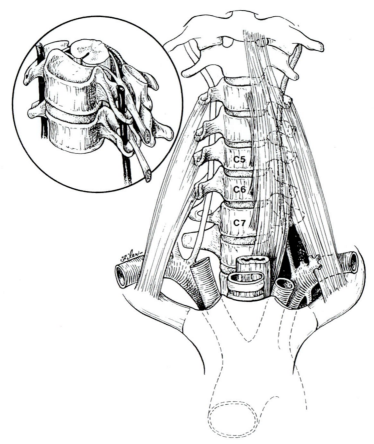

FIGURE 50-1 Schematic representation of normal vertebral artery anatomy with passage through the transverse foramina of C1 to C6. Note the midline orientation of the longus colli musculature. The *inset* depicts relationships of the artery within a transverse foramen, most notably with the exiting nerve root and associated uncovertebral joint.

Vertebral artery injury during surgical procedures of the cervical spine is a rare but devastating complication. The various procedures commonly performed by spine surgeons place the artery at risk in different ways. The vertebral artery is most susceptible to injury anteriorly at C7, laterally from C3 to C7, and posteriorly at C1 and C2. A complete understanding of normal and aberrant anatomy, strict preoperative evaluation of imaging studies, and meticulous surgical technique can minimize these risks. Despite taking all possible precautions, inadvertent injury to this vessel can still occur, thus making an understanding of treatment options following an injury a necessity for all surgeons performing these procedures. Should an injury occur, implementation of an appropriate treatment algorithm can mitigate the morbidity of this feared complication. The purpose of this chapter is to review the vertebral normal and anomalous vertebral anatomy, identify points of risk during specific cervical spine procedures, and provide a general treatment algorithm for management of intraoperative vertebral artery injuries.

Vertebral Artery Anatomy

The vertebral arteries are branches of the first portion of the subclavian arteries. These paired arteries are generally unequal in size, with the left the larger and dominant of the two.[1] The typical course of the vertebral artery allows for its classic division into four segments: V1 to V4. The first segment (V1) starts with branching of the vertebral artery from the subclavian artery and follows as it courses anterior to the transverse foramen of C7 and into the transverse foramen of C6. The second segment (V2) includes the section of the artery as it passes through the successive vertebral foramina from C6 to C1. V3 comprises the portion from the superior aspect of the arch of the atlas to the foramen magnum, whereas V4 extends from the foramen magnum to the confluence with the contralateral vertebral artery; together, they form the basilar artery[2] (Figs. 50-1 and 50-2).

Various anatomic relationships throughout the course of the vertebral artery are important to the spine surgeon. In the V2 region, the artery normally remains 1.5 mm or more lateral to the uncovertebral joint.[3] Further, the bony architecture within the region of the V2 segment dictates a mildly convergent course of the arteries through this section; the mean interforaminal distance at C6 is approximately 29 mm compared with 26 mm at C3.[4] Similarly, the mean distance from the medial edge of the longus colli to the medial edge of the vertebral artery decreases from 11.5 mm at C6 to 9 mm at C3.[5] Whereas the transverse foramina of the subaxial spine are ring shaped, the transverse foramen of C2 is an angulated canal bordered by the pedicle and lateral mass. Its inferior and lateral openings allow the artery to deviate 45 degrees laterally before continuing its ascent to enter the transverse foramen of C1.[6]

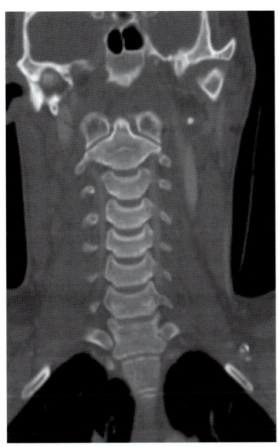

FIGURE 50-2   Coronal reconstruction of a computed tomography angiogram demonstrating normal passage and filling of bilateral vertebral arteries.

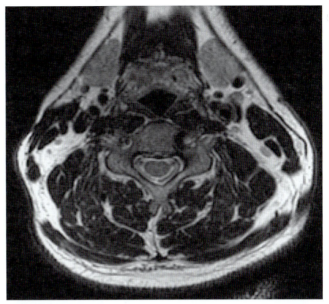

FIGURE 50-3   Axial T2-weighted magnetic resonance image demonstrating a normal right vertebral artery at the level of C4 with a medialized left vertebral artery encroaching into the C4 body. This artery would potentially be at risk during C4 corpectomy using normal anatomic landmarks.

The V3 segment becomes important to the spine surgeon mostly during the posterior approach to the atlanto-axial joint. As the artery exits the foramen of C1, it travels posteriorly and medially inside the vertebral artery groove on the superior aspect of the atlas. At a distance ranging from 8 to 18 mm from the midline, the artery abruptly changes course, traveling anteriorly and superiorly toward the foramen magnum.[6]

Anomalous Vertebral Artery Anatomy

Anatomic anomalies within the V2 segment are quite rare. However, their presence can be extremely important, particularly in patients undergoing anterior cervical spine operations. These anomalies can be divided into three major categories: intraforaminal, extraforaminal, and arterial.

Intraforaminal anomalies, or vertebral artery tortuosity, can be defined as a vertebral artery that is located medial to, or less than 1.5 mm lateral to, the uncovertebral joint.[7] In general terms, this refers to the midline migration of the vertebral artery that causes erosion into the vertebral body. Several hypotheses have been proposed to explain this phenomenon, including degenerative changes and posttraumatic changes, as well as less common causes such as infection, tumor, systemic disease, or prior surgical nonunion.[7-10] Cadaveric studies have shown the

incidence of this condition to be 2.7%, with C3 and C4 the most commonly affected levels.[11] More recent magnetic resonance imaging (MRI)–based studies showed a higher incidence, 7.6%, and found that patients with a tortuous vertebral artery tended to be older than patients without this finding[7] (Fig. 50-3).

Extraforaminal anomalies refer to a situation in which the vertebral artery runs anterior to the transverse foramen of C6 to C1. An analysis of computed tomography (CT) angiograms showed that the vertebral artery enters through the C6 transverse foramen 94.9% of the time. However, anomalous entry sites at C4, C5, and C7 occurred at 1.6%, 3.3%, and 0.3%, respectively.[12] In their MRI-based study, Eskander and associates found that only 92% of arteries entered at C6[7] (Fig. 50-4).

Arterial abnormalities are varied, but they include such findings as dual and triple lumen arteries or the presence of a hypoplastic vertebral artery. Although most of these findings have few surgical implications, vertebral artery hypoplasia affects treatment options and potential neurologic sequelae in the case of inadvertent injury. Hypoplasia occurs in approximately 10% of the population.[7]

At the atlanto-occipital joint, variations occur with greater regularity. Erosion of the C2 transverse foramen has been reported to have an incidence of 33%, occurring more commonly on the left side.[6] Of these anomalies, 20% are severe enough to preclude the safe placement of C2 instrumentation.[13] Similarly, arcuate foramina of C1 have a reported prevalence of 15.5%, with implications on exposure for C1 lateral mass screw placement.[14]

Anterior Spine Surgery

Vertebral artery injury is an uncommon complication of anterior spinal surgical procedures, namely anterior

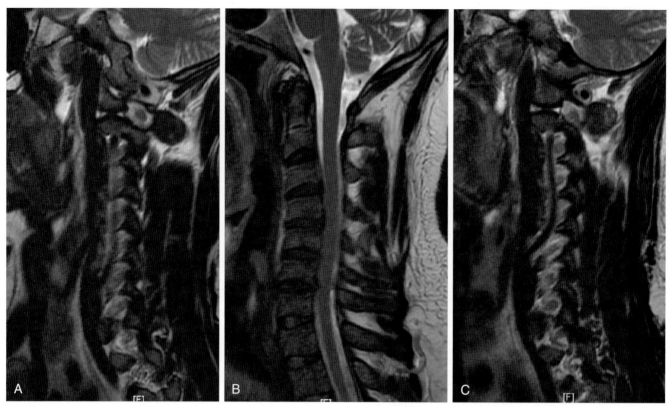

FIGURE 50-4 A to **C**, Sagittal T2-weighted magnetic resonance images of a patient with cervical stenosis. The left parasagittal image (**A**) shows the left vertebral artery passing anterior to the transverse foramen of C7 and into the transverse foramen of C6. The right parasagittal image (**C**) shows anomalous anatomy with the artery coursing anterior to the transverse foramen at C6 and into the transverse foramen at C5. The midsagittal image (**B**) is included for orientation.

diskectomy or corpectomy, such that its presence in the literature has been limited to case reports or series. The larger series cite the incidence of injury to be 0.3%.[13-16] The most common presentation of this complication is profuse bleeding intraoperatively; however, postoperative presentation with a lateral medullary infarct was also reported in a patient whose only intraoperative finding was "epidural oozing."[14]

In patients with normal vertebral artery anatomy, the artery is most susceptible to injury during anterior procedures in its position anterior to the transverse foramen of C7 or during lateral decompressive maneuvers from C3 to C6 (Fig. 50-5). Constant orientation to the anatomic midline is paramount in avoiding injury both during exposure and decompression. The midpoint between the longus colli muscles serves as a reliable intraoperative landmark of the midline, and dissection can safely be carried out over the uncovertebral joints. From C3 to C6, the artery is protected by the transverse foramen at the level of the uncovertebral joint, thus allowing for safe exposure of these structures to their lateral extent. However, care should be taken while exposing the C7 uncovertebral joint, given the anterior position of this structure at this level. The presence of an aberrant entry level, however, can place the artery at risk anteriorly at other levels if this anomaly is not recognized preoperatively. At the levels of the vertebral bodies, dissection can safely be carried to the downslope of the vertebrae.[17]

During anterior cervical diskectomy, the vertebral artery is at risk during lateral exploration of the neural foramen.

By limiting decompression laterally to the bony ridge of the uncovertebral joint, injury can be avoided. However, removal of more laterally positioned osteophytes can place the artery at risk, as can loss of orientation.[14]

When performing an anterior cervical corpectomy, the recommended width of decompression is approximately 16 mm.[18] Given that the average interforaminal distance varies from 26 to 29 mm, this amount of resection should be safe for nearly all patients at all vertebral levels. Excessive vertebral body resection laterally, however, can put the vertebral artery at risk. This can occur with asymmetric burring secondary to loss of midline orientation or as a result of oblique resection. The body wall opposite the side of surgical exposure is generally more prone to the latter, and the use of a surgical microscope is considered a further risk factor for creating an oblique corpectomy trough. Additionally, the presence of a softened lateral cortex resulting from tumor or infection has been implicated in vertebral artery injury during corpectomy.[13-15]

Recommended strategies for avoiding these complications include the use of multiple anatomic landmarks before and during decompression to ensure safe resection. Before the longus colli is dissected, the midline can be marked by using either a marking pen or electrocautery. Ensuring adequate visualization of the uncovertebral joints and planning a resection based on the use of a measuring standard of known width are important steps before beginning corpectomy. Once the decompression is started, further anatomic clues such as the lateral curvature of the vertebral body, the location of epidural veins

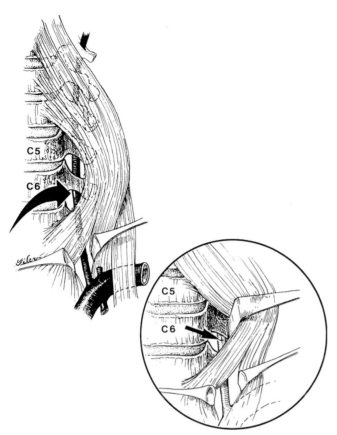

FIGURE 50-5   Schematic depicting intraoperative vertebral artery injury occurring as the artery transitions from a position anterior to the transverse foramen of C7 into the transverse foramen of C6.

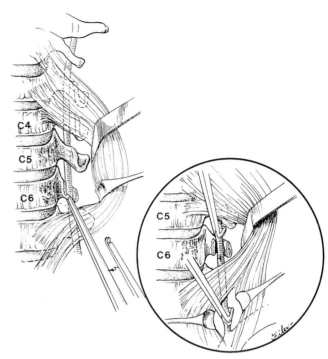

FIGURE 50-6   Schematic depicting exposure of the artery in and around the transverse foramen of C6. Note that exposure is obtained by far lateral retraction of the longus colli and opening of the transverse foramen using a Kerrison rongeur. The *inset* depicts achievement of proximal and distal control with clamps to facilitate attempted repair or ligation.

and fat, pedicle palpation, and visualization of the nerve roots can all serve as verification of orientation.[13-15]

Finally, the presence of a tortuous vertebral artery with erosion into the vertebral body can place the artery at risk despite strict adherence to the aforementioned principles.[10,16] Routine cervical MRI has been shown to be a reliable imaging modality for evaluation of this condition.[7] However, studies have shown that radiology reports of cervical spine MRI scans often fail to comment on these and other vertebral artery anomalies, and therefore all images should be scrutinized by the operating surgeon before any planned corpectomy or diskectomy.[19]

Should vertebral artery injury occur, options for management include tamponade, ligation, embolization, and repair. The therapeutic goals in treatment are threefold and progressive: (1) control of local hemorrhage, (2) prevention of immediate vertebrobasilar ischemia, and (3) prevention of cerebrovascular complications.

Initial tamponade should include the use of large pieces of hemostatic agents combined with pressure from surgical patties. The use of bone wax or other particulate materials has been discouraged, given the theoretical risk of embolization. Because of the risk of postoperative hemorrhage, delayed embolic complications, and fistula or pseudoaneurysm formation, tamponade alone has largely been abandoned as definitive treatment.[13,20,21] Additionally, arterial ligature without prior visualization is not recommended as a result of the risk of nerve root damage.[15]

Once tamponade has provided some degree of hemostasis, resuscitation by the anesthesia staff should be performed before exposure of the vertebral artery for repair or ligation. Blood loss before obtaining temporary control is considerable, with reports ranging from 2300 to 4500 mL.[15] Exposure of the artery for repair or ligation is obtained by carrying dissection of the longus colli out farther laterally over the transverse processes above and below the site of injury.[13] If the injury occurs ipsilateral to the side of exposure, this exposure can be facilitated by various maneuvers. These include partial or complete transection of the sternocleidomastoid at the level of arterial injury, distal release of the sternocleidomastoid from its insertion site, and mobilization and retraction of the carotid sheath.[15]

Once exposed, the transverse foramen can then be opened anteriorly by using either a high-speed burr or Kerrison rongeur (Fig. 50-6). Additionally, the intertransversarii muscles covering the artery between the bones are resected for exposure.[13] Temporary aneurysm clips can be applied at this point, to allow for testing of back filling through a patent circle of Willis[20] (see Fig. 50-6, *inset*). Surgical repair with the use of a 7-0 or 8-0 nonabsorbable polypropylene (Prolene) suture has been recommended as the treatment of choice if possible; however, ligation remains an option.

The decision to ligate an injured vertebral artery is not without consequence. Although most patients can tolerate unilateral vertebral artery ligation, in others it can lead to cerebellar or brainstem infarction. Patients with absence of a contralateral vertebral artery, a stenotic or hypoplastic contralateral vertebral artery, or inadequate collateralization at the circle of Willis are at risk of grave neurologic compromise with vertebral artery ligation. The reported incidence of left vertebral artery hypoplasia and absence on the left are 5.7% and 1.3%, respectively; these rates are 8.8% and 3.1% on the right. In patients without these anomalies, collateral flow can be compromised by atherosclerotic disease.[14] Overall mortality with unilateral vertebral artery ligation has been reported to be as high as 12%.[22] Other neurologic complications such as Wallenberg syndrome, cerebellar infarction, isolated cranial nerve paresis, quadriparesis, and hemiplegia have also been reported.

For these reasons, as well as the technical difficulty associated with open repair or ligation, angiography and coiling have been proposed as other treatment options, both at the time of injury or with manifestation of late complications such as pseudoaneurysm.[16,23] With angiography, the patency of collateral circulation can be confirmed before embolization. However, this treatment option depends on the skill and availability of interventional providers at the time of injury and remains viable only if patent collateral vessels exist.

In the small number of reported cases of vertebral artery injury during anterior spine surgery, outcomes vary widely, from no significant neurologic or nonneurologic complications, to cerebellar infarction, to intraoperative exsanguination and death. When successful arterial repair was performed, no investigators reported any long-term neurologic or nonneurologic complications, thus making this the treatment of choice should injury occur.

Subaxial Posterior Cervical Procedures

Posterior cervical procedures including laminoplasty and foraminotomy pose no significant risk to the vertebral artery. Posterior fixation techniques, namely, lateral mass and pedicle screw fixation for traumatic or postdecompression instability, do place the vertebral artery at theoretical risk for injury.

Numerous techniques for screw insertion have been described, and the Magerl technique is the most frequently used.[24] When screws are laterally aimed in the axial plane, the vertebral artery, although not directly visualized by the surgeon, remains safe from injury. Large series on the complications of lateral mass screw fixation have been published without a report of vertebral artery injury.[25]

Compared with lateral mass screws, subaxial cervical pedicle screws offer biomechanically improved fixation. However, their anatomic position as the medial wall of the transverse foramen places the vertebral artery at risk with a breach of the lateral pedicle wall at a level where the artery passes through the foramen. Although rare, vertebral artery injury with cervical pedicle screw placement has been reported.[26]

Atlantoaxial Fusion

During posterior atlantoaxial fusion, the vertebral artery is at risk for injury during both exposure and placement of instrumentation. During exposure of the C1 ring posteriorly, the artery is relatively unprotected in the vertebral artery groove on the superior aspect of the arch. Injury can be avoided by limiting dissection to the inferior aspect of the C1 arch; additionally, the superior aspect of the arch can safely be dissected up to 8 mm from the midline.

Instrumentation techniques for atlantoaxial fusion have evolved significantly over time. Historically, posterior wiring procedures dominated, but they were subsequently replaced by Magerl transarticular screw fixation. The Magerl technique gained popularity because of the potential for spinal cord damage during sublaminar wire placement; in addition, it offered a more rigid construct and significantly improved fusion rates over wiring.[27] The technique, however, placed the vertebral artery in significant peril, with published rates of vertebral artery injury as high as 8.2%.[28]

The ultimate goal of Magerl screw placement is safe screw passage through the C2 pars and into the lateral mass of C1. Before planning Magerl screw fixation, a surgeon must scrutinize cervical spine CT images for anomalous passage of the vertebral artery through the C2 lateral mass. Anatomic studies have shown that 20% of vertebrae have a vertebral artery course that precludes safe passage of a 3.5-mm screw.[29] In patients with anatomy conducive to screw placement, vertebral artery injury can still occur at the inferior and lateral aspects of the safe zone. As a result, a trajectory passing through the most medial and dorsal aspects of the pars minimizes the risk of vertebral artery injury.

Further identified risk factors for vertebral artery injury in patients with anatomy amenable to transarticular screw placement are (1) incomplete reduction before screw placement, (2) obliteration of the anterior tubercle of the atlas by prior transoral surgery, (3) failure to recognize an enlarged vertebral artery in the axis pedicle and lateral mass, and (4) a damaged or deficient atlantoaxial lateral mass (e.g., rheumatoid arthritis).[29,30]

For these and other reasons, C1-C2 posterior screw-rod fixation (Harms) has gained considerable popularity over transarticular screw fixation. Although the vertebral artery remains at risk during both C2 pedicle and C1 lateral mass screw placement, these risks can be mitigated to a greater extent. Intraoperative visualization of the C1 lateral mass screw entry point is key to proper screw placement, but it can be hampered by bleeding of the nearby venous plexus. Adequate hemostasis during this portion of the procedure is paramount, and the risk of vertebral artery injury is further lessened by medial angulation of the C1 lateral mass screw by approximately 10 degrees.[31]

Similar to transarticular screw placement, the risk of vertebral artery injury with the placement of a C2 pedicle screw can be minimized by accentuating medial and cephalad angulation during implant positioning. Although vertebral artery anomalies can preclude safe placement of segmental C2 fixation, this technique offers the flexibility bypassing that segment and extending the fusion to C3.[31]

Should vertebral artery injury occur during transarticular fixation or C2 instrumentation, the general recommendation is to tamponade bleeding through screw placement or by using bone wax to fill the drilled hole. In these cases, angiography and coiling are potentially useful postoperative adjuncts. If the artery is injured during exposure and can be visualized, direct repair is recommended.[30]

Conclusions

Vertebral artery injury is a rare but potentially devastating or even life-threatening complication of cervical spine surgery. The various procedures commonly performed by spine surgeons place the artery at risk in different ways. However, a complete understanding of normal and aberrant anatomy, strict preoperative evaluation of imaging studies, and meticulous surgical technique can minimize these risks. Should an injury occur, implementing an appropriate treatment algorithm can mitigate the morbidity of this feared complication.

REFERENCES

1. Moore KL, Dally AF: *Clinically oriented anatomy*, ed 4, Philadelphia, 1999, Lippincott Williams & Wilkins.
2. Heary RF, Albert TJ, Ludwig SC, et al.: Surgical anatomy of the vertebral arteries, *Spine (Phila Pa 1976)* 18:2074–2080, 1996.
3. Bohlman HH: Cervical spondylosis with moderate to severe myelopathy: a report of seventeen cases treated by Robinson anterior cervical discectomy and fusion, *Spine (Phila Pa 1976)* 2:151–162, 1997.
4. Vaccaro AR, Ring D, Scuderi F, et al.: Vertebral artery location in relation to the vertebral body as determined by two-dimensional computed tomography evaluation, *Spine (Phila Pa 1976)* 19:2637–2641, 1994.
5. Pushchak TJ, Vaccaro AR, Rauschning W, et al.: Relevant surgical anatomy of the cervical, thoracic, and lumbar spine. In Betz RR, Zeidman SM, editors: *Principles and practice of spine surgery*, Philadelphia, 2003, Mosby.
6. Madawi AA, Solanki G, Casey AT, et al.: Variation of the groove in the axis vertebra for the vertebral artery: implications for instrumentation, *J Bone Joint Surg Br* 79:820–823, 1997.
7. Ebraheim NA, Xu R, Ahmad M, et al.: The quantitative anatomy of the vertebral artery groove of the atlas and its relation to the posterior atlantoaxial approach, *Spine (Phila Pa 1976)* 23:320–323, 1998.
8. Eskander MS, Drew JM, Aubin ME, et al.: Vertebral artery anatomy: a review of two hundred fifty magnetic resonance imaging scans, *Spine (Phila Pa 1976)* 35:2035–2040, 2010.
9. Slover WP, Kiley RF: Cervical vertebral erosion caused by tortuous vertebral artery, *Radiology* 84:112–114, 1995.
10. Lindsey RW, Piepmeier J, Burkus JK: Tortuosity of the vertebral artery: an adventitious finding after cervical trauma, *J Bone Joint Surg Am* 67:806–808, 1985.
11. Tumialan LM, Wippold FJ, Morgan RA: Tortuous vertebral artery injury complicating anterior cervical spinal fusion in a symptomatic rheumatoid cervical spine, *Spine (Phila Pa 1976)* 29:E343–348, 2004.
12. Curylo LJ, Mason HC, Bohlman HH, et al.: Tortuous course of the vertebral artery and anterior spinal decompression: a cadaveric and clinical case study, *Spine (Phila Pa 1976)* 25:2860–2864, 2002.
13. Madawi AA, Casey A, Solanki G, et al.: Radiological and anatomical evaluation of the atlantoaxial transarticular screw fixation technique, *Neurosurgery* 86:961–968, 1997.
14. Young JP, Young PH, Ackerman MJ, et al.: The ponticulus posticus: implications for screw insertion into the first cervical lateral mass, *J Bone Joint Surg Am* 87:2495–2498, 2005.
15. Hong JT, Park DK, Lee MJ, et al.: Anatomical variations of the vertebral artery segment in the lower cervical spine: analysis by three-dimensional computed tomography angiography, *Spine (Phila Pa 1976)* 33:2422–2426, 2008.
16. Smith MD, Emery SE, Dudley A, et al.: Vertebral artery injury during anterior decompression of the cervical spine: a retrospective review of ten patients, *J Bone Joint Surg Br* 75:410–415, 1993.
17. Golfinos JG, Dickman CA, Zabramski JM, et al.: Repair of vertebral artery injury during anterior cervical decompression, *Spine (Phila Pa 1976)* 12:2552–2556, 1994.
18. Burke JP, Gerszten PC, Welch WC: Iatrogenic vertebral artery injury during anterior cervical spine surgery, *Spine J* 5:508–514, 2005.
19. Eskander MS, Connolly PJ, Eskander JP, et al.: Injury of an aberrant vertebral artery during a routine corpectomy: a case report and literature review, *Spinal Cord* 47:773–775, 2009.
20. Bae HW, Delamarter RB: Cervical vertebrectomy and plating. In Zdeblick TA, Bradford DS, editors: *Master techniques in orthopaedic surgery: the spine*, Philadelphia, 2004, Lippincott Williams & Wilkins.
21. Farmer JC: Anterior cervical corpectomy. In Abert TJ, Vaccaro AR, editors: *Spine surgery: tricks of the trade*, ed 2, New York, 2009, Thieme.
22. Aubin ME, Eskander MS, Drew JM, et al.: Identification of type 1 interforaminal vertebral artery anomalies in cervical spine MRIs, *Spine (Phila Pa 1976)* 35:E1610–1611, 2010.
23. Pfeifer BA, Friedberg SR, Jewell ER: Repair of injured vertebral artery in anterior cervical procedures, *Spine (Phila Pa 1976)* 19:1471–1474, 1994.
24. Golueke P, Sclafani S, Phillips T, et al.: Vertebral artery injury: diagnosis and management, *Trauma* 27:856–865, 1987.
25. Shintani A, Zervas NT: Consequence of ligation of the vertebral artery, *Neurosurgery* 36:447–450, 1972.
26. Choi JW, Lee JK, Moon KS, et al.: Endovascular embolization of iatrogenic vertebral artery injury during anterior cervical spine surgery: a report of two cases and review of the literature, *Spine (Phila Pa 1976)* 31:E891–E894, 2006.
27. Ebraheim N: Posterior lateral mass screw fixation: anatomic and radiographic considerations, *Univ Penn Orthop J* 12:66–72, 1999.
28. Heller JG, Silcox H, Sutterlin CE: Complications of posterior cervical plating, *Spine (Phila Pa 1976)* 20:2442–2448, 1995.
29. Abumi K, Shono Y, Ito M, et al.: Complications of pedicle screw fixation in reconstructive surgery of the cervical spine, *Spine (Phila Pa 1976)* 25:962–969, 2000.
30. Jeanneret B, Magerl F: Primary posterior C1/2 fusion in odontoid fractures: indications, technique, and results of transarticular screw fixation, *J Spinal Disord* 5:464–475, 1992.
31. Neo M, Fujibayashi S, Miyata M, et al.: Vertebral artery injury during cervical spine surgery, *Spine (Phila Pa 1976)* 33:779–785, 2008.

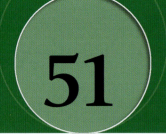

51

Spinal Cord and Nerve Injuries in the Cervical Spine

Melvin D. Helgeson and Alexander R. Vaccaro

Chapter Synopsis	Nerve injuries and spinal cord injuries following cervical spine surgery can be devastating to the patient, family, and surgeon, but with adequate counseling preoperatively and appropriate management postoperatively, the impact can be lessened. Surgical technique can help to minimize these complications, but even the best surgical techniques do not entirely prevent serious complications. Promptly recognizing a neurologic complication and managing it accordingly are vital to ensuring the best possible outcome. The purpose of this chapter is to provide an overview of the possible spinal cord and individual nerve injuries, methods to avoid them, and management should they occur.
Important Points	Spinal cord injury occurs in less than 1% of anterior and posterior cervical spine surgical procedures.
	Spinal cord and nerve injuries can occur during any phase of the perioperative period.
	Spinal cord monitoring, careful intubation, monitoring of perioperative blood pressure, and a high clinical index of suspicion are vital.
	Specific nerve injuries are associated with anterior or posterior approaches and procedures.
	A high index of suspicion remains important for diagnosis, management, and outcome of these injuries.
Clinical and Surgical Pearls	If possible, mean arterial pressures should be maintained at more than 85 mm Hg in patients with "at risk" spinal cords.
	If signaling changes occur during intraoperative monitoring, then the last procedure performed should be reversed if possible.
	Identification and protection of the superior thyroid artery may help reduce the risk of superior laryngeal nerve injury during anterior cervical approaches.
	Although anatomically the course of the recurrent laryngeal nerve is more predictable on the left, clinically the incidence of injury to the recurrent laryngeal nerve has not been lower with left-sided approaches.
	Protection of the C2 nerve root during posterior C1 and C2 procedures may help reduce the risk of occipital neuralgia.
Clinical and Surgical Pitfalls	Excessive cervical extension during intubation, even in the patient without spinal fractures and mechanical instability, can result in neurologic injury in patients with severe stenosis.
	Peripheral nerve injuries can result from intraoperative positioning and taping of the shoulders.
	Patients with C5 nerve root palsies should be enrolled in physical therapy programs to maintain range of motion.
	Because of the location of most cervical osteotomies at C7 to T1, the C8 nerve root is vulnerable to injury.

Neurologic complications during cervical spine surgery remain a source of concern for patients when they are making a decision about a surgical procedure. Patients depend on surgeons to be both honest and informative about all the potential risks involved in surgery. One of the most common questions from patients when they are considering a surgical procedure is "Can I be paralyzed?" This question is often very difficult to answer because the actual incidence varies depending on the procedure and underlying disease; however, the simple answer is always yes. A risk of permanent neurologic injury always exists during surgical procedures, and patients absolutely need to be aware of this risk preoperatively. The purpose of this chapter is to provide an overview of the possible spinal cord injuries (SCIs) and individual nerve injuries, methods to avoid them, and management should they occur.

Spinal Cord Injuries

Iatrogenic SCIs are fortunately relatively rare occurrences in anterior and posterior cervical spine surgery, with a reported incidence less than 1%.[1-5] An injury may occur during any phase of the perioperative period including intubation, head positioning, decompression, instrumentation, fracture reduction, and deformity correction, or it can be associated with hypotensive episodes resulting in decreased spinal cord perfusion. Additionally, postoperative SCIs can be directly associated with the surgical procedure (e.g., hematoma or seroma).[6]

Besides the routine surgical precautions used to avoid direct trauma and damage to the spinal cord during decompression and instrumentation, several additional strategies can be employed to decrease the incidence of iatrogenic SCI. These include spinal cord monitoring, careful intubation, close monitoring of perioperative blood pressures, and maintaining a high clinical index of suspicion. Although the use of high-dose steroids remains controversial,[6a] it is briefly discussed here as well because it is an option, but it is no longer the standard of treatment for SCIs.

Although controversial, spinal cord monitoring during the surgical management of cervical radiculopathy is not routinely necessary. However, it is used more commonly during anterior or posterior procedures for myelopathy. The techniques employed for monitoring vary widely, and because this is the topic of a separate chapter (see Chapter 11), it is discussed only briefly here. Based on the anatomy of the spinal cord, direct trauma to the anterior spinal cord may be best monitored using motor-evoked potentials (MEPs) in procedures performed anteriorly or with evidence of ossification of the posterior longitudinal ligament.[4] Conversely, direct trauma posteriorly may lead to a change in the dorsal sensory tracts and somatosensory-evoked potentials (SSEPs). The authors' facility routinely uses MEPs and SSEPs for all cervical decompressions.

Because of reports of SCI occurring during intubation and neck extension,[7] debate has centered on when to begin intraoperative spinal cord monitoring. The authors' institution routinely obtains preintubation baseline monitoring.

This monitoring should be individualized to the patient's disorder and the experience of the surgical and anesthetic teams. In these cases, the surgical monitoring team must work closely with the anesthetic team to plan preintubation monitoring. Once preintubation baseline monitoring is obtained, subsequent monitoring after intubation, before positioning, and after positioning can be compared with these baseline values.

In addition to close coordination with the neuromonitoring team, the role of the anesthesia department is particularly crucial during intubation and for perioperative blood pressure control. In patients with any possibility of mechanical instability, with severe stenosis, or with an inability to tolerate neck extension, fiberoptic intubation, rather than direct laryngoscopy, should be considered. Ultimately, this decision should be made in conjunction with the anesthesiologist, but anesthesiologists rely on surgeons to inform them of patients who are at increased risk for neurologic compromise with neck extension. A review of all cases reported to the American Society of Anesthesiologists Closed Claims database found that SCIs caused by intubation were more likely to be associated with stenosis and spondylosis than they were with instability.[7] Furthermore, this study also showed that 16% of the SCIs were associated with hypotensive episodes.[7] In patients with an "at risk" spinal cord, the authors prefer to keep patients' mean arterial pressure (MAP) higher than 85 mm Hg throughout the procedure and especially during the decompression.

Although every effort should be made to avoid injury to the spinal cord, management after SCI is recognized should be prompt and aggressive (Fig. 51-1). Intraoperatively, SCIs are usually detected by monitoring, and when these injuries occur every member of the surgical team should determine the best course of action. As a rule, the last step in the procedure should be reversed if possible. For example, if the alert occurs during anterior graft placement, then the graft should be removed. Continued communication with the anesthesia team is also paramount to ensure that MAP is being maintained.

Although the data are controversial, the use of steroids could be considered an option. The authors' institution generally administers steroids in accordance with the National Acute Spinal Cord Injury Study (NASCIS) II protocol. Additionally, every patient is managed postoperatively in a monitored setting, and MAP requirements are continued for 3 to 5 days. If evidence of spinal cord compression evolves postoperatively, epidural hematoma should be assumed, emergency magnetic resonance imaging (MRI) should be obtained, and emergency surgical intervention should be pursued if indicated (Fig. 51-2).

In conclusion, the keys to managing an intraoperative or postoperative SCI are early recognition, communication with the entire surgical team, and prompt and appropriate response. Unfortunately, despite careful planning and appropriate management, neurologic injury remains a known complication of cervical spine surgery, but the response to the event can affect patients' outcomes.

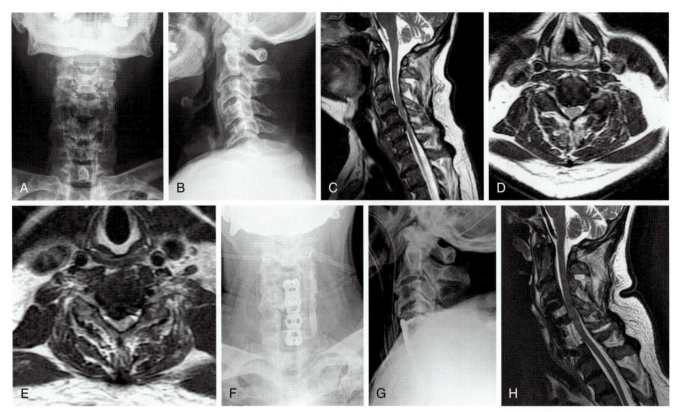

FIGURE 51-1 A 67-year-old man who presented to an outside hospital with central cord syndrome managed nonoperatively and then presented to the authors 2 months later with persistent neurologic deficit. Anteroposterior and lateral plain radiographs (**A** and **B**) and sagittal and axial T2-weighted magnetic resonance imaging (MRI) scans were obtained (**C** to **E**), revealing diffuse idiopathic skeletal hyperostosis and severe cord compression with myelomalacia. The patient was taken to the operating room for C6 corpectomy and C4-C7 anterior cervical decompression and fusion. Intraoperatively, during the decompression, complete loss of motor-evoked potentials occurred and persisted despite verifying the absence of visible compression on the spinal cord. The anesthesia department continued mean arterial pressure requirements at more than 90 mm Hg, and the patient was started on the National Acute Spinal Cord Injury Study II steroid protocol. The case was finished by inserting the bone graft, placing the plate, and closing the wound (**F** and **G**). When the patient awoke from anesthesia in the operating room, his neurologic examination was consistent with the neuromonitoring. Therefore, he was immediately taken to the MRI scanner to rule out another source of neurologic compromise (**H**). When he was fully alert, his neurologic examination improved to 2/5 strength in bilateral lower extremities and over the next 2 days improved to 4/5 strength. His motor deficit in the right upper extremity persisted.

Nerve Injuries

Anterior Cervical Spine

One of the most common procedures performed by spine surgeons comprises anterior cervical decompression and fusion. Given the significant number of cases performed annually, multiple different complications are reported in the literature. Specifically, anterior cervical spine surgery can be complicated by individual nerve injuries, most occurring with the approach to the spine.

Hypoglossal Nerve Injury

Injury to the hypoglossal nerve is a very rare complication, but this nerve is most at risk with anterior approaches to the upper cervical spine.[8] Additionally, this injury has been a reported risk with transarticular screws penetrating the anterior cortex of C1 and bicortical C1 lateral mass screws. The hypoglossal nerve or the twelfth cranial nerve (CN XII) traverses the hypoglossal canal in the occiput and then courses with the carotid sheath until it emerges into the submandibular region innervating the muscles of the tongue. In a study by Haller and colleagues, the investigators found the hypoglossal nerve to be anatomically nearest the midline at C2 to C3 and not at risk when approaching levels caudal to C3 to C4.[9] When the hypoglossal nerve is damaged, the patient presents with deviation of the tongue toward the side of the injured nerve. Unfortunately, very little can be done once the nerve is injured. The recovery rate of hypoglossal nerve injury is unknown, but of the reported cases, several have returned to function.

Superior Laryngeal Nerve Injury

The superior laryngeal nerve is likely the most vulnerable nerve associated with the anterior approach to the cervical spine. It divides into the internal and external branches; the internal branch is within 1 cm of C3 to C4, and the external branch is susceptible to approaches from C3 to C4 to C6 to C7.[9] Additionally, no apparent difference in anatomy exists between the left and right sides. Although both nerves are very difficult to identify, the external branch is smaller in diameter. Unfortunately, this branch may be more important because it supplies motor function to the cricothyroid muscle, an important muscle in maintaining tension in the vocal cords. Patients with injury to this nerve frequently present with pitch changes in their voice, decreased range, hoarseness, or voice fatigue, all problematic in singers.[10]

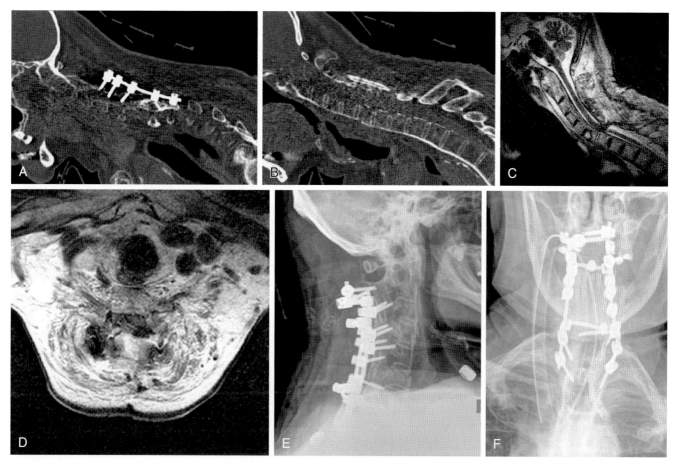

FIGURE 51-2 An 84-year-old man with ankylosing spondylitis who fell and sustained a C6 fracture requiring stabilization. Subsequently, his instrumentation failed (**A** and **B**), so he was taken to the operating room for revision instrumentation. However, during positioning but after fiberoptic intubation, the patient was noted to have a complete drop in his motor-evoked potentials to bilateral lower extremities. Therefore, he was taken on an emergency basis to the magnetic resonance imaging (MRI) scanner to evaluate for any spinal cord compression and target a decompression. MRI revealed severe spinal canal compromise (**C** and **D**). Therefore, the patient was taken back to the operating room for decompression and revision instrumentation (**E** and **F**). Postoperatively, he was maintained on mean arterial pressure requirements, steroids were initiated, and a halo was placed to support the fixation. His postoperative neurologic examination revealed full strength and sensation.

The internal branch is predominantly sensory, and patients can present with the sensation of a foreign body in the throat and a frequent need to clear the throat. Additionally, injury to the internal branch may manifest with loss of the laryngeal cough reflex that can result in aspiration.[11] The easiest method to identify the nerves clinically is to locate the superior thyroid artery. Although both branches of this nerve course through the approach, the external branch appears to be more posteriorly located in relation to the superior thyroid artery. Therefore, many surgeons believe it is very important to attempt to identify the superior thyroid artery with high cervical approaches and avoid any trauma to the tissue surrounding it.

Ligating or cauterizing the superior thyroid artery is clearly problematic, but injury to the superior laryngeal nerve is occasionally unavoidable with high approaches, and patients should be counseled preoperatively about this complication. If patients present postoperatively with any of the foregoing symptoms, the authors refer them to otolaryngology colleagues for evaluation with consideration for indirect laryngoscopy or videostroboscopy. Unless a concomitant injury to the recurrent laryngeal nerve (RLN) is present, the vocal cords will still function.

Therefore, injection medialization is usually contraindicated, although patients may benefit from voice or speech therapy.

Recurrent Laryngeal Nerve Injury

RLN injury is one of the most commonly discussed anatomic complications of cervical spine surgery, with the debate focused on the left-sided versus the right-sided approach. The basic argument for a left-sided approach is that the RLN has a more predictable course as it loops around the ligamentum and aortic root. Conversely, the right RLN loops around the subclavian artery and courses, from a lateral to medial direction, into the tracheoesophageal groove at a more cephalad location. Although anatomic studies have determined this to be true, in clinical application no significant difference in RLN palsy occurs between left-sided and right-sided approaches. Proponents of a right-sided approach argue that it is more comfortable for right-handed surgeons, avoids the thoracic duct traversing the left side, and reduces the risk to the esophagus, which lies slightly more to the left.

Damage to the RLN can be asymptomatic, but if clinical symptoms develop, patients usually present with hoarseness or, more rarely, silent or clinical aspiration. The management of RLN injury is usually an otolaryngology evaluation if symptoms persist for more than 6 weeks after anterior cervical diskectomy and fusion. After 6 weeks, injection medialization may be considered into the vocal cord if it is still not functioning properly. The injection medialization procedure is performed by an otolaryngologist who injects the vocal fold with an absorbable gelatin powder, fat, collagen, or other substrate to move the vocal fold into a more medial location and allow better phonation and protection of the airway.[12]

Sympathetic Nerve Injury

The cervical sympathetic chain consists of the superior, middle (intermediate), and inferior (stellate) ganglia, which course along the posteromedial aspect of the carotid sheath and the anterolateral aspect of the longus colli muscle. This nerve chain is at risk with anterior approaches to the cervical spine and when injured patients present with Horner syndrome (anhydrosis, miosis, and ptosis). The sympathetic chain is more at risk with lower cervical approaches, and at the C6 level it is only 11.6 mm lateral to the medial border of the longus colli.[13]

The incidence of Horner syndrome with anterior cervical approaches has been reported to be approximately 1%.[14] To avoid injury to the sympathetic chain, transverse cuts in the longus colli muscle are not recommended. Additionally, any retractor that is on the superficial side of the longus colli should be blunt, with ideal placement of self-retaining retractors deep to the muscle. Similar to other nerve injuries, the treatment strategy for Horner syndrome is expectant observation for return of function. If the injury occurred from blunt trauma (i.e., retractor), then function is very likely to return, although it can take up to 6 months.

Nerve Root Injury

The most common nerve root injury associated with both anterior and posterior cervical spine surgery is injury of the C5 nerve root. Multiple reports have theorized that this complication results from the drift of the spinal cord into a decompressed part of the spine.[15] Therefore, when discussing this complication relative to the anterior spine, the incidence appears to be increased with larger, multilevel decompressive procedures (i.e., corpectomy).

However, any of the cervical nerve roots can be at risk from direct trauma during foraminal decompressions for radiculopathy. Therefore, in particular, caution is recommended when the Kerrison rongeur is placed into a tight neuroforamen. Once the nerve root exits the foramen, it traverses in an anterior direction, and it must be identified when dissecting laterally with the decompression.

If C5 nerve palsy or new neurologic deficit develops postoperatively, advanced imaging should be considered to assess for evidence of any compressive disorder. Additionally, if C5 palsy manifests with additional nerve root involvement, the authors obtain an electromyogram to rule out brachial neuritis, which can be confused with C5 palsy. With both these diagnoses, it is important to enroll patients in a physical therapy program and maintain shoulder range of motion. Perhaps one of the most disappointing situations is one in which the shoulder becomes stiff or frozen from inactivity, and when strength returns, the patient is no longer able to use the shoulder.

Peripheral Nerve Injury

Peripheral nerve injuries associated with cervical spine surgery most frequently result from improper positioning. The most common injuries are to the ulnar nerve from direct compression and the brachial plexus from traction with shoulder taping. Intraoperative neuromonitoring can help avoid this complication when baseline monitoring is obtained before positioning and then compared with findings after positioning. Because of the difficulty of imaging the lower cervical spine, the shoulders frequently must be aggressively taped to obtain adequate imaging.

Obtaining MEPs before taping and draping can assist with determining whether the tape needs to be relaxed. If an alert occurs with taping, the authors relax the tape, extend the dissection over the anterior spine to a level that can be adequately imaged, and then count down to the level of disease. When a neuromonitoring alert occurs with the ulnar nerve, the medial aspect of the elbow must be checked. The authors routinely wrap the elbows in gel pads to protect the nerve, and it is important to ensure that all lines traversing the elbow are kept away from the medial aspect of the elbow. If a peripheral deficit persists postoperatively, it should be followed clinically for at least 6 weeks, to await the return of function. If no improvement is noted at 6 weeks, the authors refer the patient to the neurology department for electromyographic testing.

Posterior Cervical Spine

In contrast to anterior spinal approaches, the posterior approach to the cervical spine does not encounter any significant nerves when the procedure is performed appropriately. However, posterior decompressive procedures may have a higher incidence of injury to the spinal cord and nerve roots because they are more exposed to direct trauma. Individual nerve injuries, proceeding from cephalad to caudal, include C2 nerve root injury, third occipital nerve injury (C3), C5 nerve root injury, and C8 nerve root injury. Injury to the third occipital nerve is most commonly associated with the exposure, whereas injuries to the C2, C5, and C8 nerve roots are more common with instrumentation, decompression, and osteotomy procedures, respectively.

C2 Nerve Root Injury

A more recently described technique for fixation into C1 is placement of C1 lateral mass screws. To avoid injury to the vertebral artery as it courses along the cephalad aspect of the C1 arch, the safest placement of C1 lateral mass screws is along the caudal aspect of the arch and into the lateral mass. Unfortunately, this procedure places the C2 nerve root ganglion at risk, and multiple reports of injury to this nerve have been noted.[16] Most surgeons recommend protecting this nerve when drilling for or placing the C1 lateral mass screw to avoid occipital neuralgia postoperatively; however, intentional sacrifice of the nerve has also been suggested.[17,18] Postoperative neuralgia can result from excessive traction on the nerve root or from using a fully threaded screw. Therefore, the authors avoid excessive traction during placement, and the use of partially threaded screws may theoretically reduce the risk of direct root irritation. If patients present with postoperative occipital neuralgia, symptomatic treatment remains the best option, similar to injury of the third occipital nerve.

Third Occipital Nerve Injury

During the approach to the upper cervical spine, staying along the midline raphe is important, to avoid excessive bleeding and injury to the third occipital nerve. The third occipital nerve originates from the dorsal root of C3 and then traverses from a lateral to medial direction until it reaches the external occipital protuberance, where it can be as close as 3 mm from the midline.[19] The third occipital nerve is located medial to the greater occipital nerve (a branch from C2), and therefore it is more susceptible to injury during dissection or retraction.

The third occipital nerve is vulnerable during approaches to the occipitocervical junction, and injury to it can be unavoidable in some cases. Therefore, patients must be counseled about the risk of occipital neuralgia postoperatively. In addition to staying midline with the exposure, avoiding excessive retraction on the tissues also has been advocated to decrease the traction on the third occipital nerve. If patients present with persistent pain postoperatively, symptomatic treatment is the best course of action, with consideration of injections in consultation with pain management colleagues as indicated.

C5 Nerve Root Injury

The most common nerve injury with posterior cervical spine surgery is C5 nerve palsy. Although C6, C7, and C8 nerve palsies have been reported, C5 is by far the most common and therefore the focus of this discussion. The incidence of C5 palsy following cervical spine surgery appears to be close to 5%; decompressive procedures for myelopathy have the highest rate of this complication.[20] The incidence of injury to C6, C7, and C8 is much less than 1%, and only case reports are discussed in the literature.

Several theories potentially explain nerve root palsies, including direct trauma or a traction phenomenon from displacement of the spinal cord. Unfortunately, the exact etiology is uncertain; therefore, avoidance and treatment strategies for C5 palsy are less focused or beneficial. Patients with C5 palsy generally present in a delayed fashion (within 1 week) postoperatively, sometimes even as long as 1 month postoperatively. The most common presentation is with deltoid and biceps weakness. However, if this weakness is preceded by or associated with severe pain, the differential diagnosis must include brachial neuritis.[21]

When a patient presents with a new postoperative deficit postoperatively, the authors routinely obtain a MRI scan to rule out any compressive disorder that can explain the clinical findings. If no compression is noted, patients are treated symptomatically with physical therapy and pain control. Given the lack of deltoid function and the possibility of a traction phenomenon, patients with C5 palsy are given a sling for comfort. Additionally, many surgeons do not routinely administer steroids to patients with isolated nerve palsy, although some do. Most patients recover within 6 months, but if the result of manual motor testing is less than 2 out of 5, these patients will show the least potential for full recovery.[20]

C8 Nerve Root Injury

Postoperative C8 nerve injuries are almost exclusively reported with cervical osteotomies. The most common location for cervical corrective osteotomy is the C7-T1 level because of the normal course of the vertebral artery (entering the foramen at C6), the relatively larger spinal canal, and the lower potential for a significant deficit should C8 be injured.

One of the key technical aspects of cervical osteotomy is to ensure that the C8 nerve roots are mobile and adequately decompressed. Despite adequate decompression, however, C8 nerve injuries do occur. In the largest reported series of cervical osteotomies (131 patients), the incidence of C8 nerve injury was 14%.[22] With more recent advances in neuromonitoring, compression of the C8 nerve root can be identified intraoperatively, and further decompression of the nerve root can be performed if necessary. Furthermore, if the symptoms of C8 compression develop postoperatively, a computed tomography scan should be obtained to evaluate the foramen and space available for the C8 nerves. If adequate decompression has been performed, C8 nerve palsies can be treated symptomatically with physical therapy and pain control. If the nerve is adequately decompressed, recovery can be expected.

Conclusions

Nerve injuries and SCIs following surgical procedures of the cervical spine can be devastating to the patient, family, and surgeon, but with adequate counseling preoperatively and appropriate management postoperatively, the impact can be lessened. Surgical technique can help to minimize these complications, but even the best surgical techniques do not entirely prevent serious complications. Promptly recognizing a neurologic complication and managing it accordingly are vital to ensuring the best possible outcome.

REFERENCES

1. Cramer DE, Maher PC, Pettigrew DB, et al.: Major neurologic deficit immediately after adult spinal surgery: incidence and etiology over 10 years at a single training institution, *J Spinal Disord Tech* 22:565–570, 2009.
2. Daniels AH, Riew KD, Yoo JU, et al.: Adverse events associated with anterior cervical spine surgery, *J Am Acad Orthop Surg* 16:729–738, 2008.
3. Emery SE, Bohlman HH, Bolesta MJ, et al.: Anterior cervical decompression and arthrodesis for the treatment of cervical spondylotic myelopathy: two to seventeen-year follow-up, *J Bone Joint Surg Am* 80:941–951, 1998.
4. Hilibrand AS, Schwartz DM, Sethuraman V, et al.: Comparison of transcranial electric motor and somatosensory evoked potential monitoring during cervical spine surgery, *J Bone Joint Surg Am* 86:1248–1253, 2004.
5. Tew JM Jr, Mayfield FH: Complications of surgery of the anterior cervical spine, *Clin Neurosurg* 23:424–434, 1976.
6. Lee JY, Schwartz DM, Anderson DG, et al.: Epidural hematoma causing dense paralysis after anterior cervical corpectomy: a report of two cases, *J Bone Joint Surg Am* 88:198–201, 2006.

6a. Ito Y, Sugimoto Y, Tomioka M, et al.: Does high-dose methylprednisolone sodium succinate really improve neurological status in patient with acute cervical cord injury?: a prospective study about neurological recovery and early complications, *Spine (Philadelphia 1976)* 34:2121–2124, 2009.

7. Hindman BJ, Palecek JP, Posner KL, et al.: Cervical spinal cord, root, and bony spine injuries: a closed claims analysis, *Anesthesiology* 114:782–795, 2011.

8. Sengupta DK, Grevitt MP, Mehdian SM: Hypoglossal nerve injury as a complication of anterior surgery to the upper cervical spine, *Eur Spine J* 8:78–80, 1999.

9. Haller JM, Iwanik M, Shen FH: Clinically relevant anatomy of high anterior cervical approach, *Spine (Phila Pa 1976)* 36:2116–2121, 2011.

10. Kochilas X, Bibas A, Xenellis J, et al.: Surgical anatomy of the external branch of the superior laryngeal nerve and its clinical significance in head and neck surgery, *Clin Anat* 21:99–105, 2008.

11. Kiray A, Naderi S, Ergur I, et al.: Surgical anatomy of the internal branch of the superior laryngeal nerve, *Eur Spine J* 15:1320–1325, 2006.

12. Rubin AD, Sataloff RT: Vocal fold paresis and paralysis, *Otolaryngol Clin North Am* 40:1109–1131, 2007. viii-ix.

13. Civelek E, Karasu A, Cansever T, et al.: Surgical anatomy of the cervical sympathetic trunk during anterolateral approach to cervical spine, *Eur Spine J* 17:991–995, 2008.

14. Bertalanffy H, Eggert HR: Complications of anterior cervical discectomy without fusion in 450 consecutive patients, *Acta Neurochir (Wien)* 99:41–50, 1989.

15. Hashimoto M, Mochizuki M, Aiba A, et al.: C5 palsy following anterior decompression and spinal fusion for cervical degenerative diseases, *Eur Spine J* 19:1702–1710, 2010.

16. Conroy E, Laing A, Kenneally R, et al.: C1 lateral mass screw-induced occipital neuralgia: a report of two cases, *Eur Spine J* 19:474–476, 2010.

17. Goel A, Desai KI, Muzumdar DP: Atlantoaxial fixation using plate and screw method: a report of 160 treated patients, *Neurosurgery* 51:1351–1356, 2002. discussion 1356–1357.

18. Squires J, Molinari RW: C1 lateral mass screw placement with intentional sacrifice of the C2 ganglion: functional outcomes and morbidity in elderly patients, *Eur Spine J* 19:1318–1324, 2010.

19. Tubbs RS, Mortazavi MM, Loukas M, et al.: Anatomical study of the third occipital nerve and its potential role in occipital headache/neck pain following midline dissections of the craniocervical junction, *J Neurosurg Spine* 15:71–75, 2011.

20. Sakaura H, Hosono N, Mukai Y, et al.: C5 palsy after decompression surgery for cervical myelopathy: review of the literature, *Spine (Phila Pa 1976)* 28:2447–2451, 2003.

21. Park P, Lewandrowski KU, Ramnath S, et al.: Brachial neuritis: an under-recognized cause of upper extremity paresis after cervical decompression surgery, *Spine (Phila Pa 1976)* 32:E640–E644, 2007.

22. Simmons ED, DiStefano RJ, Zheng Y, et al.: Thirty-six years' experience of cervical extension osteotomy in ankylosing spondylitis: techniques and outcomes, *Spine (Phila Pa 1976)* 31:3006–3012, 2006.

Tracheoesophageal Injuries

52

Abimbola A. Obafemi, Moshe M. Yanko, and Steven C. Ludwig

CHAPTER PREVIEW

Chapter Synopsis	The anterior approach to the cervical spine has gained worldwide acceptance by spine surgeons to address a variety of pathologic conditions of the cervical spine. Injuries to the trachea and esophagus are rare, but they can result from direct or indirect injury and manifest with early or late clinical findings. Radiographic imaging such as plain radiography, computed tomography or magnetic resonance imaging, and esophagography/swallow studies can help confirm the diagnosis. Because false-negative results can occur, however, a high index of suspicion is necessary. If unrecognized, these injuries can be the source of significant morbidity and mortality, but when they are diagnosed and aggressively treated through a multidisciplinary team approach, a successful outcome can be achieved.
Important Points	Depending on the level approached, injury to various nerves innervating the tracheoesophageal structures can occur during anterior cervical surgical procedures.
	The diagnosis of tracheoesophageal injuries is based on both imaging modalities and endoscopic studies. Because false-negative results can occur, however, a high index of suspicion is necessary.
	A multidisciplinary team approach including otolaryngology or thoracic surgeons, infectious disease specialists, and nutritional support should be considered.
Clinical and Surgical Pearls	Patients undergoing revision cervical spine surgery should have a preoperative evaluation to determine the status of the superior laryngeal nerve.
	In the case of esophageal perforations, consideration for placement of a percutaneous endoscopic gastrostomy tube can provide enteric nutrition while bypassing the perforated esophagus.
	Primary closure of the esophageal perforation should be considered in both acute and delayed presentations.
	A multidisciplinary team including otolaryngology or thoracic surgeons, infectious disease specialists, and nutritional support should be considered.
Clinical and Surgical Pitfalls	Surgical approaches to the upper cervical spine place the superior laryngeal nerve, along with its associated structures, at risk.
	Asymptomatic perforations of the trachea and esophagus have been reported; therefore, a high index of clinical suspicion is required for the diagnosis of tracheoesophageal injuries.
	False-negative results of diagnostic studies have been reported and can occur. This is another reason that a high index of clinical suspicion is required for the diagnosis of tracheoesophageal injuries.
	Determination of the resolution period for tracheoesophageal perforations can be challenging.

The anterior approach to the cervical spine is a well-established surgical dissection technique that has been used successfully for the treatment of pathologic conditions of the cervical spine, including traumatic conditions, degenerative abnormalities, deformities, infections, and neoplastic diseases.[1] By virtue of the approach, it provides access to the anterior cervical spinal column and avoids the need for dissecting through the cervical posterior stabilizing elements, including the paraspinal muscles and ligamentum nuchae. However, with this approach, the anterior structures of the neck (e.g., the trachea and esophagus) are at risk for both direct injury (perforation) and indirect injury (traction or compression). This chapter reviews injuries to the tracheoesophageal structure during surgical procedures of the cervical spine.

The anterior cervical approach, championed by Robinson and Smith,[2] uses the interval between the sternocleidomastoid muscle and the neck strap muscles. This approach requires dissection through the deep cervical fascia. The trachea and esophagus are then retracted medially, and the carotid sheath is retracted laterally. The deeper surgical plane poses risks of injuring vital structures, including nerves, blood vessels, and lymphatic vessels, and it risks perforating the trachea and esophagus. For patients who have undergone an anterior cervical approach, one of the most common problems encountered during the postoperative period is dysphagia. Some studies reported that during the postoperative period, these patients presented with dysphagia 47% of the time.[1,3]

Nerve Injuries

Based on the operative level, nervous structures that can be at risk during anterior cervical dissection are the hypoglossal nerve, the superior laryngeal nerve, and the recurrent laryngeal nerve. Palsy of these nerves can manifest in the following ways: as dysphagia, which is difficulty swallowing; as dysphonia, which is an impairment of sound production as the passive vocal cords interact with the exhaled airstream; and as hoarseness, which is a breathy or harsh voice[1,4-6] (Table 52-1).

At the C1 arch level or in the anterior triangle of the neck, the hypoglossal nerve is at risk as it exits the hypoglossal foramen and passes along the anterior aspect of the C1 arch. Except for the palatoglossus muscle, all motor innervation to the tongue muscles is provided by the hypoglossal nerve; therefore, palsy of the nerve causes ipsilateral tongue deviation with difficulty swallowing as the ability to move the food toward the back of the mouth is impaired.[1,4-6]

At the C3-C4 level, the superior laryngeal nerve, along with closely associated structures (e.g., the carotid bifurcation, upper pole of the thyroid, and superior thyroid artery) are at risk. The superior laryngeal nerve is a branch of the vagus nerve (cranial nerve X) that originates in the carotid sheath before it splits into a sensory (internal) branch and a motor (external) branch. The sensory branch innervates both ipsilateral and contralateral larynges, thus preventing aspiration. The motor branch innervates the cricothyroid, a muscle that tenses the

Table 52-1 Structures at Risk During Anterior Approach to Cervical Spine

Vertebral Level	Structure(s) at Risk	Clinical Correlate
C2	HN	Dysphagia, dysarthria, ipsliateral tongue deviation
C2–C3	HN	Dysphagia, dysarthria, ipsliateral tongue deviation
C3	HN, ISLN, STA, SLA	Dysphagia, dysarthria, ipsliateral tongue deviation, impaired cough reflex
C3–C4	ISLN, STA, SLA	Impaired cough reflex
C4	ISLN, ESLN, STA, SLA	Impaired cough reflex, hoarseness, voice fatigability, impaired high-pitch phonation
C4–C5	ESLN, STA, SLA	Hoarseness, voice fatigability, impaired high-pitch phonation
C5	ESLN, STA, SLA	Hoarseness, voice fatigability, impaired high-pitch phonation
C5–C6	ESLN, STA	Hoarseness, voice fatigability, impaired high-pitch phonation
C6	ESLN, STA	Hoarseness, voice fatigability, impaired high-pitch phonation

ESLN, External superior laryngeal nerve; *HN,* hypoglossal nerve; *ISLN,* internal superior laryngeal nerve; *SLA,* superior laryngeal artery; *STA,* superior thyroid artery.
Adapted from Haller JM, Iwanik M, Shen FH: Clinically relevant anatomy of high anterior cervical approaches. *Spine (Phila Pa 1976)* 36:2116-2121, 2011.

vocal cords to produce the high-pitched sounds of singing. Palsy of the motor (external) superior laryngeal nerve branch manifests as a monotonous voice, whereas palsy of the sensory (internal) superior laryngeal nerve may be silent because the pharynx has contralateral innervation. Therefore, patients undergoing revision surgical procedures of the cervical spine should have a preoperative evaluation with electromyography, strobovideolaryngoscopy, or both, to determine the status of the superior laryngeal nerve.[1]

The recurrent laryngeal nerve is vulnerable to traction injury as it loops around the great vessels—the aorta on the left and the subclavian artery on the right—before ascending into the tracheoesophageal groove in the neck (Fig. 52-1). Other postulated causes of recurrent laryngeal nerve injury include direct trauma, pressure neurapraxia from a fixed inflated endotracheal cuff, and stretch from aggressive retractor use; the right recurrent laryngeal nerve is suggested to be more vulnerable than the left because of its more lateral point of fixation on the brachiocephalic trunk.[1]

Direct Esophageal Injuries

Direct injuries to the esophagus that occur secondary to cervical spine surgery are considered rare, with an incidence ranging from 0% to 3.4%[4-11] and a mortality rate of up to 6%.[12] The most common levels at which these injuries occur are adjacent to the C5-C6 and C6-C7 disks. Compared with operations performed for degenerative conditions, operations performed for traumatic injuries have a higher rate of perforations.[6,7,9] Most esophageal perforations are recognized during the surgical procedure.[6,10,13] However, it is not

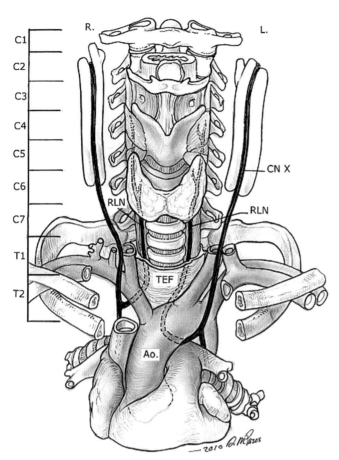

FIGURE 52-1 Schematic demonstrating course of recurrent laryngeal nerve (RLN) on each side. Tracheoesophageal fascia (TEF) is partially peeled away. *Ao.*, Aorta; *CN*, cranial nerve; *L.*, left; *R.*, right. (From Haller JM, Iwanik M, Shen FH. Clinically relevant anatomy of recurrent laryngeal nerve. *Spine (Phila Pa 1976)* 37:97-100, 2012.)

uncommon for perforations to be evident during the early postoperative course or even months to years after the surgical procedure.

Causes of esophageal injuries vary with the acuity and chronicity of their presentation. Acute esophageal perforations usually are related to intraoperative manipulations, direct trauma from sharp instruments, and malplacement of retractor blades.[6-10] Conversely, delayed esophageal perforation usually occurs secondary to implant or bone graft erosion (Fig. 52-2).

Clinically, the presenting symptoms of esophageal perforations commonly include neck or throat pain, swelling, induration, surgical wound infection, fistula, dysphagia, odynophagia, dysphonia, aspirations, hoarseness, subcutaneous emphysema, and signs of systemic infection.[6-10,13-16] Asymptomatic cases have also been reported.[7] As a general consideration, any findings of neck abscess after cervical surgical procedures should include the differential diagnosis of suspected esophageal perforation.

The diagnosis is based on both imaging modalities and endoscopic studies.[6,7,9,10,13] However, considering that false-negative results are known to occur with both modalities, ruling out an esophageal injury should also be based on clinical judgment. Plain radiography of the cervical spine and chest can serve as an initial tool for

assessing the correct placement of implants and grafts, overall spinal alignment, and the presence of excessive prevertebral anterior soft tissue swelling, in addition to any evidence of subcutaneous emphysema. Computed tomography can provide further and more accurate information regarding malplaced or dislodged hardware, subcutaneous emphysema, and the existence of prevertebral abscess.

A barium contrast-enhanced esophagram can reveal the location of the perforation, but false-negative results have occurred in 25% of tested patients[7] (Fig. 52-3). Esophageal endoscopy can provide more reliable information regarding the presence, location, and extent of the esophageal perforation. If an esophageal perforation is found, it is highly recommended that a percutaneous endoscopic gastrostomy tube be placed. Placement of the tube allows continuation of enteric nutrition by bypassing the perforated esophagus. Consultations with otolaryngology and thoracic surgeons should be conducted to establish a surgical plan for possible repair and/or management. In cases of cutaneous fistula, obtaining a fistulogram by injecting contrast dye can assist with finding the relationships among the locations of the perforation, fluid collection, surgical incision, and fistula.

Smaller perforations may be amenable to a more conservative approach. This treatment can include percutaneous drainage of the fluid collection, intravenously administered broad-spectrum antibiotics, and placement with alimentation delivered through a nasogastric tube. In the presence of abscess, the basic principles of treatment include surgical drainage of the abscess, débridement of any nonvital tissue, extensive irrigation of the infected space, and primary closure of the perforation. Discontinuing oral intake, with parenteral nutrition administered through a nasogastric tube or percutaneous endoscopic gastrostomy tube, and administering broad-spectrum antibiotic therapy are required.[6,79,10,17] The esophagus can be stented with a soft silicone tube while the perforation is allowed to heal. This technique is thought by some investigators to minimize the risk of esophageal constriction and scarring.

Depending on the underlying spinal disorder, timing of the diagnosis, clinical appearance of the surgical working zone, and patient host factors, removal of the instrumentation should be considered. However, in clinical situations in which the implant can be directly linked to the esophageal injury, the surgeon should remove the instrumentation and consider further reconstructive options.

Primary closure of the esophageal perforation should be attempted for both acute and delayed presentations. The repair should include débridement of the perforated edges and primary closure by suture repair. For larger and chronic injuries to the esophagus, more complex repairs by reconstruction may be required. Preoperative consultations with head and neck surgeons, thoracic surgeons, and plastic surgeons may be necessary. Options for these clinical situations may require the use of artificial patches, small bowel transplantation, or muscle flaps, including the sternocleidomastoid muscle, longus colli muscle, omental flap, or pedicled pectoralis major muscle flap.[6,12,15,18,19]

Repeated irrigation and débridement every few days may be necessary, depending on the clinical course and

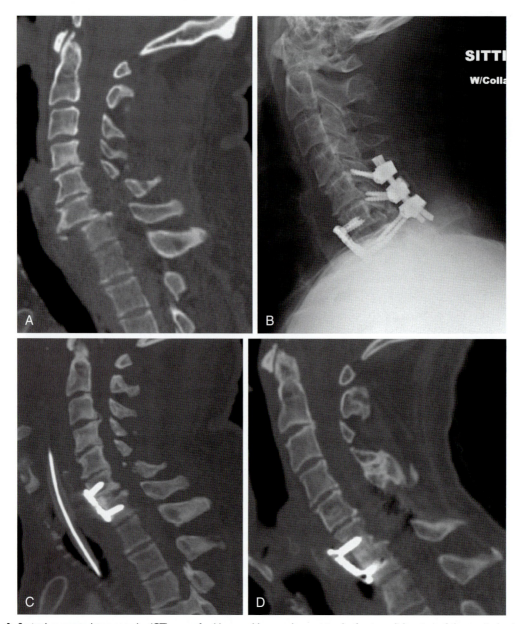

FIGURE 52-2 **A,** Sagittal computed tomography (CT) scan of a 66-year-old man who sustained a fracture-dislocation of the cervical spine with associated paraparesis. The patient underwent anterior-posterior open reduction, decompression, and stabilization of the fracture-dislocation. Immediate postoperative lateral radiograph (**B**) and sagittal CT scan (**C**) confirm reduction of the fracture-dislocation with acceptable alignment. **D,** The patient subsequently underwent a fusion procedure, but he presented 4 years later with persistent dysphagia and an esophageal leak secondary to graft subsidence and direct esophageal erosion secondary to a prominent anterior cervical plate. (Images courtesy Francis H. Shen, MD.)

the surgeon's judgment. An infectious disease specialist should be consulted for management of the appropriate choice and duration of antibiotic treatment.

Determination of the resolution period for the perforation can be challenging. The first clue should be a reduction of postoperative wound drainage. The postoperative drain should be continued for a minimum of 7 to 10 days after repair. After risks for aspiration have been ruled out, a trial of drinking water, with or without contrast dye or methylene blue, can be the next step. Before initiating oral intake, repeat endoscopy can be considered to document adequate esophageal healing when resolution of the perforation is questionable, based on clinical examination. Food ingestion can be started at a later date in a gradual or monitored manner.

Direct Tracheal Injuries

Iatrogenic disruptions and injuries to the trachea are extremely rare. A review of the literature reveals iatrogenic tracheal injuries related to orotracheal intubations, tracheotomy or tracheostomy, and interventional bronchoscopy as the most common causes.[20,21] Case reports have noted tracheal injuries during thyroid tumor resection and explorative surgical procedures for trauma to the neck.[22-24]

Although the trachea is more anterior to the esophagus and spine, the possible causes of direct injury can be the same as those discussed for the esophagus. Direct injuries include perforations from the self-retaining retractor, inadvertent dissection by a sharp surgical instrument, and erosions caused by implant dislodgment.

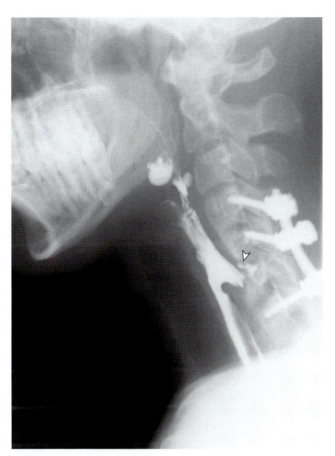

FIGURE 52-3 Barium contrast–enhanced esophagram of an 18-year-old man who sustained a traumatic cervical burst fracture. Imaging demonstrates pooling with extravasation of contrast material beyond the esophagus (*arrowhead*) that confirms the presence of a leak. (Image courtesy Francis H. Shen, MD.)

Symptoms related to tracheal injuries vary and include dyspnea, hemoptysis, soft tissue or mediastinal emphysema, and pneumothoraces. The diagnosis of a tracheal injury may be delayed because of slow or mildly progressing symptoms. The gold standard method for diagnosing these injuries is tracheobronchoscopy. This technique allows for accurate diagnosis of the extent and location of the laceration. Treatments vary. Superficial lacerations and tears are treated conservatively, whereas full-thickness tears require surgical repair.[25] Consultations with a head and neck surgeon and a thoracic surgeon are helpful in the management of this rare but complex problem.

Surgical repair of a cervical tracheal tear can be performed through a transtracheal approach.[26,27] Recommendations in the more recent literature regarding milder tracheal injuries trend toward a more conservative mode of treatment. For uncomplicated cases with the patient under mechanical ventilation, with lacerations that are covered by the esophagus, and with no loss of the tidal volumes, a conservative approach is recommended.[21] Other reports show good results with conservative treatment, even for uncomplicated full-thickness tears.[28,29] Conservative treatment includes mainly mechanical ventilation with the endotracheal tube placed distal to the laceration and ventilation with positive end-expiratory pressure and low tidal volume.

Conclusions

The anterior approach to the cervical spine has gained worldwide acceptance by spine surgeons to address a variety of pathologic conditions of the cervical spine. Injuries to the trachea and esophagus are rare. If unrecognized, they can be the source of significant morbidity and mortality. However, when they are diagnosed and aggressively treated through a multidisciplinary team approach, a successful outcome can be achieved.

Acknowledgment

The authors thank senior editor and writer Dori Kelly, MA, for editing the manuscript.

REFERENCES

1. O'Brien J, Zarro C, Gelb D, et al.: Dysphagia, aspiration, and dysphonia related to cervical surgery, *Curr Opin Orthop* 16:184–188, 2005.
2. Robinson R, Smith G: Anterolateral cervical disc removal and interbody fusion for cervical disc syndrome, *Bull Johns Hopkins Hosp* 96:223–224, 1955.
3. Smith-Hammond C, New K, Pietrobon R, et al.: Prospective analysis of incidence and risk factors of dysphagia in spine surgery patients: comparison of anterior cervical, posterior cervical, and lumbar procedures, *Spine (Phila Pa 1976)* 29:1441–1446, 2004.
4. Capen DA, Garland DE, Waters RL: Surgical stabilization of the cervical spine: a comparative analysis of anterior and posterior spine fusions, *Clin Orthop Relat Res* (196):229–237, 1985.
5. Romano PS, Campa DR, Rainwater JA: Elective cervical discectomy in California: postoperative in-hospital complications and their risk factors, *Spine (Phila Pa 1976)* 22:2677–2692, 1997.
6. Vrouenraets BC, Been HD, Brouwer-Mladin R, et al.: Esophageal perforation associated with cervical spine surgery: report of two cases and review of the literature, *Dig Surg* 21:246–249, 2004.
7. Gaudinez RF, English GM, Gebhard JS, et al.: Esophageal perforations after anterior cervical surgery, *J Spinal Disord* 13:77–84, 2000.
8. Graham JJ: Complications of cervical spine surgery: a five-year report on a survey of the membership of the Cervical Spine Research Society by the Morbidity and Mortality Committee, *Spine (Phila Pa 1976)* 14:1046–1050, 1989.
9. Newhouse KE, Lindsey RW, Clark CR, et al.: Esophageal perforation following anterior cervical spine surgery, *Spine (Phila Pa 1976)* 14:1051–1053, 1989.
10. Orlando ER, Caroli E, Ferrante L: Management of the cervical esophagus and hypofarinx [sic] perforations complicating anterior cervical spine surgery, *Spine (Phila Pa 1976)* 28:E290–E295, 2003.
11. Tew JM Jr, Mayfield FH: Complications of surgery of the anterior cervical spine, *Clin Neurosurg* 23:424–434, 1976.
12. Dakwar E, Uribe JS, Padhya TA, Vale FL: Management of delayed esophageal perforations after anterior cervical spinal surgery, *J Neurosurg Spine* 11:320–325, 2009.
13. Kelly MF, Spiegel J, Rizzo KA, Zwillenberg D: Delayed pharyngoesophageal perforation: a complication of anterior spine surgery, *Ann Otol Rhinol Laryngol* 100:201–205, 1991.
14. Fountas KN, Kapsalaki EZ, Machinis T, Robinson JS: Extrusion of a screw into the gastrointestinal tract after anterior cervical spine plating, *J Spinal Disord Tech* 19:199–203, 2006.
15. Pichler W, Maier A, Rappl T, et al.: Delayed hypopharyngeal and esophageal perforation after anterior spine fusion: primary repair reinforced by pedicled pectoralis major flap, *Spine (Phila Pa 1976)* 31:E268–E270, 2006.
16. Pompili A, Canitano S, Caroli F, et al.: Asymptomatic esophageal perforation caused by late screw migration after anterior cervical plating: report of a case and review of relevant literature, *Spine (Phila Pa 1976)* 27:E499–E502, 2002.

17. van Berge Henegouwen DP, Roukema JA, de Nie JC, van der Werken C: Esophageal perforation during surgery on the cervical spine, *Neurosurgery* 29:766–768, 1991.

18. Haku T, Okuda S, Kanematsu F, et al.: Repair of cervical esophageal perforation using longus colli muscle flap: a case report of a patient with cervical spinal cord injury, *Spine J* 8:831–835, 2008.

19. Navarro R, Javahery R, Eismont F, et al.: The role of the sternocleidomastoid muscle flap for esophageal fistula repair in anterior cervical spine surgery, *Spine (Phila Pa 1976)* 30:E617–E622, 2005.

20. Gómez-Caro Andrés A, Moradiellos Díez FJ, Ausín Herrero P, et al.: Successful conservative management in iatrogenic tracheobronchial injury, *Ann Thorac Surg* 79:1872–1878, 2005.

21. Schneider T, Storz K, Dienemann H, Hoffmann H: Management of iatrogenic tracheobronchial injuries: a retrospective analysis of 29 cases, *Ann Thorac Surg* 83:1960–1964, 2007.

22. Chauhan A, Ganguly M, Saidha N, Gulia P: Tracheal necrosis with surgical emphysema following thyroidectomy, *J Postgrad Med* 55:193–195, 2009.

23. Golger A, Rice LL, Jackson S, Young EM: Tracheal necrosis after thyroidectomy, *Can J Surg* 45:463–464, 2002.

24. Jacqmin S, Lentschener C, Demirev M, et al.: Postoperative necrosis of the anterior part of the cervical trachea following thyroidectomy, *J Anesth* 19:347–348, 2005.

25. Marty-Ané CH, Picard E, Jonquet O, Mary H: Membranous tracheal rupture after endotracheal intubation, *Ann Thorac Surg* 60:1367–1371, 1995.

26. Angelillo-Mackinlay T: Transcervical repair of distal membranous tracheal laceration, *Ann Thorac Surg* 59:531–532, 1995.

27. Jacobs JR, Thawley SE, Abata R, et al.: Posterior tracheal laceration: a rare complication of tracheostomy, *Laryngoscope* 88:1942–1946, 1978.

28. Carbognani P, Bobbio A, Cattelani L, et al.: Management of postintubation membranous tracheal rupture, *Ann Thorac Surg* 77:406–409, 2004.

29. Sippel M, Putensen C, Hirner A, Wolff M: Tracheal rupture after endotracheal intubation: experience with management in 13 cases, *Thorac Cardiovasc Surg* 54:51–56, 2006.

Dural Tear · 53

Jeffrey T. P. Luna and Tony Y. Tannoury

CHAPTER PREVIEW

Chapter Synopsis	Dural tear is not uncommon in cervical spine surgery, and the incidence varies depending on the disorder addressed and the procedure performed. Because the potential complications associated with a persistent cerebrospinal fluid (CSF) leak can be devastating, surgeons must have both intraoperative and postoperative treatment options available to them. Repair should involve appropriate measures to promote healing of the dural tear. Although direct dural repair is the preferred treatment for CSF leak, this technique is not always technically possible. In these cases, intraoperative adjuncts in combination with postoperative measures can be used to decrease the pressure gradient across the dural tear to help facilitate healing. The purpose of this chapter is to discuss dural tears during cervical spine surgery and review treatment strategies and their results.
Important Points	In a canine dural repair model, fibroblastic bridging was found to occur on day 6 and was complete by day 10.
	Collagen matrix onlay grafts attach by surface tension and act as a fibroblast scaffold for biologic repair.
	Numerous "sealant glues" are available, but results of their effectiveness vary.
	Dural drain output is adjusted based on the patient's clinical findings and neurologic status.
Clinical and Surgical Pearls	All accessible dural tears are repaired primarily.
	Dural grafting and chemical sealants can be used to augment primary repair.
	A lumbar drain is used for persistent leaks.
	Proper layered wound closure is vital to help obliterate the potential space.
Clinical and Surgical Pitfalls	The incidence of dural tears may be higher in patients with an ossified posterior longitudinal ligament.
	Primary closure of small dural tears may convert a low-pressure defect into high-pressure pinholes from the suture needle.
	Careful monitoring of patients with indwelling lumbar drains is imperative because of the potentially devastating risks associated with overdrainage of CSF.

Cerebrospinal fluid (CSF) leak from an incidental dural tear is not uncommon in cervical spine surgery. Various studies have reported an overall prevalence ranging from 0.5% to 3%.[1-3] However, for cervical spine operations in patients with ossification of the posterior longitudinal ligament (OPLL), the incidence is much higher, ranging from 4.3% to 32%.[3,4] Hannallah and associates reported that the presence of OPLL was the greatest risk factor for the development of a CSF leak after anterior

decompression surgical procedures, and patients with OPLL were 13.7 times more likely to have a CSF leak than were patients without this condition.[1]

Dural tears can occur in certain procedures during cervical spine dissection and decompression. The use of an electrocautery device during a posterior exposure, a pituitary rongeur during anterior diskectomy, a Kerrison rongeur during resection of the posterior longitudinal ligament and posterior foraminotomy, and elevation of the lamina during laminoplasty may all inadvertently tear the dura. As previously mentioned, anterior decompression with resection of the OPLL has been associated with the highest risk of producing a dural tear.[1]

The development of meningitis, spinocutaneous fistula, or pseudomeningocele has been associated with CSF leaks in the cervical spine.[5,6] In addition, patients with inadequately treated dural tears can present with delayed wound healing, postural headaches, vertigo, posterior neck pain, nausea, diplopia, photophobia, tinnitus, and blurred vision. These symptoms are caused by a persistent CSF leak from the subarachnoid space. The subsequent decrease in CSF pressure leads to a loss of buoyancy and caudal displacement of the intracranial contents.[7,8]

Because of the potential complications that may stem from an unresolved CSF leak, the surgeon must have a strategy to manage CSF leaks both intraoperatively and postoperatively. Repair should involve appropriate measures to promote healing of the dural tear. Cammisa and co-workers reported that when CSF leaks were recognized and treated appropriately, patients experienced no complications such as persistent recurrent headaches, meningitis, pseudomeningocele, cutaneous fistula, or neurologic deficit after an average follow-up of 22.4 months.[5] Various techniques have been described to manage dural tears and CSF leaks. These include the following: primary closure with microsurgical suturing or microdural stapling; augmentation with collagen matrix, fat and fascia graft, and other biologic grafts such as equine or bovine pericardium; reinforcement with the use of fibrin glue or chemical sealants; and insertion of lumbar and wound drains.[1,3,4,7,9]

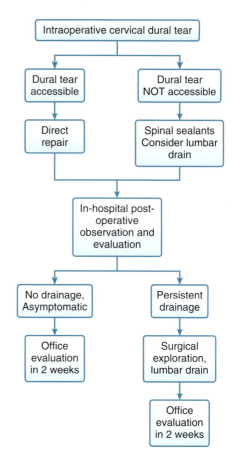

FIGURE 53-1　Treatment algorithm for cervical dural tears.

Intraoperative Strategy in the Treatment of a Cerebrospinal Fluid Leak

Primary Dural Repair

Management begins intraoperatively with proper identification of the dural tear (Fig. 53-1). Ideally, all accessible dural tears are repaired primarily. If a violation of the dura is recognized during the surgical procedure and is amenable to direct repair, then primary closure with microsurgical suture is attempted. Primary repair techniques aim to provide a watertight seal of the dural tear. However, in some cases, the lack of dural elasticity or gapping resulting from resection of adherent or ossified dura precludes watertight closure with sutures. In these instances, primary repair with a microsuturing technique may fail because of the resultant pinhole-sized tears from suture needles that allow CSF to leak through the dura. The potential risk of using primary suture closure for small incidental dural tears is conversion of a low-pressure defect to high-pressure pinholes from suture needles.[3] For this reason, intraoperative adjuncts such as collagen matrix (Duragen, Integra LifeSciences Corporation, Plainsboro, N.J.), autogenous fascia, and equine or bovine pericardium can be used to decrease the pressure gradient across the dural tear (Fig. 53-2). Cain and colleagues studied the biology of dural tear repair in a

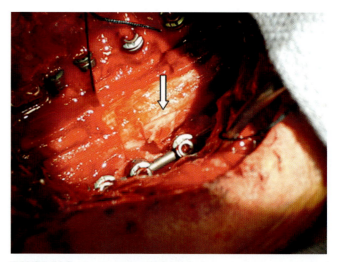

FIGURE 53-2　Intraoperative photograph demonstrating a primary dural repair augmented with bovine pericardium (*arrow*).

canine model.[10] These investigators found that fibroblastic bridging of the dural defect starts on the sixth day, and by the tenth day the defect is healed.

Dural Grafting and Chemical Sealants

Dural grafting can be used when repair is not amenable to microsuturing. The successful use of a collagen matrix onlay sutureless graft during primary repair of dural tears has been reported.[11] The onlay graft is placed

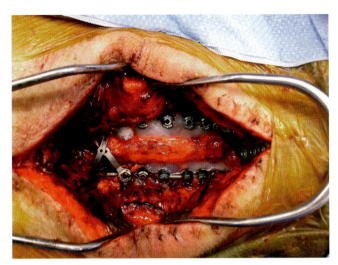

FIGURE 53-3 Intraoperative photograph demonstrating application of fibrin sealant.

over the defect and attaches by surface tension to the dura, where it provides a low-pressure absorptive surface to diffuse any CSF and acts as a site for biologic dural repair. The hemostatic properties of collagen initiate clot formation, resulting in an immediate chemical seal. The collagen matrix is a chemoattractant and provides a scaffold for fibroblasts to infiltrate and deposit new collagen, thereby reconstituting new dura. Fascial grafts can also be used to repair dural leaks primarily. Joseph and associates reported successful repair using fascial graft in combination with gelatin sponge, lumbar CSF drainage, and bed rest.[4]

Secondary augmentation of these dural repairs predominantly includes the addition of chemical materials such as sealants or fibrin glues. These substances are mainly used to enhance the primary dural repair after microsuturing or dural grafting, or they are applied to CSF leaks not amenable to primary repair (Fig. 53-3). The two sealants included DuraSeal (Confluent Surgical, Inc., Waltham, Mass.) and BioGlue (CryoLife, Kennesaw, Ga.), whereas the two human plasma-based fibrin glues included EVICEL (Johnson & Johnson Wound Management, Ethicon, Inc., Somerville, N.J.) and Tisseel (fibrin sealant; Baxter Healthcare, Deerfield, Ill.).

Results of the effectiveness and safety of sealants and fibrin glues vary. Epstein reported that although DuraSeal is approved by the U.S. Food and Drug Administration for intracranial and spinal application, two instances of paralysis have been described in the literature.[9] BioGlue has been used with good results but is classified by the manufacturer as neurotoxic. EVICEL, one of the fibrin glues, appeared in just two animal studies, whereas Tisseel, the other fibrin glue, has been used in many large clinical series with acceptable outcomes and without adverse events. In other studies, fibrin glue increased the strength of the repair of the sutured dura sevenfold and was also found to be effective as a stand-alone sealant.[12,13] Smaller tears that have low likelihood of leaking can be covered with a small piece of Gelfoam (Pfizer, New York, N.Y.), and the surgical procedure can be continued in an otherwise normal fashion.[1,4]

Lumbar Drains

The management of dural tears is governed by the size and degree of the CSF leak. If uncertainty exists about the propensity of an inaccessible dural leak to continue to drain, one should lean toward placing a lumbar CSF shunt or drain (Codman Lumbar External Drainage System, Johnson & Johnson, Raynham, Mass.). The use of a lumbar drain for cervical CSF leaks has been described.[1,3,4] It is the simplest device for decreasing intrathecal CSF pressure.

The lumbar drain is typically inserted postoperatively and is left in situ for 4 to 5 days, with drainage at a rate of 5 to 15 mL/hour, initially titrated at 10 mL/hour. This time frame is based on histologic evidence of dural sealing, which takes approximately 4 days to complete.[12,13] The rate of flow is adjusted, depending on the patient's clinical presentation and neurologic status.[13] The rate is reduced if postural headaches develop. The collection system (automatic pressure/volume-regulated pump versus gravity-assisted collection bag) attached guides whether a patient must be managed in the intensive care unit with close observation or in the general medical-surgical ward. Mobilization is generally restricted because of concerns about overdrainage and the risk of tonsillar herniation, tearing of epidural veins within the cranium, and rise of the gradient across the dural tear. Stool softeners and antiemetics are prescribed to avoid intrathecal peaks during Valsalva maneuvers.[3]

Wound Closure and Drains

Although controversial, insertion of a postoperative wound drain can also be performed. The drains are kept on gravity suction with use of a Jackson-Pratt bulb (Baxter Healthcare, Deerfield, Ill.) that is fully expanded so that it will not hold suction. The drains are usually discontinued on postoperative day 1 or 2. It is also important not to overlook proper wound closure. Wound closure should be aimed at layer by layer suturing to appose soft tissues adequately and thereby decrease the incidence of potential dead space. It is the authors' preference to have all patients with a dural tear confined to bed rest for at least one night. They are also all given antiemetics and stool softeners in an attempt to avoid the increased intrathecal pressure associated with emesis and Valsalva maneuvers.

Postoperative Management

Bed Rest

Traditional management has been mandatory bed rest for at least 48 hours following repair, with or without placement of a drain. With the muscle-splitting approach and the decreased potential (dead) space created during minimally invasive spinal surgery, the likelihood of symptoms such as spinal headaches or CSF fistulas is less. Although the duration of bed rest varies, postoperative management involves early mobilization less than 48 hours after the surgical procedure. Than and colleagues reported that early postoperative mobilization appears to be a reasonable option and results in shorter hospitalization.[14] Once stable, patients are typically seen in the office 2 weeks following discharge from the hospital.

Conclusions

Dural tear is not uncommon in cervical spine surgery, and the incidence varies depending on the disorder addressed and the procedure performed. Because the potential complications associated with a persistent CSF leak can be devastating, surgeons must have both intraoperative and postoperative treatment options available to them. Repair should involve appropriate measures to promote healing of the dural tear. Although direct dural repair is the preferred treatment for CSF leak, this technique is not always technically possible. In these cases, intraoperative adjuncts in combination with postoperative measures can be used to decrease the pressure gradient across the dural tear to help facilitate healing. The addition of a lumbar drain can be used to decrease intrathecal CSF pressure; however, care should be taken to avoid overdrainage and its associated complications.

REFERENCES

1. Hannallah D, Lee J, Khan M, et al.: Cerebrospinal fluid leaks following cervical spine surgery, *J Bone Joint Surg Am* 90:1101–1105, 2008.
2. Williams BJ, Sansur CA, Smith JS, et al.: Incidence of unintended durotomy in spine surgery based on 108,478 cases, *Neurosurgery* 68:117–123, 2010. discussion 123–124.
3. REFERENCE DELETED IN PROOFS..
4. Joseph V, Kumar GS, Rajshekhar V: Cerebrospinal fluid leak during cervical corpectomy for ossified posterior longitudinal ligament: incidence, management, and outcome, *Spine (Phila Pa 1976)* 34:491–494, 2009.
5. Cammisa FP Jr, Girardi FP, Sangani PK, et al.: Incidental durotomy in spine surgery, *Spine (Phila Pa 1976)* 25:2663–2667, 2000.
6. Fountas KN, Kapsalaki EZ, Johnston KW: Cerebrospinal fluid fistula secondary to dural tear in anterior cervical discectomy and fusion: case report, *Spine (Phila Pa 1976)* 30:E277–E280, 2005.
7. Guerin P, El Fegoun AB, Obeid I, et al.: Incidental durotomy during spine surgery: incidence, management and complications: a retrospective review, *Injury* 43:397–401, 2012.
8. McCullogh JA, Young PH: Complications of cervical spine microsurgery. In McCullogh JA, Young PH, editors: *Essentials of spinal microsurgery*, Philadelphia, 1997, Lippincott-Raven, pp 209–215.
9. Epstein NE: Dural repair with four spinal sealants: focused review of the manufacturers' inserts and the current literature, *Spine J* 10:1065–1068, 2010.
10. Cain JE Jr, Lauerman WC, Rosenthal HG, et al.: The histomorphologic sequence of dural repair: observations in the canine model, *Spine (Phila Pa 1976)* 16:S319–S323, 1991.
11. Narotam PK, Jose S, Nathoo N, et al.: Collagen matrix (DuraGen) in dural repair: analysis of a new modified technique, *Spine (Phila Pa 1976)* 29:2861–2867, 2004. discussion 2868–2869.
12. Cain JE Jr, Dryer RF, Barton BR: Evaluation of dural closure techniques: suture methods, fibrin adhesive sealant, and cyanoacrylate polymer, *Spine (Phila Pa 1976)* 13:720–725, 1988.
13. Cain JE Jr, Rosenthal HG, Broom MJ, et al.: Quantification of leakage pressures after durotomy repairs in the canine, *Spine (Phila Pa 1976)* 15:969–970, 1990.
14. Than KD, Wang AC, Etame AB, et al.: Postoperative management of incidental durotomy in minimally invasive lumbar spinal surgery, *Minim Invasive Neurosurg* 51:263–266, 2008.

54

Wound Complications

Geoffrey E. Stoker, Jacob M. Buchowski, and Albert S. Woo

CHAPTER PREVIEW

Chapter Synopsis	Wound complications, namely infection and dehiscence, are some of the most common adverse events following spinal surgical procedures. These complications can incur substantial morbidity and financial burden. Risk factor modification and prevention represent a burgeoning paradigm. Yet evidence-based guidelines for diagnosing and treating these problems are few. A working knowledge of wound healing physiology, proper surgical technique, a high index of suspicion, and sound clinical judgment must all be exercised in concert to optimize patients' outcomes.
Important Points	Although they occur with low frequency, cervical wound infections can lead to sepsis and death.
	Potentially modifiable risk factors include active infection, malnutrition, obesity, diabetes, smoking, and corticosteroid treatment, among others.
	Regardless of risk factors, prophylactic antibiotics are a proven means of preventing surgical site infections.
	Diagnosing wound infection is challenging because acute signs and symptoms mimic those observed after uncomplicated spinal surgery. Thus, a high degree of clinical suspicion is necessary.
	When a wound infection is identified, expeditious treatment is warranted.
	Management generally consists of broad-spectrum antibiotics with antistaphylococcal coverage, vigilant wound care, and formal surgical débridement for more extensive and subfascial manifestations.

As operative capabilities have improved in conjunction with perioperative medical management, increasingly older patients with more comorbidities have become viable candidates for spine surgery. Unfortunately, the risk of wound complications inherent in modern procedures is amplified in these patients. This fact is particularly salient in the cervical spine, where infection or hematoma can involve the trachea and proximal spinal cord. Thus, it is imperative that risk factors are identified, modified when possible, and thoroughly explained to patients. Appropriate technique should be exercised, and a high index of suspicion must be maintained postoperatively. Timely diagnosis is the only way to treat complications optimally and to avoid medicolegal repercussions reliably. With a decided focus on surgical site infections (SSIs), this chapter reviews strategies for the avoidance and management of cervical spine wound complications.

Preoperative Complications

Prevalence

Contemporary antisepsis and antibiotics have dramatically reduced the prevalence and morbidity of SSIs across all disciplines. Spine surgery is no exception, with wound infection rates as low as 0.2% and 1.6% reported in the anterior cervical setting. In a reported series, 132 of 3174 (4.2%) patients undergoing any spinal procedure developed infection.[1] At the authors' center, acute SSIs complicated only 1.0% of 1001 consecutive posterior cervical cases.[2] Despite these low figures, SSI is one of the most common adverse events in spine surgery. Furthermore, the prevalence of methicillin-resistant *Staphylococcus aureus* (MRSA) is rising, thus making risk factor modification invaluable.

Demographic and Medical Risk Factors

Alcohol consumption, cigarette smoking, and intravenous drug abuse represent behavioral risk factors for SSI.[3] Smoking intervention even a month before the surgical procedure may prove beneficial. Indwelling venous catheters serve as reservoirs for nosocomial organisms. To diminish such colonization, patients hospitalized for extended periods may be allowed to return home before elective procedures. Trauma victims and those admitted to an intensive care unit are at high risk, but their medical status often obviates interim discharge. Fortunately, the comorbidities associated with trauma can be addressed. Most importantly, active infection should be treated as long as the spinal disorder permits.

Ironically, both malnutrition and obesity predispose patients to SSI.[1,2,4] Because malnutrition hampers antibody production, hyperalimentation is an attractive preventive measure. A lymphocyte count lower than 1500 mm^{-3}, albumin lower than 3.5 g/dL, or transferrin lower than 226 mg/dL should raise concern. The role of obesity is less clear. Whereas the dissection required for a corpulent neck entails a wide field for inoculation, adipose tissue is relatively immunoprivileged. Despite these mechanisms, the correlation of body mass to infection is perhaps more aptly described by comorbidity. The glucose level of uncontrolled diabetes (>200 mg/dL) retards leukocyte function and has been linked to a variety of complications including SSI.[1,4] Optimizing glucose concentrations preoperatively is ideal.

Intuitively, immunosuppression augments the likelihood of infection. Causes include certain malignant diseases, cancer chemotherapeutics, drugs to combat graft-versus-host disease, and acquired immunodeficiency syndrome with a CD4 count lower than 200 mm^{-3} or a viral load greater than 10,000 mL^{-1}. Rheumatoid arthritis is an especially relevant medical risk factor.[2] The disease itself promotes cervical instability, and antirheumatic agents hinder wound healing. Tapering of iatrogenic causes of immunosuppression and dehiscence demands careful risk-to-benefit discussions, often with an internal medicine specialist. For instance, an approximately 2-month window (6 weeks before and 2 weeks after surgical procedures) exists around which radiation therapy may be scheduled to maximize healing.[5]

Radiation therapy and prior spine operations also increase scar tissue and intraoperative hemorrhage, which predisposes to hematoma.[6] This can cause airway compression and serve as a nidus for infection. Evidence for the use of antifibrinolytic agents in major spine surgery has accumulated, although these agents are seldom indicated in the cervical surgical setting. Moreover, hypervascular tumor embolization may be appraised before resection.

Antibiotic Prophylaxis

Antibiotic prophylaxis is widely supported in spine surgery.[7] Depending on body habitus, a dose of 1 to 2 gs of first-generation cephalosporins is favored, given that these drugs cover *S. aureus* and *Staphylococcus epidermidis*, which are constituents of normal skin flora and are common causes of SSI.[7,8] Intravenous administration of cefazolin between 30 and 60 minutes before incision is generally regarded as optimal timing.[4] Patients who have sustained traumatic soft tissue injury should be evaluated for gram-negative and polymicrobial infection before the drug is chosen. In patients with a cephalosporin allergy, clindamycin and vancomycin are considered. Vancomycin may also be a prudent choice for patients at risk of MRSA colonization, but it is rarely contraindicated because of potential toxicity in renal failure. Gram-negative coverage is recommended during transoral exposure. With the exception of immunodeficiency, broad-spectrum cocktails should be avoided to reduce the selection of bacterial resistance.

Intraoperative Complications

Surgical Risk Factors

Because preoperatively administered antibiotics are inevitably cleared from the body, repeat doses are warranted at the 3- to 4-hour threshold.[1] Blood loss greater than 1 L correspondingly depletes the serum of antibiotics.[1] Conceivably a proxy for anemia, allogeneic transfusion is a risk factor for SSI. The risk of allogeneic bone graft, alternatively, may result from inflammatory changes incited by the foreign tissue. Microscopes and undue nonessential personnel may also increase contamination.

A greater incidence of spinal wound infection has been found with posterior approaches and more than three surgical levels.[2,4] Because cervical disease is frequently addressed with less invasive anterior cervical diskectomy and fusion, cervical operations have a lower rate of SSI.[4] Furthermore, anterior dissection is carried out through avascular planes, whereas posterior exposure entails muscle stripping, and necrotic tissue is often spared from débridement for the sake of wound coverage. Instrumentation provides a substrate for biofilms, and persistent micromotion may cause inflammation and edema. Recombinant human bone morphogenetic protein-2 has been implicated in the development of seroma as well and should not be used in the anterior cervical spine unless it is overwhelmingly necessary.[9] Dehiscence resulting from instrumentation prominence can provide an entry route for pathogens. Implants and graft may be padded with muscle or fat. Similarly, esophageal perforations and transoral exposures communicate with the gastrointestinal tract. In these cases, antibiotics should be modified.

Antisepsis and Technique

Thorough hand and forearm scrubbing and double gloving are mandatory. Nearby hair should be shaved with an electric trimmer. At the authors' center, the skin and surrounding drapes are pre-prepared with alcohol foam.[2] The surgical site is then cleansed with either povidone-iodine or chlorhexidine-alcohol solution.[10,11] Occlusive membranes may complete the preparation. Intraoperatively, meticulous hemostasis is crucial. To this end, bipolar electrocautery, Gelfoam, and Surgicel are all valuable. Self-retaining retractors are periodically loosened to maintain perfusion, and the wound is generously irrigated.

During closure, necrotic tissue should be débrided, but large defects may preclude coverage. Integument compromised by corticosteroids or radiation therapy is predisposed to dehiscence even in the absence of infection. The authors advise soliciting the assistance of a plastic surgeon for soft tissue flap transfer. In any case, elimination of dead space and watertight closure are essential. Before posterior closure, 500 mg of topical, intrawound vancomycin powder is applied, and a subfascial drain is placed.[2] Superficial drains are added in patients with more than 2 cm of subcutaneous adipose tissue.

Postoperative Complications

General Care

Postoperatively, the same risk factors identified and addressed before the surgical procedure continue to play a role. Previously bedridden patients with spinal cord injury should be monitored for decubitus ulcers and incontinence. All patients should be mobilized and encouraged to walk as soon as possible. Prophylactic antibiotics are customarily readministered every 6 hours and are terminated within 24 hours. Drains, barring evidence of infection, are removed within 48 hours. Dressing changes are dictated by the condition of the wound, as noted on daily inspection. Therefore, the signs and symptoms of wound complications must be explained to the patient and relatives, who should be instructed to contact the hospital or present to an emergency department immediately if such problems are heralded.

Clinical Presentation

Because SSIs can manifest with a broad continuum of signs and symptoms, some far more overt than others, a high index of suspicion is essential. Acute superficial SSI occurs in the epidermis and dermis within 3 to 4 weeks, usually before full healing.[8] As such, characteristic swelling, warmth, erythema, and drainage often become quite apparent. Pain is a ubiquitous symptom. It may arise after initial relief and seem incongruent with other signs. These features can be difficult to discern from the normal recuperative response to surgery. When the signs and symptoms persist after day 3, suspicion is raised. Other red flags include prolonged or putrid drainage, purulence, expanding erythema, and constitutional signs and symptoms such as fever, chills, malaise, and lethargy.

Differentiating deep from superficial infections is also challenging in the acute stage. Conversely, the evident nature of superficial SSI may mask an occult deep infection below the fascia overlying the platysma and paraspinal muscles. The signs mimic those of a superficial infection but may not manifest as early[8]; multilayer closure contributes to an initially benign appearance. Patients commonly present with increasing pain and drainage, which proves recalcitrant to routine care. Left untreated, myonecrosis and cellulitis may develop. Local problems eventually give way to systemic sequelae, possibly culminating in septic shock. The diagnosis of deep SSI is further complicated when it occurs months or years after successful healing (Fig. 54-1). Pain and tenderness may be the only ostensible findings.

Besides frank infection, wound complications can cause significant morbidity through mass effects. In the cervical spine, abscess, hematoma, and seroma pose risks to the trachea and esophagus. Swelling with dysphagia or labored breathing must be investigated on an emergency basis. Retropharyngeal infection, conversely, can promote dysphagia without true abscess formation. The lack of pain and erythema in the presence of sterile hematoma or seroma allows the clinician to worry less about SSI. Abscess and hematoma may form in the spinal canal as well, creating spinal cord compression and neurologic deficit.

Diagnostics

When SSI cannot be ruled out based on physical findings, blood workup ensues, ideally during episodes of fever. After uncomplicated surgical procedures of the spine, up to 6 weeks of erythrocyte sedimentation rate (ESR) elevation has been reported, thus limiting its utility.[12] This rise is characterized by a peak within the first or second week. A spike thereafter is worrisome. In general, C-reactive protein (CRP) peaks within 2 days, uniformly returns to baseline within 2 weeks, and is considered the most sensitive marker for SSI.[12,13] Serial measurement is simple and reliable.[13] CRP and ESR normalization may be further delayed by instrumentation. In a large series, CRP and ESR were elevated in 98% and 94% of SSI cases, respectively.[8] In contrast, white blood cell count may be abnormally high in less than 50% of cases and even less robust in superficial SSI.

Radiology plays a less important role in diagnosis than in determining whether infection has invaded the bony vertebral column. Besides shadows of abscess and necrotizing gas formation, changes on plain films may not be observed for 3 to 6 weeks. These signs include peri-implant radiolucency, end plate dissolution, and disk collapse. Screw pull-out and instability may be harbingers of such structural changes. Computed tomography can detect bony abnormalities sooner and may facilitate aspiration, but this modality is more useful when infection has spread to the spine. Magnetic resonance imaging is the gold standard modality for soft tissue. Normal and pathologic soft tissue edema, however, gives rise to similar Modic I changes. A peripheral ring of gadolinium enhancement may be the only factor delineating infectious from benign fluid collections.

Culture analysis ascertains drug sensitivity, Gram staining, and anaerobic versus aerobic metabolism. Culture of wound drainage may be obscured by skin flora contamination, blood culture results are often negative, and deep aspiration through an untreated superficial infection may seed subfascial SSI. Latent infections with periprosthetic glycocalyx will likely produce negative culture results as well. Furthermore, spinal aspiration failure rates as high as 30% have been reported. Positive yields approach 100% with tissue acquired from a reopened wound. Thus, when open treatment is planned, prior culture is unnecessary. Ultimately, intervention must not be postponed for the sake of radiologic or microbiologic corroboration. If SSI is identified or even suspected, immediate intervention is preferred over expectant management.

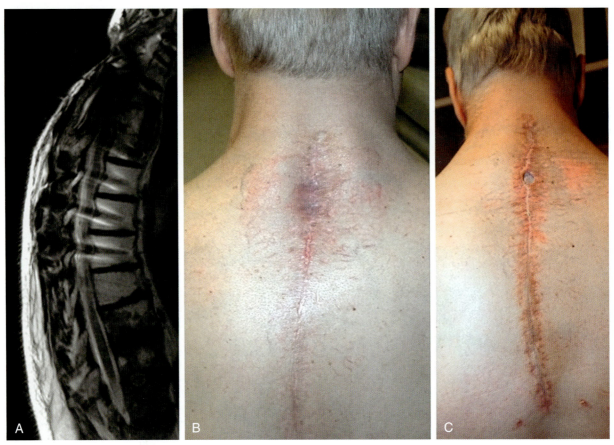

FIGURE 54-1 **A,** This 45-year-old man's magnetic resonance scan showed metastasis involving T3 and paraspinal muscles, as well as diffuse postradiation fatty marrow replacement. **B,** Four months following revision posterior instrumented fusion, he developed fluctuance beneath his incision. The fluid was aspirated, and cultures were consistent with coagulase-negative *Staphylococcus*. Given the likelihood of a deep surgical site infection, irrigation and débridement with seroma capsulectomy and trapezius advancement were performed. **C,** Postoperatively, minor superficial dehiscence occurred.

Management

Indications for surgical débridement include persistent drainage or constitutional signs, dehiscence, epidural abscess, neurologic deficit, instrumentation failure, and spinal instability. When these conditions are not met, conservative intervention consists of a 6-week trial of oral broad-spectrum antibiotics with vigilant wound care and ESR and CRP surveillance.[8] If a positive culture result is obtained, the antibiotic regimen is tailored accordingly. Long-term suppression may be prudent in the presence of instrumentation. These decisions should be made in concert with an infectious disease service.

If the indications for open treatment are met or conservative therapy fails, as is likely with subfascial SSI, the wound must be promptly explored. Antibiotics should be withheld for at least 24 hours before any specimen is excised for culture. These drugs can be reinstituted immediately thereafter and modified according to the results. A limited superficial SSI in a healthy individual may be treated with simple reopening, irrigation, and drainage.[8] Whether in limited exploration or formal surgical débridement, one must ensure that the subfascial compartment appears spared of infection. Local tissue culture is then obtained, and the deep space is aspirated. Wet-to-dry dressing with healing by secondary intention may be appropriate, along with an antibiotic course similar to that described earlier. When these measures fail or if organisms are cultured from the subfascial space, operative débridement is undertaken.

Even in formal débridement, the deep space may be left closed if compelling evidence indicates that it has been spared of infection. If not, the entire wound is reopened along the original surgical planes. The next objective is thorough, sharp débridement of all devitalized soft tissue and bone. Muscles are closely scrutinized for myonecrosis; electrocautery-induced muscle contractions suggest viability. The integrity of the esophagus should be assessed. Any tear should be oversewn, and a consultation with an ear, nose, and throat specialist should be considered. Necrotic or loose bone graft is débrided and replaced. If osteolysis or débridement has compromised fixation or stability, the construct is revised, preferably with titanium. Maintaining stability is the third major goal. With débridement complete, the defect is pulsatile lavage irrigated with copious (5 to 10 L) antibiotic-laden saline.[14] Repeat washout and débridement may be scheduled at 48 and 72 hours if multiple or highly virulent organisms are cultured, if diffuse myonecrosis is noted, and if the patient is immunocompromised or at otherwise high risk of future infection or dehiscence.[3] Culture specimens should be obtained at each successive procedure because wound flora often changes. Some investigators have suggested using antibiotic-impregnated cement beads in such cases. Nevertheless, these decisions are largely based on the surgeon's preference.

Various methods are used to effect wound closure, the last main objective of surgical management. Ideally, primary closure is attained over drains at each level. These drains may be removed when output drops to less than 20 mL/day. Repeat surgery is warranted if purulence reemerges. Large wounds with extensive deep infection or myonecrosis or wounds in immunocompromised patients may be left open to heal and granulate with daily wet-to-dry dressing changes. Alternatively, a vacuum-assisted closure (VAC) sponge can be placed. The negative pressure imparted by these devices is postulated to increase perfusion, mechanically stimulate cells, and remove inhibitory signals from the local interstitium. However, the use of VAC is contraindicated in the anterior cervical setting and in patients with bleeding diatheses or a local fistula.

As stated earlier, plastic surgeons are valuable allies for complex final closure. A discussion of muscle, myocutaneous, and fasciocutaneous flap advancement is beyond the scope of this text, but every spine surgeon should be cognizant of their advantages. These techniques afford coverage and padding of prominent implants and bone. Arguably more important, these flaps augment vascularity, thus allowing leukocytes and antibiotics to permeate the physiologically challenged tissue. Once again, organism-specific drugs follow broad-spectrum antibiotics, and long-term suppression decisions are made based on the host's immune status, the microbes, and the presence of implants.[3]

CLINICAL CASE

A 59-year-old woman had instrumented fusion and radiation therapy 2 years earlier for T4 and T5 renal cell carcinoma metastasis. Imaging revealed T5 fracture and retropulsion, which explained her myelopathy. She underwent posterior reconstruction from T1 to T10 (Fig. 54-2, *A*).

One month postoperatively, the patient presented with wound necrosis but no purulence. The next day, formal débridement was performed with vacuum-assisted closure (VAC) device placement. Preplanned repeat débridement was performed 2 days later.

At 5-week follow-up, a small focus of dehiscence, which overlay a cavity extending to the trapezius, was observed (Figs. 54-2, *B*, and 54-3, *A*). When the patient presented 2 days later for VAC application, the defect was markedly enlarged. Implant exposure was noted, with minimal granulation, but neither erythema nor induration. C-reactive protein (8 mg/dL) and erythrocyte sedimentation rate (62 mm/hour) values were elevated, but results of culture were negative. The infectious disease department recommended oral doxycycline suppression. Over the next several weeks, the dehiscence worsened (Fig. 54-3, *B*). Despite the patient's nausea and vomiting, as well as numerous attempts to notify the patient of the situation's gravity, she refused to follow up at the authors' center.

The patient eventually returned after 10 weeks. She had an open wound with right latissimus exposure and skin retraction (Fig. 54-3, *C*). No evidence of infection was noted. The plastic surgery department performed next-day extensive débridement and bone biopsies (Fig. 54-4, *A*). Instrumentation was intact and retained. A superficial portion of the right trapezius was dissected and flipped on a hinge of medial muscle. This flap was sutured to the contralateral trapezius, thus spanning the defect (Fig. 54-4, *B*). Skin was undermined and mobilized to effect coverage. Biopsy specimens grew no organisms, and lifelong oral doxycycline suppression therapy was prescribed. At 1-month follow-up, the drain was removed, and the incision was intact (Fig. 54-4, *C*). At the most recent, 8-month follow-up, the wound had healed, and the patient expressed satisfaction with her result.

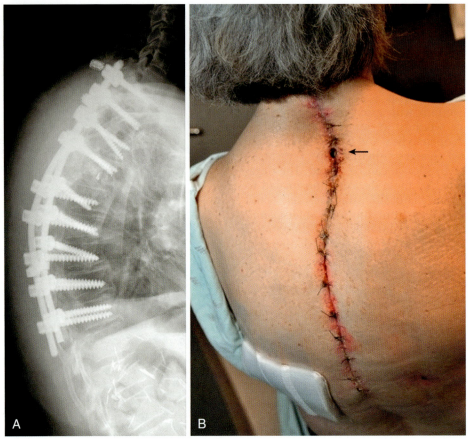

FIGURE 54-2 A, This 59-year-old woman underwent revision posterior reconstruction from T1 to T10 for pathologic fracture of T5 with resultant myelopathy. **B,** One-month postoperative clinical photographs showed a small focus of dehiscence (*arrow*).

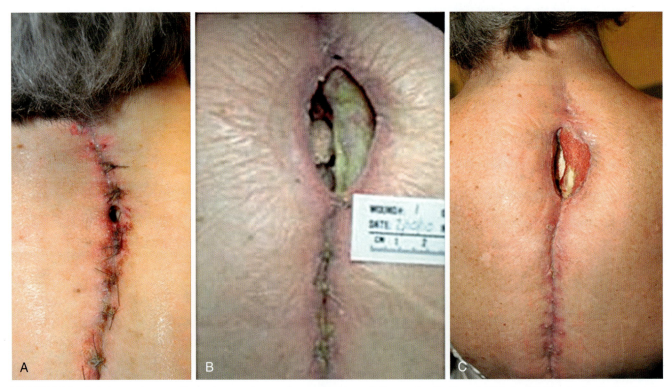

FIGURE 54-3 A, A deep cavity extending to the trapezius muscle was noted beneath the opening. **B,** Approximately 1 week after leaving the hospital, the patient's daughter e-mailed a photograph demonstrating further wound breakdown and exposure of underlying graft material. **C,** When the patient returned for follow-up, the defect was 6 cm long and 3 cm wide but without signs of infection.

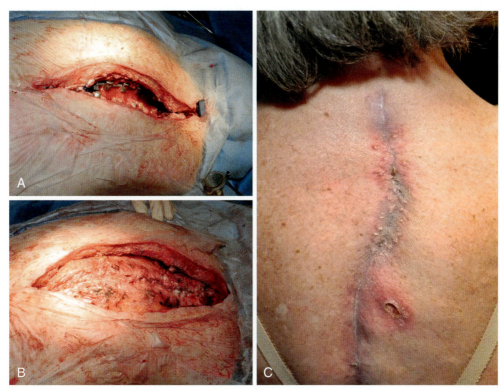

FIGURE 54-4 A, The patient's wound was widely reopening along the original surgical plane. **B,** A trapezius flap was rotated across the wound defect to cover and pad all prominent instrumentation and graft material. **C,** One month following wound reconstruction, the incision was healed. Because of minimal persistent output, the patient's drain was removed.

Conclusions

Postoperative wound complications can incur substantial morbidity. Abscess and sterile seroma can injure the neural elements or trachea. Causative organisms may disseminate to afflict vital organs, with the potential for mortality. Moreover, the financial ramifications of wound complications and their burden on our health care system are significant. The total cost of subfascial SSI treatment has been estimated at $20,000. A half-gram of vancomycin powder, in contrast, costs less than $20. Considering this and the dearth of evidence-based guidelines for the diagnosis and treatment of SSI, the importance of prevention cannot be overstated and yet will only grow as nosocomial infection reimbursement policies evolve in the United States.

REFERENCES

1. Pull ter Gunne AF, Cohen DB: The incidence, prevalence, and analysis of risk factors for surgical site infection following adult spinal surgery, *Spine (Phila Pa 1976)* 34:1422–1428, 2009.
2. Pahys JM, Pahys JR, Cho SK, et al.: Methods to decrease postoperative infections following posterior cervical spine surgery, *J Bone Joint Surg Am* 95:549–554, 2013.
3. Thalgott JS, Cotler HB, Sasso RC, et al.: Postoperative infections in spinal implants: classification and analysis—a multicenter study, *Spine (Phila Pa 1976)* 16:981–984, 1991.
4. Olsen MA, Nepple JJ, Riew KD, et al.: Risk factors for surgical site infection following orthopaedic spinal operations, *J Bone Joint Surg Am* 90:62–69, 2008.
5. Ghogawala Z, Mansfield FL, Borges LF: Spinal radiation before surgical decompression adversely affects outcomes of surgery for symptomatic metastatic spinal cord compression, *Spine (Phila Pa 1976)* 26:818–824, 2001.
6. Awad JN, Kebaish KM, Donigan J, et al.: Analysis of the risk factors for the development of post-operative spinal epidural haematoma, *J Bone Joint Surg Br* 87:1248–1252, 2005.
7. Barker FG 2nd: Efficacy of prophylactic antibiotic therapy in spinal surgery: a meta-analysis, *Neurosurgery* 51:391–400, 2002. discussion 400–401.
8. Pull ter Gunne AF, Mohamed AS, Skolasky RL, et al.: The presentation, incidence, etiology, and treatment of surgical site infections after spinal surgery, *Spine (Phila Pa 1976)* 35:1323–1328, 2010.
9. Cahill KS, Chi JH, Day A, Claus EB: Prevalence, complications, and hospital charges associated with use of bone-morphogenetic proteins in spinal fusion procedures, *JAMA* 302:58–66, 2009.
10. Bibbo C, Patel DV, Gehrmann RM, Lin SS: Chlorhexidine provides superior skin decontamination in foot and ankle surgery: a prospective randomized study, *Clin Orthop Relat Res (438)* 204–208, 2005.
11. Darouiche RO, Wall MJ Jr, Itani KM, et al.: Chlorhexidine-alcohol versus povidone-iodine for surgical-site antisepsis, *N Engl J Med* 362:18–26, 2010.
12. Thelander U, Larsson S: Quantitation of C-reactive protein levels and erythrocyte sedimentation rate after spinal surgery, *Spine (Phila Pa 1976)* 17:400–404, 1992.
13. Kang BU, Lee SH, Ahn Y, et al.: Surgical site infection in spinal surgery: detection and management based on serial C-reactive protein measurements, *J Neurosurg Spine* 13:158–164, 2010.
14. Cheng MT, Chang MC, Wang ST, et al.: Efficacy of dilute betadine solution irrigation in the prevention of postoperative infection of spinal surgery, *Spine (Phila Pa 1976)* 30:1689–1693, 2005.

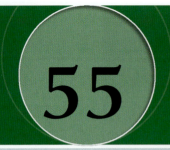

55

Adjacent Segment Disease

Conor Regan and Moe R. Lim

CHAPTER PREVIEW

Chapter Synopsis	Adjacent level disease is a relatively frequent clinical finding in cervical spine surgery. An overall rate of approximately 3% per year can be expected in patients who have undergone cervical surgical procedures. Whenever possible, nonoperative treatment should be attempted, but it may be less successful than in de novo cervical spondylotic syndromes. Anterior cervical diskectomy and fusion at the adjacent level or posterior procedures provide good clinical outcomes, whereas disk arthroplasty requires further study. The purpose of this chapter is to review the biomechanical and technical considerations, as well as the history, examination, imaging, and treatment for adjacent segment disease.
Important Points	Adjacent level *degeneration* is radiographic evidence of degenerative change and may or may not be associated with symptomatic adjacent segment *disease*.
	The incidence of adjacent segment disease remains relatively constant at 3% per year after cervical spine surgery.
	Furthermore, the incidence of adjacent segment disease remains the same after both fusion and motion-preserving cervical spine surgery.
	Adjacent segment disease may be related to biomechanical and technical considerations or may be the natural history of cervical disk degeneration, or both.
Clinical and Surgical Pearls	Nonoperative management remains the mainstay of treatment whenever possible for adjacent segment disease, although it may be less effective for spondylotic disease.
	Anterior cervical plate placement less than 5 mm from the adjacent disk space may increase adjacent segment disease.
	In cases of revision anterior cervical surgical procedures, preoperative otolaryngology consultation is strongly recommended to evaluate for occult recurrent laryngeal nerve injury on the side of the index procedure.
Clinical and Surgical Pitfalls	Incorrect needle localization at the time of the index surgical procedure may increase adjacent segment degeneration rates.
	Fusion of the cervical spine in a kyphotic alignment may increase the rate of adjacent level degeneration.

Adjacent level or adjacent segment *disease* was defined by Hilibrand and colleagues as the development of new radiculopathy or myelopathy referable to a motion segment adjacent to the site of a previous anterior arthrodesis of the cervical spine[1] (Table 55-1). Adjacent level *degeneration*, conversely, refers only to radiographic evidence of degenerative changes, whereas adjacent level ossification disease (ALOD) refers to anterior ossification at an adjacent level with or without degenerative changes within the disk space.

Adjacent segment disease is a relatively common phenomenon following cervical spine surgery. In their landmark article, Hilibrand and associates showed a relatively constant incidence of 3% per year for the development of adjacent segment disease following anterior cervical diskectomy and fusion (ACDF).[1] These investigators demonstrated that adjacent segment disease requiring treatment was associated with fusion adjacent to C5 to C6 or C6 to C7 and in patients with preexisting radiographic

Table 55-1 Radiographic Grading of Adjacent Segment Disease

Grade	Radiographic Findings	MRI Findings
I	Normal	Normal
II	Narrowing of disk space without posterior osteophytes	Signal change in intervertebral disk
III	Narrowing of disk space with posterior osteophytes	Disk protrusion without cord or nerve root compression
IV	Narrowing of disk space with posterior osteophytes	Spinal cord compression

MRI, Magnetic resonance imaging.

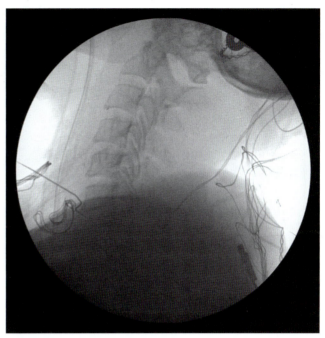

FIGURE 55-1   Needle localization of C6 and C7 in preparation for C6-7 anterior cervical diskectomy and fusion.

degeneration at the adjacent level. The incidence found by Hilibrand and co-workers has been corroborated by other investigators.[2]

Despite general agreement among investigators regarding the risk of adjacent segment disease, consensus on its cause is lacking. Many investigators believe that adjacent segment disease is the direct result of surgical intervention. Several biomechanical and clinical findings support the idea of iatrogenic adjacent segment disease. Other investigators, however, believe that adjacent segment disease follows the natural history of cervical spondylosis.

Natural history cohort studies suggest a correlation of ACDF with adjacent segment degeneration. Matsumoto and associates compared magnetic resonance imaging (MRI) findings in 64 patients who had undergone ACDF with MRI findings in 201 asymptomatic volunteers.[3] At a mean follow-up of approximately 12 years, the ACDF-treated group had significantly greater adjacent level decrease in disk signal intensity, disk herniation, disk space narrowing, and foraminal stenosis.

Biomechanical and Technical Considerations

Several biomechanical studies demonstrated increased disk pressure and hypermobility in disks adjacent to cervical fusion. Eck and associates performed C5-C6 ACDF on six cadaveric specimens and measured adjacent intradiskal pressure and segmental motion during range-of-motion testing.[4] In flexion, intradiskal pressure increased by 73.2% at the cranial adjacent level and 45.3% at the caudal level. Segmental motion increased at the adjacent levels in both extension and flexion. These results support the idea that adjacent segment disease is caused by increased adjacent disk pressure and shear forces compared with the normal state.

In addition to these biomechanical findings, several technical surgical issues have been found to play a role in adjacent segment degeneration, but not necessarily disease. Faldini and colleagues retrospectively evaluated 107 patients after single-level ACDF. At a mean of 16 years of follow-up, the group who underwent fusion initially in segmental kyphosis (postoperative sagittal alignment <0°) had a radiographic adjacent segment degeneration rate of 60%. In contrast, the patients who underwent fusion in lordosis (postoperative sagittal alignment >0°)

exhibited a rate of 27%.[5] Katsuura and co-workers retrospectively evaluated 42 patients after ACDF at a mean of 9.8 years. These investigators found an adjacent segment radiographic degeneration rate of 77% in patients fused in kyphosis.[6]

Another technical issue believed to be predictive of accelerated adjacent level degeneration is incorrect-level intraoperative needle localization (Fig. 55-1). A retrospective analysis of 87 consecutive patients following 1- or 2-level ACDF showed a 3-fold increase in adjacent level radiographic degeneration in patients who had incorrect-level needle localization. Patients who were correctly marked intraoperatively at the time of index ACDF had an adjacent segment degeneration rate of 32% at 2-year follow-up versus 60% in those who were incorrectly marked.[7]

Anterior cervical plate position may also be another technical issue related to adjacent segment abnormalities. Adjacent level ossification disease (ALOD) is defined as the development of anterior ossification at a level adjacent to a fusion and has been shown to be correlated with plate placement less than 5 mm from the adjacent disk space (Fig. 55-2). Park and colleagues retrospectively evaluated 118 patients at a mean follow-up of 25.7 months. ALOD developed in 59% of the cephalad levels and 29% of the caudal levels. Placement of the plate more than 5 mm from the adjacent disk space reduced ALOD rates from 67% to 24% at the cephalad level and from 45% to 5% at the caudal level.[8]

In contrast to the contention that adjacent segment disease is iatrogenically caused by fusion, several other lines of evidence support the notion that the disease is caused by the natural history of cervical spondylotic disease. Reitman and associates,[9] as well as Kolstad and associates,[10] performed motion analysis in patients before

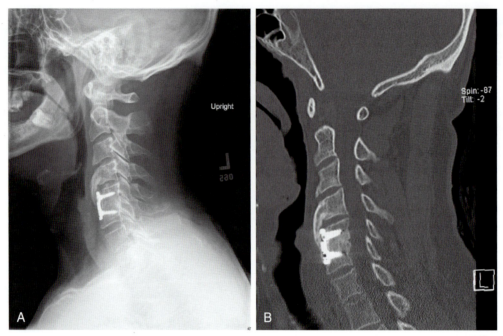

FIGURE 55-2 Lateral radiograph (**A**) and computed tomography scan (**B**) of a patient with grade 4 adjacent level ossification development after C5-C6 anterior cervical diskectomy and fusion.

and after ACDF by using either dynamic fluoroscopy or flexion and extension radiographs. Despite previous cadaveric findings, neither group of investigators found a significant increase in adjacent level motion after ACDF, thus refuting the claim of iatrogenically increased shear at the adjacent level after fusion. Fuller and co-workers used stereophotogrammetry to show that, although the presence of a fusion results in increased motion in the remaining segments, the motion is spread evenly over the spine rather than concentrated at the adjacent level.[11] This finding suggests that all levels, and not just the adjacent level, are at an increased risk for symptomatic spondylotic disease.

Natural History Considerations

Several clinical studies also support the natural history hypothesis. The study by Hilibrand and associates does show an incidence of 3% per year for adjacent segment disease.[1] However, these authors found that the highest rate of adjacent segment disease occurred at C5 to C6 or C6 to C7 and only rarely occurred at C2 to C3 or C7 to T1. These are the same levels most likely to degenerate and require an index surgical procedure. Another interesting finding was that the rate of adjacent segment disease was lower in patients undergoing multilevel fusion than in those with single-level index procedures. If the cause of adjacent segment disease is iatrogenically increased adjacent level pressure and shear, then multilevel fusions should accelerate adjacent segment disease because of the higher shear forces adjacent to a longer construct. Instead, longer fusions tend to decrease adjacent segment disease, probably by treating the levels most likely to undergo symptomatic degeneration in the first place.

Other clinical studies also refute the iatrogenic argument. In a retrospective study of 864 patients who had undergone posterior laminoforaminotomy, Henderson and co-workers evaluated the presence of adjacent segment disease at a mean of 2.8 years of follow-up. These investigators also found a rate of approximately 3% per year, even though posterior laminoforaminotomy is a motion-sparing procedure.[2] Lunsford and colleagues compared patients who had undergone anterior cervical diskectomy versus those who had undergone ACDF. Regardless of fusion state, these investigators found an adjacent segment disease rate of 2.5% per year in their patients.[12] Both these clinical studies refute the idea that adjacent segment disease is caused by fusion and resultant adjacent level increased stress.

Although fusion per se has not been shown to be associated with adjacent segment disease, proponents of cervical total disk replacement have argued that maintaining index level motion may decrease its risk. Unfortunately, the available evidence does not suggest that adjacent segment disease is decreased in total disk replacement versus ACDF, although middle- to long-term data are not currently available.[13]

Given the amount of available evidence arguing for both the iatrogenic and natural history theories, it is not surprising that the cause of adjacent segment disease remains unclear. However, evidence is sufficient to establish risk factors for the development of significant adjacent level disease. These risk factors include an index procedure adjacent to C5 to C6 or C6 to C7 and the presence of neurologic compression or radiographic changes at the adjacent level at the time of the index surgical procedure. Technical issues such as incorrect needle localization and index level fusion in kyphotic alignment increase rates of adjacent level degeneration, but not necessarily clinically relevant disease.

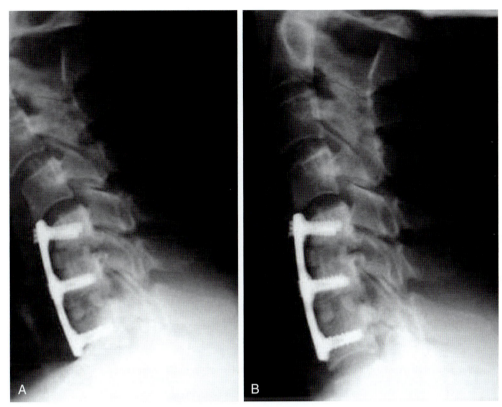

FIGURE 55-3   Lateral radiographs of the cervical spine in flexion (**A**) and extension (**B**) showing failure (pseudarthrosis).

History

Patients with adjacent segment disease present with new radiculopathic or myelopathic symptoms after an interval of improvement. Pain, numbness, or weakness in a specific nerve root distribution is suggestive of radiculopathy. A history of worsening balance or loss of hand coordination is suggestive of myelopathy. It is important to determine whether the symptoms result from neural compression at the adjacent level or from recurrent compression at the index level.

Physical Examination

The physical examination of the cervical spine is performed as described elsewhere in this text. Careful attention should be paid to a thorough neurologic examination to determine the problematic level. Physical examination findings such as the Lhermitte or Hoffmann sign, poor balance, or hand intrinsic wasting indicate myelopathy and should provoke further imaging.

Imaging

Imaging in patients with adjacent segment disease should include standard anteroposterior and lateral radiographic views of the cervical spine, as well as lateral radiographs in full flexion and extension. Flexion and extension radiographs can reveal instability at the adjacent level and can help to rule out nonunion at the index level. The distance between adjacent spinous processes of the fused level is measured in the flexion and extension views (Fig. 55-3). A change of more than 1 to 2 mm from flexion to extension suggests nonunion.[14]

In patients with radiculopathy or myelopathy as determined by the history and physical examination, MRI or computed tomography (CT) myelogram is warranted to further elucidate neural compression. MRI images can often be difficult to interpret because of metallic artifact from adjacent hardware, but improvements in MRI techniques have somewhat alleviated these effects. CT myelogram is appropriate in patients who cannot undergo MRI (e.g., patients with pacemakers). CT myelogram can also give more detailed information about the possible presence of pseudarthrosis at the index level.

Treatment

Treatment for adjacent segment disease can broadly be outlined as nonoperative or operative. If operative treatment is indicated, the treating surgeon can decide between an anterior and a posterior approach and between fusion and a motion-sparing procedure.

Nonoperative Treatment

Nonoperative treatment for adjacent segment disease has not been particularly well studied in the literature. Although several investigators have described successful treatment of de novo radiculopathy and mild myelopathy by using conservative measures, only two studies have

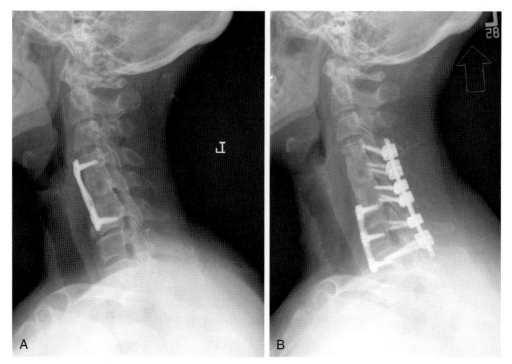

FIGURE 55-4 Preoperative radiograph (**A**) of a patient with adjacent segment disease at C6 to C7. He underwent revision anterior cervical diskectomy and fusion at C6 to C7 and subsequently went on to nonunion at this level. He ultimately required a posterior fusion from C4 to T1 (**B**) 2 years later for neck pain relief.

specifically addressed nonoperative treatment of adjacent segment disease.

Hilibrand and associates showed that only 13 of 46 patients (28%) followed for more than 2 years with adjacent segment disease responded to conservative measures, whereas 59% required surgical treatment.[1] An additional 6 patients either refused surgical treatment or where not considered operative candidates because of medical comorbidities. Ishihara and colleagues found a slightly more encouraging success rate. They followed 112 patients for more than 2 years after ACDF, during which time 19 of 112 patients (17%) developed adjacent segment disease. Of the patients with adjacent segment disease, 63% responded to conservative measures, and 37% underwent revision surgery, mostly for worsening myelopathy.[15]

Nonoperative standard care encompasses multiple modalities. These modalities include isometric neck exercises, home- or office-based traction, nonsteroidal antiinflammatory medications, physical therapy, selective nerve root blocks or epidural injections, education booklets, and limited use of braces or collars.

Because of the relative dearth of high-quality evidence for or against any nonoperative modality, it is difficult to give patients an accurate prognosis. However, success rates of nonoperative therapy for adjacent segment disease, varying in the literature from 28% to 63%, seem to be generally lower than for de novo cervical spondylotic disease, and patients should be counseled accordingly.

Operative Treatment

If nonoperative treatment fails, radiculopathy or myelopathy caused by adjacent level disease can be treated operatively much in the same manner as de novo disease. In the case of rapidly progressive myelopathic symptoms, a more aggressive timetable for operative treatment is warranted to prevent irreversible neurologic changes. Relevant considerations in the operative treatment of adjacent segment disease include anterior versus posterior approaches, fusion versus motion-preserving procedures, and single-level versus multilevel surgical procedures.

The anterior approach to the cervical spine has been used with good outcomes in the literature. Evidence indicates that the use of revision ACDF at segments adjacent to a fusion has a good outcome, but longer fusion segments may predispose to adjacent level nonunions (Fig. 55-4).[16] Great care should be taken when performing a revision anterior approach because of scarring of the intermuscular planes and close proximity of vital structures. If an anterior approach through the contralateral aspect of the neck is chosen, strong consideration should be given to preoperative otolaryngology consultation to rule out occult recurrent laryngeal nerve injury on the index side. Injury to the recurrent laryngeal nerve can occur in 1.5% to 6% of patients after ACDF, with resultant paralysis of the posterior cricoarytenoid muscle. Although paralysis of this muscle unilaterally is usually benign, bilateral paralysis can lead to severe airway difficulties and the need for tracheostomy.

Another possible reason to avoid an anterior approach is suspected pseudarthrosis at the index level. Posterior decompression and fusion can provide a high fusion rate and avoid revision ACDF at the index level. Patients with multilevel spondylotic compression may also benefit from a posterior approach to address multiple levels of disease (Figs. 55-5 and 55-6). This is especially true in

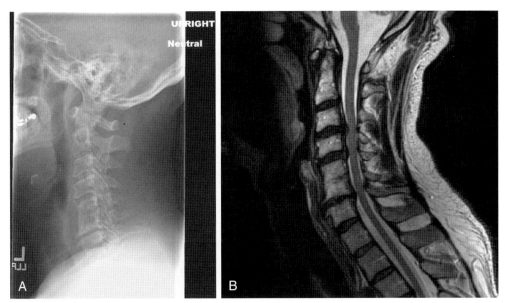

FIGURE 55-5   Lateral radiograph (**A**) and midline sagittal T2-weighted magnetic resonance imaging (**B**) of a 42-year-old man with Charcot-Marie-Tooth disease with a history of C5-C6 anterior cervical diskectomy and fusion without instrumentation who developed progressive weakness, loss of balance, and loss of hand function.

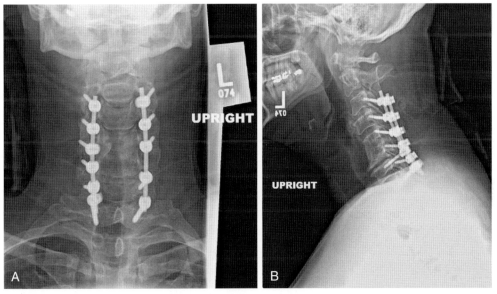

FIGURE 55-6   Anteroposterior (**A**) and lateral (**B**) radiographs of the patient in Figure 55-5 treated with C3-T1 laminectomy and fusion to address multilevel disease after C5-C6 anterior cervical diskectomy and fusion. Left C6-C7 foraminotomy was performed to address preoperative left C7 radiculopathy.

patients with ossification of the posterior longitudinal ligament.

Posteriorly based nonfusion options include laminoforaminotomy for single-level radiculopathic symptoms and laminoplasty for multilevel disease. Laminoforaminotomy has been shown to be a safe and reliable procedure for the treatment of radiculopathic symptoms as an index procedure.[2] Although no clinical series have described laminoforaminotomy in adjacent level disease, the procedure may be a viable option to treat symptomatic adjacent segment disease.

In patients with compressive myelopathy, laminoforaminotomy alone is not sufficient. In the presence of single-level or, more commonly, multilevel disease,

laminoplasty has been shown to be a reliable treatment in index disease.[17,18] No currently available series have addressed laminoplasty in the setting of adjacent segment disease, but given the similar pathologic process present in index and adjacent segment disease–related myelopathy, laminoplasty may be a reasonable option. Contraindications to laminoplasty include cervical kyphosis, which does not allow the spinal cord to drift posteriorly and be indirectly decompressed, and significant preoperative neck pain. The rate of postoperative neck pain after laminoplasty is high, and patients should be counseled accordingly.

A final consideration is the role of disk arthroplasty at levels adjacent to a fusion. Given the relatively recent advent of cervical disk arthroplasty, clinical data are currently not sufficient to recommend for or against arthroplasty at a level adjacent to a fusion, although some data suggest feasibility.[19] Biomechanical data do show an advantage to a hybrid construct of fusion and arthroplasty in terms of decreased loads to attain a predetermined range of motion,[20] but it is unclear whether this finding will be clinically relevant for patients. More clinical data are needed to determine whether arthroplasty at a symptomatic adjacent level is the optimal approach for adjacent segment disease.

Conclusions

Adjacent level disease is a relatively frequent clinical condition in cervical spine surgery. An overall rate of approximately 3% per year can be expected in patients who have undergone surgical procedures, whether motion-preserving operations or fusion. Nonoperative treatment should be attempted, but it may be less successful than in de novo cervical spondylotic syndromes. ACDF at the adjacent level or posterior procedures provide good clinical outcomes, whereas disk arthroplasty requires further study as treatment for adjacent segment disease.

REFERENCES

1. Hilibrand AS, Carlson GD, Palumbo MA, et al.: Radiculopathy and myelopathy at segments adjacent to the site of a previous anterior cervical arthrodesis, *J Bone Joint Surg Am* 81:519–528, 1999.
2. Henderson CM, Hennessy RG, Shuey HM Jr, Shackelford EG: Posterior-lateral foraminotomy as an exclusive operative technique for cervical radiculopathy: a review of 846 consecutively operated cases, *Neurosurgery* 13:504–512, 1983.
3. Matsumoto M, Okada E, Ichihara D, et al.: Anterior cervical decompression and fusion accelerates adjacent segment degeneration: comparison with asymptomatic volunteers in a ten-year magnetic resonance imaging follow-up study, *Spine (Phila Pa 1976)* 35:36–43, 2010.
4. Eck JC, Humphreys SC, Lim TH, et al.: Biomechanical study on the effect of cervical spine fusion on adjacent-level intradiscal pressure and segmental motion, *Spine (Phila Pa 1976)* 27:2431–2434, 2002.
5. Faldini C, Pagkrati S, Leonetti D, et al.: Sagittal segmental alignment as predictor of adjacent-level degeneration after a Cloward procedure, *Clin Orthop Relat Res*(469)674–681, 2011.
6. Katsuura A, Hukuda S, Saruhashi Y, Mori K: Kyphotic malalignment after anterior cervical fusion is one of the factors promoting the degenerative process in adjacent intervertebral levels, *Eur Spine J* 10:320–324, 2001.
7. Nassr A, Lee JY, Bashir RS, et al.: Does incorrect level needle localization during anterior cervical discectomy and fusion lead to accelerated disc degeneration? *Spine (Phila Pa 1976)* 34:189–192, 2009.
8. Park JB, Cho YS, Riew KD: Development of adjacent-level ossification in patients with an anterior cervical plate, *J Bone Joint Surg Am* 87:558–563, 2005.
9. Reitman CA, Hipp JA, Nguyen L, Esses SI: Changes in segmental intervertebral motion adjacent to cervical arthrodesis: a prospective study, *Spine (Phila Pa 1976)* 29:E221–E226, 2004.
10. Kolstad F, Nygaard ØP, Leivseth G: Segmental motion adjacent to anterior cervical arthrodesis: a prospective study, *Spine (Phila Pa 1976)* 32:512–517, 2007.
11. Fuller DA, Kirkpatrick JS, Emery SE, et al.: A kinematic study of the cervical spine before and after segmental arthrodesis, *Spine (Phila Pa 1976)* 23:1649–1656, 1998.
12. Lunsford LD, Bissonette DJ, Jannetta PJ, et al.: Anterior surgery for cervical disc disease. Part 1. Treatment of lateral cervical disc herniation in 253 cases, *J Neurosurg* 53:1–11, 1980.
13. Jawahar A, Cavanaugh DA, Kerr EJ 3rd, et al.: Total disc arthroplasty does not affect the incidence of adjacent segment degeneration in cervical spine: results of 93 patients in three prospective randomized clinical trials, *Spine J* 10:1043–1048, 2010.
14. Cannada LK, Scherping SC, Yoo JU, et al.: Pseudoarthrosis of the cervical spine: a comparison of radiographic diagnostic measures, *Spine (Phila Pa 1976)* 28:46–51, 2003.
15. Ishihara H, Kanamori M, Kawaguchi Y, et al.: Adjacent segment disease after anterior cervical interbody fusion, *Spine J* 4:624–628, 2004.
16. Hilibrand AS, Yoo JU, Carlson GD, et al.: The success of anterior cervical arthrodesis adjacent to a previous fusion, *Spine (Phila Pa 1976)* 22:1574–1579, 1997.
17. Steinmetz MP, Resnick DK: Cervical laminoplasty, *Spine J* 6(Suppl):274S–281S, 2006.
18. Hale JJ, Gruson KI, Spivak JM: Laminoplasty: a review of its role in compressive cervical myelopathy, *Spine J* 6(Suppl):289S–298S, 2006.
19. McAfee PC, Pimenta L, Cappuccino A, et al.: Prospective series of 92 cervical arthroplasties in 73 patients adjacent to prior fusions, *Spine J* 8(Suppl):76S–77S, 2008.
20. Lee MJ, Dumonski M, Phillips FM, et al.: Disc replacement adjacent to cervical fusion: a biomechanical comparison of hybrid construct versus two-level fusion, *Spine (Phila Pa 1976)* 36:1932–1939, 2011.

Nonunions and Implant Failures of the Cervical Spine

56

Rick C. Sasso and M. David Mitchell

CHAPTER PREVIEW

Chapter Synopsis	Nonunions and implant failures of the cervical spine indicate a failure to stabilize the spine biomechanically. The most difficult failures to reconstruct are multilevel corpectomy procedures. The assessment and reconstructive methods that are needed are discussed in this chapter.
Important Points	The goals of revision surgery should be to obtain adequate decompression, restore sagittal balance, and achieve solid fusion.
	The failure rate of cervical corpectomy increases as the number of levels increases.
	Biomechanical stability of multilevel anterior cervical corpectomy is greatly aided by the addition of concomitant posterior fusion.
Clinical and Surgical Pearls	A 36-inch full-length standing lateral radiograph provides useful information in determining sagittal alignment and for planning reconstructions after implant failure.
	In patients with a kyphotic sagittal alignment, the surgeon must determine whether the deformity is fixed or reducible.
	Biomechanically, an anterior cervical plate moves the instantaneous axis of rotation anteriorly in a long graft construct.
Clinical and Surgical Pitfalls	Use of an anterior junctional or buttress plate alone, particularly in multilevel reconstructions with strut grafts, is a high risk for implant failure and graft dislodgment.
	Direct laryngoscopy to assess the function of the direct recurrent nerve is recommended in patients undergoing a revision anterior cervical surgical procedure through a contralateral approach.
	Use of spinal cord monitoring should be strongly considered in revision cervical surgery.

The literature shows that sound biomechanical constructs of the cervical spine decrease the percentage of nonunions and implant failures.[1,2] Therefore, it is essential that the surgical procedures selected increase the biomechanical strength of a construct while addressing the cervical spine dysfunction. The most common failures occur when treating cervical dysfunction with multilevel anterior corpectomy reconstructions and the least common occur with single-level anterior cervical corpectomy procedures.[3-5a]

When developing a surgical plan for the management of spinal disorders, the goals of the intervention should include obtaining adequate decompression, restoring sagittal balance, and creating long-lasting stability by achieving solid fusion. Inherently, one should attempt cervical reconstruction to create a biomechanically

desirable construct with as minimal an operation as possible. Regardless, all operations should also minimize causes of implant failure. The purpose of this chapter is to review the causes, diagnosis, and management for pseudarthrosis and implant failures in the cervical spine.

Etiology and Biomechanics of Cervical Implant Failure

Most commonly, implant failure is either caused by the development of pseudarthrosis or is secondary to excessive biomechanical loads. Multilevel cervical corpectomy has a reported rate of failure of 9% and 50% for two-level and three-level anterior cervical corpectomy plated

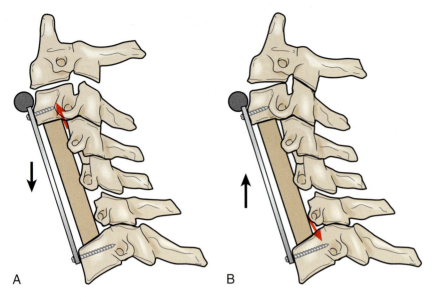

A

B

FIGURE 56-1 A, Schematic modeling a three-level corpectomy reconstruction with a strut graft and anterior cervical plate. Notice that with anterior cervical plating the instantaneous axis of rotation (IAR) is moved anteriorly to the cervical plate so that with cervical flexion and under flexion loads, the strut graft is relatively unloaded. **B,** Conversely, with cervical extension and under extension loads, the graft is placed under extreme compression. This can place the strut graft, vertebral end plates, and cervical plate at increased risk of failure.

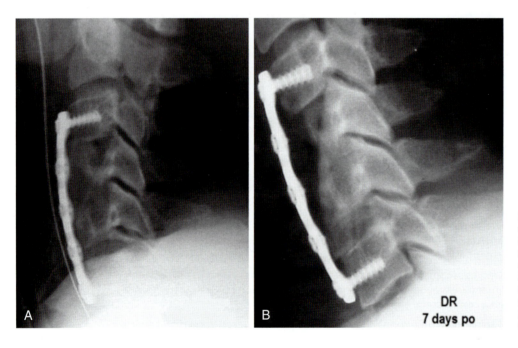

FIGURE 56-2 A, Lateral cervical radiograph 1 day after multilevel corpectomy and anterior cervical instrumentation. The autogenous iliac crest strut graft is well placed. **B,** Radiograph 1 week postoperatively (po) showing the strut graft kicking anteriorly at the caudal aspect and posteriorly into the spinal canal at the cephalad end.

reconstructions, respectively.[2] Other studies have demonstrated a failure rate of 6% with two-level corpectomy and anterior plating increasing to a 71% failure rate with three-level corpectomy and anterior plating.[6] Regardless, the failure rate of cervical anterior corpectomy appears to increase as the number of corpectomy levels increases. Furthermore, the addition of an anterior cervical plate has not eliminated this complication.

Biomechanically, the addition of an anterior cervical plate moves the instantaneous axis of rotation anteriorly in a long graft construct. The resulting forces cause reversal of the loading pattern when compared with what is seen in the uninstrumented constructs. The addition of an anterior cervical plate leads to paradoxical unloading of the graft in flexion and increased compression of the graft in extension[7] (Fig. 56-1). Theoretically, this motion

can result in graft cavitation through the caudal vertebral body and loosening of the plate from the lowest vertebral body. Loose anterior cervical plates are at risk for kicking out anteriorly, typically at the lowest level. Conversely, the proximal portion of the graft is at risk for dislodgment posteriorly into the spinal canal, with resulting spinal cord compression (Fig. 56-2).

Junctional (buttress) plates span only the superior, inferior, or both ends of the strut graft and act as a buttress plate against graft kick-out. However, attempts at using an anterior cervical junctional plate alone in multilevel reconstructions with strut grafts without posterior instrumentation have been shown to increase the risk of failure. Complications associated with strut graft dislodgment can be devastating and include, among other things, catastrophic neurologic compromise and tracheal

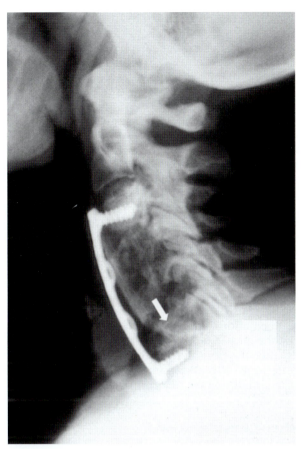

FIGURE 56-3 Lateral radiograph of a three-level corpectomy reconstruction with autogenous iliac crest bone graft and a constrained anterior cervical plate. Radiographs suggest graft fracture. Surgical revision confirmed fracture of the strut graft (*arrow*) and solid fusion of both the cephalad and caudal graft-host junctions.

and esophageal injury.[8] As a result, junctional plates are no longer routinely used alone and are typically used in conjunction with posterior fixation.

The presence of cervical strut or interbody graft pseudarthrosis does not always lead to symptoms. However, if fusion fails to occur, then implant failure is possible. Although uncommon, even long strut grafts that heal at their cephalad and caudal ends can still fracture in the body of the strut graft itself (Fig. 56-3). Other reported complications include plate and screw breakage or dislodgment. The decision to proceed with operative revision of these implant failures is determined by the patient's symptoms and should be individualized to the patient's need and the surgeon's preference and experience.[8a]

Imaging

To visualize an implant failure, a lateral radiograph is frequently the most useful, but computed tomography (CT) scans with sagittal and coronal reconstructions are helpful in detecting the presence of pseudarthrosis and fracture of the long strut grafts. Although the presence of fractured spinal implants on a plain radiograph or CT scan in itself is not definitive for pseudarthrosis, it is strongly suggestive. The presence of movement of the implant on dynamic flexion and extension films, however, confirms the definitive diagnosis of implant instability and associated pseudarthrosis.

A 36-inch full-length standing lateral radiograph including the cervical, thoracic, and lumbar regions gives useful information for determining the sagittal alignment and for planning surgical reconstructions after implant failure. A plumb line from C2 and its measurement to where it falls in relation to the sacral promontory aids in understanding the global sagittal balance. If the sagittal balance is markedly displaced anteriorly to the sacral promontory, then the surgeon should consider extending the cervical salvage reconstruction caudally into the upper thoracic spine to lessen the biomechanical stresses produced when correcting this large amount of kyphotic deformity.

Salvage and Revision Techniques

As the number of levels of anterior cervical diskectomy and fusion (ACDF) increases, most studies indicate an increase in the rate of pseudarthrosis. The most successful procedure for the management of symptomatic pseudarthrosis after single-level ACDF is posterior spinal fusion with instrumentation using modern screw-rod systems.[9] However, not all single-level ACDF pseudarthroses are necessarily symptomatic, so proper patient selection is important. Diagnostic procedures such as posterior cervical facet blocks, which can help determine whether local anesthesia of the motion segment results in pain relief, can aid in making the assessment.

Alternatively, anterior revision surgery can be performed, which frequently consists of resection of the pseudarthrotic levels and strut grating with anterior cervical plating. The literature suggests that the anterior revision rate failure of 44% is found to be much higher than the posterior revision rate failure of 2%.[9] Similar findings have been reported by Brodsky and associates, whose anterior revision fusion rate was 76% and posterior revision fusion rate was 94%.[10] Furthermore, in these studies the posterior fusion group did better clinically.

Correction of strut graft failure of three or more levels requires careful evaluation of the neurologic and biomechanical issues. If early detection of a long anterior construct nonunion is noticed on postoperative films, then a simple posterior stabilization procedure may be performed. Because this approach is usually through virgin soft tissue posteriorly, it avoids the dangers of a revision anterior approach. This approach is possible only if the proper sagittal balance is present.

Unfortunately, in cases of an anterior multilevel construct and the presence of a large kyphotic deformity, the bending moments may challenge the corrective forces of the posterior instrumentation and may increase the incidence of posterior implant failures. In these cases, a combination of anterior-posterior surgical approach may be required (Fig. 56-4). First the anterior strut graft is replaced, and additional corpectomy procedures are performed if damage from cavitation is significant. An anterior or junctional plate is added if needed. A biomechanically sound posterior fixation is then performed to reduce the risk of subsequent failure (Fig. 56-5).

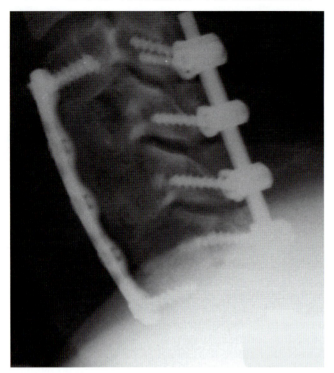

FIGURE 56-4 Lateral cervical radiograph demonstrating a revision with an anterior reconstruction followed by posterior lateral mass fixation.

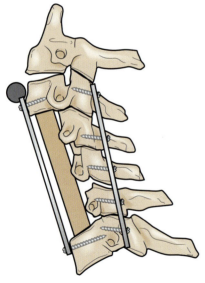

FIGURE 56-5 Schematic modeling of a three-level corpectomy reconstruction with a strut graft and combined anterior plate and posterior instrumentation. In this clinical situation, unlike in isolated anterior cervical plate fixation, the instantaneous axis of rotation is moved posteriorly, thus loading the strut graft in a more physiologic manner during flexion and extension.

Special Considerations for Kyphotic Conditions

In patients with a salvage situation and a kyphotic deformity, the surgeon must determine whether the kyphotic deformity is fixed or reducible. If the deformity is reducible on flexion and extension radiographs or in traction, then the deformity is not fixed. In these cases, if an acceptable

reduction of the kyphosis can be obtained, then this can be addressed with either a posterior alone procedure or an anterior-posterior procedure. In the case of a fixed cervical kyphotic deformity, care should be taken to identify the location of the fixed deformity.

If the deformity is fixed posteriorly, then consideration should be given to performing a posterior cervical release and reduction first, followed by anterior revision of the strut graft. This gives the surgeon the ability to address and correct the fixed kyphosis directly. This procedure is then followed by posterior fixation, which is typically with lateral mass screws and bone grafting. This method has been referred to as a "back-front-back" technique.

Conversely, if the anterior construct appears to have fused in a kyphotic deformity and is inhibiting an adequate posterior kyphotic correction, then an anterior release is performed first. This procedure is then followed by the appropriate posterior procedure, which frequently includes reduction, bone grafting, and posterior instrumentation with or without associated decompression. The next step consists of anterior strut grating with or without instrumentation. This "front-back-front" technique may allow for greater reduction of the fixed kyphotic deformity after the posterior laminectomy. Furthermore, the laminectomy also allows for direct visualization of the spinal cord during the reduction maneuver.

Other Considerations

The incidence of intraoperative and postoperative complications of any salvage operations is higher that of other cervical spine procedures because of the need to operate through previously operated tissues. Therefore, any technique that minimizes the complexity is most useful. In case of revision anterior cervical procedures, preoperative direct laryngoscopy to assess the status of the recurrent laryngeal nerve is important, particularly if a contralateral anterior cervical approach is being considered. In addition, it cannot be stressed enough that the potential for catastrophic complications is very real in these revision procedures. If possible, spinal cord monitoring should be considered as well. Therefore, the risks, benefits, alternatives, and postoperative expectations should be discussed at length with the patient and the patient's family before any intervention is undertaken.

Conclusions

Salvage operations for the cervical spine are complex. Therefore, whenever possible, obtaining the most biomechanically successful procedure at the time of the index procedure is ideal. Implant failures will continue to occur despite our best operations. In the event that a revision surgical procedure is necessary, a careful history and examination and appropriate imaging will help identify the disorder that needs to be addressed. Typically, most pseudarthroses can be managed with posterior fusion with instrumentation. However, in most cases in which a fixed kyphotic deformity exists, an anterior or circumferential procedure is frequently required. In these cases, successful reconstruction requires careful systematic assessment of the deformity. Considerations include the cause of the deformity, the rigidity of the deformity anteriorly or posteriorly, and the degree to which the sagittal balance is affected. Ultimately, the technique recommended should be individualized to the specific patient's disorder and the surgeon's experience and preference.[11]

REFERENCES

1. Riew D, Sethi N, Devney J, et al.: Complications of buttress plate stabilization of cervical corpectomy, *Spine* 24:2404–2410, 1999.
2. Vaccaro A, Falatyn S, Scuderi G, et al.: Early failure of long segment anterior cervical plate fixation, *J Spinal Disord* 11:410–415, 1998.
3. Sukoff M, Harris J, Denenny D, Czaykowski V: Cervical corpectomy: indications, review of literature, technique, rationale for its use, and presentation of 82 consecutive cases, *Neurosurg Q* 7: 209–220, 1997.
4. Epstein N: The management of one-level anterior cervical corpectomy with fusion using Atlantis hybrid plates: a preliminary experience, *J Spinal Disord* 13:324–328, 2000.
5. Wang J, McDonough P, Kanim L: Increased fusion rates with cervical plating for three-level anterior cervical discectomy and fusion, *Spine* 26:643–647, 2001.
5a. Liu Y, Qi M, Chen H, et al.: Comparative analysis of complications of different reconstructive techniques following anterior decompression for multilevel cervical spondylotic myelopathy, *Eur Spine J* 21:2428–2435, 2012.
6. Sasso R, Ruggiero R, Reilly T, Hall P: Early reconstruction failures after multilevel cervical corpectomy, *Spine* 28:141–142, 2003.
7. DiAngelo D, Foley K, Vossel K, et al.: Anterior cervical plating reverses load transfers through multilevel strut-grafts, *Spine* 25:783–795, 2000.
8. Vanichkackorn J, Vaccaro A, Silveri C, Albert T: Anterior junctional plate in the cervical spine, *Spine* 23:2462–2467, 1998.
8a. Xu Wei-bing, Shen Wun-Jer, Lv Gang, et al.: Reconstructive techniques study after anterior decompression of multilevel cervical spondylotic myelopathy, *J Spinal Disord Tech* 22:511–515, 2009.
9. Carreon L, Glassman S, Mitchell C: Treatment of anterior cervical pseudoarthrosis: posterior fusion versus anterior revision, *Spine J* 6:154–156, 2006.
10. Brodsky A, Momtaz K, Sassard W, Newman B: Repair of symptomatic pseudarthrosis of anterior cervical fusion: posterior versus anterior repair, *Spine* 10:1137–1143, 1992.
11. Helgeson M D, Albert T J: Surgery for failed cervical reconstruction, *Spine* 37:E323–E327, 2012.

Page numbers followed by *f* indicate figures; *t*, tables; *b*, boxes.